P9-AQQ-538

Conditioning

REPRESENTATION OF INVOLVED NEURAL FUNCTIONS

ADVANCES IN BEHAVIORAL BIOLOGY

Recent Volumes in this Series

Volume 17 ENVIRONMENTS AS THERAPY FOR BRAIN DYSFUNCTION
Edited by Roger N. Walsh and William T. Greenough

Volume 18 NEURAL CONTROL OF LOCOMOTION
Edited by Richard M. Herman, Sten Grillner, Paul S. G. Stein, and Douglas G. Stuart

Volume 19 THE BIOLOGY OF THE SCHIZOPHRENIC PROCESS
Edited by Stewart Wolf and Beatrice Bishop Berle

Volume 20 THE SEPTAL NUCLEI
Edited by Jon F. DeFrance

Volume 21 COCAINE AND OTHER STIMULANTS
Edited by Everett H. Ellinwood, Jr. and M. Marlyne Kilbey

Volume 22 DISCRIMINATIVE STIMULUS PROPERTIES OF DRUGS
Edited by Harbans Lal

Volume 23 THE AGING BRAIN AND SENILE DEMENTIA
Edited by Kalidas Nandy and Ira Sherwin

Volume 24 CHOLINERGIC MECHANISMS AND PSYCHOPHARMACOLOGY
Edited by Donald J. Jenden

Volume 25 CHOLINERGIC MECHANISMS: Phylogenic Aspects, Central and Peripheral Synapses, and Clinical Significance
Edited by Giancarlo Pepeu and Herbert Ladinsky

Volume 26 CONDITIONING: Representation of Involved Neural Functions
Edited by Charles D. Woody

A Continuation Order Plan is available for this series. A continuation order will bring delivery of each new volume immediately upon publication. Volumes are billed only upon actual shipment. For further information please contact the publisher.

Conditioning

REPRESENTATION OF INVOLVED NEURAL FUNCTIONS

Edited by
Charles D. Woody
Center for the Health Sciences
University of California, Los Angeles
Los Angeles, California

PLENUM PRESS—NEW YORK AND LONDON

Library of Congress Cataloging in Publication Data

Main entry under title:

Conditioning: representation of involved neural functions.

(Advances in behavioral biology; v. 26)
"Proceedings of a Symposium Conditioning: Representation of Involved Neural Functions, held October 25–27, 1981, at Asilomar, California"—T.p. verso.
Includes bibliographical references and index.
1. Conditioned response—Congresses. 2. Neurophysiology—Congresses. I. Woody, C. D. (Charles D.) II. Symposium on Conditioning: Representation of Involved Neural Functions (1981: Asilomar, Calif.) III. Series. [DNLM: 1. Conditioning (Psychology)—Physiology—Congresses. W3 AD215 v. 26/ BF 319 S989c 1981]
QP416.C66 1982 152′.3224 82-9857
ISBN 0-306-41028-1 AACR2

Proceedings of a Symposium on Conditioning: Representation of Involved Neural Functions, held October 25–27, 1981, at Asilomar, California

A Division of Plenum Publishing Corporation
233 Spring Street, New York, N.Y. 10013

Printed in the United States of America

To
Dr. Herbert Jasper and colleagues
for leading the way

PREFACE

I would like to thank all those who contributed to the success of this symposium and its proceedings by providing the material herein. The purpose of the symposium was to examine current knowledge of the brain's function in supporting conditioned behavior. The research of those assembled has led to much of this knowledge. It is a pleasure to acknowledge the organizational help of Drs. D. Alkon, D. Cohen, J. Disterhoft, T. Thach, R. Thompson, and L. Voronin, and also the UCLA Brain Research Institute, the UCLA Mental Retardation Research Center, and Dolores Squires, who assisted faithfully in the administrative organization of the symposium. Special thanks are also due the publisher and publishing editor, James Busis, for lending us their expertise in the preparation of camera-ready material and its rapid publication.

C.D. Woody

CONTENTS

THE ROLE OF THE HIPPOCAMPUS IN THE ACQUISITION OF LEARNED BEHAVIOR

CELLULAR BASIS OF CONDITIONING

INSTRUMENTAL CONDITIONING AND ELECTROPHYSIOLOGICAL STUDIES IN PRIMATES

NICTITATING MEMBRANE AND EYEBLINK CONDITIONING

CONDITIONING: OTHER PREPARATIONS, OTHER LOCI, AND OTHER APPROACHES

ROLE OF THE HIPPOCAMPUS IN REVERSAL LEARNING OF THE RABBIT NICTITATING MEMBRANE RESPONSE

Theodore W. Berger and William B. Orr

Psychobiology Program
Departments of Psychology and Psychiatry
Univ. of Pittsburgh, Pittsburgh, PA 15260

SUMMARY

The effect of hippocampal lesions on two-tone discrimination reversal of the rabbit nictitating membrane response was examined. Animals with hippocampal and neocortical damage or just neocortical damage were compared with operated controls. No differences between the three groups were seen in acquisition rates during initial discrimination learning, with all animals reaching criterion within 3-5 training sessions. The effect of hippocampal damage was apparent only during reversal learning. Hippocampal lesioned animals required more than four times as many sessions to reach reversal criterion than did either operated controls or neocortically damaged rabbits. These data show a selective effect of hippocampectomy on reversal learning, and have implications for the functional significance of hippocampal cellular plasticity which takes place during classical conditioning of the nictitating membrane response.

INTRODUCTION

Over the past several years, the rabbit nictitating membrane (NM) preparation (Gormezano, 1972) has been used to examine the electrophysiological activity of the mammalian hippocampus during classical conditioning. These studies have shown that pyramidal cells of the hippocampus proper substantially increase frequency of firing over the course of learning (Berger et al., 1976; Berger and Thompson, 1978c). In addition to a heightened frequency, hippocampal pyramidal neurons exhibit a distinctive pattern of discharge during conditioning trials (Berger & Thompson, 1978a; Berger et al.,

1980). Briefly, the distribution of action potentials within a trial parallels the amplitude of the conditioned membrane response during that trial (see Figure 1). A number of control procedures have demonstrated that these changes in cell firing are specifically related to behavioral learning, and are not simply a result of repetitive sensory stimulation (i.e., sensitization) or movement on the part of the organism (Berger and Thompson, 1978a). It has also been shown that the hippocampal plasticity described by these studies occurs in more than one animal species (Patterson et al., 1979), more than one type of learning paradigm (Thompson et al., 1980), and with the use of visual as well as auditory CS modalities (Coates and Thompson, 1978). In this sense, hippocampal cellular plasticity during NM conditioning is a general phenomenon which should reflect some fundamental property of hippocampal function.

The initial impetus for examining cellular responsivity of the hippocampal brain region during NM conditioning came from the large literature which exists on the role of the hippocampus in animal learning (see reviews by Douglas, 1967; Kimble, 1968; Isaacson, 1974), and in particular, from clinical evidence indicating that bilateral damage to the hippocampus in humans results in severe anterograde amnesia (Milner, 1970). Studies from several laboratories, however, have shown that -- despite the dramatic changes in hippocampal activity which occur as a result of NM conditioning -- lesions of the rabbit hippocampus do not retard behavioral learning in the nictitating membrane paradigm (Schmaltz and Theios, 1972; Solomon and Moore, 1975). The latter NM lesion results are actually not surprising given the existing hippocampal lesion literature. It is well established that hippocampal damage in animals does not prevent learning simple discriminations (Douglas, 1967; Kimble, 1968; O'Keefe and Nadel, 1978), and that humans with hippocampal damage can successfully learn and show retention on a number of simple tasks while being severely deficient when challenged with more complex mnemonic demands (Sidman et al., 1968; Milner, 1970).

It would be more appropriate, then, to re-examine the effects of hippocampal damage on classical conditioning of the NM response during more complex learning tasks known to be affected by hippocampectomy. One learning task which has consistently been shown sensitive to hippocampal damage in animals is reversal of a previously learned discrimination (see Hirsh, 1974 for review). In short, while learning of the initial discrimination is unaffected by hippocampal lesion, reversal of that discrimination is consistently retarded. Human amnesics (more specifically, Korsakoff patients) have also been shown to be incapable of reversal learning on a verbal task (Warrington and Weiskrantz, 1974). The purpose of the following experiment was to test the

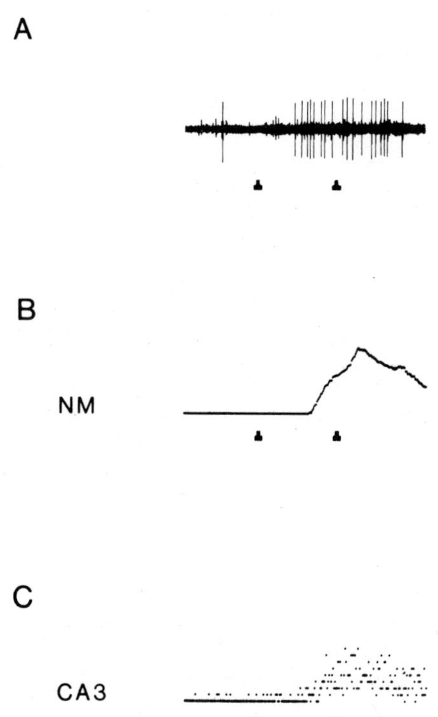

Fig. 1. Example of conditioned hippocampal pyramidal cell response during a one-tone discrimination task. Upper trace shows hippocample pyramidal cell discharge during a single conditioned trial. Middle trace shows averaged conditioned nictitating membrane (NM) response for 109 trials. Lower trace shows peristimulus time histogram for the same 109 trials. First cursor indicates CS (tone) onset; second cursor indicates UCS (airpuff) onset. From Thompson et al., 1980.

possibility that hippocampal damage would prevent discrimination reversal in the rabbit NM preparation as well, and if so, suggest the functional significance of unit changes occurring during NM conditioning.

METHODS

Three groups of male, New Zealand White rabbits were used in the present study. One group received aspiration lesions of the hippocampus and the parietal neocortex overlying the dorsal hippocampus (N=4). A second group received aspiration lesions of just the parietal neocortex overlying the dorsal hippocampus (N=4), while a third group of operated controls (N=4) was given a midline incision. All surgical procedures were performed under halothane anesthesia. Following hippocampal or neocortical aspiration, brain tissue was washed with a dilute solution of Thrombin until all bleeding ceased. Lesioned areas were gently packed with wet Gelfoam and bone wax used to cover skull-removed regions. Extreme care was taken to minimize damage to the temporal neocortical areas overlying posterior-ventral hippocampus. All animals, including controls, were permanently implanted with plastic headstages for holding a UCS delivery system and an NM measurement potentiometer used during conditioning sessions. Skull screws and dental acrylic were used to implant the headstages. Three weeks were allowed for recovery.

Animals were conditioned within a sound-proff chamber while held in a Plexiglas restrainer (see Gormezano, 1972). Eyeclips were used to hold the eyelids open throughout training, and a nylon loop was sewn into the nictitating membrane for response measurement. For each training session, the loop was connected to the arm of a potentiometer mounted on headgear worn by the subject. Variations in the potentiometer output were measured both on a polygraph and a storage oscilloscope. One-half millimeter of NM movement was required for response criterion.

After two days of habituating to restraint in the conditioning chamber, two-tone discrimination training was begun. Either a 1K Hz or a 10K Hz (counterbalanced design) 850 msec tone was used as the CS+ or the CS- (85 dB SPL). Corneal airpuff (100 msec duration) served as the UCS. The inter-trial-interval was a pseudo-random 20-40 sec, averaging 30 sec., and the ISI was 750 msec., with tone and airpuff terminating simultaneously. Twelve blocks of 16 trials per block (8 CS+ and 8 CS-) were administered each day until behavioral criterion was reached. Criterion for discrimination conditioning was $\geq$ 85% CR rate to the CS+ and $\leq$ 15% CR rate to the CS-, as measured during the last half of each session (i.e., the last 96 trials). The day following criterion performance on discrimination, reversal training was begun by switching the tones serving as CS+ and CS-. Criterion performance for reversal learning was $\geq$ 90% CR rate for the new CS+ and < 50% CR rate for the new CS-, or until 56 sessions (8 weeks reversal training) were completed.

Following completion of reversal training, animals were overdosed with Nembutal and perfused transcardially with 0.9% saline followed by 10% formalin. The brains were removed and stored in perfusate until sectioned on a cryostat, using tissue-embedding medium to provide support for lesioned brain areas. Tissue was later stained with cresyl violet and examined microscopically for the extent of brain damage.

RESULTS

Histological results showed that all hippocampal animals received extensive damage to the hippocampus and subiculum proper, with the lesions always including the rostral pole of the hippocampus and continuing through to posterior-ventral hippocampal regions. The lesions sometimes extended into the fornix, but never reached any portion of the septum. Likewise, thalamic nuclei were never seen to be lesioned or compressed. The most temporal end of the hippocampus was always left intact, and in general, approximately 15% of the hippocampal formation was left undamaged. The entorhinal cortex was also left undamaged in all cases. A description of lesions to the subiculum proper would be identical to that given for the hippocampus in extent, though the presubiculum was only minimally damaged in all cases. Some damage to the cingulum occurred in all cases, though usually near the rostral end of the hippocampus only. Cell body regions of temporal neocortex were entirely free from lesions, though some damage to the white matter was apparent in two cases.

Neocortical lesions did not involve any part of the hippocampus or the angular bundle, nor did they extend into the cingulum. Though some damage to the alveus overlying the dorsal hippocampus cannot be ruled out, it was not apparent. Tissue of operated control animals appeared entirely normal.

Behavioral effects of the lesions were fairly straight-forward. Animals in all groups -- operated controls, neocortical lesions and hippocampal lesions -- learned the initial two-tone discrimination at the same rate. The trials-to-criterion measure used was the total number of trials inclusive of the session in which the animal reached criterion performance. All animals reached discrimination criterion within three to five sessions, with the mean number of trials for normals equalling 768 (± 157 S.D.); neocorticals, 720 (± 96 S.D.); and hippocampals, 768 (± 157 S.D.). No statistical differences in trials to criterion on

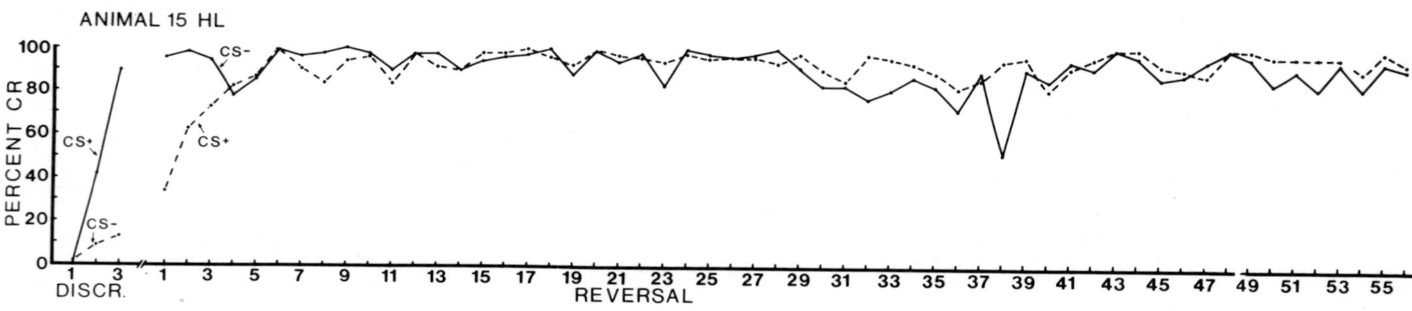

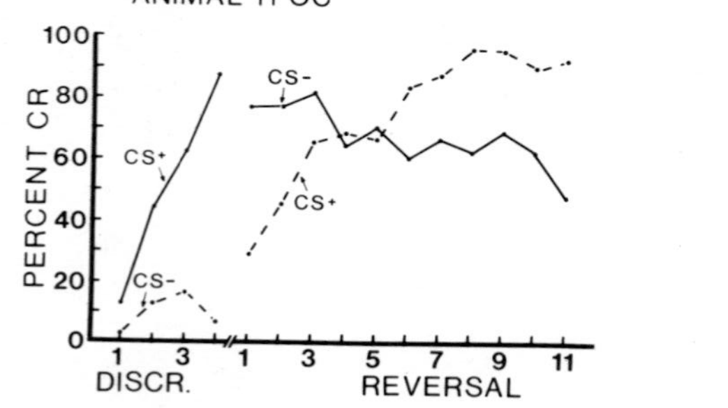

Fig. 2. Conditioned NM response rates during two-tone discrimination (Discr.) and reversal learning for one operated control (OC) animal and one hippocampal lesioned (HL) animal. For both animals, a 1K Hz tone served as the CS+ during discrimination training and the CS- during reversal training. All values represent CR rates for the last half of each training session.

initial discrimination were evident (neocorticals vs. hippocampals, t = 0.52, NS; normals vs. hippocampals, t = 0.00, NS). Neocortical lesions also had no effect on discrimination conditioning (normals vs. neocorticals, t = 0.52, NS).

In contrast, reversal learning was severely affected by hippocampal but not neocortical damage. One hippocampal lesioned animal was finally terminated after eight weeks (56 sessions) of reversal training without reaching criterion (see Fig. 2, HL). The other three animals in the group did eventually reverse behavioral responding to the CS+ and CS–, but required an average of four times as many trials as either normal or neocortically lesioned rabbits (normals vs. hippocampals, t = 7.04, $p < .001$, corticals vs. hippocampals, t = 7.27, $p < .001$). The mean number of trials to criterion equalled 2064 (± 480 S.D.) for operated controls, 1920 (± 415 S.D.) for cortically lesioned animals and 8352 (± 1721 S.D.) for the hippocampal lesioned group (see Fig. 3). No differences in reversal learning were seen between normal and neocortically damaged animals (t = 0.45, NS).

In all hippocampal lesion cases, failure at reversal learning resulted from continued responding to the new CS– (the initial CS+) rather than low levels of responding to the new CS+ (the initial CS–). Animals in all groups, including hippocampal lesions, readily increased CR rates to the new CS+ in the reversal phase of training (see Figure 2).

DISCUSSION

The present study demonstrates that hippocampectomy severely impairs reversal learning of the rabbit nictitating membrane response. Initial two-tone discrimination learning, however, develops at a normal acquisition rate with hippocampal damage, so that hippocampal lesions selectively disrupt only the mnemonic function required for reversal learning. This result is consistent with previous demonstrations of hippocampal damage disrupting reversal but not initial discrimination learning in a variety of species and types of learning tasks (Teitelbaum, 1964; Kimble and Kimble, 1965; Niki, 1966; Douglas and Pribram, 1966; Winocur and Olds, 1978).

The behavioral requirements for successful reversal learning involve two criteria (see Methods) -- an increased CR rate to the new CS+ (the previous CS–) and a decreased CR rate to the new CS– (the previous CS+). It is apparent from the present analysis that hippocampectomy prevents animals from reaching the latter criterion, but not the first. That is, hippocampal damaged animals are successful at learning to respond to the new CS+, but fail to stop responding to the new CS– and as a result, fail to fully reverse. At first consideration, this deficit may appear

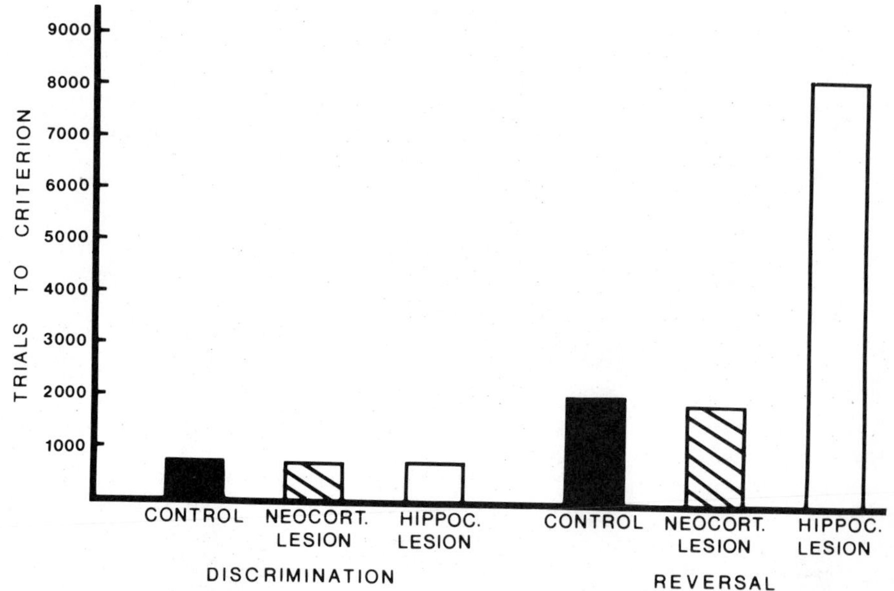

Fig. 3. Number of trials to criterion for operated control (solid), neocortical lesioned (stripe) and hippocampal lesioned (open) animals during discrimination and reversal conditioning.

analogous to previous demonstrations of increased resistance to extinction after hippocampal lesions (Douglas, 1967; Kimble, 1968; Altman et al., 1973). There are a number of reasons for believing, however, that increased resistance to extinction is an inadequate explanation for failure at reversal learning in the present task (and in others as well). First, while disruption of an inhibitory process (of one type of another) has been theorized to occur with hippocampal lesions, a characterization of hippocampal function in terms of inhibition *per se* is not well supported empirically (see Nadel et al., 1974). Secondly, most available evidence fails to support the conclusion that increased resistance to extinction of conditioned NM responding occurs after hippocampal lesions. Solomon and Moore (1975) and Solomon (1977) have reported no differences in extinction rates between normal and lesioned animals. Schmaltz and Theios (1972) have reported increased resistance to extinction with the rabbit NM preparation, but only after repeated re-acquisition and re-extinction training. Consistent with the Solomon and Moore studies, Schmaltz and Theios' animals showed normal CR rates on the initial extinction test. Powell and Buchanan (1980) have reported increased resistance to extinction in the rabbit eyeblink preparation, but only two extinction sessions were reported for comparison of normal vs. lesioned animals. In total, little if any increased resistance to extinction of the NM response appears to occur after hippocampal lesions, and so is unlikely to account for the reversal failure reported here.

Because of the selective effect of hippocampectomy on reversal but not discrimination NM learning, one might predict that hippocampal unit activity exhibits cellular plasticity only during reversal learning as well. This clearly is not the case, however, as hippocampal pyramidal cell firing changes substantially during a one-tone discrimination NM task (Berger et al., 1976; Berger and Thompson, 1978a,c). This apparent discrepancy may indicate that hippocampal cellular activity is significantly different during discrimination vs. reversal phases of conditioning. Disterhoft and Segal (1978) and Deadwyler (Deadwyler et al., 1979) have recorded hippocampal unit responses in rat during reversal conditioning and found differential discharge rates to the CS+ and CS-. In both studies, however, hippocampal units responded differentially during discrimination learning as well. These unit recording results, together with the lesion data, indicate that while hippocampal neurons exhibit enhanced firing rates to CS+ stimuli during both discrimination and reversal training, enhanced hippocampal responsiveness is behaviorally relevant only during reversal learning. While admittedly speculative, one possibility is that neural elements of other brain structures -- particularly those efferent to the hippocampus -- determine whether hippocampal activity is causally related to behavior. If the cellular activity of hippocampal efferent targets (e.g., cingulate) is enhanced only during reversal learning, the differential responsiveness of hippocampal neurons to the CS+ and CS- could be "gated" through to exert a greater synaptic influence on the excitability of other brain systems more immediately responsible for motor behavior. This possibility is currently being investigated.

ACKNOWLEDGEMENTS

Supported by grants from the McKnight Foundation, NSF (BNS 80-21395) and NIMH (MH00343). We gratefully thank Dolores Shirk for manuscript preparation.

REFERENCES

Altman, J., Brunner, R.L. and Bayer, S.A., 1973, The hippocampus and behavioral maturation, Behav. Biol., 8:557-596.

Berger, T.W., Alger, B. and Thompson, R.F., 1976, Neuronal substrate of classical conditioning in the hippocampus, Science, 192:483-485.

Berger, T.W., Laham, R.I. and Thompson, R.F., 1980, Hippocampal unit-behavior correlations during classical conditioning, Brain Res., 193:229-248.

Berger, T.W. and Thompson, R.F., 1978a, Neuronal plasticity in the limbic system during classical conditioning of the rabbit nictitating membrane response. I. The hippocampus, Brain Res., 145:323-346.

Berger, T.W. and Thompson, R.F., 1978b, Neuronal plasticity in the limbic system during classical conditioning of the rabbit nictitating membrane response. II. Septum and mammillary bodies, Brain Res., 156:293-314.

Berger, T.W. and Thompson, R.F., 1978c, Identification of pyramidal cells as the critical elements in hippocampal neuronal plasticity during learning, Proc. nat. Acad. Sci. (Wash.), 75:1572-1576.

Coates, S.R. and Thompson, R.F., 1978, Comparing neural plasticity in the hippocampus during classical conditioning of the rabbit nictitating membrane response to light and tone, Neurosci. Abstracts, 4:792.

Deadwyler, S.A., West, M. and Lynch, G., 1979, Activity of dentate granule cells during learning: differentiation of perforant path input, Brain Res., 169:29-43.

Disterhoft, J. and Segal, M., 1978, Neuron activity in rat hippocampus and motor cortex during discrimination reversal, Brain Res. Bull., 3:583-588.

Douglas, R.J., 1967, The hippocampus and behavior, Psych. Bull., 67:416-442.

Douglas, R.J. and Pribram, K.H., 1966, Learning and limbic lesions, Neuropsychol., 4:197-220.

Gormezano, I., 1972, Investigations of defense and reward conditioning in the rabbit, In: Classical Conditioning II: Current Research and Theory, A.H. Black and W.F. Prokasy (Eds.), Appleton-Century-Crofts, New York: pp. 151-181.

Hirsh, R., 1974, The hippocampus and contextual retrieval of information from memory: A theory, Behav. Biol., 12:421-444.

Isaacson, R.L., 1974, The Limbic System, Plenum, New York.

Kimble, D.P., 1968, Hippocampus and internal inhibition, Psych. Bull., 70:285-295.

Kimble, D.P. and Kimble, R.J., 1965, Hippocampectomy and response perseveration in the rat, J. comp. Physiol. Psych., 60:474-476.

Milner, B., 1970, Memory and the medial temporal regions of the brain, In: Biology of Memory, K.H. Pribram and D.E. Broadbent (Eds.), Academic, New York: pp. 29-50.

Nadel, L., O'Keefe, J. and Black, A., 1975, Slam on the brakes: A critique of Altman, Brunner and Bayer's response-inhibition model of hippocampal function, Behav. Biol., 14:151-162.

Niki, H., 1966, Response perseveration following hippocampal ablation in rat, Jap. Psych. Res., 8:1-9.

O'Keefe, J. and Nadel, L., 1978, The Hippocampus as a Cognitive Map, Oxford University Press, New York.

Patterson, M.M., Berger, T.W. and Thompson, R.F., 1979, Neuronal plasticity recorded from cat hippocampus during classical conditioning, Brain Res., 163:339-343.

Powell, D.A. and Buchanan, S., 1980, Autonomic-somatic relationships in the rabbit (Oryctolagus cuniculus): Effects of hippocampal lesions, Physiol. Psych., 8:455-462.

Schmaltz, L.W. and Theios, J., 1972, Acquisition and extinction of a classically conditioned response in hippocampectomized rabbits (Orcytolagus cuniculus), J. comp. Physiol. Psych., 79:328-333.

Sidman, M., Stoddard, L.T. and Mohr, J.P., 1968, Some additional quantitative observations of immediate memory in a patient with bilateral hippocampal lesions, Neuropsychologia, 6: 245-254.

Solomon, P.R., 1977, The role of the dorsal hippocampus in blocking and conditioned inhibition of the rabbit's nictitating membrane response, J. comp. Physiol. Psych., 91:407-417.

Solomon, P.R. and Moore, J.W., 1975, Latent inhibition and stimulus generalization of the classically conditioned nictitating membrane response in rabbits (Oryctolagus cuniculus) following dorsal hippocampal ablations, J. comp. Physiol. Psych., 89:1192-1203.

Teitelbaum, H., 1964, A comparison of the effects of orbitofrontal and hippocampal lesions upon discrimination learning and reversal in cat, Exp. Neurol., 9:452-462.

Thompson, R.F., Berger, T.W., Berry, S.D., Hoehler, F.K., Kettner, R.E. and Weisz, D.J., 1980, Hippocampal substrate of classical conditioning, Physiol. Psych., 8:262-279.

Warrington, E.K. and Weiskrantz, L., 1974, The effect of prior learning on subsequent retention in amnesic patients, Neuropsychologia, 12:419-428.

Winocur, G. and Olds, J., 1978, Effects of context manipulation on memory and reversal learning in rats with hippocampal lesions, J. comp. Physiol. Psych., 92:312-321.

LONG TERM MODULATION OF INTRINSIC MEMBRANE PROPERTIES OF HIPPOCAMPAL NEURONS

L.S. Benardo and D.A. Prince

Department of Neurology
Stanford University Medical Center
Stanford, CA 94305

SUMMARY

We studied the mechanisms of action of acetylcholine (ACh) and dopamine (DA) on hippocampal CA1 pyramidal cells of the *in vitro* slice preparation. ACh caused an initial hyperpolarization in half the cells studied which was eliminated when synaptic transmission was blocked and was therefore presynaptic in origin. Muscarinic excitation was evoked in all neurons and consisted of slow depolarization and a voltage-sensitive increase in membrane resistance (R_N) which resulted from antagonism of a voltage-dependent K^+ conductance. R_N increases lasted hours after a single ACh application and concomitant changes in cell firing mode from single spikes to burst generation occurred. This long term effect was Ca^{2+} dependent. DA application resulted in spontaneous hyperpolarization and an increase in the amplitude and duration of the afterhyperpolarizations (AHPs) which normally follow repetitive spiking. These effects were long-lasting and associated with up to a 22% decrease in R_N. DA-induced hyperpolarizations persisted in cells impaled with Cl^--containing electrodes and had a reversal potential of about -87 mV, findings consistent with an increased K^+ conductance. Mn^{2+} blocked the spontaneous or evoked hyperpolarizations produced by DA (1 μM), however larger volume DA applications were effective even in low Ca^{2+}, Mn^{2+}-containing solutions. Intracellular EGTA blocked all DA actions. DA effects were mimicked by DA agonists and by intra- or extracellular application of cAMP, and blocked by DA antagonists. We conclude that DA actions are mediated by effects on intracellular [Ca^{2+}] which in turn modulates a Ca^{2+}-activated K^+ conductance. The long term nature of these actions may relate to receptor coupled increases in cAMP.

ACh and DA are neuromodulators which produce long term alterations in intrinsic cell properties and would be expected to effectively alter the influences of other afferent systems. The implications for learning and memory are discussed.

INTRODUCTION

Most of our basic knowledge concerning synaptic transmission comes from classical studies of the neuromuscular junction, where transmitter actions characteristically produce short latency, brief, postsynaptic events. However these transient changes seem inadequate as neurophysiological substrates for such higher cortical functions as learning and memory, processes which are known to develop slowly and which must involve very long lasting alterations in cellular activities. Certain classes of neurochemicals have been shown to mediate synaptic effects of long latency and slow decay, which alter subsequent neuronal responses. These agents have been appropriately termed neuromodulators.[1] Until recently however, the nature of neuromodulator actions in the mammalian cortex had not been well studied, primarily because of the technical difficulties posed by such experiments. Development of the _in vitro_ slice preparation and its application to studies of cellular mechanisms of transmitter action[2,3] has largely overcome these obstacles.

The hippocampus has proven particularly amenable to this technique since many of the anatomical and physiological relationships observed _in vivo_ are preserved _in vitro_.[4,5,6,7] Since the hippocampus has been implicated by many investigators in the processes of learning and memory,[8,9,10,11] it would be especially important to investigate the actions of putative transmitter agents on this structure, particularly those which might have long duration effects. Such studies would provide greater insight into possible mechanisms subserving the complex functions of this cortical area. In the experiments discussed here we have examined the mode of action of two such agents, namely acetylcholine and dopamine. The data indicate that both of these substances qualify as neuromodulators in the hippocampus and that they must play an important role in normal hippocampal physiology.

METHODS

Experiments were conducted using 350μ thick guinea pig hippocampal slices prepared and maintained _in vitro_ as described elsewhere.[7,12] The composition of the perfusion solution was (in mM): NaCl, 124; KCl, 5; NaH_2PO_4, 1.25; $MgSO_4$, 2; CaCl, 2; $NaHCO_3$, 26; glucose, 10. When Mn^{2+} was added to the bathing medium,

Cl^- was substituted for phosphate and sulfate. The temperature of the media in the tissue chamber was maintained at 37°C. Intracellular recordings from CA1 cells were usually obtained with beveled or unbeveled 4 M K acetate filled microelectrodes having resistances of 30-175 MΩ. Neurons with resting membrane potentials of at least -55 mV and action potentials of 70 mV or greater were selected for study. Current was applied through the recording electrode using an active bridge circuit and continuous monitoring and adjustment of bridge balance.

Drugs were applied extracellularly by iontophoresis, direct drop application, or by superfusion.[13] When it was necessary to apply certain drugs intracellularly, cells were impaled with drug-containing microelectrodes from which the agent could either diffuse passively or be electrophoresed.

RESULTS

Cholinergic System

Data from studies of neocortical neurons[14] and those from recent experiments in the hippocampal slice[13,15] indicate that the muscarinic action of ACh produces a decrease in neuronal input resistance (R_N), an effect also described in other preparations,[16,17] and one which would be characteristic for the action of a neuromodulator.[1] Further, cholinergic excitation is known to be associated with lasting changes in neuronal metabolism,[18] an action compatible with induction of long-term changes in neuronal excitability. These findings prompted a detailed analysis of cholinergic muscarinic actions in the hippocampus which we will summarize here.

ACh effects on membrane potential and input resistance: ACh was applied to 45 CA1 hippocampal pyramidal cells, recorded intracellularly from slices bathed in normal Ringer's solution. Approximately 1-3 seconds following drug application, an initial hyperpolarization occurred in 15 of 33 cells studied quantitatively. This hyperpolarization had a mean amplitude 3.1 ± 1.8 (S.D.) mV (range 2-10 mV), and a duration of from 2-30 seconds. In 9 neurons, the increase in membrane potential (V_m) was associated with a reduction in membrane input resistance (R_N) which had a mean of 21 ± 9% (S.D.). The recording of Fig. 1A1-2 shows an example of these effects. One explanation for these findings would be a direct cholinergic inhibition as previously concluded from extracellular studies of ACh action on cortical units.[19] Our data lead to a different conclusion however. Coincident with the ACh-induced changes in R_N and V_m, we often observed spontaneous hyperpolarizing potentials (Fig. 1B2). This suggests that cholinergic excitation of presynaptic inhibitory interneurons mediates the

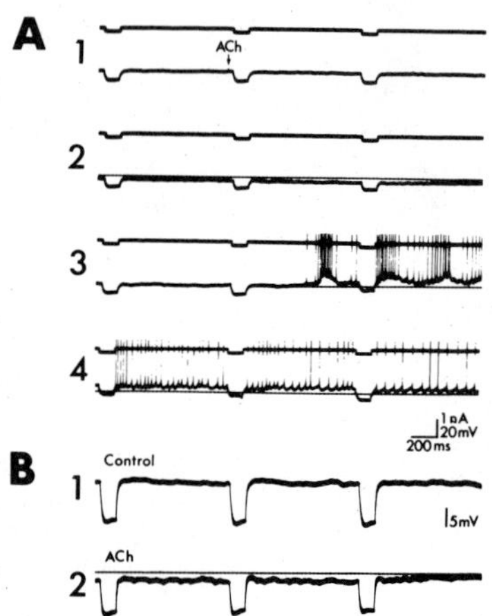

Fig. 1. Sequential noncontinuous segments showing response of a hippocampal pyramidal neuron to ACh. A1: droplet of ACh (50 mM) applied at arrow. A2: initial hyperpolarization of 4 mV lasted 9 seconds and was associated with a 27.5% decrease in R_N. A3-A4: subsequent 10 mV depolarization coincident with a rise in R_N and development of intermittent bursts and repetitive firing. B: higher gain, filtered (bandwidth, DC-100 Hz) records from same cell. B1: control baseline activity. B2: same segment as A2, demonstrating spontaneous hyperpolarizing events during initial slow hyperpolarization. Spikes cut off in photography. Spike height: 80 mV. Upper traces in A: current monitor. Time calibration in A4 for all segments of A-B. Voltage and current calibration in A4 for A1-4. Voltage calibration in B1 for B1-2. Baselines in A2-4, B2: resting V_m = -65 mV.

initial hyperpolarization. Such an interpretation is further supported both by the finding that ACh can excite cells which have the physiological characteristics of inhibitory interneurons, and by the observation that initial hyperpolarizations are not seen when evoked synaptic transmission is blocked.

Following the initial hyperpolarizing ACh response, R_N and V_m returned to control values for a brief period (usually 1-2 seconds), after which a slow depolarization occurred (10 mV at peak in Fig. 1A3). Membrane depolarization was also observed in cells not showing an initial hyperpolarization. A mean depolarization of 14.3 ± 10.8 (S.D.) mV from a mean resting V_m of -64.4 ± 5.6 (S.D.) mV occurred within 120 seconds after ACh exposure. The depolarizing phase of ACh action was variable but could last several minutes. Depolarizing responses were associated with marked increases in spike discharge. The cell in Fig. 1 showed no spontaneous activity prior to ACh, but following drug application it developed a peak firing rate of 65 Hz which declined to about 15 Hz within six seconds. The repetitive spiking and intermittent bursting shown in Fig. 1 are representative of the increases in activity seen in other hippocampal pyramidal cells after ACh application. Comparable depolarizations in control neurons did not produce similar increases in spike frequency or burst responses. Following complete or partial repolarization, cell firing rate remained higher than under control conditions.

An increase in R_N was consistently observed following ACh application. In cells responding with depolarizations, the shift in R_N accompanied the decreases in V_m but persisted much longer (see below). Increases in R_N ranged up to about 300% of the control values measured at resting V_m, with a mean increase of 60% (n = 33). Peak R_N changes occurred at a mean V_m of -51.4 mV, which was above the firing threshold.

Since R_N in hippocampal pyramidal cells normally increases with depolarization,[20] it was necessary to examine R_N at various levels of V_m before and after ACh exposure in the same cell to determine how much of the change in R_N could be attributed to ACh action, versus depolarization *per se*. The results of such an experiment in one neuron are shown in Fig. 2. This is a plot of R_N, determined from the voltage response of the membrane to constant current hyperpolarizing pulses (ordinate) against steady state membrane potential which was varied with DC current (abscissa). Under the control conditions the apparent R_N increased with depolarization as previously reported.[20] Increases in voltage-dependent conductances for Ca^{2+} and Na^+ occur during depolarization, and underlie the apparent increase in resistance recorded at lower potentials (i.e. anomalous inward rectification). Depolarization also activates K^+ conductance in these neurons, however this is insufficient to overcome the apparent resistance elevation due to

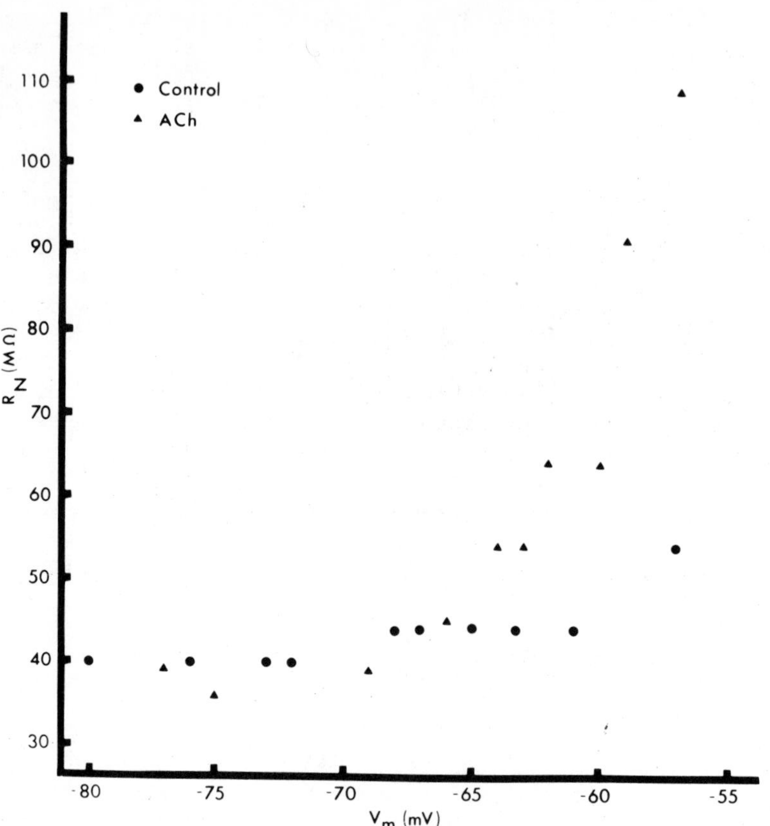

Fig. 2. Plot of R_N versus V_m for one neuron before (●) and following (▲) ACh application. Under control conditions R_N increases from 40 MΩ to 54 MΩ as V_m is depolarized from -80 mV to -57 mV (spike threshold). However following ACh delivery R_N increases from 40 MΩ to 109 MΩ at V_ms from -77 mV to -57 mV, demonstrating the prominent voltage-sensitive nature of ACh action. Resting V_m: -65 mV.

inward movement of charge carried by Na^+ and Ca^{2+}. Following ACh application, resistance was noted to increase significantly in the region of anomalous rectification. Increases at hyperpolarized levels were also sometimes seen, perhaps reflecting a voltage-insensitive component of ACh action. To quantify the voltage-sensitive ACh induced R_N increases, R_N was measured in each neuron at both a hyperpolarized and a depolarized membrane potential, that is at -75 and -60 mV respectively, before and after ACh application. The mean R_N at -75 mV before and after ACh exposure was 39.6 MΩ and 42.1 MΩ ($n = 11$), respectively. This increase in R_N in the population amounted to only a 6% change, and was insignificant. Mean R_N values at -60 mV were 49.3 MΩ and 63 MΩ before and after ACh addition (n = 11), respectively, corresponding to a statistically significant increase in R_N of 28% ($p < 0.05$). From these measurements ACh appears to act, at least in part, on a voltage-sensitive conductance (g), thereby enhancing depolarizing anomalous rectification. Such effects might be due to an enhancement of gNa or gCa, or a decrease in gK.

Ionic mechanisms of ACh effects: Subsequent experiments were designed to investigate the ionic mechanisms for the ACh-induced R_N increases and slow depolarization. In order to accomplish this, the responses to ACh were monitored in the presence of blockers of voltage-dependent conductances. Table 1 summarizes the results of these experiments. Exposure of slices to Mn^{2+}-containing solutions blocked evoked chemical synaptic transmission[21,22] and thus served to eliminate possible presynaptic actions of ACh. In addition the blockade of voltage-dependent gCa in hippocampal pyramidal cells by Mn^{2+} allowed an assessment of the contribution of gCa to the ACh-induced R_N increases, and depolarization. Under these conditions little or no depolarization followed ACh application. Thus Ca^{2+} contributes significantly to the depolarizing component of the ACh response, either through its mediation of synaptic activity or through its direct effects as a charge carrier for inward current in CA1 hippocampal pyramidal cells. ACh did induce substantial increases in R_N in Mn^{2+} solutions, even though V_m did not change. As shown in Table 1, when R_N was compared at -75 mV before and following ACh application an insignificant decrease was measured. By contrast, when R_N measured at -60 mV was compared before and after ACh a significant increase of 29% ($p < 0.05$) was obtained. Except for its duration (see below), this voltage-dependent increase in R_N was very similar to that observed in normal medium. Persistence of such increases in R_N in Mn^{2+} solutions suggests that ACh effects on gCa are not responsible for the observed changes.

As previously shown,[20] voltage-dependent conductances for both Ca^{2+} and Na^+ contribute to the anomalous rectification seen during depolarization of CA1 hippocampal pyramidal cells. In order to eliminate any possible contribution of gNa to the effects of ACh on R_N, slices were exposed to both tetrodotoxin (TTX) and Mn^{2+} prior to ACh application. Under these conditions ACh caused little if any change in membrane potential. A representative plot of R_N versus V_m from one neuron exposed to Mn^{2+}-TTX solution is shown in Fig. 3. In this cell R_N decreased as V_m was depolarized, i.e. delayed rectification was present. This effect began at membrane potentials in the -65 mV to -60 mV range and extended to the lowest membrane potential studied. Rectification over this range of membrane potentials was quite substantial, amounting to 50% in the example shown. Upon addition of ACh, R_N values were increased relative to control at various levels of membrane potential. Rectification was still present, but its activation appeared to be shifted to lower potentials, perhaps as a consequence of

Table 1. Summary of ACh effects on input resistance (R_N) and membrane potential (V_m).

Condition		$\frac{R_N \text{ after ACh at } -60 \text{ mV}}{R_N \text{ before ACh at } -60 \text{ mV}}$	$\frac{R_N \text{ after ACh at } -75 \text{ mV}}{R_N \text{ before ACh at } -75 \text{ mV}}$	ΔV_m after ACh
Normal	(n=11)	1.28 ± 0.18*	1.06 ± 0.10	+14.3 ± 10.8 mV (n=33)*
Mn^{2+}	(n=5)	1.29 ± 0.18*	1.02 ± 0.06	+ 2.0 ± 3.5 mV
Mn^{2+}-TTX	(n=10)	1.31 ± 0.33*	1.05 ± 0.06	+ 1.4 ± 2.1 mV
TTX	(n=6)	1.32 ± 0.20*	1.16 ± 0.18	+ 6.2 ± 3.1 mV*

Numbers are means ± S.D. ΔV_m = change in resting membrane potential (+ = depolarization); R_N = input resistance determined from measurement with constant-current pulses. Asterisks indicate that values for cells before and after ACh differ significantly at $p < 0.05$.

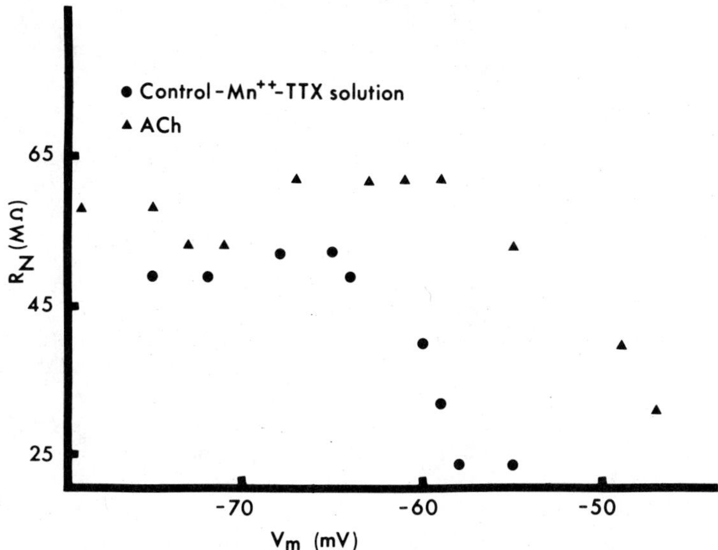

Fig. 3. Plot of R_N versus V_m of a single cell before (●) and after (▲) ACh exposure in medium containing Mn^{2+} and TTX. Rectification is evident in the control condition where R_N decreases about 50% as the cell is depolarized from -75 mV to -55 mV. After ACh application R_N increases, and rectification is still observed but its activation is shifted to lower V_ms. Voltage-dependent action of ACh is prominent at V_ms < -63 mV. Resting V_m: -61 mV.

superimposed R_N increases in the range of V_ms from -65 mV to the most depolarized levels tested. Under these conditions, as shown in Table 1, ACh still produced a voltage-dependent increase in R_N, prominent at -60 mV, but insignificant at -75 mV.

These experiments indicate that the voltage-dependent component of ACh action persists after gCa and gNa are blocked. Other data suggest that ACh effects are produced by blockade of a specific gK. For example, although membrane rectification was prominent in cells exposed to Mn^{2+}-TTX both before and after ACh, rectification was less pronounced, and became apparent only at more depolarized levels following ACh. These findings indicate that there are two components of voltage-dependent K^+ conductance whose activation ranges overlap to some extent, only one of which is decreased by ACh. The ACh-sensitive component is most likely independent of the delayed rectifier, since no concurrent effects on spike duration were seen, though these neurons are known to show spike broadening after exposure to agents such as TEA which blocks delayed rectification.[23] The ACh effect in pyramidal neurons seems analogous to the action of ACh in bullfrog sympathetic ganglion cells reported by Brown and Adams.[17] ACh appears to act on a voltage-dependent K^+ current pharmacologically distinguishable by its sensitivity to muscarinic agonists. This K^+ current has been termed the M-current by Brown and Adams.[17] Recent experiments employing a single electrode voltage clamp in CA1 neurons support our conclusion that M-current is present in these cells.[24]

If Ca^{2+} entry was responsible for the depolarization of V_m after ACh application, as suggested by the results obtained in Mn^{2+}-containing solutions, an activation of the Ca^{2+} mediated gK known to be present in these neurons[21] would be expected to terminate the ACh evoked depolarization and cause an increase in membrane conductance. Such effects were not seen. Therefore we wondered whether ACh might depress Ca^{2+}-activated gK in addition to its action on voltage-dependent gK. Following gNa blockade with TTX, the actions of ACh on Ca^{2+} activated gK were investigated by measuring the conductance following a presumed Ca^{2+} spike, evoked with intracellular current before and after ACh application (Fig. 4). As shown, under control conditions a significant increase in conductance followed a single Ca^{2+} spike (Fig. 4A). ACh application in stratum radiatum caused a depolarization and increased R_N (Fig. 4B). Single Ca^{2+} spikes, evoked under these conditions were not followed by increases in conductance (cf. Figs. 4B1 and 4B2). This effect was transient, lasting about 30 seconds, after which an increase in conductance could again be seen following elicitation of a Ca^{2+} potential (Fig. 4C).

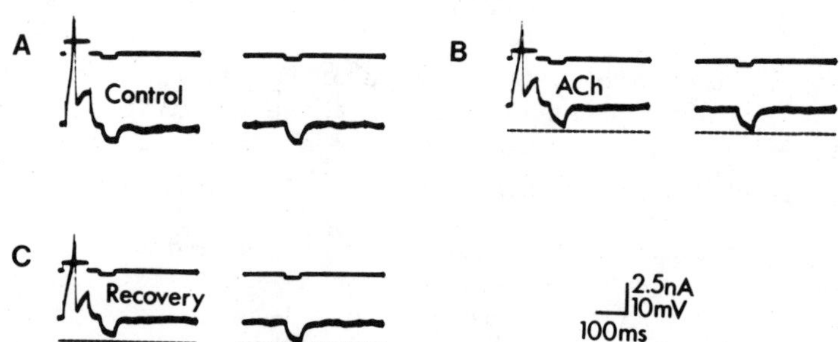

Fig. 4. ACh-induced blockade of conductance increase following single presumed Ca spike. A: control sweeps showing a 17% increase in conductance following TTX-resistant spike. B: 30 sec after application of ACh to the stratum radiatum, the same cell shows depolarization, increased R_N, and a loss of the conductance increase following directly evoked slow spike. Depolarizing current intensity was decreased from A to B so that only single spike was evoked. C: 15 sec after B. Some recovery of the post-spike conductance. Calibration in C for all sweeps.

Long time-course effects of ACh: Of particular relevance to the general topic of this symposium is the long-term nature of the effects of ACh on neuronal behavior. The increases in R_N described above, which followed a single ACh application, had a prolonged time course and were associated with a parallel increase in cell excitability. CA1 neurons characteristically fire single spikes in response to various stimuli.[27,28] However following ACh application these cells became capable of prolonged depolarizations and burst generation, and this change in firing mode could last for hours. Figure 5A shows a typical orthodromic control response to stratum radiatum stimulation which consisted of a suprathreshold EPSP followed by an IPSP. Approximately 60 seconds after ACh application this same cell fired a spike doublet in response to orthodromic stimulation at the same intensity (Fig. 5B), and within an additional 30 seconds the same stimulus evoked a well-formed burst (Fig. 5C). In other experiments we found that this bursting could be widespread and synchronous in the population as indicated by the development of multiphasic field potentials which occurred spontaneously and in response to orthodromic stimulation. Bursts were similar to those seen after application of convulsant agents.[29] Since identical bursts could be elicited by brief (1 msec) depolarizing intracellular current pulses, and blocked with hyperpolarizing DC current, ACh-induced bursting did not seem to be due to presynaptic effects in a given neuron, although synaptic mechanisms were obviously involved in synchronizing the population. It is possible that ACh-induced depression of inhibitory synaptic activities contributes to synchronization and burst generation.[31] Once burst firing became evident in a region of the slice previously exposed to ACh, a complete return to the mode of single spike generation was not observed during experiments which lasted many hours.

These significant changes in the neuronal firing pattern were accompanied by persistent increases in R_N. Additional experiments were done to further explore these long duration changes in behavior. Since Ca^{2+} entry is known to activate intracellular metabolic events which have a long time course in other preparations,[32] we examined the duration of ACh-induced changes in R_N in slices treated with Mn^{2+}, a Ca^{2+} blocker. As noted above, changes in R_N still occurred under these circumstances however their time course was brief, measured in seconds, compared to the increases in R_N following ACh application in normal medium.

These results suggest that the ACh-induced long duration increases in R_N are dependent upon activation of intracellular processes by Ca^{2+}. To further test the hypothesis that ACh was producing a tonic modulation of the properties of CA1 pyramidal neurons, we produced selective blockade of presumed tonic ACh activity using bath application of atropine (10^{-6}-10^{-7} M) or

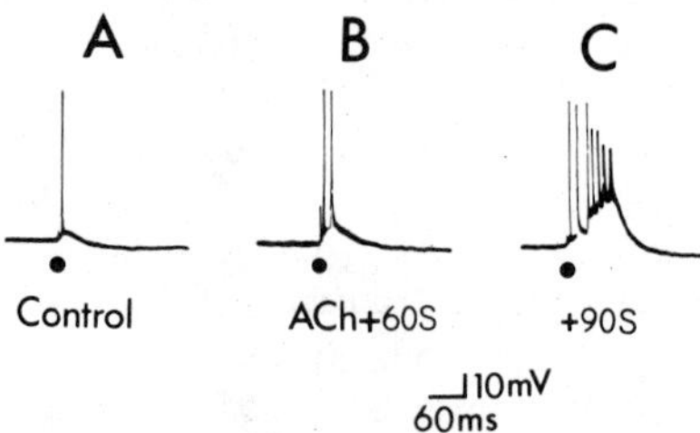

Fig. 5. Development of orthodromically evoked burst generation in a pyramidal neuron following ACh application. A: control response to stimulation of stratum radiatum (●), showing the usual EPSP-IPSP sequence. ACh (1 mM) was applied between A and B giving rise to a 10 mV depolarization from a resting V_m of -60 mV, and a 12% increase in R_N. B: sixty sec following ACh delivery after the cell had repolarized. Orthodromic stimulus at the same current intensity evoked a spike doublet. C: 30 sec after B, same orthodromic stimulus evoked a fully developed burst response which could be blocked by hyperpolarizing current (not shown).

scopolamine (10^{-6} M). Under these conditions all responses to ACh were blocked, suggesting that they were mediated by ACh interaction with muscarinic receptors. But in addition to blocking ACh effects, atropine and scopolamine alone induced changes in membrane properties of hippocampal pyramidal cells which required at least 1 hr to fully develop. The mean R_N of the population of neurons exposed to atropine was 21.9 ± 7.7 (S.D.) MΩ (n = 24), at a mean resting potential of -63.4 ± 6.7 (S.D.) mV. This R_N value was significantly reduced ($p < 0.001$) in comparison to control values of 37.6 ± 8.7 (S.D.) MΩ (n = 74) at a mean resting potential of 66.2 ± 7.3 (S.D.) mV obtained in normal medium. As previously mentioned, control recordings in hippocampal pyramidal cells characteristically show that there is a range of membrane potential extending from about -70 mV to the firing threshold over which an apparent increase in R_N, or anomalous inward rectification, occurs.[20] However following exposure to atropine, none of the 24 neurons studied showed prominent anomalous rectification in the depolarizing direction, presumably because of the increase in voltage-dependent gK which developed after muscarinic blockade. These effects of muscarinic antagonists on the resting R_N and its response to membrane depolarization are opposite to those of exogenously applied ACh, which both increases R_N at rest and exaggerates a voltage-sensitive component of R_N during depolarization. Whereas muscarinic blockade of ACh responses began after minutes, the changes in membrane properties seemed to develop slowly after 1-2 hrs of perfusion with atropine or scopolamine. These data suggest that there is a tonic action of ACh on membrane properties, which is not directly antagonized by muscarinic receptor blockade. It appears that ACh receptor interaction initiates some type of secondary process which in turn alters R_N. It may be that the latency between the initiation of muscarinic blockade by atropine, and its effects on R_N represents the time required for dissipation of this secondary process.

Because of reports that ACh actions are mimicked by guanosine 3'5 cyclic monophosphate (cGMP) in some[33,34] but not other[35,36,37] preparations, we attempted to reproduce the ACh effects on R_N both by extracellular application of dibutyryl cGMP (up to 10^{-3} M) or by direct intracellular iontophoresis of cGMP (10^{-3}-10^{-4} M in K acetate). Neither method produced changes similar to those of ACh applications, even though techniques were identical to those used in other experiments which showed significant effects of adenosine 3'5' cyclic monophosphate (cAMP) applications (see below).

Dopaminergic System

Our interest in studying the action of DA on hippocampal pyramidal neurons relates to the paucity of information on the physiological effects of this agent on cortical neurons. Recent reports show that DA containing terminals are present in the hippocampus[38,39] and that DA stimulates hippocampal cAMP by activating a DA receptor.[40,41,42] It has been proposed that alterations in intracellular cAMP induce important long-term effects on membrane excitability properties.[18] We therefore focused these studies on the nature of DA action, and on potential long duration effects.

The initial response to DA in 16 of 21 CA1 hippocampal pyramidal neurons consisted of a small hyperpolarization which occurred within 3-40 sec of application (Fig. 6A). These hyperpolarizations were often not associated with a prominent change in R_N, although decreases in R_N were seen in cells which showed the largest hyperpolarizing responses. A second effect of DA was to augment the afterhyperpolarizations which are known to occur in hippocampal pyramidal neurons as a consequence of repetitive spike activity.[21,26,43] These slow afterhyperpolarizations (AHPs) normally can last up to 1-2 seconds following repetitive spike discharges. Under control conditions, when depolarizing current pulses were delivered at frequencies of about 1 Hz and at sufficient intensities to elicit 2-10 action potentials, we found that the slow AHPs which followed each group of spikes summated until a steady membrane

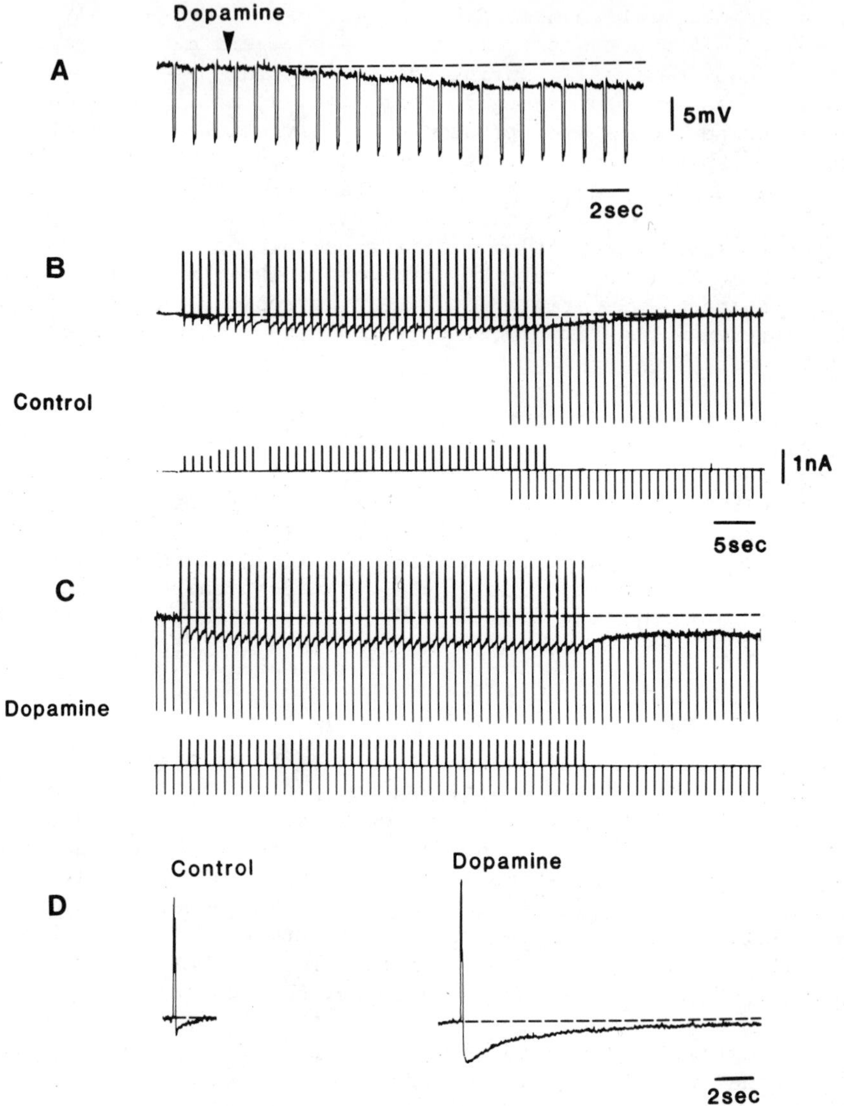

Fig. 6. Dopamine actions on hippocampal neurons. A: hyperpolarizing response of a cell to application of 10^{-5} M DA. The voltage response to constant-current hyperpolarizing pulses shows that no detectable change of input resistance accompanies this hyperpolarization. Resting potential: -60 mV. B: in another neuron under normal conditions a 1 Hz train of 120 msec duration depolarizing current pulses, of sufficient intensity to elicit 2-10 spikes, results in membrane hyperpolarization associated with a decrease in resistance. When depolarizing pulses are discontinued the membrane repolarizes and resistance recovers to the control level. C: after DA application onto the cell of B the membrane potential hyperpolar-

potential was reached. In the control state V_m consistently recovered to the baseline level within seconds after such stimulation was discontinued (Fig. 6B). Following DA application however, the slow AHPs evoked by the same depolarizing current pulses were larger and the steady summated hyperpolarization was maintained even after pulses were discontinued, i.e., there was no recovery of V_m (or R_N) to the prestimulus baseline potential (Fig. 6C). Once this effect was observed it was also noted that slow AHPs following a single evoked spike train were augmented as well. Such AHPs were of larger amplitude than control responses and could last up to 18 seconds (cf. Fig. 6D, "Control" and "Dopamine"). The DA effect on AHPs were detectable within seconds after application fo the agent, reached a maximum over several minutes, and persisted for at least 1 hr following a single application.

The maximum total hyperpolarization recorded subsequent to DA delivery (i.e. the spontaneous increase in V_m (Fig. 6A) plus stimulated summated AHPs (Fig. 6C)) was 7.7 ± 6.0 (S.D.) mV (n = 13). These peak increases in V_m were associated with decreases in R_N of 19-42%. Similar changes in R_N could not be produced by hyperpolarization alone, i.e., they were not related to membrane rectification.

A reversal potential for the DA hyperpolarization was estimated from plots of voltage versus applied current before and after DA application. The mean reversal potential obtained from intersection

ized by a few millivolts (not shown) and was then depolarized to a control level (dashed line) with DC current. A train of depolarizing pulses comparable to that in B was delivered. R_N decreased during the train and membrane potential and resistance at the end of the train of depolarizing pulses did not recover to prestimulus levels. Control resting potential: -56 mV. D: examples of slow afterhyperpolarizations in control and DA-treated neurons, elicited by depolarizing current pulses which evoke 5-6 spikes. Dashed lines: baseline resting potentials. These segments and those in subsequent figures except 2A are from a strip chart recorder. Spike amplitudes are amputated or attenuated by low frequency response. Voltage calibration in A for all segments. Calibrations in B for B and C.

of voltage-current lines was -86.8 ± 11.1 (S.D.) mV (n = 8). A reversal potential at this negative level would be more consistent with DA action to increase a K^+, rather than a Cl^- conductance. Estimates of the K^+ equilibrium potential obtained from reversal of slow AHPs[26] are very close to the above value for the DA hyperpolarization, whereas the equilibrium potential for chloride obtained from the reversal potential of GABA-induced hyperpolarization in hippocampal pyramidal cells is about -70 mV.[44] The conclusion that chloride is not involved in DA action was further supported by the observation that DA-induced increases in V_m were equally prominent in neurons impaled with KCl-containing microelectrodes, even when IPSPs, known to be primarily Cl^- mediated,[19,45] were reversed.

Thus the increases in conductance during the spontaneous or triggered hyperpolarizations which follow DA application are consistent with increases in K^+ permeability. Augmentation of AHPs following repetitive spikes could be due to activation of a pump by DA, an action similar to that described for norepinephrine,[46] or to some enhancement of the slow AHP which is known to be due to a Ca^{2+} activated gK in hippocampal pyramidal cells.[21,25,26] Support for the latter explanation is offered by the findings that DA-enhanced AHPs are associated with conductance increases, as are slow AHPs in control neurons, and that the reversal potentials for control and DA augmented AHPs occur at similar very negative V_m levels. In addition, DA-enhanced AHPs are blocked by Mn^{2+}, a Ca^{2+} antagonist, as are control slow AHPs.[21,25] If the DA-enhanced slow AHP were due in part to a Na^+-K^+ pump activation,[47] we would have expected persistence of at least a component of this potential when trains of spikes were evoked in Mn^{2+} solutions. This was not the case, however. Stimulus-evoked slow AHPs were entirely blocked in Mn^{2+} solutions. However these experiments did show that spontaneous hyperpolarizations associated with conductance increases could still be observed after application of larger volumes of DA to some neurons in Mn^{2+} solutions, suggesting that Ca^{2+} entry _per se_ was not required for this DA effect.

We propose that the most likely explanation for the spontaneous and stimulus-evoked hyperpolarizations and increased conductance produced by DA would be an action of this agent to induce or enhance the Ca^{2+} dependent K^+ conductance in hippocampal CA1 pyramidal neurons. Such an effect could be due to processes which increase intracellular Ca^{2+} concentration as proposed for neocortical neurons following dinitrophenol injection[48] and for cockroach neurons following DA application.[49] For example, the DA induced initial hyperpolarization could result from release of Ca^{2+} from intracellular stores, and/or decreased Ca^{2+} buffering. These actions combined with tonic Ca^{2+} entry, which presumably occurs at resting potential,[20] would cause a prolonged increase in gK. The persistence of DA-induced hyperpolarization in Mn^{2+} solution would be consistent with a DA-mediated release of Ca^{2+} from intracellular stores. The cumulative hyperpolarization which follows repetitive stimulus-induced spike trains would thus derive from prolonged increases in intracellular Ca^{2+} concentration following Ca^{2+} influx, which in turn would activate a long lasting change in gK. Such a mechanism is consistent with hypotheses regarding the dependence of membrane K^+ permeability on intracellular Ca^{2+} concentration.[50] One test of the above hypothesis would be to enhance buffering of intracellular Ca^{2+} by loading neurons with a Ca^{2+} chelator. This maneuver is known to block the normal Ca^{2+}-dependent K^+ conductance and the slow AHP in hippocampal pyramidal neurons[26,51] and would therefore be expected to depress DA effects as well. As is illustrated in Fig. 7, EGTA injection into these cells depresses both DA-induced hyperpolarization and enhancement of AHPs. Thus DA effects on intracellular Ca^{2+} seem to be the most likely explanation for the neuronal behaviors described above.

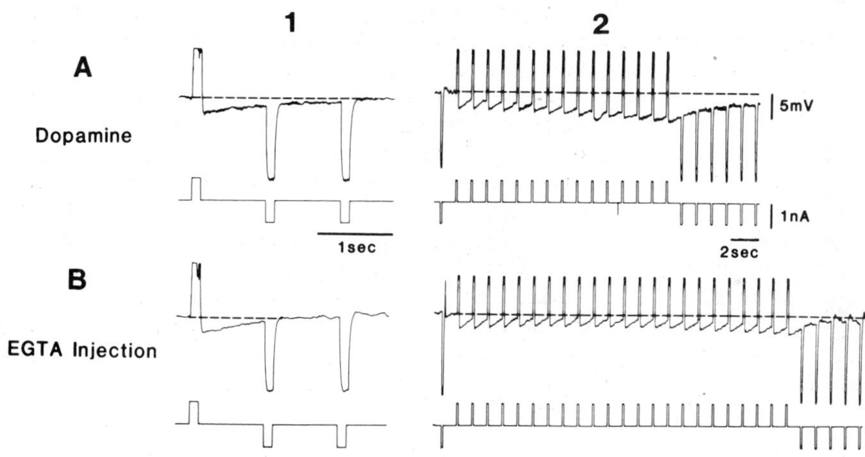

Fig. 7. Actions of intracellular EGTA on DA effects. A-B: records obtained from cell impaled with EGTA containing microelectrode following application of DA (10^{-5} M). A1: before EGTA iontophoresis a slow afterhyperpolarization lasting 2 sec follows a single depolarizing current pulse. A2: a train of depolarizing current pulses causes a decrease in resistance, and a hyperpolarization of membrane potential which does not recover to prestimulus level. B: following 1 min, 1.5 nA hyperpolarizing DC current to electrophorese EGTA. B1: single depolarizing current pulse elicits a slow afterhyperpolarization lasting 1 sec. B2: response of neuron to train of depolarizing current pulses similar to those of A2. Slow afterhyperpolarizations are of reduced amplitude and duration. Membrane potential recovers to prestimulus level following train. Dashed line = resting potential in A-B: -61 mV. Calibrations in A for A-B.

Since other investigators have demonstrated DA-stimulated increases in hippocampal cAMP, it might be proposed that the long duration DA actions described above are in some way mediated by an increase in intracellular cAMP. To test this hypothesis we applied 8-bromoadenosine 3'5'-cyclic monophosphate (10^{-4}M) by bath perfusion or adenosine 3'5'-cyclic monophosphate (10^{-3} M) by intracellular iontophoresis. The effects were similar to those of DA, i.e. AHPs were augmented and spontaneous increases in V_m developed associated with decreases in R_N.

In order to determine whether the DA actions detailed above were specific to activation of DA receptors, we studied the effects of application of DA agonists apomorphine and epinine, and receptor blockers chloropromazine and flupenthixol. The agonists closely mimicked the action of DA, while the antagonists blocked DA effects.

DISCUSSION

The cholinergic and dopaminergic inputs to the hippocampus have several common properties. In both cases, the cell bodies of origin are remote from the target structure and project diffusely to the cellular elements in the hippocampus.[40,52] Our data indicate that both agents can produce prolonged effects upon neuronal properties lasting many minutes or even hours; such effects could fundamentally alter neuronal responses to other inputs. These actions can be defined as modulatory in nature,[1] and appear to be mediated through effects on intracellular processes rather than typical receptor-ionophore interactions. The modulation induced by these agents has as its final common path a prolonged effect on K^+ channels. In the case of ACh, long duration excitatory effects are mediated predominantly by blockade of a voltage-dependent gK, whereas DA appears to act indirectly to enhance an ion-activated gK, producing inhibitory effects.

Our results suggest that there is tonic release of ACh which can lead to modulation of R_N over a wide range of values. Cell responses to other inputs would predictably be under control of this powerful biasing system, so that cholinergic activation or inactivation might give rise to heterosynaptic facilitation or disfacilitation, respectively. If some degree of specificity is maintained between septal cholinergic neurons and their target cells in the hippocampus, cell behavior of individual neurons or groups of neurons could be influenced in a very complex manner.* This could have very important implications for learning and memory.

---

*In this chapter we have chosen to emphasize the postsynaptic actions of ACh. This agent probably has significant presynaptic actions as well which would make for even more complex effects on net hippocampal excitability.

It has often been suggested that long term potentiation is involved in these processes[53] and, interestingly, extracellular recordings *in vivo* show that ACh application or inactivation of the cholinergic pathway augment facilitation.[56] Thus it is reasonable to speculate that the role of the cholinergic system is to prime the hippocampus to receive information from other specific inputs, and that this action is important in facilitating long term information storage. In this context it is interesting that when the cholinergic system is blocked chemically by atropine, amnesia results[57] and when the cholinergic cells of origin are ablated, conditioning is retarded.[58] Such maneuvers would be associated with a pronounced change in the basic membrane properties of hippocampal pyramidal neurons.[13] Previous studies have suggested that cholinergic mechanisms may play a role in epileptogenesis.[59,60] The modulation of excitability by ACh described above might play an important role in the pathological as well as physiological processes, given the propensity of ACh treated populations of pyramidal neurons to generate synchronous epileptiform bursts. The known connectivity in the hippocampal septal system would cause the excitatory output of pyramidal neurons to further increase the release of ACh from medial septal nucleus neurons back onto hippocampal pyramidal cells, thus forming a positive feedback loop, and potentially leading to development of ictal activity.

One of the most intriguing aspects of DA effects on hippocampal pyramidal cells is the finding that this agent promotes long term alterations in cell behavior which are contingent upon and triggered by cell firing. However, unlike ACh, DA induces an increase in conductance which tends to make cells less excitable. Our results suggest that DA, by augmenting AHPs, may significantly influence the cyclical excitability which at times characterizes hippocampal pyramidal cell activity (e.g., generation of theta activity;[53] intrinsic burst generation;[4,25] and epileptogenesis[29]) through its facilitation of afterhyperpolarizations. The precise role of DA actions in learning and memory are of course poorly understood. Although the DA system in the hippocampus is known to be a very sparse projection and might therefore be regarded as somewhat unimportant, our data indicate that DA acts on hippocampal pyramidal cells at concentrations at least as low as 1 μM, has long term, possibly cumulative actions, and therefore may have a powerful influence on hippocampal neuronal activities *in vivo*. As in the case of the cholinergic septo-hippocampal system, hippocampal output could influence the excitability of remote dopaminergic somata and produce feedback modulation of pyramidal cell activities.

ACKNOWLEDGMENTS

This work was supported by NIH grants NS 12151 and NS 06477 from the NINCDS to DAP and NSF Predoctoral Fellowship to LSB.

REFERENCES

1. I. Kupferman, Modulatory actions of neurotransmitters, Ann. Rev. Neurosci. 2:447-465 (1979).
2. R. Dingledine, J. Dodd, and J.S. Kelly, The in vitro brain slice as a useful neurophysiological preparation for intracellular recording, Neurosci. Meth. 2:323-362 (1980).
3. P. Andersen and I.A. Langmoen, Intracellular studies on transmitter effects on neurones in isolated brain slices, Quart. Rev. of Biophys. 13:1-18 (1980).
4. E.R. Kandel and W.A. Spencer, Electrophysiology of hippocampal neurons. II. Afterpotentials and repetitive firing. J. Neurophysiol. 24:243-259 (1961).
5. E.R. Kandel, W.A. Spencer, and J.F. Brinley, Jr., Electrophysiology of hippocampal neurons. I. Sequential invasion and synaptic organization, J. Neurophysiol. 24:225-242 (1961).
6. W.A. Spencer and E.R. Kandel, Electrophysiology of hippocampal neurons. III. Fast prepotentials, J. Neurophysiol. 24: 272-285 (1961).
7. P.A. Schwartzkroin, Characteristics of CA1 neurons recorded intracellularly in the hippocampal in vitro slice preparation, Brain Res. 128:53-68 (1975).
8. J.D. Green, The hippocampus, Physiol. Rev. 44:561-608 (1964).
9. R.F. Thompson, M.M. Patterson, and T.J. Teyler, Neurophysiology of learning, Ann. Rev. Psychol. 23:73-104 (1972).
10. R.L. Isaacson, The Limbic System, Plenum Press, New York (1974).
11. R.L. Isaacson and K.H. Pribram, The Hippocampus (2 Vols.), Plenum Press, New York (1975).
12. C. Yamamoto, Intracellular study of seizure-like afterdischarges elicited in thin hippocampal sections in vitro, Exp. Neurol. 35:154-164 (1972).
13. L.S. Benardo and D.A. Prince, Acetylcholine induced modulation of hippocampal pyramidal neurons, Brain Res. 211:227-234 (1981).
14. K. Krnjevic, R. Pumain, and L. Renaud, The mechanism of excitation by acetylcholine in the cerebral cortex, J. Physiol. 215:447-465 (1971).
15. J. Dodd, R. Dingledine, and J.S. Kelly, The excitatory action of acetylcholine on hippocampal neurones of the guinea pig and rat maintained in vitro, Brain Res. 207:109-127 (1981).
16. F.F. Weight and J. Votava, Slow synaptic excitation in sympathetic ganglion cells: evidence for synaptic inactivation of potassium conductance, Science 170:755-758 (1970).
17. D.A. Brown and P.R. Adams, Muscarinic suppression of a novel voltage-sensitive K^+ current in a vertebrate neurone, Nature, Lond. 283:673-676 (1980).
18. I. Kupferman, Role of cyclic nucleotides in excitable cells, Ann. Rev. Physiol. 42:629-641 (1980).

19. K. Krnjevic, Chemical nature of synaptic transmission in vertebrates, Physiol. Rev. 54:419-540 (1974).
20. J.R. Hotson, D.A. Prince, and P.A. Schwartzkroin, Anomalous inward rectification in hippocampal neurons, J. Neurophysiol. 42:889-895 (1979).
21. J.R. Hotson and D.A. Prince, A calcium activated hyperpolarization follows repetitive firing in hippocampal neurons, J. Neurophysiol. 43:409-419 (1980).
22. M.J. Gutnick and D.A. Prince, Dye-coupling and possible electrotonic coupling in the guinea pig neocortex, Science 211: 67-70 (1981).
23. P.A. Schwartzkroin and D.A. Prince, Effects of TEA on hippocampal neurons, Brain Res. 185:169-181 (1980).
24. J.V. Halliwell, P.R. Adams, and D.A. Brown, "M" and "F" currents in voltage-clamped hippocampal pyramidal cells, Biophys. J. 33:90a (1981).
25. R.K.S. Wong and D.A. Prince, Participation of calcium spikes during intrinsic burst firing in hippocampal neurons, Brain Res. 159:385-390 (1978).
26. B.E. Alger and R.A. Nicoll, Epileptiform burst afterhyperpolarization: calcium-dependent potassium potential in hippocampal CA1 pyramidal cells, Science 210:1122-1124 (1980).
27. D.A. Prince and P.A. Schwartzkroin, Non-synaptic mechanisms in epileptogenesis, in: Abnormal Neuronal Discharges, N. Chalazonitis and M. Boisson, eds., Raven Press, New York (1978).
28. R.K.S. Wong, D.A. Prince, and A.I. Basbaum, Intradendritic recordings from hippocampal neurons, Proc. Nat. Acad. Sci. (Wash.) 76:986-990 (1979).
29. P.A. Schwartzkroin and D.A. Prince, Penicillin-induced epileptiform activity in the hippocampal in vitro preparation, Ann. Neurol. 1:463-469 (1977).
30. R.J. Valentino and R. Dingledine, Presynaptic inhibitory effect of acetylcholine in the hippocampus, J. Neurosci. 1:784-792 (1981).
31. R.K.S. Wong and D.A. Prince, Dendritic mechanisms underlying penicillin-induced epileptiform activity, Science 204: 1228-1231 (1979).
32. J.W. Phillis, The role of cyclic nucleotides in the CNS, Can. J. Neurol. Sci. 4:151-195 (1977).
33. F.F. Weight, G. Petzhold, and P. Greengard, Guanosine 3',5'-monophosphate in sympathetic ganglia: increase associated with synaptic transmission, Science 186:942-944 (1974).
34. C.D. Woody, B.E. Swartz, and E. Gruen, Effects of acetylcholine and cyclic GMP on input resistance of cortical neurons in awake cats, Brain Res. 158:373-395 (1978).

35. N.J. Dun, K. Kaibara and A.G. Karczmar, Muscarinic cGMP induced membrane potential changes: differences in electrogenic mechanisms, Brain Res. 150:658-661 (1978).
36. K. Krnjevic, Intracellular actions of a transmitter, in: Iontophoresis and Transmitter Mechanisms in the Mammalian Central Nervous System, R.W. Ryall and J.S. Kelly, eds., Elsevier, Amsterdam (1978).
37. F.F. Weight, P.A. Smith, and J.A. Schulman, Postsynaptic potential generation appears not to be associated with synaptic elevation of cyclic nucleotides in sympathetic neurons, Brain Res. 158:197-202 (1978).
38. L.W. Swanson and B.K. Hartman, The central adrenergic system. An immunofluorescence study of the location of cell bodies and their efferent connections in the rat utilizing dopamine-β-hydroxylase as a marker, J. Comp. Neurol. 163: 467-505 (1975).
39. S. Bischoff, B. Scatton, and J. Korf, Biochemical evidence for a transmitter role of dopamine in the rat hippocampus, Brain Res. 165:161-165 (1979).
40. T. Hokfelt, A. Ljungdalal, K. Fuxe, and O. Johansson, Dopamine nerve terminals in the rat limbic cortex: aspects of the dopamine hypothesis of schizophrenia, Science 184:177-179 (1974).
41. B. Scatton, H. Simon, M. LeMoal, and S. Bischoff, Origin of dopaminergic innervation of the rat hippocampal formation, Neurosci. Lett. 18:125-131 (1980).
42. A. Dolphin and J. Bockaert, β-adrenergic receptors coupled to adenylate cyclase in cat brain: regional distribution, pharmacological characteristics and adaptive responsiveness, in: Recent Advances in the Pharmacology of Adrenoreceptors, E. Szabadi et al., eds., Elsevier, Amsterdam (1981), in press.
43. R.K.S. Wong and D.A. Prince, Afterpotential generation in hippocampal pyramidal cells, J. Neurophysiol. 45:86-97 (1981).
44. P. Andersen, R. Dingledine, L. Gjerstad, I.A. Langmoen, and A. Mosfeldt-Laursen, Two different responses of hippocampal pyramidal cells to application of gamma-aminobutyric acid, J. Physiol. Lond. 305:279-296 (1980).
45. B.E. Alger and R.A. Nicoll, Enkephalin blocks inhibitory pathways in the vertebrate CNS, Nature 281:315-317 (1979).
46. M. Segal, The action of norepinephrine in the rat hippocampus: intracellular studies in the slice preparation, Brain Res. 206:107-128 (1981).
47. J.K.S. Jansen and J.G. Nicholls, Conductance changes, an electrogenic pump and the hyperpolarization of leech neurones following impulses, J. Physiol. Lond. 229:635-655 (1973).
48. J.M. Godfraind, H. Kawamura, K. Krnjevic, and R. Pumain, Actions of dinitrophenol and some other metabolic inhibitors on cortical neurones, J. Physiol. Lond. 215:199-222 (1971).

49. B.L. Ginsborg, C.R. House and M.R. Mitchell, On the role of calcium in the electrical responses of the cockroach salivary gland cells to dopamine, J. Physiol. Lond. 303:325-335 (1980).
50. R.W. Meech, Calcium-dependent potassium activation in nervous tissue, Ann. Rev. Biophys. Bioeng. 7:1-18 (1978).
51. P.A. Schwartzkroin and C.E. Stafstrom, Effects of EGTA on the calcium-activated afterhyperpolarization in hippocampal CA3 pyramidal cells, Science 210:1125-1126 (1980).
52. G.S. Lynch, G. Rose and C.M. Gall, Anatomical and functional aspects of the septo-hippocampal projections, in: Functions of the Septo-Hippocampal System, K. Elliot and J. Whelan, eds, Elsevier, Amsterdam (1978).
53. K. Elliot and J. Whelan, Functions of the Septo-Hippocampal System, Elsevier, Amsterdam (1978).
54. C. Yamamoto and N. Kawai, Presynaptic action of acetylcholine on thin sections from the guinea-pig dentate gyrus in vitro, Exp. Neurol. 19:176-187 (1967).
55. J. Hounsgaard, Presynaptic inhibitory action of acetylcholine in area CA1 of the hippocampus, Exp. Neurol. 62:787-797 (1978).
56. J.F. DeFrance, J.C. Stanley, J.E. Marchand, and R.B. Chronister, Cholinergic mechanisms and short-term potentiation, in: Functions of the Septo-Hippocampal System, K. Elliot and J. Whelan, eds., Elsevier, Amsterdam (1978).
57. I.R. Phines and M. Nickerson, Atropine, scopolamine, and related antimuscarinic drugs, in: The Pharmacological Basis of Experimental Therapeutics, L.S. Goodman and A. Gilman, eds., MacMillan, New York (1975).
58. S.D. Berry and R.F. Thompson, Medial septal lesions retard classical conditioning of the nictitating membrane response in rabbits, Science 205:209-210 (1979).
59. J.H. Ferguson and H.H. Jasper, Laminar DC studies of acetylcholine activated epileptiform discharge in cerebral cortex, Electroenceph. Clin. Neurophysiol. 30:377-390 (1971).
60. A.G. Nasello and E.S. Marichich, Effects of some cholinergic, adrenergic and serotonergic compounds, glutamic acid, and GABA on hippocampal seizures, Pharmacology 9:233-239 (1973).
61. D.A. Prince, B.W. Connors, and L.S. Benardo, Transitions from interictal to ictal epileptiform discharge, in: International Symposium on Status Epilepticus (1981), in press.

VISUAL AND AUDITORY CUES SUPPORT PLACE FIELD ACTIVITY OF HIPPOCAMPAL UNITS IN THE RAT

Phillip J. Best and Alvin J. Hill

Department of Psychology
University of Virginia
Charlottesville, Virginia 22901

SUMMARY

The firing rates of hippocampal units vary as a function of the animal's position in space. For example, on an elevated radial maze a particular cell might show enhanced activity on one arm. In intact rats, if the maze is rotated within the environment, the place field of the cell persists with respect to the environment and not to the maze. Lesions of the fornix or entorhinal cortex reduce the robustness of place field activity and severely disrupt persistence with respect to the environment.

In blind and deaf rats hippocampal cells have place fields. Following maze rotation the place fields of most cells (11 of 15) remain on the original arm of the maze. In the other (4) cells the place fields persist with respect to the environment, but spinning the rat, to disturb vestibular function, disrupts this environmental persistence. Thus removal of sensory information has similar effects on hippocampal place cell activity as does lesions of hippocampal connections.

INTRODUCTION

Conditioning does not occur in a vacuum. The cognitive processing that accompanies the association of the conditioned stimulus (CS) and the unconditioned stimulus (UCS) is much more complex than the automatic elicitation of an arbitrarily chosen behavioral response. A wide variety of overt behavioral responses and more covert internal variables can be modified during conditioning, and the measurable changes in these responses can occur at different rates. Yet, in studies of the neurobiological substrates of conditioning a CS and UCS are paired in a specific environment and a single behavioral response is measured as an index of the strength of conditioning.

The fact that unit activity in the hippocampus (or any other structure) shows reliable changes during conditioning, which precede and correlate with a particular behavioral response, does not necessarily indicate that the hippocampus provides the neural substrate of that conditioned response. Instead, the hippocampus could be the neural substrate for one or more of the other conditioned behavioral or internal responses. In fact, the conditioned responses of hippocampal cells could merely reflect the myriad of changes conditioning hath wrought in other structures. For example, conditioning can result in changes in the arousal response to the CS, and the conditioned hippocampal activity could be merely reflecting those changes in arousal (see Best and Best, 1976).

Much more is learned by an animal during a conditioning procedure than the mere association of the contiguous CS and UCS. The conditioning paradigm teaches the animal about the particular environment in which conditioning has occurred. In fact the environment supports conditioning. Thus, an animal conditioned in one environment will show very weak responses to the same CS in a different environment.

Although the importance of space, context, and environment in animal behavior and especially in learning processes was recognized by early behavioral investigators (Pavlov, 1927; Tolman, 1932), their role was deemphasized for a long time. Place learning was once considered to be merely a variant of cue learning (Restle, 1957). Recent theories of classical conditioning recognize the important role of spatial, contextual, environmental cues in the conditioning process (Rescorla and Wagner, 1972), but until very recently they have been assigned a very passive role.

Lesions of the hippocampus or of its connections produce severe enduring performance deficits in spatial discrimination tasks. However, when these tasks are changed so they can be learned by nonspatial cues the deficits are alleviated (O'Keefe et al., 1975; Olton et al., 1978). Whereas lesions of the hippocampus do not interfere with simple learning they do interfere with aspects of learning that may be very sensitive to the role of contextual cues, such as blocking and latent inhibition (Solomon, 1979; O'Keefe, Nadel, and Willner, 1979). Therefore the apparent role of hippocampus in learning may be more related to an important role in the processing of environmental, contextual, spatial stimuli (O'Keefe and Nadel, 1978).

One of the first indications that the hippocampus may be involved in spatial processing is a report by O'Keefe and Dostrovsky (1971) that some hippocampal pyramidal cells showed augmented firing patterns in different places in the testing apparatus independent of the animal's behavior. Subsequent studies under a variety of conditions indicate that the overwhelming majority of hippocampal pyramidal cells show drastic changes in firing rate when the animal is in a particular place in a test environment (O'Keefe, 1976; Olton, Branch, and Best, 1978; Best and Ranck, in press). Some cells fire faster when an animal moves through a place field than when an animal is stationary in the field. However these cells do not show a change in activity during movement outside of its place field. The place field for a cell appears to be established very rapidly in a novel environment (Hill, 1978). Place fields seem to be determined by multiple distal, spatial, contextual cues and not by local cues on the test apparatus (O'Keefe and Conway, 1978).

We have been investigating place field activity of hippocampal neurons in an attempt to determine the nature of the sensory information that supports place cell activity and the pathways of this information to the hippocampus. We record cellular activity as the animal traverses an elevated radial arm maze in which the arms radiate from a central platform like the spokes of a wheel (Olton and Samuelson, 1976). This apparatus has been extensively used in behavioral studies in intact and lesioned rats. The apparatus is useful for us because it provides an organized space with clearly differentiated subunits.

In intact rats, over 90% of the hippocampal pyramidal cells show clearly delineable place field activity on this maze (Olton, Branch, and Best, 1978; Miller and Best, 1980). An example of place field activity on an 8 arm radial maze is illustrated in figure 1A. The arms are numbered in serial clockwise order. Note that the cell fires much faster when the animal is on arm #1 than on the other arms.

One way to determine the type of sensory information the place field of the cell is dependent upon is to rotate the maze and compare the place field before and after rotation. The maze can be rotated 90° such that arm 3 now occupies the position originally occupied by arm 1. If the place field of the cell is determined by local maze cues, such as odor or floor texture, the field should still be on arm 1 following rotation. However, if the place field is determined by nonmaze cues, such as cues

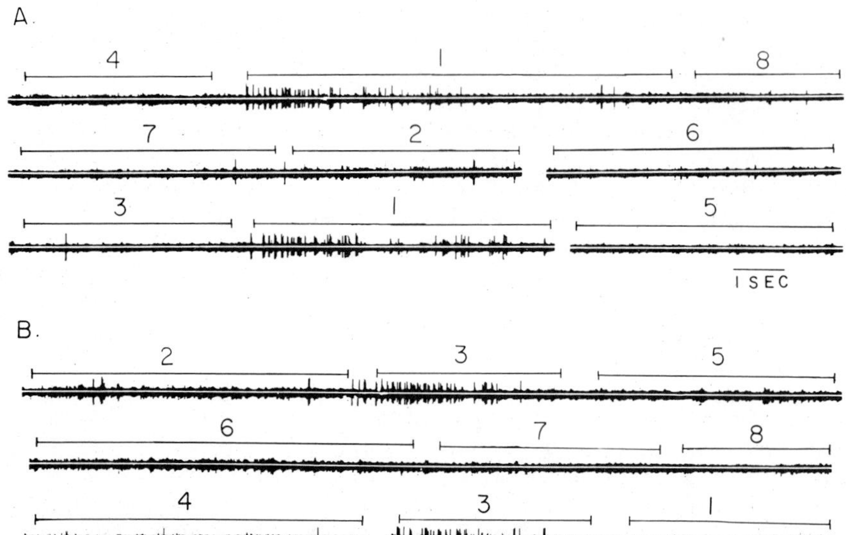

Figure 1. Hippocampal unit activity in an intact rat. The number bars above the signal represent the arms of the maze.
A: Maze is in initial position; place field is on arm 1.
B: Maze has been rotated 90°, arm 3 occupies position of arm 1; place field on arm 3. (From Miller and Best, 1980)

from the surrounding environment or the vestibular system, the field should be found on arm 3 following rotation. Figure 1B illustrates the effects of 90° maze rotation on the place field of the cell in figure 1A. Note that the place field is now on arm 3. The place field persists with respect to the environment and not the local maze cues. Such environmental or spatial persistence has been found in every place cell we have recorded in intact rats (Miller and Best, 1980). This result is consistent with the observations that the behavior of intact rats on the radial arm maze is not altered by rotation of the maze in a fixed environment (Olton and Samuelson, 1976).

Since lesions of the hippocampus or its connections severely debilitate performance on the radial arm maze and other spatial tasks, we decided to ask if such lesions disrupt place cell activity. We examined place cell activity in rats which had undergone bilateral electrolytic lesions of the entorhinal cortex or of the dorsal fornix. Neither lesion totally obliterated place field activity, but both lesions interfered with spatial firing patterns (see Table 1).

Table 1. The effects of lesions on place cell activity, spatial persistence and robustness.

	No. Cells	Place	Persist	Robustness
Intact	24	100 %	100%	201%
Fornix	35	80%	57%	90%
Entorhinal	30	43%	3%	58%

Fewer cells in the lesioned rats showed place fields, and the robustness of the place fields in these cells was reduced. (Robustness is calculated as increase in firing rate in place field as a percent of mean firing rate.) Further, the number of place cells which showed spatial persistence was severely reduced. The entorhinal lesions produced a greater deficit. In fact, only one place cell in a rat with entorhinal lesions showed spatial persistence. Five cells showed a place field on the same physical arm before and after rotation, and seven failed to show significant place field activity after rotation.

Since anatomical studies have indicated that the entorhinal cortex is a source of afferents that carry sensory information to hippocampus (Jones and Powell, 1970; Van Hoessen and Pandya, 1975), entorhinal lesions may produce their effects primarily by disrupting these inputs. The present experiment was designed to determine whether peripheral sensory deprivation could duplicate the effects of entorhinal lesions on behavior and/or on spatial firing in hippocampus. Observations were made using rats deprived of vision and hearing, since these modalities were thought most likely to mediate distant (i.e., extramaze) cues.

METHODS

Male Sprague-Dawley rats were implanted with seven 62 u nichrome wire electrodes in dorsal hippocampus following the procedure of Best, Knowles, and Phillips (1978). Electrodes were positioned on the basis of unit activity monitored during implantation. They were then led through small holes drilled in a 9-pin Amphenol connector and secured against the connector pins with steel screws. The connector was then cemented to the rat's skull. An opaque rubber mask was attached during experimental sessions to deprive rats of vision (Hill, 1979).

Unit recordings were made as rats ran on a 6-arm elevated radial maze similar to that used by Miller and Best (1980). At the end of each arm was a small plastic dish. Twenty percent sucrose solution could be injected into each dish through polyurethane tubing from a syringe mounted outside the shielded recording chamber. The rats were kept water deprived. Unit signals were amplified by an FET source follower which was attached to the connector on the rat's head, a Grass P15B AC preamplifier and an AC solid-state amplifier. Unit activity was recorded on the audio channel of a Sony AV 3650 videotape recorder. The rat's behavior was recorded on the video portion of the tape.

Two days following surgery, each rat was masked, brought into the recording chamber and placed on the 6-arm maze. All arms were initially baited with sucrose, and were rebaited on an arbitrary schedule. The rat was allowed to run freely on the maze while firing rates were monitored from the implanted electrodes. When a cell was observed that showed good isolation and clear spatial firing activity, it was recorded, along with the rat's behavior, until the animal had run down each arm of the maze at least 6 times.

The rat was then removed from the maze and held wrapped in a soft cloth. The maze was rotated by 60° or 120° clockwise or counterclockwise and the rat was replaced. Recording was continued until the rat had again run down each arm at least 6 times. A second rotation was performed for some cells. If the cell's field showed spatial persistence following the first rotation, the rat was held wrapped in the cloth and spun rapidly by hand in a small horizontal circle for 20-30 seconds before being replaced on the maze.

The data were reduced to a mean firing rate for each arm of the maze (sum of rates on each visit/total visits to that arm) and a grand mean firing rate (sum of rates on all visits to all arms/total visits to all arms). Criteria for a spatial unit were 1) mean firing rate on an arm exceeding grand mean by at least 3 standard errors and 2) firing rate exceeding grand mean on a significant ($p < .05$) number of visits as determined by a sign test.

RESULTS

Fifteen spatial cells were recorded from 9 animals. Four cells showed spatial persistence. That is, these cells fired in the same locations relative to the recording chamber before and after the first maze rotation. The fields of the remaining 11 cells shifted relative to the recording chamber. For 7 cells spatial fields shifted with the maze and occupied the same arms before and after maze rotation. For the remaining 4 cells, the fields shifted in the direction of maze rotation, but to a lesser degree. That is, if the maze was rotated 120° clockwise the cell fired on the arm 60° in that direction.

Complete recordings (at least 6 visits per arm) were made after a 2nd maze rotation from 3 non-persistent cells. In each case, the spatial field again followed the physical arm of the maze. Complete recordings were made after a 2nd maze rotation from 3 persistent cells. These rats were spun before being replaced on the maze. Spinning produced clear and immediate behavioral effects: counterturning, tail rotation, disequilibrium. Nevertheless, rats usually resumed running on the maze within one or two minutes. In each case spatial persistence was disrupted.

Results for a persistent cell are illustrated in Figure 2. The data are represented by vector diagrams. The length of each vector represents the mean firing rate on each arm. The radius of the circle corresponds to the grand mean during that run. The large arrow indicates the direction of arm #1 of the maze. The cell fired rapidly only on arm #3 in the initial configuration. After maze rotation (without spin), spatial firing persisted in the same spatial location, occurring only on arm #1. Figure 2c shows the result of the second rotation (with spin). The cell still fired on arm #1, now in a new position. That is, its field followed the maze.

It was possible to record from two persistent cells, on the day after the initial recording session. On Day 2, the maze was placed in its original orientation (arm #1 "south"). Recordings were made in the initial configuration, after maze rotation with spin, and after maze rotation without spin, in that order. For both cells spatial fields followed the maze after rotation when the rat was spun, but persisted in the new location after maze rotation when the rat was not spun. In other words, the order of the manipulations did not affect the results. At the beginning of Day 2, the place fields of both cells had "reset" to their initial Day 1 locations. Referring to Figure 2c, at the end of Day 1 the cell fired on arm #1 in position "north." At the beginning of the

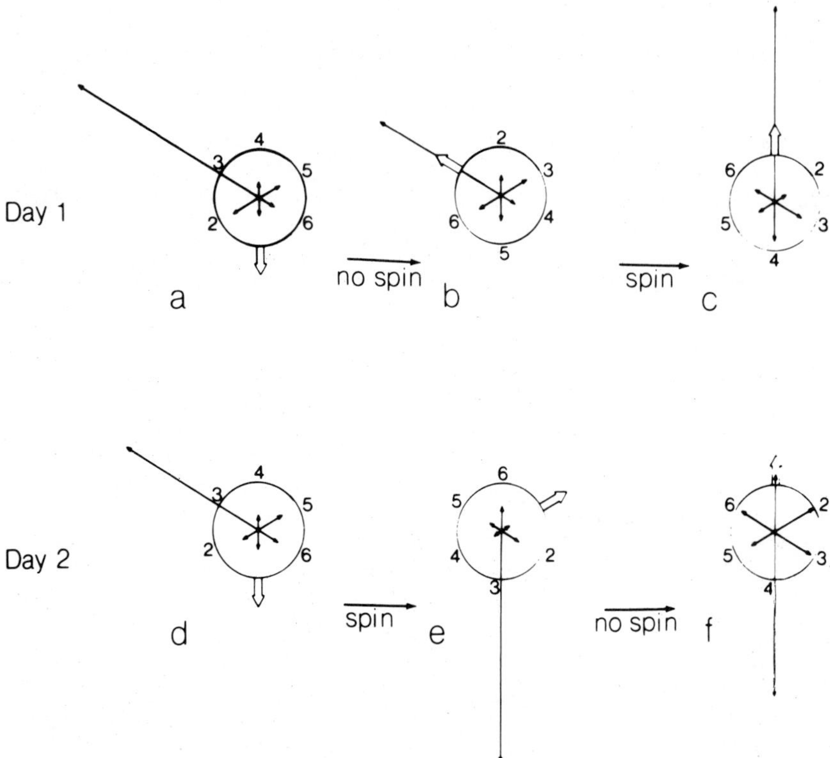

Figure 2. Vector representation of firing rates for a spatially presistent cell. The length of each vector represents mean firing rate over all visits to the arm. The radius of the circle represents the grand mean rate. The wide arrow is arm #1. Day 1: a) initial orientation; b) after maze rotation 120° clockwise; c) after second maze rotation 60° clockwise with animal spun. Day 2: d) initial orientation; e) after maze rotation 120° counterclockwise with spin; f) after second maze rotation 120° counterclockwise.

next day, with the maze in its original configuration, the cell fired on arm #3 in position "northwest" (2d), just as it had at the beginning of Day 1 (2a). The effect involved an overnight change relative to both intramaze and extramaze cues.

DISCUSSION

Hippocampal cells in rats deprived of sight and hearing have well defined place fields. All 15 units in this study showed a definite place field after maze rotation which could be related in a logical way to the field observed before maze rotation. That is, fields did not shift at random about the maze or change drastically in size or disposition. In intact animals all place cells are spatially persistent after maze rotation (Miller and Best, 1980). In animals deprived of vision and hearing in this experiment most place cells (11/15) are not persistent (i.e. follow the maze). The results suggest that in intact animals visual and/or auditory extramaze cues are the principal basis of place firing. The intra-maze cues to which non-persistent cells respond in the blind/deaf animals probably include kinesthetiz/tactile and olfactory cues.

The place fields of 4 units showed spatial persistence following maze rotation. In these cases the rat (and the cell) must have had some afferent referent to the fixed environment. It is possible that the animals were still receiving some auditory or visual information. However, the disruption of spatial persistence by spinning the animals implies that the vestibular system was supporting the prior spatial persistence of these cells.

The effect of sensory deprivation on hippocampal place cell activity, namely disruption of spatial persistence, is similar to the effects of entorhinal lesions. However, entrohinal lesions produce more severe deficits on unit activity and on behavior. We did not observe the behavioral performance impairments in the sensory deprived rats that have been observed in rats with entorhinal lesions (Miller and Best, 1980; Olton et al., 1978).

It seems clear that entorhinal cortex contributes more to spatial behavior than merely relaying sensory information to the hippocampus. It may provide the hippocampal outputs necessary for appropriate spatial behavior or it may make an important contribution to the processing of spatial information.

REFERENCES

Best, M. R., and Best, P. J., 1976, The effects of state of consciousness and latent inhibition on hippocampal unit activity during conditioning, Exp. Neurol., 51:564.

Best, P. J., Knowles, W. D., and Phillips, I. M., 1978, Chronic brain unit recording for pharmacological applications, J. Pharmacol. Methods, 1:161.

Best, P. J., and Ranck, J. B., Jr., Reliability of the relationship between hippocampal unit activity and sensory-behavioral events in the rat, Exp. Neurol., in press.

Hill, A. J., 1978, First occurrence of hippocampal spatial firing in a new environment, Exp. Neurol., 62:282.
Hill, A. J., 1979, Unpublished doctoral dissertation.
Jones, E. G., and Powell, T. P. S., 1970, An anatomical study of converging sensory pathways within the cerebral cortex of the monkey, Brain, 93:793.
Miller, V. M., and Best, P. J., 1980, Spatial correlates of hippocampal unit activity are altered by lesions of the fornix and entorhinal cortex, Brain Res., 194:311.
O'Keefe, J., 1976, Place units in the hippocampus of the freely moving rat, Exp. Neurol., 51:78.
O'Keefe, J., and Conway, D. H., 1978, Hippocampal place units in the freely moving rat: why they fire when they fire, Exp. Brain Res., 31:573.
O'Keefe, J., and Dostrovsky, T., 1971, The hippocampus as a spatial map: Preliminary evidence from unit activity in the freely moving rat, Brain Res., 34:171.
O'Keefe, J., and Nadel, L., 1978, "The Hippocampus as a Cognitive Map," Claranden Press, Oxford.
O'Keefe, J., Nadel, L., Keightly, S., and Kell, D., 1975, Fornix lesions selectively abolish place learning in the rat, Exp. Neurol., 48:152.
O'Keefe, J., Nadel, L., and Willner, J., 1979, Tuning out irrelevance? Comments on Solomon's temporal mapping view of the hippocampus, Psychol. Bull., 86:1280.
Olton, D. S., Branch, M., and Best, P. J., 1978, Spatial correlates of hippocampal unit activity, Exp. Neurol., 58:387.
Olton, D. S., and Samuelson, R. J., 1976, Remembrance of places plased: Spatial memory in rats, J. Exp. Psych.: Animal Behav. Processes, 2:97.
Olton, D. S., Walker, J. A., and Gage, F. H., 1978, Hippocampal connections and spatial discrimination, Brain Res., 139:295.
Pavlov, J., 1927, "Conditioned Reflexes," Oxford University Press, London.
Rescorla, R. A., and Wagner, A. R., 1972, A theory of Pavlovian conditioning: variations in the effectiveness of reinforcement and nonreinforcement, in: "Classical Conditioning II: Current Research and Theory," A. H. Black and W. F. Prokasy, eds., Appleton-Century-Crofts, New York.
Restle, F., 1957, Discrimination of cues in mazes: a resolution of the place vs response question, Psychol. Rev., 64:217.
Solomon, P. R., 1979, Temporal versus spatial information processing theories of hippocampal function, Psychol. Bull., 86:1272.

Tolman, E. C., 1932, "Purposive Behavior in Animals and Men," Century, New York.

Van Hoesen, G. W., and Pandya, D. N., 1975, Some connections of the entorhinal (area 28) and peripheral (area 35) cortices of the rhesus monkey, Brain Res., 95:1.

Vernier, V. G., and Alleva, F. R., 1968, The bioassay of kanamycin auditory toxicity, Archives Internationales de Pharmacodynamie, 176:59.

HIPPOCAMPAL PLASTICITY AND EXCITATORY NEUROTRANSMITTERS

Carl W. Cotman, Graham E. Fagg and Thomas H. Lanthorn

Department of Psychobiology, University of California

Irvine, California 92717

SUMMARY

The identification of excitatory transmitters used at specific pathways in the CNS is a major, but as yet largely unsolved problem which is of critical importance for analyzing the mechanisms of learning and memory. The hippocampus appears to be involved in several aspects of learning and is an excellent model system for the study of these processes. Much evidence favors the idea that glutamate is the transmitter of the perforant path, the major cortical input to the hippocampus. Thus, glutamate release in the dentate gyrus is Ca^{2+}-dependent and stimulated by depolarization; removal of the perforant path reduces this release as well as the high affinity uptake of glutamate. The glutamate analogue, L-2-amino-4-phosphonobutyric acid, selectively blocks synaptic transmission at the lateral but not medial perforant path. The dose required to reduce transmission by 50% is about 3 μm, making this drug the most potent antagonist of excitatory amino acid transmission in the brain. The action is selective to the L-isomer and shorter or longer chain derivatives are less effective. The transmitters of the Schaffer collateral/commissural input to CA1 neurons appear to be glutamate and aspartate based on release and uptake data. An effective antagonist for this pathway has not been found at the present time. The transmitter of the mossy fiber system is unknown, although evidence exists which suggests the involvement of a kainic acid-like molecule. Plasticity studies using L-APB show that paired pulse potentiation in the lateral perforant path is enhanced in the presence of the drug, probably due to interactions with presynaptic release mechanisms.

INTRODUCTION

At the present time, most studies on conditioning have focused on the development of appropriate models for the process and the elucidation of the brain loci where plastic changes occur. Major advances toward these objectives have been made and one of the next frontiers is the elucidation of mechanisms underlying these changes.

Studies on the mechanisms of learning would be greatly facilitated if the transmitters of the relevant pathways were known and if specific antagonists of synaptic transmission along these pathways were available. Most transmitters identified for specific pathways are inhibitory. Comparatively little is known about the transmitters and pharmacological properties of excitatory pathways in the CNS. However, excitatory pathways certainly play a major role in behavioral plasticity and it is important to know their transmitters.

Over the past several years we have sought to identify the excitatory transmitters in one part of the brain, the hippocampus, with the long range goal of using this information to investigate plasticity mechanisms in this structure. In this article we summarize the current state of knowledge on hippocampal excitatory transmitters, their pharmacological properties and plasticity. Particular emphasis is placed on the perforant path input to the dentate gyrus. Detailed reviews of acidic amino acid transmission have appeared elsewhere (Cotman, Foster, Lanthorn, 1981; Cotman and Nadler, 1981; Watkins and Evans, 1981).

OVERVIEW OF NEUROTRANSMITTERS: SURVEY BASED ON UPTAKE AND RELEASE DATA

Figure 1 summarizes the transmitter candidates for various hippocampal pathways based on uptake and release studies. Entorhinal, Schaffer collateral-commissural, and mossy fiber projections have been singled out for study because (a) they are the major excitatory pathways in the hippocampus and (b) they can be manipulated with relative ease. It is evident that the acidic amino acids are major transmitter candidates.

The initial clues that glutamate and aspartate might be excitatory transmitters in the hippocampus came from iontophoretic data on hippocampal pyramidal neurons (Biscoe and Straughan, 1966) and from *in vivo* experiments demonstrating the release of glutamate from the hippocampus following stimulation of the entorhinal cortex (Crawford and Conner, 1973). However, despite all the evidence pointing toward glutamate and aspartate as excitatory transmitters in the CNS, neither could be associated conclusively with a particular

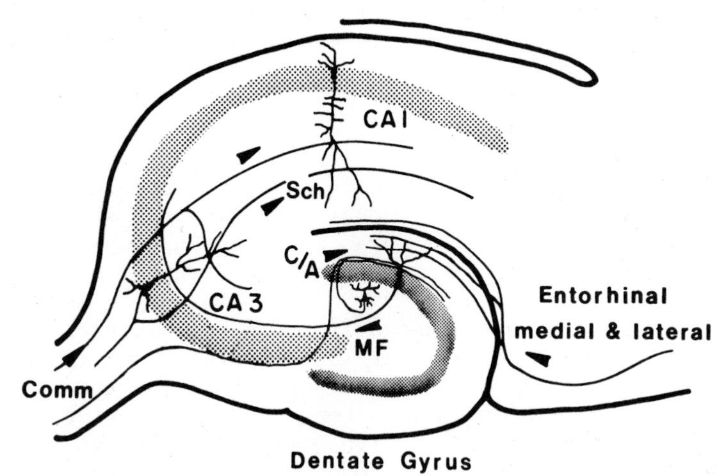

Projection		Putative Transmitter
Entorhinal fibers:	to dentate gyrus	Glutamate
	to CA1	Unknown
Commissural-associational (C/A) fibers:	to dentate gyrus	Aspartate
Schaffer-commissural (Sch, Comm) fibers	to CA1	Glutamate, Aspartate
Mossy fibers (MF)	to CA3	Unknown

Figure 1. Proposed assignment of transmitters to the major excitatory hippocampal projections. Diagram of transverse hippocampal slice shows location of excitatory pathways. Shaded areas denote pyramidal and granule cell body layers of Ammon's horn and the dentate gyrus. Arrows indicate the normal direction of impulse flow. Comm, commissural fibers to CA1 region; C/A, commissural-associational fibers to the molecular layer of the dentate gyrus; Sch, Schaffer collateral fibers; MF, mossy fibers.

pathway and more definitive tests were needed to establish them as transmitters. We therefore sought a more suitable approach. The tissue content of glutamate or aspartate did not seem to be a reliable indicator of a transmitter role, since this probably reflected the size of metabolic stores more than that of any transmitter store. Nor were there any enzymes thought to be uniquely associated with glutamate or aspartate transmitter systems. No definitive pharmacological tools were available. Furthermore, there was no evidence that a high affinity transport carrier for acidic amino acids uniquely marked boutons that used these amino acids as transmitters. In this regard, the demonstration of such a transport carrier in glial membranes showed that uptake alone could not be used as a definitive test (see Fagg and Lane, 1979).

We therefore concluded that only by demonstrating release of the amino acid by boutons of a particular pathway and then obtaining evidence that this amino acid mediated the postsynaptic response to stimulation of the pathway could a convincing argument be made that glutamate or aspartate acted as transmitters. Investigations along these lines have provided solid and consistent evidence that glutamate and aspartate are transmitters in the hippocampus.

Most of our release experiments have been carried out using thin tissue slices prepared from the various hippocampal subfields. Slices were incubated in a physiological salt solution, and the release of glutamate and/or aspartate was evoked by an appropriate stimulus, such as the introduction of high K^+ or veratridine into the medium. The Ca^{2+}-dependence of the evoked release was always assessed, since this appears to be a property characteristic of most stimulus-secretion coupling systems (Rubin, 1970).

Tissue slices prepared from dentate gyrus released glutamate, aspartate and GABA, but only glutamate appeared to originate from the perforant path fibers. Thus, bilateral removal of the entorhinal cortex reduced the Ca^{2+}-dependent release of glutamate from dentate slices by an average of 46 percent within 8-9 days, but did not affect efflux in the absence of Ca^{2+} (Nadler et al., 1976, 1978). Release of glutamate from slices of regio superior was not significantly changed. Ca^{2+}-dependent release of aspartate from dentate slices was not decreased, but actually increased. In subsequent studies, Ca^{2+}-dependent release of endogenous glutamate (as well as glutamate synthesized from radio-labelled glucose or glutamine) from slices of dentate molecular layer similarly decreased after removal of the ipsilateral entorhinal cortex (there are few crossed perforant path fibers) (Hamberger et al., 1978; 1979a,b). These results suggested that perforant path fibers release glutamate but not aspartate as their transmitter.

In the same experiments we were also able to determine the effect of entorhinal cortical lesions on the high affinity uptake of radiolabelled glutamate and measuring the accumulation of radioactivity. Bilateral entorhinal cortex ablation significantly reduced the quantity of glutamate accumulated by dentate slices, but not by slices of regio superior. It did not affect the uptake of all amino acids, however, since the same denervated tissue accumulated a normal quantity of radiolabelled GABA. These results suggested that the perforant path boutons possess a high affinity transport carrier for acidic amino acids [the carriers for glutamate and aspartate in the hippocampal formation appear to be identical (Sandoval et al., 1978)]. Similar data have been obtained using other biochemical and histochemical techniques (Storm-Mathisen, 1977a,b, 1978; Storm-Mathisen and Iversen, 1979). Autoradiographic analysis of glutamate uptake in the molecular layer showed that the synaptic field of the lateral perforant path accumulated more glutamate than the termination field of the medial part (Cotman, 1980).

Perforant path boutons therefore appear capable of both releasing and accumulating glutamate. Accordingly, we postulated glutamate as a transmitter of the perforant path fibers. Release and uptake experiments have also been performed on the commissural projection to CA1. The data favor the notion that both glutamate and aspartate are released from these fibers. On the other hand, the mossy fiber transmitter is probably neither glutamate or aspartate because reduction in granule cell number by X-irradiation during development increases rather than decreases release. The mossy fiber transmitter may be a kainic acid-like molecule since kainate receptors are particularly concentrated at this termination field (Foster et al., 1981a). A more comprehensive discussion of evidence derived from release data has been published previously (Cotman and Nadler, 1981).

While the data point toward acidic amino acids as strong candidates for transmitters in specific hippocampal pathways, certain issues are unresolved. For example, the measurement of release has not yet included a precise fractionation of pathways (e.g. lateral vs. medial perforant path), the demonstration of exocytotic release from vesicular storage pools under physiological conditions, and the release of acidic compounds other than glutamate or aspartate. Most importantly, however, release studies do not reveal whether or not the postsynaptic response is identical to that expected for the acidic amino acid candidate. Accordingly, we have begun a detailed pharmacological analysis on hippocampal pathways. The identification of glutamate-using pathways would be greatly facilitated by the discovery of specific antagonists.

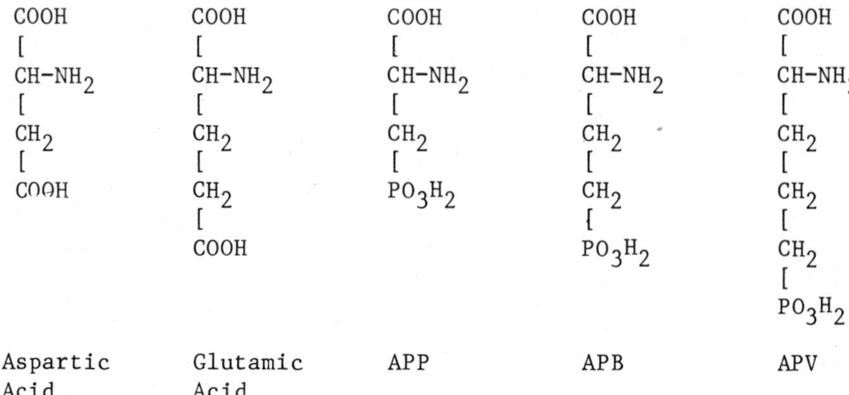

Figure 2. Structures of aspartic and glutamic acids and the phosphonic acid analogues described in the text.

PHARMACOLOGICAL PROPERTIES

We have employed the hippocampal slice preparation for studying the pharmacology of hippocampal synaptic transmission. Recent studies have shown that the glutamate analogue 2-amino-4-phosphonobutyric acid (L-APB, see Fig. 2) is an effective antagonist of perforant path synaptic transmission. Apparently the perforant path contains two pharmacologically-distinct components (see Koerner and Cotman, 1981). In examining dose-response relationships in the perforant path, it was clear that micromolar concentrations of APB partially inhibited synaptic transmission and that further increasing the dose had little additional effect. This suggested that perhaps the perforant path consisted of two components, a very sensitive one and another insensitive one. Since the perforant path is anatomically segregated into components from the lateral and medial entorhinal cortex we guessed that this might account for our results.

Figure 3 shows the log dose response curves for the lateral and medial termination fields of the perforant path (outer and middle portions of the molecular layer of the dentate gyrus, respectively). The middle portion of the dentate gyrus requires a 500-fold higher concentration of L-APB for 50% inhibition than the outer part. Both kinds of response originate from fibers of the perforant path, because they can both be activated by stimulating the slices where the perforant path traverses the subiculum. Mathematical analysis of the data suggests that the response in the outer molecular layer

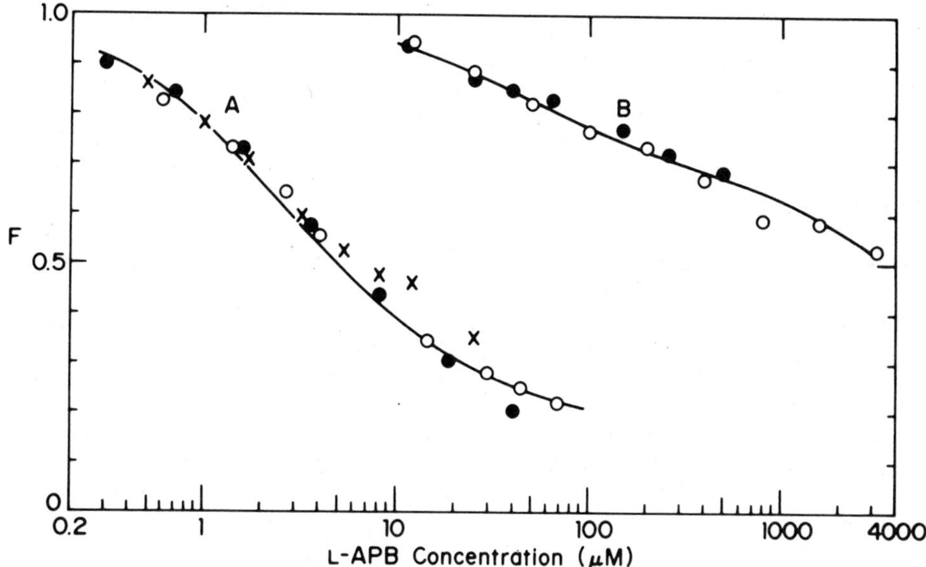

Figure 3. Dose-response curves for the effect of L-APB on the perforant path-evoked field potentials in (A) the outer and (B) the middle molecular layer of the rat dentate gyrus. F, fractional response.

includes some drug resistant synapses. This is probably due to contamination with synapses of the middle molecular layer, as it varies depending on electrode placement and orientation of the plane of the slice. If this contamination is taken into account, about 75% of the response for the outer molecular layer can be attributed to a component for which L-APB acts as an antagonist with an apparent K_I of 2.5 μM (Koerner and Cotman, 1981).

The responses to the enantiomer D-APB and to the homologues D,L-2-amino-3-phosphonopropionic acid (DL-APP, an analogue of aspartic acid, see Fig. 2) and D,L-2-amino-5-phosphonovaleric acid (DL-APV) were also tested. For the outer molecular layer, 65 μM D-APB reduced the response 30%; this is 40-fold less potent than L-APB. The actual difference may be even greater since these compounds were prepared by resolution of the racemate, and each one may be contaminated with a small amount of its enantiomer. Also for the outer molecular layer, 200 μM DL-APV antagonized the evoked response by 33% (100-fold less potent than L-APB) while 200 μM DL-APP inhibited 4% (2,000-fold less potent). It is noteworthy that DL-APP, with a smaller extended length which might fail to span a glutamate receptor, was least potent while the longer homologue DL-APV exhibited a small but readily measurable antagonist action (see also Table 2).

These data on the relative effects of L-APB, its enantiomer and higher and lower homologues on synapses of the lateral perforant path comprise the most compelling evidence to date that a close structural analogue of L-glutamic acid (see Fig. 2) can exert a highly specific inhibition of a defined mammalian neuronal pathway. Also, with an apparent K_I of 2.5 μM, L-APB is the most potent antagonist currently known for a major brain excitatory amino acid pathway. These results contrast strongly with those obtained for the same drugs against an N-methyl-D-aspartate-sensitive pathway in the spinal cord. In that system, DL-APV inhibits at micromolar concentrations, DL-APB is 100 times less potent, and the D-isomers are most active (Davies et al., 1980; Watkins et al., 1980). However, recent as yet unpublished data by Watkins and coworkers (private communication) support our results. The monosynaptic dorsal root-evoked ventral-root response in the frog spinal cord is blocked by L-APB at micromolar concentrations and D-APB is less effective. D-APV is a powerful antagonist only of the polysynaptic response in the spinal cord.

Thus, these data indicate the existence of a previously undescribed amino acid receptor in the CNS. It appears that these APB-sensitive sites do not fit precisely into previous classification schemes of excitatory amino acid receptors. They probably are a major new class or perhaps a subclass distinct from those already described (see Watkins and Evans, 1981; Cotman, Foster, Lanthorn, 1981).

The pharmacology at the Schaffer collateral system is distinct from that of the lateral perforant path (Table 1). L-APB is ineffective and so far a powerful antagonist has not been identified. The only compound we have found which reduces synaptic transmission at this pathway is baclofen (Lanthorn and Cotman, 1981). Baclofen is believed to act by reducing transmitter release at acidic amino acid synapses (Potashner, 1978). The mossy fiber system has not yet been studied in sufficient detail, although the analogue gamma-D-glutamylglycine appears to be a relatively effective antagonist.

Table 1. Antagonism of Schaffer collateral-evoked responses by acidic amino acid analogues.

Compound	Apparent K_I (mM)
DL-APB	9
L-APB	10
D-APB	4
DL-APV	8
D-α-aminoadipate	9
D-α-aminosuberate	3
Diaminopinelate	10

BIOCHEMICAL PROPERTIES OF L-APB RECEPTORS

The properties of L-APB receptors can be further characterized using biochemical methods which measure the binding of radiolabelled glutamate to isolated synaptic membranes. In this way it is possible to determine the affinity of the glutamate-receptor interaction in synaptic membranes and the sensitivity of the binding to ions and various drugs. In early work, DL-APB was a rather weak blocker of L-glutamate binding and the other phosphonic acid derivatives were not very different (Foster and Roberts, 1978; Biziere et al., 1980; unpublished observations). This contrasted, of course, to our physiological data. The usual binding assay medium differs greatly from that used for hippocampal slice physiology, both in its cation and anion content. We have now found that by changing the ionic composition of the assay buffer to correspond more closely to that used in the physiological salt solution (e.g., see Foster et al., 1981b), L-APB is a good antagonist of binding and D-APB is about 1/15 as potent. Also, APV is less effective than APB and APP is essentially completely ineffective. This change in pharmacological specificity appeared to be due to the introduction of a new population of glutamate binding sites (Fagg et al., 1981; and unpublished observations).

The results are very important because they demonstrate that *in vitro* binding data can correspond to physiological data. The K_I values show a striking parallel between binding and physiological measures (Table 2).

Table 2. Inhibitory Potency of Phosphonic Acid Derivatives

Compound	K_I Value at: L-glutamate binding sites µM	K_I Value at: Lateral perforant path-granule cell synapse µM
DL-APP	>1000	5000
DL-APB	18	ND
DL-APV	39	250
L-APB	5	2.5
D-APB	75	100

ND: not determined
Each value is the mean from 2-4 separate experiments.

L-APB-sensitive receptors appear to be a major class of receptor in the brain since our experiments were carried out using synaptic membranes isolated from the entire forebrain and APB inhibits about 80% of the glutamate binding. Moreover, APB-sensitive receptors now have been reported in the spinal cord (Evans et al., 1981) and retina (Slaughter and Miller, 1981).

USE OF L-APB FOR STUDYING PERFORANT PATH PLASTICITY

The perforant path is well known for its plastic properties, displaying habituation, paired pulse potentiation, and long term potentiation. Paired pulse potentiation (homosynaptic facilitation) is a form of short term plasticity where the magnitude of the synaptic response is enhanced as a function of preceding activity. At the perforant path, facilitation occurs over an interstimulus interval of 20-500 msec with optimal interstimulus interval at about 35 msec. Paired pulse potentiation is generally believed to be a presynaptic phenomenon involving an accumulation of Ca^{2+} ions inside the presynaptic terminal following the first pulse (see Zucker, this volume). If the same mechanism is used at the perforant path and if L-APB only acts as a postsynaptic receptor antagonist, the drug should have no effect on paired pulse potentiation. A reduction in the number of available postsynaptic receptors would reduce the evoked response to both pulses equally. Paired pulse potentiation was examined in the presence and absence of the drug in the bath. In the absence of APB, the second pulse increased up to 1.5 fold, depending somewhat on the stimulus intensity delivered (Fig. 4). In the presence of the drug, paired pulse potentiation was further enhanced over a wide range of stimulus intensities. This enhancement is not readily consistent with the expected mode of action of L-APB on postsynaptic receptors. Perhaps L-APB has two modes of action -- one presynaptic and the other postsynaptic. Presynaptic endings in the CNS often have autoreceptors which mediate feedback inhibition of transmitter release. Hence, blocking these autoreceptors would be predicted to result in a larger second response. However, it is also possible that L-APB is acting presynaptically and somehow interacting with the control of Ca^{2+} ion fluxes. We are currently evaluating these and other possibilities. We expect that L-APB will help to elucidate new mechanisms underlying short term plasticity in hippocampus.

Habituation at the perforant path has previously been shown to meet the essential criteria for behavioral habituation and thus is an appropriate synaptic analogue of non-associative learning. Detailed analysis of habituation at the perforant path produced the surprising result that while the medial perforant path showed the expected characteristics of habituation, the lateral perforant path did not habituate over the same stimulus conditions (Lanthorn et al., in preparation). Thus the perforant path shows a complex

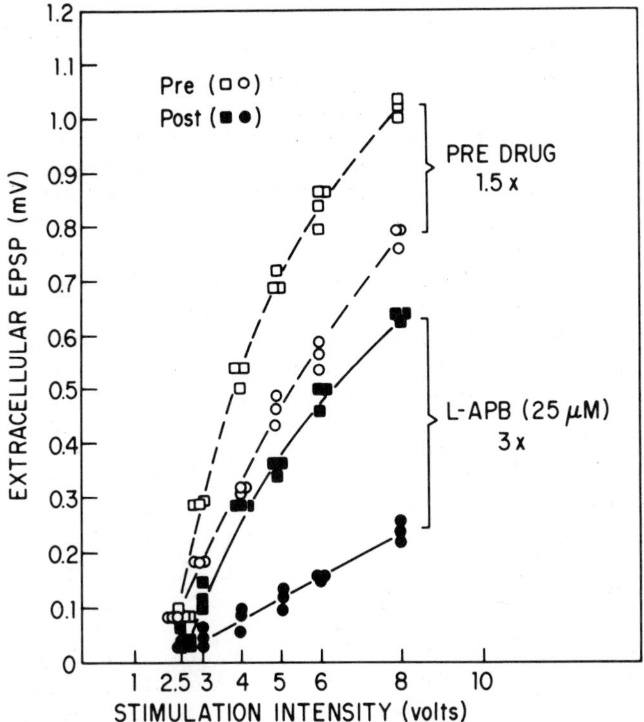

Figure 4. Effect of L-APB on paired-pulse potentiation of the lateral perforant path response. Responses were judged to be lateral perforant path responses when the response to the second of a pair of stimulus pulses, 35 or 350 msec apart, was larger than the first. The amplitude of the first (o •) and second response (□ ■) to two pulses at an interpulse interval of 35 msec are shown. Prior to addition of L-APB (□ o) the second response was about 1.5 times the first response at all stimulus intensities. In the presence of L-APB (■ •) the second response was potentiated to a greater extent (about 3 times) (Harris et al., unpublished observations).

input/output function. The major anatomical difference between the medial and lateral pathways is that the lateral circuit involves the subiculum to a much greater extent than the medial one. This links the lateral pathway primarily into the limbic system via the Papez circuit whereas the medial pathway appears more specialized for cortical association inputs. Perhaps for hippocampal function it is necessary to maintain a relatively constant background of limbic information (such as internal body state) and thus habituation is not displayed. The action of L-APB on long term potentiation has not been studied at the present time.

CONCLUSION

The past several years have produced major advances toward understanding excitatory transmitters in the hippocampus. Glutamate and aspartate have emerged as major candidates at the perforant path and Schaffer/commissural systems. This is based on multiple criteria -- release, uptake, and the electrophysiological properties of the target neurons. It is clear, however, that multiple receptors for acidic amino acids exist on hippocampal neurons as evidenced by the selectivity of L-APB only for lateral perforant path and the different pharmacologies of perforant path- and Schaffer collateral/commissural-evoked responses. This is encouraging in the sense that pharmacological agents can be developed which will probably be sufficiently selective to be useful for the detailed dissection of complex pathways. Selective drugs can provide new and unexpected findings on the plastic properties of central pathways as, for example, the action of L-APB on paired pulse potentiation.

ACKNOWLEDGEMENTS

We should like to express our appreciation to Ms. Susanne Bathgate for assistance with the preparation of this manuscript. The work described in this paper was supported in part by grants NS08957 and MH19691 from the National Institutes of Health.

REFERENCES

Biscoe, T. J., and Straughan, D. W., 1966, Micro-electrophoretic studies on neurones in the cat hippocampus, J. Physiol. (Lond.), 183:341-359.

Biziere, K., Thompson, H., and Coyle, J. T., 1980, Characterization of specific, high affinity binding sites for L-[^{3}H]glutamic acid in rat brain membranes, Brain Res. 183:421-423.

Cotman, C. W., 1980, Acidic amino acids as excitatory transmitters, In: Regulatory Mechanisms of Synaptic Transmission, (R. Tapia and C. W. Cotman, Eds.), Plenum Press, New York, pp. 43-57.

Cotman, C. W., Foster, A. C., and Lanthorn, T. L., 1981, An overview of glutamate as a neurotransmitter. In: Glutamate as a Neurotransmitter, (G. DiChiara and G. L. Gessa, Eds.), Raven Press, New York, pp. 1-27.

Cotman, C. W., and Nadler, J. V., 1981, Glutamate and Aspartate as hippocampal transmitters: biochemical and pharmacological evidence, In: Glutamate: Transmitter in the Central Nervous System, (P. J. Roberts, J. Storm-Mathisen and G. A. R. Johnston, Eds.), John Wiley & Sons, New York, pp. 117-154.

Crawford, I. L., and Conner, J. D., 1973, Localization and release of glutamic acid in relation to the hippocampal mossy fibre pathway, Nature, 244:442-443.

Davies, J., Francis, A. A., Jones, A. W., and Watkins, J. C., 1981, 2-amino-5-phosphono valerate (2APV), a potent and selectve antagonist of amino acid-induced and synaptic excitation, Neurosci. Lett. 21:77-81.

Evans, R. H., Jones, A. W., and Watkins, J. C., 1981, Depressant action of the L-glutamate analogue (+)2-amino-4-phosphonobutyrate, Br. J. Pharmacol., in press.

Fagg, G. E., and Lane, J. D., 1979, The uptake and release of putative amino acid neurotransmitters, Neuroscience 4:1015-1036.

Fagg, G. E., Foster, A. C., Mena, E. E., Koerner, J. F., and Cotman, C. W., 1981, Calcium ions and the pharmacology of acidic amino acid receptor sites, Trans. Am. Soc. Neurochem. 12:122.

Foster, A. C., and Roberts, P. J., 1978, High affinity L-[^{3}H]glutamate binding to postsynaptic receptor sites in rat cerebellar membranes, J. Neurochem. 31:1467-1477.

Foster, A. C., Mena, E. E., Monaghan, D. T., and Cotman, C. W., 1981a, Synaptic localization of kainic acid binding sites, Nature 289:73-35.

Foster, A. C., Mena, E. E., Fagg, G. E., and Cotman, C. W., 1981b, Glutamate and aspartate binding sites are enriched in synaptic junctions isolated from rat brain, J. Neurosci. 1:620-625.

Hamberger, A., Chiang, G., Nylen, E. S., Scheff, S. W., and Cotman, C. W., 1978, Stimulus evoked increase in the biosynthesis of the putative neurotransmitter glutamate in the hippocampus, Brain Res. 143:549-555.

Hamberger, A. C., Chiang, G. H., Nylen, E. S., Scheff, S. W., and Cotman, C. W., 1979a, Glutamate as a CNS transmitter. I. Evaluation of glucose and glutamine as precursors for the synthesis of preferentially released glutamate, Brain Res. 168:513-530.

Hamberger, A. C., Chiang, G. H., Nylen, E. S., Scheff, S. W., and Cotman, C. W., 1979b, Glutamate as a CNS transmitter. II. Regulation of synthesis in the releasable pool, Brain Res. 168:531-541.

Koerner, J. R., and Cotman, C. W., 1981, Micromolar L-2-amino-4-phosphonobutyric acid selectively inhibits perforant path synapses from lateral entorhinal cortex, Brain Res. 216:192-198.

Lanthorn, T. L., and Cotman, C. W., 1981, Baclofen selectively inhibits excitatory synaptic transmission in the hippocampus. Brain Res., in press.

Lanthorn, T. H. et al., The effects of L-2-amino-4-phosphonobutyrate on synaptic plasticity in the perforant path, in preparation.

Nadler, J. V., Vaca, K. W., White, W. F., Lynch, G. S., and Cotman, C. W., 1976, Aspartate and glutamate as possible transmitters of excitatory hippocampal afferents, Nature 260:538-540.

Nadler, J. V., White, W. F., Vaca, K. W., Perry, B. W., and Cotman, C. W., 1978, Biochemical correlates of transmission mediated by glutamate and asparate. J. Neurochem. 31:147-155.

Potashner, S. J., 1978, Baclofen: effects on amino acid release, Can. J. Physiol. Pharmacol. 56:150-154.

Rubin, R. P., 1970, The role of calcium in the release of neurotransmitter substances and hormones, Pharmacol. Rev. 22:389-248.

Sandoval, M. E., Horch, P., and Cotman, C. W., 1978, Evaluation of glutamate as a hippocampal neurotransmitter: glutamate uptake and release from synaptosomes, Brain Res. 142:285-299.

Slaughter, M. M., and Miller, R. F., 1981, 2-amino-4-phosphonobutyric acid: a new pharmacological tool for retina research. Science 211:182-185.

Storm-Mathisen, J., 1977a, Glutamic acid and excitatory nerve endings: reduction of glutamic acid uptake after axotomy, Brain Res. 120:379-386.

Storm-Mathisen, J., 1977b, Localization of transmitter candidates in the brain: the hippocampal formation as a model, Prog. Neurobiol. 8:119-181.

Storm-Mathisen, J., 1978, Localization of putative transmitters in the hippocampal formation, with a note on the connections to septum and hypothalamus, In: Functions of the Septo-Hippocampal System, CIBA Foundation Symposium 58:49-86.

Storm-Mathisen, J., and Iversen, L. L., 1979, Uptake of [^{3}H]glutamic acid in excitatory nerve endings: light and electron microscopic observations in the hippocampal formation of the rat, Neuroscience 4:1237-1253.

Watkins, J. C., Davies, J., Evans, R. H., Francis, A. A. and Jones, A. W., 1981, Pharmacology of receptors for excitatory amino acids, In: Glutamate as a Neurotransmitters, (G. Di Chiara, and G. L. Gessa, Eds.), Raven Press, New York, pp. 263-273.

Watkins, J. C. and Evans, R. H., 1981, Excitatory amino acid transmitters, Ann. Rev. Pharmacol. Toxicol. 21:165-204.

NEURAL ACTIVITY IN THE DENTATE GYRUS OF THE RAT DURING THE ACQUISITION AND PERFORMANCE OF SIMPLE AND COMPLEX SENSORY DISCRIMINATION LEARNING

Sam A. Deadwyler, Mark O. West and Edward P. Christian

Department of Physiology and Pharmacology
Bowman Gray School of Medicine
Winston-Salem, NC 27103

SUMMARY

Neural activity recorded in the outer molecular layer of the dentate gyrus changes during the course of simple and differential auditory discrimination learning. Such neural activity in the form of time-locked evoked potentials to the conditioned auditory stimulus has been correlated with 1) the acquisition, extinction and reconditioning of a simple discrimination task, and 2) maintained performance of a complex differential discrimination task. Several tests examining the possible influences of behavioral variables have indicated that the above neural activity is not generated by gross changes in the behavior of the animal during the different phases of conditioning. The sensory evoked neural activity in the dentate gyrus has been shown to reflect the inputs of two major hippocampal afferents, the septo-hippocampal fibers, and the perforant path. Recent experiments suggest that such activity may represent not only processes which are directly related to the conditioned status of the auditory stimulus in terms of its behavioral significance, but also the pattern of events which has just preceded that stimulus.

INTRODUCTION

It has been suggested by a number of investigators over several years that the hippocampus participates in brain activities which underlie memory and learning.[1-7] Several lines of evidence support this assumption including recent reports from the animal[8,9] and human literature.[10,11] At the animal level extensive analyses have been made of changes in hippocampal unit discharges which accompany the conditioning of behavioral responses. Although this approach is certainly not new in the history of experimental attempts to discover the functions of the hippocampus,[1,17,18] new information deriving from these experiments has refined the possible roles that various hippocampal cell groups might play in conditioning and other behavioral processes.[12-16]

As a result of this increased interest in the hippocampus, it has also become apparent that hippocampal cells have more than one behavioral and/or functional correlate.[19] A change in firing rate during conditioning may therefore be only one attribute, or even a part of the same attribute of a given hippocampal unit.[20] Furthermore, it has also been tentatively established that not all cell types within the hippocampus have the same behavioral and conditioning correlates.[16,21,22] Finally, it is not at all certain how "necessary" some of these observed changes in hippocampal unit activity are for the maintenance and execution of the implied functional process manifested in the behavioral or conditioning correlate.[23]

While the above approach to the study of hippocampal involvement in learning and memory will no doubt continue to be productive, several questions concerning the operation of hippocampal mechanisms in such processes may remain unanswered. An alternative to the above method of study involves the delineation of known synaptic events within a given homogeneous hippocampal cell population under various different manipulations known to produce substantial changes in the behavior of the animal. Once such synaptic events are reliably identified in the behaving animal it then becomes possible to gain information as to their functional significance. Using this strategy, investigation of not only when the hippocampus becomes involved in a given behavioral task but also how such involvement is brought about by the extrinsic and intrinsic hippocampal pathways becomes feasible. In the past we have employed this strategy in an attempt to describe the functional characteristics of the dentate granule cells[24,25] and the two major afferent fiber systems to the dentate gyrus and hippocampus, the septo-hippocampal projection and the connections from the entorhinal cortex.[26] This approach has yielded considerable information regarding the basis of granule cell activation by sensory stimuli within a variety of different experimental circumstances.

Sensory Evoked Potentials in the Dentate Gyrus

When unrestrained water deprived rats have been trained to make a simple operant response (nosepoke) in the presence of an auditory stimulus (1 or 4 kHz tone) to obtain a water reward, a distinct time-locked averaged evoked potential (AEP) can be recorded from the outer molecular (OM) layer of the dentate gyrus. We have termed this potential the OM AEP,[26] and it consists of two main components: 1) an "unconditioned", short duration negative wave, N_1, the amplitude of which is inversely related to the acquired conditioned status of the auditory stimulus, and 2) a "conditioned" longer duration negative wave, N_2, which is positively correlated with the conditioned status of the tone stimulus during stable discrimination performance. The two components of the OM AEP are not mutually exclusive, and in several phases of conditioning they often appear together in 50 trial averages. The earlier N_1 component has a latency of 20 msec from tone onset and a duration which seldom

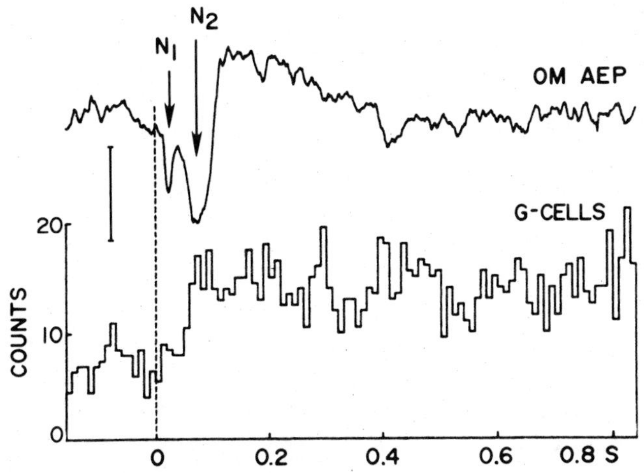

Fig. 1. OM AEP and post-stimulus histogram (PSH) showing granule cell (g-cell) unit discharge to tone onset (dashed line) during criterion performance of a discimination task. The OM AEP and PSH are summed over 50 trials recorded during the same session. Calibration: 300 μV. Timebase: 1.0 sec.

exceeds 20 msec. N_2 has an onset latency which is slightly longer (40 msec) and a duration of 50-70 msec. Very often there is a late positive-going slowwave in the OM AEP which has a peak at 150-250 msec (Figure 1). The discharge pattern of the dentate granule cells (g-cells) coincides with the N_2 component of the OM AEP. The g-cell burst duration varies from 150 msec to 1.0 sec in overtrained conditioned animals (Figure 1).

It has been shown that the N_1 component of the OM AEP exhibits a depth profile consistent with its restriction to the zone of synaptic termination of perforant path fibers. The N_2 component is maximal in amplitude in the terminal zone of the commissural/associational fibers.[24,26] Lesions which either destroy the entorhinal cortex or interrupt the angular bundle eliminate the occurrence of N_1 but leave N_2 unchanged. Conversely, destruction of the medial septal nucleus produces no change in N_1, but N_2 appears in the OM AEP of unconditioned animals and does not decrease in amplitude during extinction as is the case with intact or entorhinal lesioned animals.[26]

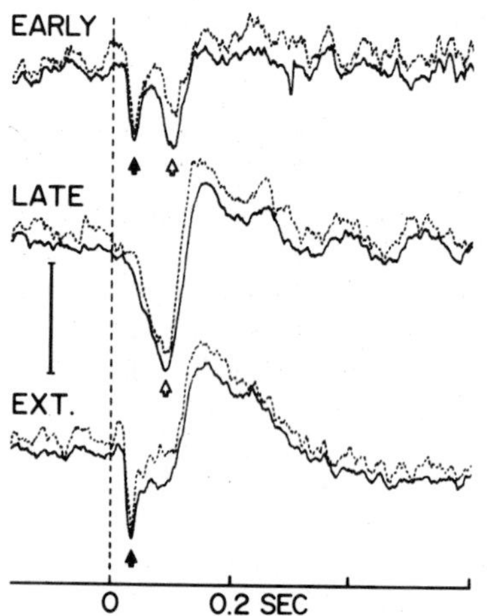

Fig. 2. Composites of OM AEPs obtained during performance of the single tone discrimination task for "early", "late", and extinction (Ext.) sessions. Four 50-trial averages were combined to obtain each trace (dotted lines show standard deviation). Black arrows N_1. White arrows N_2. Tone onset at dashed vertical line. Calibration: 300 μV.

The OM AEP and Simple Discrimination Learning

Rats trained to respond in a simple (single tone) auditory discrimination paradigm exhibit OM AEPs which begin to emerge from the background EEG over a series of 2-5 daily 100 trial sessions.[24] The N_1 component is large in the early phases of acquisition and N_2 is small, and less consistent (Figure 2). As criterion performance on this task (i.e., responding only in the presence of the tone) is achieved, the N_2 component increases in amplitude; with overtraining the N_1 component is reduced in amplitude but N_2 remains stable (Figure 2). During extinction the reverse change in amplitude of these two components is evidenced; that is, N_1 becomes large, and N_2 decreases markedly as behavioral responding to the auditory stimulus ceases to occur (Figure 2). Reconditioning reestablishes the two component configuration of the OM AEP concomitant with resumption of discriminative behavioral responding.[26] These changes in OM AEP configuration are accompanied by increased g-cell unit discharges at tone onset during conditioning (Figure 1) and a decrease in tone evoked g-cell discharges during behavioral extinction.[27] Such discharges do not reflect either the gross body movements of the animal, or the occurrence of hippocampal theta rhythm.[28]

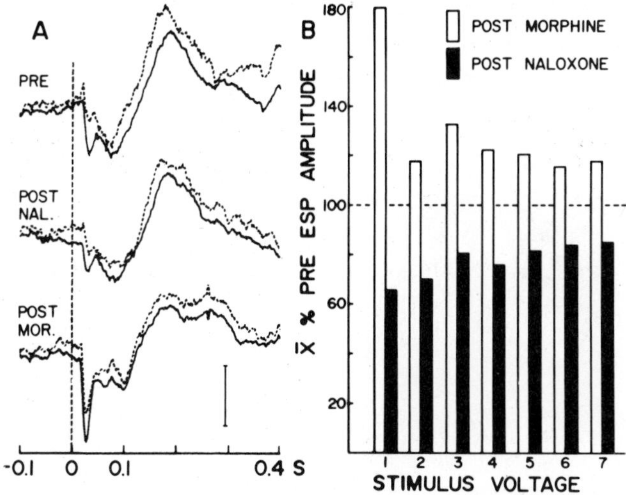

Fig. 3. A. Composite OM AEPs (4 separate daily 50-trial averages in each) obtained to positive tone during criterion performance of differential discrimination task following saline (PRE), naloxone (NAL), or morphine (MOR) injections (IP). Tone onset at dashed line. Calibration: 300 µV. B. Mean percent change in amplitude of perforant path extracellular synaptic potential (ESP) following morphine or naloxone administration.

The conditioned behavior of the animal as well as the configuration of the OM AEP are both modified by moderate doses of opiates and opioid peptides. Morphine and the opioid peptide FK 33-824 produce a large increase in N_1 and a decrease in N_2 which is followed by a termination of the conditioned behavior.[29] These changes resemble those produced by behavioral extinction but the animal remains conditioned as shown by the immediate resumption of discriminative responding following an injection of the opiate antagonist naloxone. In addition to the increase in N_1 and decreased behavioral responding, there is an increase in the amplitude of the perforant path elicited extracellular synaptic potential following opiate administration which is reversed by naloxone (Figure 3). These latter findings suggest that the establishment and maintenance of the conditioned behavior is mediated in part by opioid modulation of perforant path synapses.

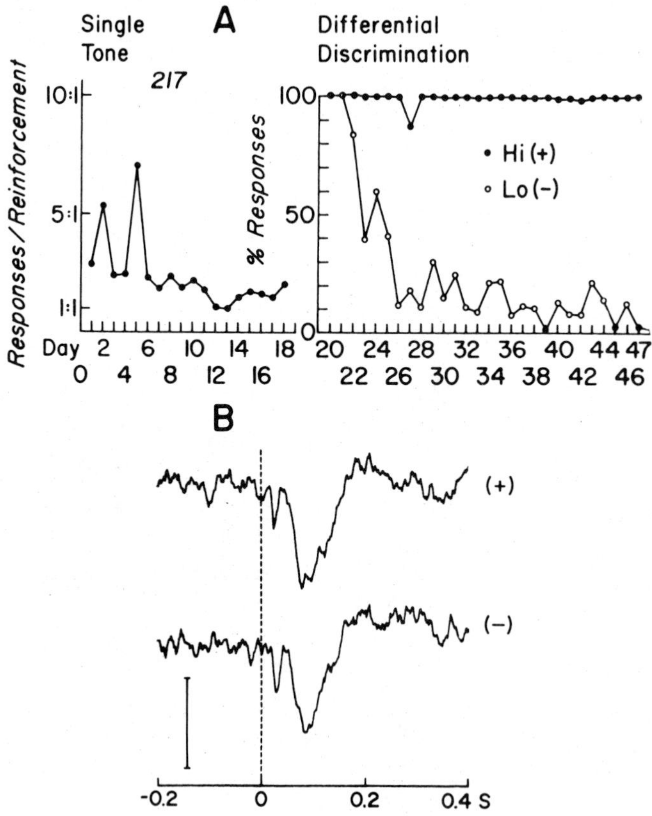

Fig. 4. A. Behavioral record of one animal (217) during acquisition of differential discrimination. B. OM AEPs to both tones obtained on day 47. Averages of 50 positive (+) and 50 negative (-) trials. Tone onset at dashed line. Calibration: 300 μV.

The OM AEP and Differential Discrimination Performance

During performance of a differential discrimination task where responding in the presence of only one of two randomly presented tones is reinforced, tone elicited g-cell discharges are differentiated to the positive and negative tones.[25] The OM AEP has a dual component configuration similar to that exhibited during simple discrimination learning and performance. However, there are two additional features of the OM AEP which are unique to the differential discrimination paradigm. As criterion performance is achieved on the differential discrimination task, the N_1 component remains large and stable across sessions, and does not decline as in simple discrimination learning. Secondly an identical OM AEP occurs to the negative (non-reinforced) tone, even though behavioral responses to the negative tone occur on less than 15% of these trials (Figure 4). Thus in 50 trial averages of the OM AEP, there is no differentiation to positive and negative tones corresponding to the conditioned differential behavior (Figure 4).

More detailed analyses of these data however revealed that the similarity between positive and negative OM AEPs during differential discrimination performance was produced by variations in N_1 on successive trials during the random presentation of positive and negative tones. Individual tone evoked potentials were sorted by computer according to 1) the auditory stimulus which elicited them (positive or negative tone), and 2) the nature of the trial sequence which preceded a particular tone. Trials were sorted and averaged on the basis of whether 1-5 similar or dissimilar trials preceded the presentation of a given tone. Twenty-four daily 100 trial sessions were sorted and summed in this manner for the animal whose behavioral record is shown in Figure 4. Since both tones were presented according to a Bernoulli sequence, longer runs of similar or dissimilar trials occurred less often than shorter runs. OM AEPs preceded by shorter sequences therefore contained more trials than OM AEPs preceded by longer sequences. However, the OM AEP amplitudes shown in Figure 5 can be compared directly since each potential is normalized to the number of trials which went into the average.

The results of these analyses show why combined averages of all positive and all negative trials within or across sessions (Figure 4) failed to indicate a consistent source of variation in the OM AEP. Clearly, both the type of preceding trial sequence (positive or negative) and the length of that trial sequence (1-5) substantially influenced the configuration of the OM AEP (Figure 5). As the prior sequence of trials tended to deviate from a simple alternation series to runs of 2 or more similar or dissimilar trials, the amplitude of the N_1 component in the OM AEP on subsequent trials varied accordingly. This was most dramatically illustrated by OM AEPs which occurred following long "runs" of (4-5) trials in which the opposite tone occurred. On these occasions the OM AEP configuration and the N_1 amplitude resembled that generated by the prior sequence of dissimilar trials (bottom and top traces in Figure 5). Thus, for example, the OM AEP was more characteristic of a negative tone, even though elicited by a positive tone, if it was preceded by a series of negative tone trials. The amplitude of the N_1 component varied from being barely detectable following prior runs of positive trials, to 250 μV in amplitude following prior runs of negative trials (Figure 5). These fluctuations in N_1 amplitude were not significantly different as a function of positive or negative tone presentation; they were, however, highly significant ($p \leq .001$ by two-way ANOVA) as a function of prior trial sequence.

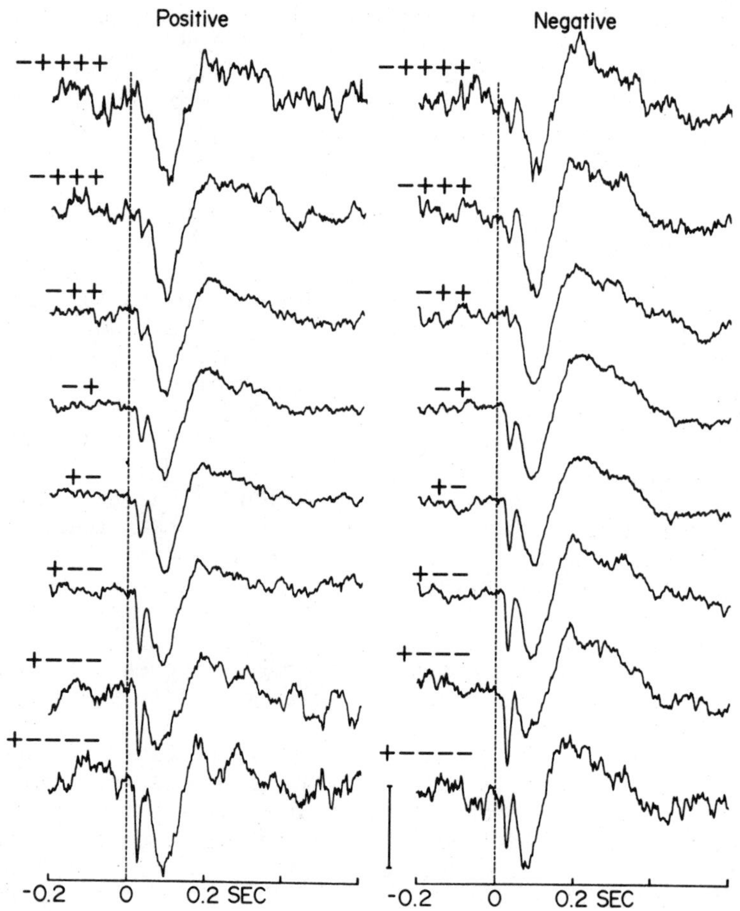

Fig. 5. OM AEPs to positive (left column) and negative (right column) tones, sorted on the basis of preceding trial sequence (indicated at the left of each trace). Dashed lines indicate tone onset. Calibration: 300 μV.

The N_2 component of the OM AEP showed very little amplitude variation related to prior trial sequence, although it was significantly larger on positive trials than on negative trials when compared across all sequences. Thus N_2 varied along a dimension different from that of the N_1 component, reflecting more the behavioral significance of the stimulus rather than the bias produced by the prior trial sequence. N_1 and N_2 continued to vary along the reinforcement-extinction continuum in a manner identical to that observed in simple discrimination learning. When the differential discrimination behavior of the animal shown in Figure 5 was extinguished N_1 became very large and the N_2 component was reduced to minimal amplitude (Figure 2).

CONCLUSION

The above results illustrate at least two important features of the input pathways to the hippocampus and their involvement in conditioning and learning processes. First the processes represented by these potentials can be dissociated from the behavioral context in which they occur (i.e., differential discrimination learning) even though in some situations there appears to be a tight coupling between the electrical events and behavioral performance of the discrimination task (i.e., simple discrimination learning). Second, the type of neural information represented by these electrical events may not be accurately deciphered by techniques which do not take into account the influence of sequential dependencies and stimulus likelihood on neural responses to conditioned sensory stimuli. The latter considerations may be of appropriate concern for analyses of behavioral performance on tasks which require the retention of specific sensory information from the immediate past.[9,11] It may be necessary under such circumstances for the subject to be able to update and/or disregard sensory information to maintain a high performance level from trial to trial.[8] If such neural mechansims are involved in the solution of complex discrimination problems, then the data presented here implicate hippocampal circuitry as being critical for the maintenance of these functions.

ACKNOWLEDGEMENTS

We would like to express our gratitude to Dr. J. H. Robinson for writing the computer software utilized in these analyses. The assistance of Janice Conner and especially Stephanie Burgoyne is appreciated. This research was supported by NSF Grant BNS 78-09787 and NIDA Grant DA-02048 to S.A.D.

REFERENCES

1. Olds, J., The central nervous system and the reinforcement of behavior, Am. Psychol. 24:114 (1969).
2. Adey, W.R., Neurophysiological correlates of information transaction and storage in brain tissue, in: "Progress in Physiology and Psychology," J. Sprague and E. Stellar, eds., Academic Press, New York (1966).
3. Graystan, E., K. Lissak, I. Madaas, and H. Donhoffer, Hippocampal electrical activity during the development of conditioned reflexes, EEG Clin. Neurophysiol., 11:409 (1959).
4. Douglas, R.J., The development of hippocampal function: implications for theory and for therapy, in: "The Hippocampus," vol 2, K. Pribram and R. Isaacson, eds., Plenum Press, New York, (1975).
5. Kilmer, W. and T.A. McLardy, A diffusely preprogrammed but sharply trainable hippocampus model, Intern. J. Neurosci. 2:241 (1971).
6. Marr D., Simple memory: A theory for archicortex. Philo. Trans. Royal Soc. (London), 262:23 (1971).
7. Kimble, D.P., Hippocampus and internal inhibition, Psych. Bull. 70:285 (1968)
8. Olton, D.S. and W.A. Feustle, Hippocampal function required for nonspatial working memory, Exp. Brain Res., 41:380 (1981).
9. Moss, M., H. Mahut, and S. Zola-Morgan, Concurrent discrimination learning of monkeys after hippocampal entorhinal, or fornix lesions, J. Neurosci., 1:227 (1981).
10. Halgren, E., N.K. Squires, C.L. Wilson, J.W. Rourbaugh, T.L. Babb, and P.H. Crandall, Endogenous potentials generated in the human hippocampal formation and amygdala by unexpected events. Science, 19:803 (1980).
11. Cohen, N.J. and L.R. Squire, Preserved learning and retention of pattern-analyzing skill in amnesia: dissociation of knowing how and knowing that, Science, 210:207 (1980).
12. Thompson, R.F., T.W. Berger, C.F. Cegavsky, M.M. Patterson, R.A. Roemer, T.J. Tyler, and R.A. Young, The search for the engram, Am. Psychol., 31:209 (1976).
13. Thompson, R.F., T.W. Berger, S.D. Berry, F.R. Hoehler, F.E. Kettner, and D.J. Weisz, Hippocampal substrate of classical conditioning, Physiol. Psych., 8:262 (1980).
14. Berger, T.W. and R.F. Thompson, Identification of pyramidal cells as the critical elements in hippocampal neuronal plasticity during learning, Proc. Nat. Acad Sci., 75:1572 (1978).
15. Berger, T.W., R.I. Laham, and R.F. Thompson, Hippocampal unit-behavior correlations during classical conditioning, Brain Res., 193:229 (1980).
16. Delacour, J., Conditioned modifications of arousal and unit activity in the rat hippocampus, Exp. Brain Res., 38:95 (1980).

17. Segal, M. and J. Olds, Activity of units in the hippocampal circuit of the rat during differential classical conditioning, J. Comp. Physiol. Psychol., 82:195 (1973).
18. Segal, M., Flow of conditioned responses in limbic telencephalic system of the rat, J. Neurophysiol., 36:840 (1973).
19. Ranck, J.R., Jr., Discussion II. in: "Functions of the Septo-Hippocampal System," Ciba Foundation Symposium, New York 58:309 (1977).
20. Best, M.R. and P.J. Best, The effects of state of conciousess and latent inhibition on hippocampal unit activity in the rat during conditioning, Exp. Neurol., 51:564 (1976).
21. O'Keefe, J., and L. Nadel, "The Hippocampus as a Cognitive Map," Oxford University Press, New York (1978).
22. Ranck, J.B., Jr., Studies on single neurones in the dorsal hippocampal formation and septum in unrestrained rats. I: Behavioral correlates and firing repertoires, Exp. Neurol., 41:401 (1973).
23. Solomon, P.R., A time and place for everything? Temporal processing views of hippocampal function with specific reference to attention, Physiol. Psych., 8:254 (1980).
24. Deadwyler, S.A., M.O. West, and Lynch G., Synaptically identified slow potentials during behavior, Brain Res., 161:211 (1979).
25. Deadwyler, S.A., M.O. West, and G. Lynch, Activity of dentate granule cells during learning: Differentiation of perforant path input, Brain Res., 169:29 (1979).
26. Deadwyler, S.A., M.O. West, and J.H. Robinson, Entorhinal and septal inputs differentially control sensory-evoked responses in the rat dentate gyrus, Science, 211:1181 (1981).
27. West, M.O., J.H. Robinson, and S.A. Deadwyler, A dual component sensory evoked potential in the dentate gyrus of the chronic rat, Fed. Proc., 39:1753 (1980).
28. West, M.O., E. Christian, J.H. Robinson, and S.A. Deadwyler, Dentate granule cell discharge during conditioning: Relation to movement and theta rhythm, Exp. Brain Res., in press (1981).
29. Christian, E.P., M.O. West, J.H. Robinson, and S.A. Deadwyler. Effects of opiates on sensory evoked potentials in the dentate gyrus of the chronic rat during conditioning, Soc. Neurosci. Abstr., 7, 1981.
30. West, M.O., E. Christian, J.H. Robinson, and S.A. Deadwyler, Evoked potentials in the dentate gyrus reflect the retention of past sensory events, Neurosci. Lett. (Submitted).

MNEMONIC FUNCTION OF THE HIPPOCAMPUS: CORRESPONDENCE BETWEEN ANIMALS AND HUMANS

Raymond P. Kesner

Department of Psychology
University of Utah
Salt Lake City, Utah 84112

SUMMARY

The purpose of the present paper is to demonstrate that in humans and animals the hippocampus is equivalent in terms of mnemonic function. In both animals and humans it can be shown that disruption of normal hippocampal function results in an impairment of long-term memory (episodic or working memory) for specific events without markedly altering short-term memory or memory for rules (semantic or reference memory). It is suggested that the exact nature of the deficit following hippocampal disruption is an impairment in the encoding of long-term temporal and absolute spatial attributes of specific events. Other attributes (e.g., short-term temporal, emotional) of specific events would be encoded by other neural regions.

COMPARISON BETWEEN ANIMALS AND HUMANS: ROLE OF THE HIPPOCAMPUS

Ever since the observation that bilateral medial temporal lobe damage including the hippocampus, produced in human patients an extensive and durable amnesia for new information, it has been assumed that the hippocampus is a critical neural region involved in the mediation of normal memory processes.

The most striking feature of this amnesic syndrome seen in patients with hippocampal damage is that they appear to forget rather quickly events that occur in their daily life. Many of these events are forgotten even after a period of a few minutes. As an example they are usually unable to tell you where they are, what they had for breakfast or when they had met you previously. In contrast, they are able to converse normally at least about events that occurred prior to their brain damage, their verbal skills are intact and they can carry out mental arithmetic. Thus, one cardinal feature of the amnesic syndrome in these patients appears to be one of an impaired long-term memory (LTM) for specific events (episodic memory) with an intact short-term memory (STM). One elegant study (Baddeley and Warrington, 1970) serves to illustrate this main point. It is well known that immediate free recall of a list of words results in a serial position curve with better memory performance for the first items (primacy effect) and the last items (recency effect) compared to items located in the middle of the list. It has been proposed by some theorists (Atkinson and Shiffrin, 1968), that the primacy effect reflects information storage in LTM, while the recency effect reflects information processing in STM. Baddeley and Warrington (1970) presented ten unrelated words to amnesic and control patients followed by an immediate test of free recall. Compared to controls amnesic patients had an impaired primacy effect, suggesting a deficit in LTM, but no impairment of the recency effect suggesting a normal operating STM. A similar pattern of results was obtained in patient H. M. and patients with large left hippocampal removal (Milner, 1978). More recently there has been an increased emphasis on a second cardinal feature of amnesic patients, namely that they can reasonably learn and retain a variety of rules of specific perceptual-motor (tracking, mirror tracing, eye-lid conditioning) and pattern analyzing (mirror reading, rule-based verbal paired-associate learning, rules of card games) skills, while not remembering having previously performed the task, the specific contingencies of the task, or when and where they learned the task. This dissociation can be thought of as reflecting a distinction between episodic and semantic memory (Tulving, 1972; Kinsbourne and Wood, 1975), working and reference memory (Olton, Becker, and Handelmann, 1980), or between procedural or rule based memory ("knowing how"), and declarative or data based memory ("knowing that") (Cohen and Squire, 1980). Notice that again there is a LTM loss in the ability to utilize information contained in specific events (episodic memory or data base of knowledge of components of a task), but in this case the comparison is made between relatively intact memory for rules (semantic memory) and poor memory for specific temporal-spatial experiences that make up the rules. There are many examples of this dissociation. To mention a few more recent observations, Weiskrantz and Warrington (1979) demonstrated that amnesic patients can acquire and retain classical eye-lid conditioning, but they could neither remember performing the task nor describe the apparatus or the procedure. Cohen and Squire (1980) demonstrated that amnesic patients could acquire and retain a mirror reading skill, but between sessions could not remember repeated words that made up the reading task.

Because of a desire (a) to prove that the hippocampus is the crucial neural region that must be damaged to produce the above mentioned characteristics and (b) to provide for a possible evolutionary significance of the hippocampus with respect to memory function, it was deemed of importance to search for comparable deficits across species including rats, cats and monkeys. However, it has proven to be very difficult to interfere with normal hippocampal function in animals and reproduce the basic characteristics of the human amnesic syndrome. A number of suggestions have been made aimed at resolving this discrepancy. The first and simplest idea is that the function of hippocampus is different for animals and humans. A second possibility is that the amnesic syndrome produced by medial temporal lobe lesions is not due to hippocampal damage, but rather a function of damage to the temporal stem containing input and output pathways of temporal cortex and amygdala, but not hippocampus (Horel, 1978). This suggestion was based on an extensive review of the literature and on the experimental observation that cuts of the temporal stem in monkeys abolished a preoperatively learned visual pattern discrimination.

A third possibility is that the amnesic syndrome is due not only to hippocampal damage but due to a combination of hippocampus plus amygdala damage (Mishkin, 1978). Mishkin demonstrated in monkeys that in a delayed object matching-to-sample task neither amygdala nor hippocampal lesions alone produced a deficit, but a severe performance deficit was observed with combined amygdala plus hippocampal lesions. However, it is important to note that neither Horel nor Mishkin have observed that temporal stem or amygdala plus hippocampal lesions produce a differential disruptive effect on STM vs LTM (episodic or working memory) and on episodic or working memory vs. semantic or reference memory.

A different alternative suggests that the hippocampus is the critical neural region, but that the tasks used to test memory in animals are not necessarily functionally equivalent to those used to test human memory. For example, Iversen (1976) has argued that the major effect of hippocampal lesions leading to long-term memory deficits is excessive interference. Since most animal tests tend to be simple and very repetitive, there often is little interference and, thus, one would not expect to observe deficits. Support for Iversen's hypothesis comes both from the animal and human literature. For example, Jarrard (1975) found that animals with hippocampal lesions were similar to controls in their ability to perform a spatial alternation task at relatively long delays, but differed from controls in that they were markedly affected by interpolated motor activity. Also deficits are found in monkeys and rats with hippocampal lesions in tasks, which can be interpreted to contain a large number of interference cues, including discrimination reversal learning, transfer of training between related problems, maze learning, and sequential ordering of responses. Similar results have been found in amnesic patients in which large numbers of perserverative and criteria errors occur from learning prior paired associate lists as well as impaired reversal learning and difficulty in learning complex mazes. For a more detailed review and other points of correspondence between the animal and human literature, one should consult Iversen (1976) and Weiskrantz (1978).

Even though there appear to be many similarities between animals and humans given that functionally equivalent tasks are used, there is still a great deal of skepticism partially because of the expectation that hippocampal damaged animals should have a long-term retention deficit on all tasks (this expectation is however unrealistic given that some learning and long-term retention has been found in amnesic patients), and partially because tests have not yet been used in animals aimed at demonstrating (a) that specific event information is available in STM but not LTM, (b) that previously learned or newly acquired rules can be used for efficient performance, but that memory for the specifics generating the rule are not remembered or, (c) a combination of a and b.

In order to add further support to the idea that the operation of the hippocampus is functionally equivalent at least in rats and humans, I will present two new studies demonstrating that (a) disruption of normal hippocampal function in rats can result in a memory deficit in LTM but not STM for unique event(s) that has (have) occurred in specific places and (b) memory for the appropriate rule is intact, but specific information necessary to apply the rule is not remembered.

In the first situation, animals are first trained to perform in an Olton eight-arm radial maze. Following acquisition, reinforcement (a piece of Froot Loop cereal) is placed in only one of the eight arms on any one trial (one per day). The location of the food varied randomly from day to day. Ten seconds after finding the food, the animal is returned to the center and is contained there for a variable delay period. Following the delay, the animal must return to the same arm in order to receive a second reinforcement.

Rats can delay in this eight-choice spatial matching-to-sample task up to 20 min making only a few errors (error is defined as an entry into an arm not containing the reinforcement). On half of the trials subseizure level dorsal hippocampal stimulation was applied for 10 seconds during the consumption of the Froot Loop reinforcement on the correct arm. It is assumed that electrical stimulation serves as a temporary disruptive agent of normal dorsal hippocampal function. On the other half of the trials no brain stimulation was applied. A retention test was given either at a 1 min, 12 min or 20 min delay. Each of the six animals in the study was tested three times at each retention test delay with and without electrical brain stimulation.

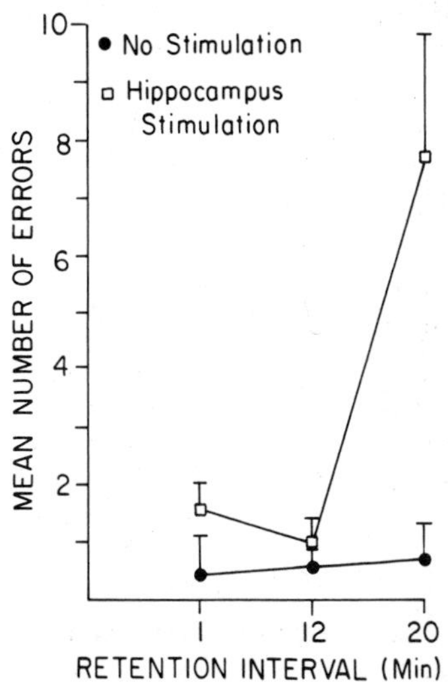

Figure 1. Effects of hippocampal stimulation on performance (mean number of errors for seven animals based on a total of three tests) as a function of time of retention test. I represents one standard error.

Results are shown in Figure 1 and clearly indicate that animals make few errors at all delays in the absence of hippocampal stimulation. Hippocampal stimulation, however, resulted in a large number of errors (memory deficit) only at the 20 min, but not at the 1 or 12 min retention test (Bierley, Kesner, and Novak, 1981). Of interest is the additional observation that hippocampal stimulation applied after the 10 sec exposure to the correct arm had no deleterious effect on performance at the 20 min. retention test. Also, amygdala stimulation does not produce a disruptive effect at the 20 min retention test. These data are consistent with previous findings in which immediate post-training hippocampal stimulation applied after an aversive or appetitive experience disrupts subsequent retention measured at long but not at short retention time intervals (Berman and Kesner, 1976; Kesner and Conner, 1974).

If one assumes that STM is operating at short-retention delays and LTM at long retention delays, then one can conclude from the results of the above mentioned studies that hippocampal disruption produces memory deficits in LTM, but not STM.

At this point one could argue that electrical stimulation of the hippocampus does not represent a comparable condition to that seen with brain damage in amnesic patients. Thus, the purpose of the next study (Kesner and Novak, 1981) was to test for the effects of hippocampal lesions on memory for order of a list of items, which represents a task in which memory for the early items has been contributed to LTM and memory for the last items has been used as an index of STM.

Rats were trained on an eight arm radial maze for Froot Loop reinforcement. After extensive training each animal was allowed on each trial (one per day) to visit all eight arms in an order that was randomly selected for that trial. The sequencing of the eight arms was accomplished by sequentially opening of Plexiglas doors (one at a time) located at the entrance of each arm. Immediately (within 20 seconds) after the animal had received reinforcement from the last of the eight arms, the test phase began. Only one test was given for each trial and consisted of opening two doors simultaneously. On a random basis either the 1st and 2nd, 4th and 5th, or 7th and 8th doors that occurred in the sequence were selected for the test. The rule to be learned leading to an additional reinforcement was to choose the arm that occurred earlier in the sequence. The results are shown in Figure 2. Based on 36 tests per animal all rats displayed a serial position curve, e.g., prominant retention (better than chance (50%) performance) for 1-2 and 7-8 positions, but no retention (chance performance) for 4-5 position. The same animals were given an additional 15 trials with 5 test trials for each 1-2, 4-5, 7-8 position, but with the test phase delayed by 10 min. Results are also shown in Figure 2 and indicate that retention of the 4-5 and 7-8 position was at chance, while retention of 1-2 position was still quite good. Thus, a 10 min delay disrupted the recency (7-8) portion of the serial position curve without markedly altering the primacy (1-2) component. It is important to note that this is the first demonstration of a prominant serial position curve in rats. Two animals then received a dorsal hippocampal lesion, while the other two animals served as sham-operated controls. Since the sham operation had no deleterious effect on the serial position

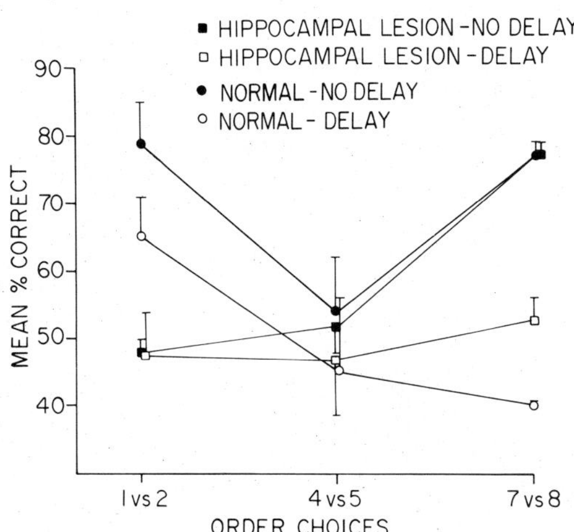

Figure 2. Serial position curves for normal and dorsal hippocampal lesion conditions with and without a retention test delay. I represents one standard error.

curve, the two animals were subsequently subjected to dorsal hippocampal lesions. All four lesioned animals were given 36 immediate tests with 12 at each choice position. The results of all four animals are shown in Figure 2. The lesioned animals displayed excellent retention only for the 7-8 position, but no retention (chance performance) for the 1-2 position. Thus, these animals showed disruption of the primacy (LTM), but not the recency (STM) component of the serial position curve. All animals were then given additional tests at 10 min delay. The results are shown in Figure 2 and clearly indicate that hippocampal lesioned animals performed at chance level at all three (1-2, 4-5, 7-8) positions indicating that they had no memory for order information. The results of this experiment are remarkably similar to the performance of amnesic patients, including H. M., on memory for a list of items (Baddeley and Warrington, 1970; Milner, 1978), in that hippocampal damage disrupted the primacy, but not the recency component of the serial position curve. Furthermore, with an additional delay between presentation and retention test the hippocampal lesioned animals demonstrated no retention similarly to what has been described clinically with amnesic patients. Thus, it is possible to reproduce one cardinal feature of the amnesic syndrome, namely a disruption of LTM for specific events with an intact STM in hippocampus damaged rats.

An additional important observation in this study was that lesioned rats could remember the previously learned rule (choose the arm that occurred earlier in the sequence) given that the retention test employed a choice between 7th and 8th item of the sequence. This suggests that hippocampal damage did not interfere with the ability to remember the rule and that the deficit in remembering the 1st and 2nd item of a particular sequence might have been due to the inability to remember the specific and unique details characteristic of appropriate encoding of the first two items. Similar results were obtained by Olton, Becker, and Handelmann (1980), who demonstrated that fimbria-fornix damaged animals would make in a 17-arm radial maze many repeated entries (errors) in arms in which food was available (working memory), but would not enter arms (no errors) in which food was never available (reference memory). Thus, the above mentioned studies provide some indirect support for the second cardinal feature of the amnesic syndrome, namely that specific rules can be learned and remembered, while forgetting when and where they had experienced the initial information.

ATTRIBUTE THEORY OF MEMORY: ROLE OF THE HIPPOCAMPUS

Given then that there exists a reasonably strong correspondence in hippocampal function between animals and humans, there should also be a common explanation for the amnesic syndrome. Milner (1970) assumed that information is processed in a dual STM and LTM system and that these systems are organized sequentially. Thus, the memory deficit was assigned to a lack of transfer of information from STM to LTM resulting in a consolidation failure within LTM. The exact nature of the consolidation deficit remained to be specified. Each of these assumptions has been challenged and further elaborations have been made in describing the nature of the deficit. First, with respect to the sequential STM-LTM assumption, a number of theoreticians have proposed that either STM and LTM systems are organized in parallel (Kesner, 1973; Warrington, 1971) or short- and long-term memory processes are organized into a single continuous system that might vary on other dimensions (Craik and Jacoby, 1975; Shiffrin and Schneider, 1977). Second, with respect to the assumption concerning the process that must be altered given some dysfunction of the hippocampus, a number of researchers have suggested that the primary deficit resides in (a) the inability to encode information properly (Butters and Cermak, 1975; Kesner, 1980), (b) excessive interference of irrelevant information (Weiskrantz, 1978; Douglas, 1967), (c) the inability to chunk information to be consolidated (Wickelgren, 1979), and (d) the inability to retrieve appropriate cues for efficient retention of information (Weiskrantz, 1978). Space limitations preclude a detailed analysis of each of these suggestions.

Finally, with respect to the nature of the memory deficit, it has been suggested that the hippocampus stores information concerning absolute space; i.e., the hippocampus represents a coding system capable of maintaining a spatial map of the subject's geographical environment (O'Keefe and Nadel, 1978). Thus, the memory deficit is due to the inability to encode absolute space or part of the environmental context. Others (Winocur and Olds, 1978; Kinsbourne and Wood, 1975) have also suggested that the memory deficit is due to inappropriate utilization of the external environmental context.

As a working hypothesis, I would like to propose that the deficit lies in the inability of hippocampal damaged animals and humans to encode and subsequently store and retrieve long-term temporal and absolute spatial attributes associated with specific episodes or events, i.e., the environmental context. Before examining this hypothesis in detail, it is first necessary to provide a background in the form of a theoretical framework and some of its underlying assumptions.

The first assumption is that long-term memory consists of a set or bundle of traces, each representing some attribute or feature of a learning experience. This assumption is not novel but, rather, has become generally accepted as a model of memory representation by many theoreticians studying human information processing (Bower, 1967; Tulving, 1972; Underwood, 1969; Wickens, 1972) and more recently in the study of animal memory (Spear, 1976). This multidimensional scaling of the memory trace contrasts with the assumption that the structure of memory consists of a monolithic trace, the strength of which can be represented by a unidimensional measure.

The second assumption is that different neural "units" subserve different attributes. The neuroanatomical "unit" of analysis [(e.g., synapse, synaptic conglomerate, synaptic assembly, neuron, neural assembly, junctional thicket, simple circuit, neural region, system, or complex system (Welker, 1976)] cannot be specificed at the present time. I will arbitrarily use neural regions such as the hippocampus, amygdala, and caudate as the initial neural units of analysis, but with more refined techniques specific subregions within each of the larger units might emerge as the more critical units of analysis. The strong version of the assumption would propose that each specific neural region stores (contains the mnemonic representation) of a specific attribute or set of attributes. The weaker version of the assumption would propose that each specific neural region processes only information represented by a specific attribute or set of attributes. The organization of these attributes will largely be determined by the anatomical and functional nature of the interconnections of the critical neural regions subserving the important attributes.

A spatial attribute within this framework involves the encoding of specific stimuli representing places or relationships between places which can be dependent or independent of the subject's own body schema. Borrowing from distinctions made by O'Keefe and Nadel (1978), I propose that mnemonic representation of space is encoded in the form of spatial attributes by at least two different systems. One system involves the encoding of personal, relative, or egocentric spatial attributes and depends upon accurate assessment of one's body orientation in space. It is exemplified by the ability to encode and remember right-left responses. The other system involves the encoding of extra-personal, absolute, or nonegocentric spatial relationships among external stimuli. It is exemplified by the ability to encode and remember maps and localize stimuli in external space. A person who is unable to encode or retrieve both personal and extrapersonal spatial attributes of specific situations would have a loss of "topographic memory"; that is, he would be unable to orient himself in space, follow or identify routes or recognize familiar places, or use spatial cues to guide his movement from one place to another.

Furthermore, it is possible that these two spatial systems are encoded independently and are subserved by different neuronal substrates. In accordance with O'Keefe and Nadel (1978), the hippocampus would primarily mediate the encoding of absolute spatial attributes, while the parietal cortex would primarily mediate the encoding of relative spatial attributes.

A temporal attribute within this framework involves the encoding of specific stimuli or sets of spatially or temporally separated stimuli as part of an episode marking or tagging its occurrence in time, that is, separating one specific episode from previous or succeeding episodes. Borrowing from distinctions made by Atkinson and Shiffrin (1968) and Kesner (1973), I propose that mnemonic representation of an event occurring at some specified point in time is encoded in the form of temporal attributes by at least two different systems. One involves the encoding of a short-term temporal attribute and depends upon the maintenance of activated neural activity for a matter of seconds (perhaps up to a few minutes). It is exemplified by the ability to retain information for short periods of time, as measured at short retention delays (seconds). The other system involves the encoding of a long-term temporal attribute and depends upon the elaboration, growth, or consolidation of activated neural traces leading to persistence of information from seconds, to hours, to days, to a life-time. It is exemplified by the ability to retain information for long periods of time, as measured at long retention delays (minutes, hours, days).

In accordance with a previous suggestion (Kesner, 1973), I would like to propose that these two systems can operate independently and are subserved by different neural structures, with the hippocampus primarily subserving the encoding of long-term temporal attributes and the midbrain reticular formation and frontal cortex primarily subserving the encoding of short-term temporal attributes of a situation. Thus, I am proposing that the hippocampus is primarily involved in the encoding of long-term temporal and absolute spatial attributes of episodes associated with specific learning situations. To the extent that encoded memories can be retrieved without the activation of long-term temporal and absolute spatial attributes (i.e., independent of specific environmental context) as exemplified by one's general knowledge of the world, the hippocampus should not play a role.

This attribute model of memory can easily account for the hippocampal syndrome in animals and humans. Since the hippocampus is limited to the processing of long-term temporal and absolute spatial attributes, deficits would be expected only when distinctive events that have occurred in specific places must be remembered at some later time (in the order of minutes, hours, days). No deficits would be expected when distinctive spatial events have to be remembered immediately or involve the operation of rules, because other neural systems are involved in the encoding of short-term temporal-spatial attributes as well as attributes associated with rule learning. Thus, the attribute model of memory can rather easily account for both normal and deficient retention of hippocampal damaged humans and animals.

This model of hippocampal mnemonic function differs from O'Keefe and Nadel's cognitive map and Winocur and Old's environmental context models in that the emphasis is not only on spatial attributes, but rather on the combination of both spatial and temporal attributes. It also differs from process (encoding, excessive interference, consolidation, retrieval) oriented models in that its main emphasis is directed towards the role of the hippocampus in mediating long-term spatial-temporal attributes of the memory trace. This mediation can take the form of encoding, storage and/or retrieval of the long-term spatial-temporal attributes, although there is a somewhat greater emphasis on the encoding process.

Obviously more research is necessary to test the model. Future directions should be aimed at (1) refining the neuroanatomical unit of analysis within the hippocampus, (2) selection of appropriate situations and procedures to maximize hippocampal involvement, so that more meaningful correlations can be found between electrophysiological and biochemical analyses of the hippocampus, and (3) using multiple measures of retention aimed at the discovery of meaningful dissociations.

REFERENCES

Atkinson, R. C., and Shiffrin, R. M., 1968, Human memory: A proposed system and its control processes, in: "Advances in the psychology of learning and motivation, research and theory (Vol. 2)," K. W. Spence and J. T. Spence, ed., Academic Press, New York.

Baddeley, A. D., and Warrington, E. K., 1970, Amnesia and the distinction between long- and short-term memory, J. Verb. Learn. and Verb. Behav., 9:176.

Berman, R. F., and Kesner, R. P., 1976, Post-trial hippocampal, amygdaloid, and lateral hypothalamic electrical stimulation: Effects upon memory of an appetitive experience, J. Comp. Phys. Psychol., 90:260.

Bierley, A. R., Kesner, R. P., and Novak, J. M., 1981, Episodic long-term memory in the rat: Time dependent effects of hippocampal stimulation (in preparation).

Bower, G., 1967, A multicomponent theory of the memory trace, in: "Advances in the psychology of learning and motivation (Vol. 1)," K. W. Spence and J. T. Spence, ed., Academic Press, New York.

Butters, N., and Cermak, L., 1975, Some analyses of amnesic syndromes in brain-damaged patients, in: "The hippocampus (Vol. 2)," R. L. Isaacson and K. H. Pribram, ed., Plenum Press, New York.

Cohen, N. J., and Squire, L. R., 1980, Preserved learning and retention of pattern-analyzing skill in amnesia: dissociation of knowing how and knowing that, Science, 210:207.

Craik, F. I. M., and Jacoby, L. L., 1975, A process view of short-term retention, in: "Cognitive theory (Vol. 1)," F. Restle, R. M. Shiffrin, N. J. Castellan, H. R. Lindman, and D. B. Pisoni, ed., Erlbaum, Hillsdale, New Jersey.

Douglas, R. J., 1967, The hippocampus and behavior, Psychol. Bull., 67:416.

Horel, J. A., 1978, The neuroanatomy of amnesia: A critique of the hippocampal memory hypothesis, Brain, 101:403.

Iversen, S. D., 1976, Do hippocampal lesions produce amnesia in animals?, Int. Rev. Neurobiol., 19:1.

Jarrard, L. E., 1975, Role of interference and retention by rats with hippocampal lesions, J. Comp. Phys. Psychol., 89:400.

Kesner, R. P., 1973, A neural system analysis of memory storage and retrieval, Psychol. Bull., 80:177.

Kesner, R. P., 1980, An attribute analysis of memory: The role of the hippocampus, Phys. Psychol., 8:189.

Kesner, R. P. and Conner, H. S., 1974, Effects of electrical stimulation of limbic system and midbrain reticular formation upon short- and long-term memory, Phys. and Behav., 12:5.

Kesner, R. P. and Novak, J. M., 1981, Memory for lists of items in rats: Role of the hippocampus, Neurosci. Abst., (In Press).

Kinsbourne, M. and Wood, F., 1975, Short-term memory processes and the amnesic syndrome, in: "Short-term memory," D. Deutsch and J. A. Deutsch, ed., Academic Press, New York.

Milner, B., 1970, Memory and the medial temporal regions of the brain, in: "Biology of memory," K. H. Pribram and D. E. Broadbent, ed., Academic Press, New York.

Milner, B., 1978, Clues to the cerebral organization of memory, in: "Cerebral correlates of conscious experience," P. A. Buser and A. Rougeul-Buser, ed., Elsevier, Amsterdam.

Mishkin, M., 1978, Memory in monkeys severely impaired by combined but not by separate removal of amygdala and hippocampus, Nature, 273:297.

O'Keefe, J. and Nadel, L., 1978, "The hippocampus as a cognitive map," Clarendon Press, Oxford.

Olton, D. S., Becker, J. T., and Handelmann, G. E., 1980, Hippocampal function: Working memory or cognitive mapping?, Phys. Psychol., 8:239.

Shiffrin, R. M. and Schneider, W., 1977, Controlled and automatic human information processing: II. Perceptual learning, automatic attending, and a general theory, Psych. Rev., 84:127.

Spear, N. F., 1976, Retrieval of memories: A psychobiological approach, in: "Handbook of learning and cognitive processes (Vol. 4)," W. K. Estes, ed., Erlbaum, Hillsdale, New Jersey.

Tulving, E., 1972, Episodic and semantic memory, in: "Organization of memory," E. Tulving and W. Donaldson, ed., Academic Press, New York.

Underwood, B. J., 1969, Attributes of memory, Psych. Rev., 76:559.

Warrington, E. K., 1971, Neurological disorders of memory, Brit. Med. Bull., 27:243.

Weiskrantz, L., 1978, A comparison of hippocampal pathology in man and other animals, in: "Functions of the septo-hippocampal system," Elsevier, Amsterdam.

Weiskrantz, L. and Warrington, E. K., 1979, Conditioning in amnesic patients, Neuropsychol., 17:187.

Welker, W. I., 1976, Brain evoluation in mammals. A review of concepts, problems, and methods, in: "Evolution of brain and behavior in vertebrates," R. B. Masteron, M. E. Bitterman, B. Campbell, and N. Hotton, ed., Erlbaum, Potomac, Maryland.

Wickelgren, W. A., 1979, Chunking and consolidation: A theoretical synthesis of semantic networks, configuring in conditioning, S-R versus cognitive learning, normal forgetting, the amnesic syndrome, and the hippocampal arousal system, Psych. Rev., 86:44.

Wickens, D. P., 1972, Characteristics of word encoding, in: "Coding processes in human memory," A. W. Melton and E. Martin, ed., V. H. Winston, Washington, D.C.

Winocur, G. and Olds, J., 1978, Effects of context manipulation on memory and reversal learning in rats with hippocampal lesions J. Comp. Phys. Psychol., 92:312.

TONIC AND PHASIC FIRING OF RAT HIPPOCAMPAL COMPLEX-SPIKE CELLS IN THREE DIFFERENT SITUATIONS: CONTEXT AND PLACE

John L. Kubie and James B. Ranck, Jr.

Department of Physiology
Downstate Medical Center, State University of New York
Brooklyn, New York 11203

The firing of hippocampal complex-spike cells has previously been demonstrated to be related to a rat's position in its environment. In this paper we examine the firing of individual complex-spike cells in three familiar environments: an Olton radial maze, an operant chamber with a DRL-16 schedule in effect, and a home box with the rat's pups. We have found that individual neurons have spatial fields in several environments, and that the position of the fields is stable within an environment but unpredictable from one environment to the next. We have also found that tonic firing rates are stable in one environment but vary dramatically and unpredictably from one situation to another. The results are interpreted in terms of a hippocampal context system.

The behavioral significance of context has been discussed intermittantly for many years in psychology. There seems to be common agreement that context is important, but we are not aware of many comprehensive discussions of the issue (see Nadel and Wilner 1980). Indeed there are no commonly accepted definitions. For instance, context has been considered to be tonic cues or background cues or part of cognitive mapping or discriminative stimuli for an operant (S^D) which signal which contingencies are in effect. Context has been considered multiple cues or single cues. It is not clear if contextual cues are qualitatively different from non-contextual stimuli. Context seems to have been discussed with increasing frequency over the last ten years. Perhaps it is beginning to come into focus.

Hirsh (1974), and Winocur and Olds (1978) have argued that the deficits seen in animals after hippocampal lesions are due to loss of the ability to use context retrieval. Kinsbourne and Wood (1975) and Winocur and Kinsbourne (1978) have argued that the amnesia of Korsakoff's syndrome is also at least partially due to a deficit in the use of contextual cues. In animals and man it is argued that lack of adequate use of context leads to inappropriate use of phasic cues. In this study we show that the tonic firing of hippocampal complex-spike cells are specific to the situation and we sugges that it is context that is significant in the tonic firing of these hippocampal neurons.

This study also addresses the issue of spatial correlates of firing of hippocampal neurons (place fields). In a given apparatus most hippocampal complex-spike neurons have been reported to have place fields, (O'Keefe 1976, Olton, Branch, and Best 1976), but surely a representation of a three-arm maze or an eight-arm maze is not built into the brain of a rat. We recorded the same neuron in three different situations. We usually found place fields in all three situations but we were not able to find anything in common among the place fields of the same neuron. We suggest that use of information from the place field firing of hippocampal neurons requires information about context and that both place and context are represented in the firing of hippocampal neurons. In the situations we have studied, context seems to be associated with tonic firing, and place with phasic firing.

METHODS

The subjects were female Long-Evans rats. They were trained to perform three tasks in three different situations.

a) Rats were trained on an eight-arm radial Olton maze (Olton and Samuelson 1976) to take eight choices of arms. The end of each arm was baited with a 45 mgm pellet. The optimal strategy is to choose eight different arms, which the rats readily learn to do. After eight choices, they were placed in a clear plastic cylinder in the center of the maze. The arms were rebaited, the cylinder was removed and eight more choices are offered. This is repeated for 10 to 20 minutes. In a well trained rat a cycle of eight choices plus rebaiting took one and a half to two minutes.

b) Rats were trained on differential reinforcement for low rates of responding with a 16 second interval (DRL-16) in a operant chamber with two pairs of bars and food dispensers. Only one pair was active at a time. The training included at least two hours of successful continuous reinforcement in the beginning of training, before the interval was progressively increased. Sometimes the active bar and dispenser was signalled by a light. The rats were well trained, receiving at least ten days of experience on DRL-16, 20 minutes per day.

The box has a wire mesh front and an open top making many distal room cues visible to the rat.

c) The subjects were all lactating when the recording took place. Lactation was maintained by replacing pups with new pups when necessary. The dams live with the pups in a large box (70 x 53 x 30 cm), which has a clear plexiglass front wall and a wire mesh roof (called the home box). The dams retrieved pups placed at various sites in the box. Forty-five mgm pellets were placed at various sites in the box for the dams to retrieve. The dams also displayed spontaneous exploratory activity.

(The performance of each of these three tasks is disrupted by lesions of hippocampus or fornix-fimbria (Becker, Walker and Olton, 1980; Clark and Isaacson, 1965; Kimble, Rogers and Hendrickson, 1967)).

Recordings were made with moveable tungsten electrodes with etched tips, or more recently with moveable 25 um nichrome wires, with cut off ends. The implantations were made at least a week before recording. The electrode was lowered until a neuron was recorded with adequate isolation. The rat was then observed in each of the three situations while recording from the neuron. The behavior was TV taped, and the electrical activity of the neuron was recorded on the audio channel of the TV tape recorder. The order in which the three situations were observed was varied. Each of the three situations was recorded in the same place in the recording room with respect to distal cues by placing the operant chamber and the home box on the Olton maze. Each situation was recorded for at least ten minutes. At least one situation was repeated. During recording in each situation the apparatus was rotated, to see if any place fields are constant with respect to local or distal cues. In each situation at the end of observing spontaneous behavior the rat was held in the experimenter's hand and moved passively throughout the apparatus.

Some features are common to all three situations: The distal cues are the same, most of the behavior is walking (and hence accompanied by hippocampal slow wave theta rhythm), eating 45 mgm pellets occurs in all, and rats are moved in the environment in the experimenter's hand.

The TV tape of the data was played back later. The neuronal electrical activity was fed into a window discriminator, which was fed into an integrator on a polygraph. The integrator was reset every five seconds. From these data histograms of rate of firing in five second bins were produced. (i.e. number of bins with zero action potentials in five seconds, one action potential in five seconds, etc).

The terms tonic and phasic are not sharply defined. We are currently searching for useful ways to distinguish tonic and phasic firing in this data, using automatic analysis. We currently find three methods of use, all of which give similar results.

a) Tonic rates are simply slow rates and phasic rates fast. We look for a break in the histogram of rates in five second intervals to determine the division.

b) If one assumes that tonic firing occurs with a Poisson distribution, then the form of this distribution (and mean firing rate) can be determined from the proportion of five second bins in which there are zero action potentials. Phasic firing is any firing not accounted for by this assumption.

c) Tonic firing is firing in regions of an environment which does not include the place field of a neuron.

RESULTS AND DISCUSSION

Twenty-four complex-spike cells were recorded in nine rats. Complex-spike cells are presumed to be hippocampal projection cells or pyramidal cells (Fox and Ranck, 1981; Berger and Thompson, 1979).

Behavior

There were no differences noted between the behavior of the rats during training and during recording. The rats were well trained and their behavior in each situation was reproduceable and successful Rats often made better than seven out of eight successful arm choices on the radial maze. The DRL-16 rewards were more than 1.5 per minute (the maximum possible is 3.7). They performed successfully on both bars. Pup retrieval was usually prompt and appropriate.

The rats perceived these three environments as distinctly different environments. The point is not trivial since all recording was actually done in the same space in the laboratory (with the same distal cues). But the fact that the rats exhibited different patterns of behavior in the different environments, and that these patterns were appropriate to the well-learned environmental contingencies demonstrate that the environmental changes were salient to the rats.

Phasic Firing

To date, almost all analysis of phasic firing has been observational and subjective. Most, if not all, clear-cut relations of phasic firing to behavior have been spatial. That is, neurons dramatically change their rates of firing when a rat is in a particular place. Our observations are entirely consistent with the earlier disruptions of spatially related unit firing of hippocampal complex-spike cells (O'Keefe 1976, Olton, Branch and Best 1978, Hill 1978, O'Keefe 1979). The place fields which were found in the operant chamber are especially significant. The use of two pairs of bar and dispenser with the animal using first one and then another is a strong test of behavior versus place. The firing is clearly spatial. This result is also remarkable because we think the deficit on DRL performance seen after hippocampal ablation is among the most difficult to explain on the basis of loss of a spatial map. This, in fact, was part of the reason for the choice of the DRL as one of the situations.

Each unit exhibited some degree of spatial firing in more than one environment. This seems to demonstrate that hippocampal cells do not simply code one position in the universe such as an arm on the eight-arm maze. Although this was an unlikely possibility, it could not be discounted from the results of previous reports.

Spatial firing was always determined by distal cues in the eight-arm maze (i.e., did not rotate with maze rotation) and by proximal cues in the home box and the operant chamber (i.e., did rotate with apparatus rotation). Spatial fields usually were maintained, and were sometimes strengthened, when the rat was held in the experimenter's hand and moved through the field. Some cells exhibited no place fields in at least one of the three environments.

A most notable finding was that the place fields were very different in the different environments. Place fields in these situations were as large as about 900 cm^2 or two arms of the Olton maze or as small as 50 cm^2. A single neuron could have a large place field in one situation and a small field in another situation. In the same situation a neuron can have single or multiple place fields. This could vary between situations. There was no constancy of the place fields of the same neuron with respect to distal cues.We have not been able to discover any organizing or over-riding principles for the positioning of a single cell's place fields across environments. This somewhat negative observation suggests that, if the rats are using place-cell firing to register their position in space, as Nadel and O'Keefe (1978) suggest, then they must also have a context system to keep the places straight.

Tonic Firing

Much of the recent focus of our interest has been on the tonic firing of neurons in the three environments. This interest in tonic firing was triggered by the unexpected observation that a few neurons appeared to practically turn off in one of the three environments. This phenomenon can be so striking that one is almost convinced that the unit is lost or dead until the rat is switched to a new environment and the firing rate dramatically increases. It occurred to us that perhaps this turning-off represented only the extreme cases of changes in tonic firing rates. This paper, which describes early stages of analysis, suggests that this is the case.

All neurons we have examined exhibit dramatic changes in mean firing rate from one situation to another. Hippocampal complex-spike cells have been noted for their low firing rates. We have observed mean firing rates within an environment ranging from .02 action potentials per second to 4 action potentials per second. The magnitude of the mean firing rate changes within a cell can be large -- over twenty fold when comparing two situations. For all neurons examined thus far mean firing rates vary at least 2.5 fold across the three situations.

Two examples of these changes in firing rates are illustrated in figures 1 & 2 which are data taken from two neurons in one rat. These figures are histograms of the percentage of five-second bins exhibiting various firing rates. Bins without any action potentials are not plotted. The faster a cell fires, the further to the right the data within the histogram should move. Tonic firing is represented by the bins to the left and phasic firing by the bins to the right. For the first unit (figure 1) the home box is associated with the highest rates of firing (2.45/sec) which includes both tonic and phasic firing. This is followed by the radial maze (0.46/sec), and the operant chamber is a distant third (0.09/sec). In the operant chamber the unit is almost silent: seventy-seven percent of the five-second bins have no spikes and the most spikes observed in a five-second bin was four. The second unit from the rat (figure 2), was recorded three days later. It illustrates a case where the operant chamber elicited the fastest unit firing (1.02/sec), followed by the home box (0.64/sec), followed by the radial maze (0.27/sec). It should be noted that none of these distributions are close to a Poisson distribution -- they are too dispersed. Such a dispersion could be caused by a mixture of tonic and phasic firing.

The mean firing rate recorded within a situation was quite stable: it varied less than fifteen percent comparing the first half of a videotape record with the last, and varied less than twenty percent when a situation was repeated at the end of a tape session.

We believe that these changes are not due to changes in the rat's behavior *per se* for two reasons: First, in our observations, which were almost entirely while rats were in a theta-mode awake state, the rats behavior itself appears to have little to do with tonic or phasic firing; and second, the three situations elicit many of the same behavior patterns, such as running and eating, yet during these behaviors differences between firing rates in the three environments were maintained. We also believe that the differences we observed

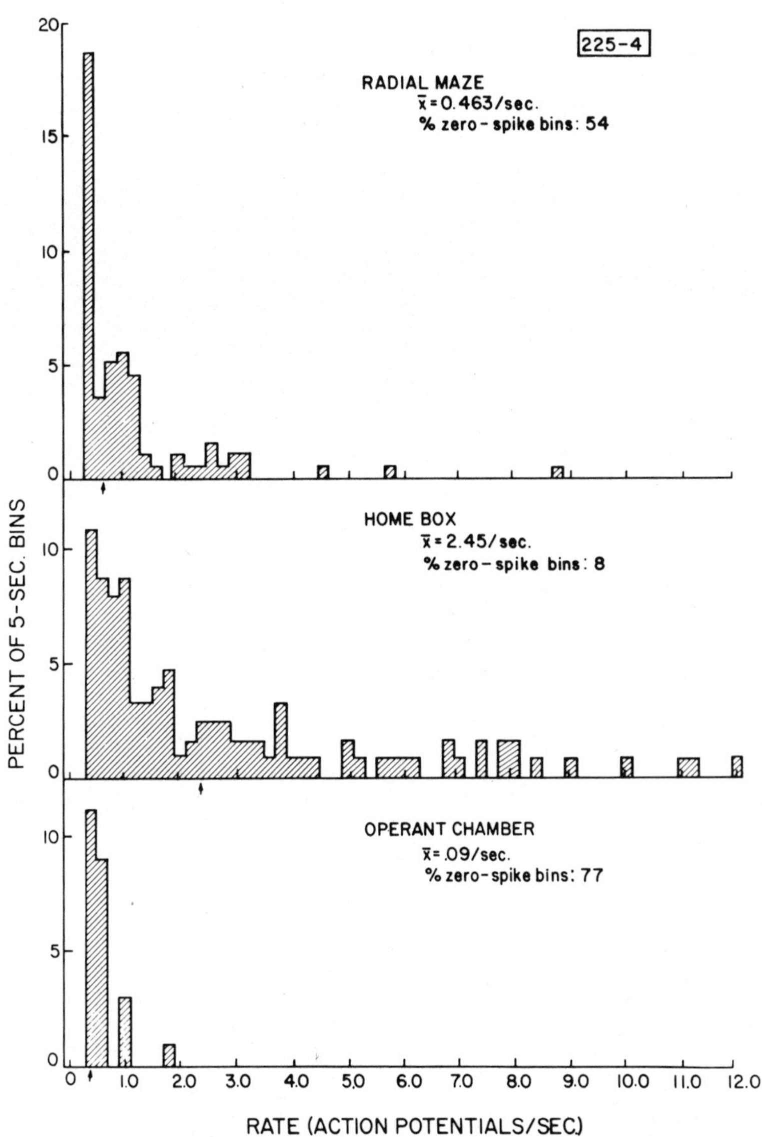

Figure 1. Firing-rate distribution for rat 225 unit 4 in each situation. Each entry in a histogram represents the firing rate for a five-second interval. Over one hundred intervals were sampled in each histogram. The zero-rate intervals are not plotted.

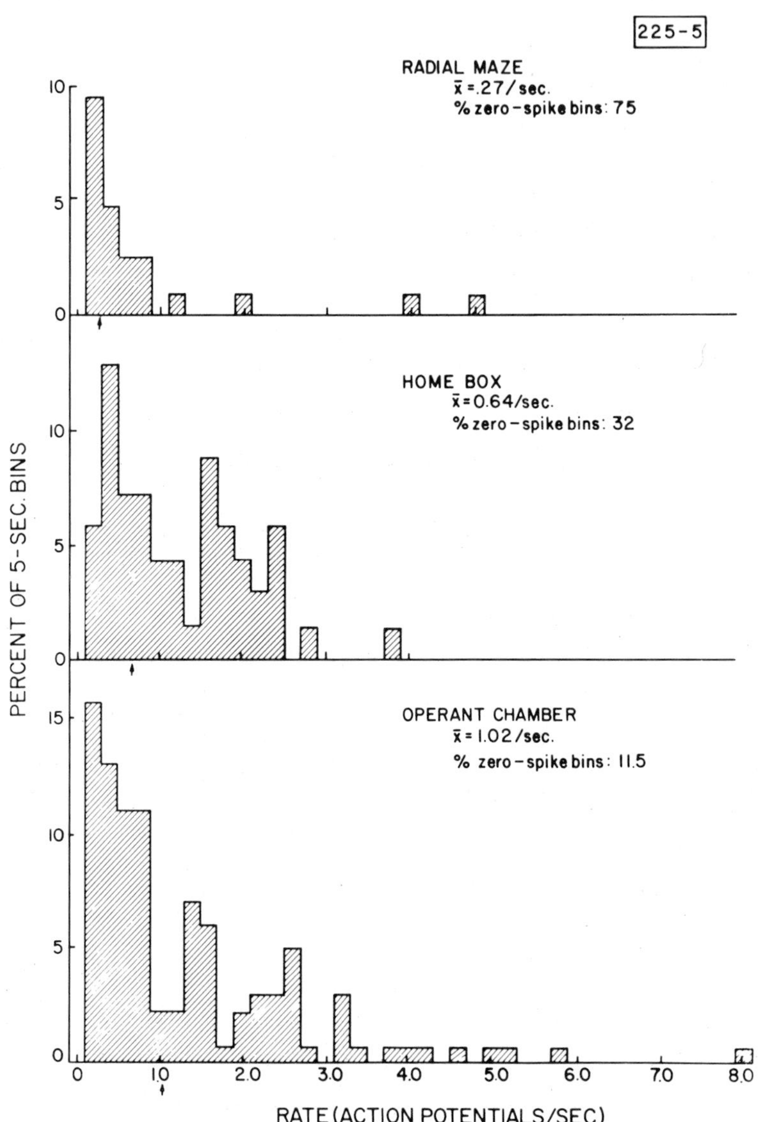

Figure 2. Firing-rate distribution for rat 225 unit 5 in each situation. The histograms are constructed with the same method as figure 1. Note the difference in the rank order of mean firing rates across situations.

are not due to a non-specific internal state of the rat such as arousal. If the firing rates of the cells were correlated with a single dimension, such as arousal, one would expect the situation associated with the highest rate would be the same in all or most neurons, and the situation with the slowest rate would be the same in all or most neurons. In fact all six possible rank orders of siturations ordered by tonic firing rates are observed in approximately equal frequency. Although this is not definitive evidence, we have not found arousal or other non-specific internal states useful constructs in analyzing tonic or phasic firing.

Using the three statistical methods to define tonic and phasic, our early estimates are that in these situations one-third to one half of hippocampal unit firing is tonic, the rest being phasic. The magnitude of change in tonic firing rate within cells across situations has a median of about five-fold and ranges from two-fold to well in excess of twenty-fold. The number of action potentials and the range over which the rate varies indicate that tonic firing is of physiological importance regardless of its behavioral significance. Changes in tonic firing rates in the nervous system have rarely been studied, with the exception of studies on sleep. Our results show that tonic firing is also an important subject of study in the hippocampus in awake animals.

Tonic firing in situation specific, but the rank order of situation by firing rate varies between neurons. There are many possible reasons these relations may exist. We suggest context may be a fundamental correlate, acknowledging that it is poorly defined. We can imagine that, in a given context, each complex-spike cell has a characteristic firing rate. The mosaic presented by the tonic firing rates of the entire sheet of hippocampal pyramidal cells could well be unique for each context and provide an across-neuron representation of each context. Such a representation of context could be the internal representation of shifting behavioral contingencies. We have noted above that in different situations there are different place fields in the same neuron. Perhaps a hippocampal context system provides the necessary information to keep these different place fields straight. Although extremely tentative, this hypothesis is important in that it concretely suggests cellular mechanisms for the hippocampal context system, a system which is suggested by lesion data. Our preliminary results clearly support the hypothesis.

ACKNOWLEDGEMENTS

This work was supported by NIH grant NS 14497 and NSF grant BNS 77-09375 and NIH fellowship 1F32NS06152. John Pomfret and Mary Ranck trained some of the rats. Claude Jeanty helped in data analysis. Drs. Sloane Wolfson and Steven E. Fox contributed valuable discussions.

REFERENCES

Becker, J.T., Walker, J.A. and Olton, D.S., 1980, Neuroanatomical bases of spatial memory. Brain Research 200: 307.

Berger, T.W. and Thompson, R.F., 1978, Identification of pyramidal cells as the critical elements in hippocampal neuronal plasticity during learning. Proc. Natl. Acad. Sci. 75:1572.

Clark, C.V.H. and Isaacson, R.L., 1965, Effects of bilateral hippocampal ablation on DRL performance. J. comp. physiol. psychol. 59:137.

Fox, S.E. and Ranck, J.B., Jr., 1981, Electrophysiological characteristics of Hippocampal Complex-spike cells and theta cells. Exp. Brain Res. 41:399.

Hill, A.J., 1978, First occurrence of hippocampal spatial firing in a new environment. Exptl. Neurol. 62:282.

Hirsch, R., 1974, The hippocampus and contextual retrieval of information from memory: A theory, Behavioral Biology 12:421.

Kimble, D.P., Rogers, L., and Hendrickson, C., 1967, Hippocampal lesions disrupt maternal, not sexual, behaviour in the albino rat. J. comp. physiol. Psychol. 48:281.

Kinsbourne, M. and Wood, F., 1975, Short-term memory processes and the amnesic syndrome. in. "Short-term Memory" J.A. Deutsch, ed. Academic Press, New York

Nadel, L. and Wilner, J., 1980, Context and conditioning. Physiol. Psych. 8:218.

O'Keefe, J., 1976, Place units in the hippocampus of the freely moving rat. Exptl. Neurol.51: 78.

O'Keefe, J., 1979, A review of the hippocampal place cells. Progress in Neurobiology, 13:419.

O'Keefe, J. and Nadel, L., 1978, "The Hippocampus as a Cognitive Map." Oxford University Press, Oxford.

Olton, D., Branch, M., and Best, P., 1978, Spatial correlates of hippocampal unit activity. Exptl. Neurol. 58:387.

Olton, D.S. and Samuelson, R.J., 1976, Remembrance of places passed: spatial memory in rats. J. exp. Psychol. Anim. Behav. Proc. 2:97.

Winocur, G. and Kinsbourne, M., 1978, Contextual cueing as an aid to Korsakoff amnesics, Neuropsychologia, 16:671.

Winocur, G. and Olds, J., 1978, Effects of context manipulation on memory and reversal learning in rats with hippocampal lesions. J. comp.physiol. Psychol. 92:312.

HIPPOCAMPAL FUNCTION AND MEMORY PROCESSES

David S. Olton

Department of Psychology
The Johns Hopkins University
Baltimore, MD 21218

SUMMARY

The experiments described here used an experimental design in which each rat was presented simultaneously with different discriminations, allowing a within-subject, within-test dissociation of performance. The results demonstrate that the rats with fimbria-fornix lesions showed a greater impairment in the discriminations requiring working memory than in discriminations requiring only reference memory. This dissociation rules out a variety of different interpretations of the behavioral impairment in the working memory discrimination and provides strong support for the idea that these lesions produce a selective difficulty in processing the temporal/personal context of the information to be remembered. Because the details of the experiments have been presented elsewhere, the emphasis here is on the concepts behind the experiments, the implications of the results, and the relationship of the results to different theories of memory.

INTRODUCTION

The hippocampus is one of the brain structures importantly involved in the processing of memory (Baker et al., in press; Gaffan, 1974, 1977; Jarrard, 1976, 1978, 1980; Kesner, 1980; Kesner et al., 1975; Milner, 1968; Mishkin, 1978; Olds, 1972; Thomas, 1978, 1979; Thomas et al., 1980; Thompson et al., 1980; Thompson et al., 1976; Winocur, 1980; Winocur and Olds, 1978). However, considerable disagreement still exists about the types of memory that require hippocampal function. Consequently, experiments designed with different types of memory requirements are useful because they can clarify more precisely the role of the hippocampal system in memory by demonstrating behavioral dissociations following damage to this structure.

Our research has been concerned with a distinction between two types of memory (Honig, 1978, 1979, in press; Olton, 1978a, 1979; Olton et al., 1979a,b, 1980). Working memory contains the temporal/personal associations necessary to determine the time at which an event occurred. Reference memory contains the logical and formal interrelationships among rules and procedures that are independent of the temporal/personal context in which the events occurred.

This distinction between working memory and reference memory is similar but not identical to other distinctions that have been used to characterize human amnesias (episodic and semantic--Kinsbourne and Wood, 1975; Rozin, 1976; Schacter and Tulving, in press; knowing that and knowing how--Cohen and Squire, 1981), particularly those following temporal lobe damage and Senile Dementia of the Alzheimer's Type (SDAT). These two human amnesias have many characteristics in common (Corkin, 1981, in press), and can be described as a failure of working memory in the presence of an intact reference memory. Although the neuropathological data from these individuals shows that the hippocampus is involved (review of SDAT in Terry and Davies, 1980, pp. 86-89; review of temporal lobe amnesia in Kolb and Whishaw, 1980, p. 322), the presence of abnormalities in many other brain areas precludes any discrete localization of the sites critical for the memory impairments. Indeed, investigations of the neurobiological bases of these syndromes may best be pursued with animals because the production of the pathology, and its evaluation, can be precisely controlled. Thus our research has used both working memory procedures and reference memory procedures to test rats with fimbria-fornix lesions in order to describe the amnesic syndrome seen following these discrete lesions in animals, and compare it to that seen following more involved neuropathology in humans.

PROCEDURE AND RESULTS

Working memory and reference memory have become operationally defined in a variety of tasks (see Honig, 1978, in press; Olton et al., 1979a,b, 1980). Of most relevance to the present report are procedures using radial arm mazes. Each maze had a central platform, and a series of arms extending away from that platform like spokes on a wheel. We have used mazes with four arms (Walker and Olton, 1979a), eight arms (Olton and Samuelson, 1976), and 17 arms (Olton et al., 1977). On each maze, the central platform was about 50 cm in diameter, and each arm was about 70 cm long, and

10 cm wide. At the far end of each arm, a hole in the end of it served as a food cup. An important feature of the mazes was the inclusion of a set of guillotine doors, one in front of each arm. These doors were lowered after each choice, confining the rat to the center of the maze and interrupting the response habits that appear when such confinement is not incorporated (Olton et al., 1977; Walker and Olton, 1979a,b).

At the beginning of the experiments, each rat was food deprived to about 85% of his *ad lib* body weight, shaped to run out the ends of the arms to get the food, and then given one to three test sessions each day. At the start of each test session, one piece of food was placed at the end of the appropriate arms. The rat was placed on the central platform with all the guillotine doors closed. The doors were opened, and the rat allowed to run out an arm. When he was on an arm, the doors to the other arms were closed. All the doors remained closed for at least five seconds. All the doors were then opened again, and the rat allowed to make another choice. This procedure continued until the rat had chosen each arm with food on it, or some criterion (based on the total number of choices made or the amount of time passed in the test session) was reached, when the test session ended and the rat returned to his home cage.

Lesions were made using standard surgical procedures for rats (see descriptions in Becker et al., 1981; Handelmann and Olton, 1981; Olton et al., 1978; Olton et al., in press; Rawlins and Olton, 1981). Radiofrequency current was used for lesions of the fimbria-fornix, amygdala, entorhinal cortex, and caudate nucleus, electrolytic current for the medial septal area, aspiration for the sulcal frontal cortex and medial frontal cortex, and kainic acid for the CA3 pyramidal cells.

Following testing, rats were anesthetized and perfused. Their brains were taken, cut while frozen in a cryostat, and stained. All brains were stained with cresyl violet for cell bodies and luxol fast blue for myelinated fibers in the area of the lesion. Most brains were stained for AChE activity in the area of the hippocampus. The procedures for these stains have been described in detail elsewhere (Becker et al., 1981; Olton et al., 1978).

In all of the behavioral analyses, emphasis has been placed on rats that have complete lesions of the structure in question, in addition to minimal destruction of surrounding tissue. In general, then, the lesions were substantial, completely destroying the appropriate structure. Detailed histological results have been presented in each of the relevant articles referenced here.

For the dissociation between working memory and reference

memory, the rats were presented with two different sets of arms (Olton and Papas, 1979). For the spatial baited set, one pellet of food was placed at the end of each arm at the beginning of each test session. The optimal strategy for the rat with respect to these arms was to choose each one once, and not return to a chosen arm during the remainder of the test session. Accurate performance on this set of arms required working memory because during the first approach to each arm, the correct response was to choose the arm, while during all subsequent approaches in that test session, the correct response was to avoid that arm. In order to determine whether or not a particular arm in the baited set should be chosen, the rat had to remember whether or not he had chosen that arm previously in that test session. The second set of arms was the spatial unbaited set. These arms never had food on them. Thus the optimal strategy for the rat was never to go to the end of these arms during any test session. Performance on these arms did not require working memory because the correct response was always the same every time the rat approached these arms; no temporal associations were necessary to determine whether these arms should be chosen.

Normal rats learned and remembered the reward contingencies for both sets of arms, avoiding the unbaited arms entirely, and choosing each of the baited arms once during each test session. Rats with lesions of the fimbria-fornix also performed the reference memory component accurately, but they had a severe impairment of choice accuracy in the working memory component, returning to arms that had already been chosen in a particular test session as readily as they went to unchosen arms. This dissociation was interpreted as indicating that the hippocampus is selectively involved in processes that require working memory, but not in those that require reference memory.

Although such a conclusion is consistent with the results of that experiment, it is compromised by two procedural aspects of that task. First, all rats were trained preoperatively to perform the task correctly. Thus all the information necessary to choose accurately in the reference memory component was obtained preoperatively (because the rat should never respond to those arms), while the information necessary to choose accurately in the working memory component had to be acquired postoperatively (the correct response on a baited arm changed as a function of whether or not that arm had been chosen previously in each test session). Consequently, the dissociation of performance in the baited and unbaited sets of arms may have been due to the difference between the relative importance of the postoperatively acquired information, rather than to the distinction between working and reference memory.

In order to test this possibility, a second experiment included a group of rats which was given lesions first, and then trained in the task (Olton et al., 1981). If the inability to learn the working memory component in the Olton and Papas (1977) experiment was due to the necessity of acquiring information postoperatively, then rats with lesions in the present experiment should fail to learn both the working memory and the reference memory components. If, however, the selective impairment in the previous study was due to the different memory requirements of the two components, then rats with lesions should show the same dissociation here, learning the reference memory component, but not learning the working memory component.

The results demonstrated the same dissociation even with postoperative acquisition of the task. Rats with fimbria-fornix lesions learned the spatial unbaited procedure and performed it well so that at the end of testing, performance in the spatial unbaited (reference memory) set of arms was good, while performance in the spatial baited (working memory) set of arms was poor. Thus the dissociation observed in the Olton and Papas (1979) experiment was due to the memory requirements of the two different sets of arms, and not to the relative importance of preoperatively acquired information as compared to postoperatively acquired information.

A second difference between the baited and unbaited discrimination in the Olton and Papas (1979) study was the relative importance of flexible responding on an arm. For the baited arms, which required working memory, the rat had to first approach, and then avoid each arm during each test session. For the unbaited arms, however, the correct response was always the same: avoid the arms. Thus the dissociation of performance in the two sets of arms might have been due to the different response requirements on those arms, rather than to the different memory requirements.

To evaluate this hypothesis, an additional set of arms was included in another experiment (Olton et al., 1981). These _cued_ arms had visual stimuli placed on them to indicate whether or not the arm was correct. At the beginning of each test session, one of the cued arms had one pellet of food placed on it. While that arm still had a food pellet (i.e., the rat had not chosen it), a white stimulus was present on the arm. When that arm no longer had food (i.e., the rat had chosen it), a black stimulus was present on the arm. Consequently, the response requirements on this arm were the same as those on the spatial baited (but uncued) arms. However, a stimulus was present to indicate whether or not the arm had food, so that the rat did not have to form any temporal associations in order to remember whether or not he had chosen the arm. Furthermore, the reinforcement status indicated by the stimuli never changed during testing, so that this information could be processed in reference memory. If the dissociation of performance observed in the Olton and Papas (1979) experiment was due to the different response requirements in the baited and unbaited sets of arms, then the rats with lesions in the present experiment should fail to perform correctly in the cued set of arms because the response requirements are the same as in the spatial baited set of arms. If, however, that dissociation was due to the difference in memory requirements, then rats with lesions in the present experiment should perform correctly in the cued set of arms because this discrimination does not require working memory.

Rats with fimbria-fornix lesions learned this cued discrimination rapidly following lesions, and showed good retention of it when trained preoperatively. Thus they performed the cued discrimination well, while at the same time performing the spatial baited discrimination at chance levels. These results again demonstrate that the dissociation observed in the Olton and Papas (1979) experiment was due to the different memory requirements in the spatial baited and spatial unbaited arms, rather than the different requirements.

DISCUSSION

These dissociations are very similar to that found in humans following damage to the temporal lobe or SDAT (Corkin, 1981, in press). Typically, these patients are able to recall information from reference memory, but are unable to use working memory. One of the clearest demonstrations of this type of dissociation was seen in the performance of a patient with temporal lobe damage on two versions of a visual discrimination (Sidman et al., 1968). The delayed matching to sample procedure was formally analogous to the spatial baited discrimination used here (except that a matching contingency was used and HM had to remember only a single item). He was unable to solve this task with more than a few seconds between the sample and the comparison stimuli. The other discrimination procedure was formally analogous to the cued discrimination used here. He was able to learn this task (although at a slower rate than would be expected for a normal person) and retain it for 24 hours (the longest test interval examined). Similar types of dissociations have been found with other test procedures (Corkin, 1981), suggesting that damage to the hippocampal system may be the critical factor responsible for the memory impairments of temporal lobe amnesics and SDAT (c.f. Terry and Davies, 1980; Kolb and Whishaw, 1980). The poor performance of aged rats in the working memory component of the radial arm maze task (Ingram et al., 1981; Wallace et al., 1980), and the involvement of the hippocampus and its cholinergic projections in these deficits (Barnes, 1979; Eckerman et al., 1980; Ingram et al., 1981; Watts et al., 1981) provide further evidence that the hippocampal system is responsible for the memory loss of SDAT.

Taken together, the dissociations of performance following fimbria-fornix lesions substantially limit the number of explanations that can be offered to explain the behavioral impairments of rats with fimbria-fornix lesions. Thus all factors that were common to the spatial baited discrimination (which the rats with lesions did not learn) and the other two discriminations (which the rats with lesions did learn) can not be relevant. The rats must have performed the sensory discriminations necessary to identify the different sets of arms; used the spatial, extramaze stimuli identifying the arms in the spatial baited and the spatial unbaited discriminations appropriately to distinguish between these two sets of arms; produced the motor responses necessary to move around correctly on the arms in the cued discrimination; remembered that food was sometimes present in the spatial baited arms, was never present in the spatial unbaited arms, and was present only in the arm with the white stimulus in the cued arms; inhibited responses to the spatial unbaited arms, to the cued arms that didn't have food on them, and to the cued arm that did have food when the food was removed and the white stimulus was no longer present; been motivated sufficiently by the presence of a food pellet to go to arms that might have food on them, and motivated sufficiently by the absence of a food pellet to avoid arms that didn't have food on them in the spatial unbaited discrimination and in the cued discrimination. In short, the only difficulty exhibited by the rats with lesions at the end of testing was remembering which of the arms in the spatial baited discrimination they had chosen previously during that test session.

These dissociations indicate that explanations based on factors such as perception, attention, use of spatial stimuli, use of a cognitive mapping strategy, response inhibition, or response flexibility are inadequate to describe the psychological processes disrupted by the lesions. Thus the most appropriate explanation seems to be the type of memory needed for accurate performance in the spatial baited discrimination as compared to the other two discriminations. As discussed earlier, working memory was required for successful choice accuracy in the spatial baited discrimination because the only way the rat could determine whether an arm in this set had been chosen was to remember whether or not he had been to that arm previously in that test session. Thus the memory of a response to that arm had to be placed in the temporal/personal context of a particular test session. In contrast, working memory was not required for accurate performance in the other two discriminations. In the spatial unbaited discrimination, the arms never had food; thus the correct response was always never to go to these arms, irrespective of the test session or the number of times that these arms had been chosen previously. In the cued discrimination, the white and black stimuli could be used in place of the rat's working memory to determine whether or not an arm should be chosen because the response requirements with respect to the white and black stimuli were always the same irrespective of the test session, or the number of times those stimuli had been approached previously. Thus when the rat had to remember the personal/temporal context of a response, as in the spatial baited discrimination, rats with fimbria-fornix lesions exhibited a severe and enduring impairment of choice accuracy in both the postoperative acquisition of the discrimination and the postoperative retention of the preoperatively learned discrimination. When the rat could use memories that did not require a personal/temporal context to determine the correct response, as in the spatial unbaited and the cued discriminations, rats with fimbria-fornix lesions were able to perform as well as control rats by the end of testing in both postoperative acquisition and postoperative retention of preoperatively learned information.

Other experiments have examined the functional organization of the connections within the septohippocampal system. Bilateral lesions in the medial septum, lateral septum, CA3 pyramidal cells, precommissural fornix, postcommissural fornix, fimbria-fornix, and entorhinal area all produced similar behavioral impairments in tasks that required working memory (Handelmann and Olton, 1981; Olton et al., 1978; Rawlins and Olton, 1981). A disconnection analysis, using unilateral lesions combined with transection of the hippocampal commissures, showed that a functional disconnection of the subcortical areas and the neocortical areas normally interconnected through the septohippocampal system also produced behavioral impairments (Olton et al., in press). Furthermore, bilateral lesions in other brain systems, such as the sulcal frontal cortex, medial frontal cortex, amygdala, caudate nucleus, and posterolateral neocortex did not have these effects (Becker et al., 1980). These data demonstrate that the entire septohippocampal system is involved in tasks that require working memory, and many other brain systems are not needed. The behavioral effects seen in working memory procedures after fimbria-fornix lesions such as those used here can, therefore, be taken as a reasonable index of the behavioral effects that would be seen after destruction of the entire hippocampus proper.

Others have suggested that the major function of the hippocampus is to allow rats to store and use cognitive maps (Black, 1975; Black et al., 1977, 1979; Nadel and O'Keefe, 1974; Nadel et al., 1975; Nadel and MacDonald, 1980; O'Keefe, 1976, 1979; O'Keefe and Black, 1978; O'Keefe and Conway, 1978; O'Keefe and Dostrovsky, 1971; O'Keefe and Nadel, 1978, 1979; O'Keefe et al., 1975). According to this *cognitive mapping theory*, lesions of the septohippocampal system should produce a selective deficit in tasks that require cognitive mapping, irrespective of the type of memory required by those tasks (see reviews in Olton et al., 1979a,b, 1980). The dissociation of performance of rats with fimbria-fornix lesions in the spatial baited discrimination and in the spatial unbaited discrimination clearly contradicts this prediction. The arms in both of these discriminations were identified and remembered on the basis of extramaze spatial stimuli (O'Keefe and Conway, 1978; Olton, 1978a, 1979; Olton and Collison, 1979; Suzuki et al., 1979). Yet the rats with lesions performed the spatial unbaited discrimination normally, but never reached criterion performance in the spatial baited discrimination. Other experiments have demonstrated that in tasks that require cognitive mapping but not working memory, rats with fimbria-fornix lesions perform normally (Becker and Olton, in press; Becker et al., 1981; Walker and Olton, 1981), while in tasks that prevent cognitive mapping but require working memory, rats with fimbria-fornix lesions perform no better than expected by chance (Olton and Feustle, 1981). Thus the major variable influencing the accuracy of choice behavior following lesions in the septohippocampal system appears to be the memory requirements of the task, rather than its spatial or cognitive mapping requirements.

Although the rats with fimbria-fornix lesions did learn to perform the spatial unbaited discrimination and the cued discrimination as well as control rats, they took longer than controls to learn both discriminations during postoperative acquisition, and to relearn the spatial unbaited discrimination during postoperative retention. These types of transient impairments have been reported in a variety of tasks that require only reference memory (Becker and Olton, in press; Becker et al., 1981; Olton and Papas, 1979; Walker and Olton, 1981), and have been called "relative" ones, to distinguish them from other, "absolute" ones, which seem to persist permanently (Olton, 1978b). The reason for these types of transient impairments is not clear. Certainly, the behavioral changes do not reflect the shift from a preferred cognitive mapping strategy to a nonpreferred (and presumably less efficient) alternative because following fimbria-fornix lesions, rats performed transfer tests as well as normal, indicating that they did use cognitive mapping strategies (Becker and Olton, in press; Becker et al., 1981; Walker and Olton, 1981). Thus the impairments may reflect a general disruption in behavior caused by brain damage, difficulties arising from a dissociated state (Rawlins, 1979), etc. The description of the hippocampus as involved in working memory has focused on the stable behavior patterns exhibited a long time after surgery, rather than the changing patterns exhibited immediately after surgery, because these are easier to interpret and should provide us with stronger conclusions about the relationship between brain structures and behavioral functions. Nonetheless, the transient behavioral changes do appear reliable following lesions of the septohippocampal system, and any theory that wishes to describe completely the functions of this system will have to be able to explain these as well. An important point in developing such an enterprise, however, is the realization that the mechanisms responsible for the relative and absolute impairments may well be different.

The distinction between working memory and reference memory has been made at an operational level; the information in working memory is useful for only a single trial, while the information in reference memory is useful for all trials. This operational distinction emphasizes the two ends of a continuum, because information can be useful for any number of trials within an experiment. These ends of the continuum provide the most appropriate starting point, because if the distinction is not useful there, then it is unlikely to be useful elsewhere. Given the dissociations demonstrated here, the differences between working memory and reference memory should be developed along a continuum rather than as dichotomous categories. Of particular interest is determining how many trials with consistent information are required for rats with septohippocampal lesions to use that information.

The idea of two different types of memory, one of which incorporates the temporal/personal context of the event being remembered, the other of which does not, has appeared in a variety of different settings: normal animals solving discriminations (Honig, 1978, 1979; Olton, in press), predators searching for prey (Kamil, 1978; Olton et al., 1981), normal people recalling information (Tulving, 1972), the performance of animals with brain damage (Olton et al., 1979a,b, 1980), and the memory deficits exhibited by humans with brain damage (Cohen and Squire, 1981; Kinsbourne and Wood, 1976; Rozin, 1976; Schacter and Tulving, in press). The exact way in which working memory codes the temporal/personal context of the item being remembered remains to be determined, but the distinction appears to be meaningful and useful in describing both the mechanisms underlying normal cognitive processes, and the functional organization of the brain.

REFERENCES

Baker, L. J., Kesner, R. P., and Michal, R. E., in press, Differential effects of a reminder cue with amygdala and hippocampus stimulation induced amnesia, J. Comp. Physiol. Psychol.

Barnes, C. A., 1979, Memory deficits associated with senescence: A neurophysiological and behavioral study in the rat, J. Comp. Physiol. Psychol., 93:74-104.

Becker, J. T., Olton, D. S., Anderson, C. A., and Breitinger, E. R. P., 1981, Cognitive mapping in rats: The role of hippocampal and frontal systems in retention and reversal, Beh. Brain Res., 3:1-22.

Becker, J. T., Walker, J. A., and Olton, D. S., 1980, Neuroanatomical bases of spatial memory, Brain Res., 200:307-320.

Black, A. H., 1975, Hippocampal electrical activity and behavior, in: "The Hippocampus, Vol. 2: Neurophysiology and Behavior," R. L. Isaccson and K. H. Pribram, eds., Plenum Press, New York.

Black, A. H., Nadel, L., and O'Keefe, J., 1977, Hippocampal function in avoidance learning and punishment, Psychol. Bull., 84:1107-1129.

Cohen, J. J., and Squire, L. R., 1981, Preserved learning and retention of pattern-analyzing skill in amnesia: Dissociation of knowing how and knowing that, Science, 210:207-210.

Corkin, S., 1981, Some relationships between global amnesias and the memory impairments in Alzheimer's Disease, Submitted manuscript.

Corkin, S., in press, Brain acetylcholine, aging, and Alzheimer's Disease: Implications for treatment, Trends in Neurosci.

Eckerman, D. A., Gordon, W. A., Edwards, J. D., MacPhail, R. C., and Gage, M. I., 1980, Effects of scopolamine, pentobarbital, and amphetamine on radial arm maze performance in the rat, Physiol. Behav., 12:595-602.

Gaffan, D., 1974, Recognition impaired and association intact in the memory of monkeys after transection of the fornix, J. Comp. Physiol. Psychol., 86:1100-1109.

Gaffan, D., 1977, Recognition memory after short retention intervals in fornix-transected monkeys, Quart. J. Exp. Psychol., 29:577-588.

Handelmann, G., and Olton, D. S., 1981, Spatial memory following damage to hippocampal CA3 pyramidal cells with kainic acid: Impairment and recovery with preoperative training, Brain Res., 217:41-58.

Honig, W. K., 1978, Studies of working memory in the pigeon, in: "Cognitive Processes in Animal Behavior," S. H. Hulse, H. Fowler, and W. K. Honig, eds., Lawrence Erlbaum, Hillsdale, N.J.

Honig, W. K., 1979, Spatial aspects of working memory, Behav. Brain Sci., 2:332-333.

Honig, W. K., in press, Working memory and the temporal map, in: "Expression of Knowledge," R. L. Isaacson and N. E. Spear, eds., Academic Press, New York.

Ingram, D. K., London, E. D., and Goodrick, C. L., 1981, Age and neurochemical correlates of radial maze performance in rats, Neurobiol. Aging, 2:41-47.

Jarrard, L. E., 1976, Anatomical and behavioral analysis of hippocampal cell fields in rats, J. Comp. Physiol. Psychol., 90: 1035-1050.

Jarrard, L. E., 1978, Selective hippocampal lesions: differential effects on performance by rats of a spatial task with preoperative versus postoperative training, J. Comp, Physiol. Psychol., 92:1119-1127.

Jarrard, L. E., 1980, Selective hippocampal lesions and behavior, Physiol. Psychol., 8:198-206.

Kamil, A. C., 1978, Learning and memory in the wild: systematic foraging by a nectar feeding bird, the Amakihi (Loxops virens), J. Comp. Physiol. Psychol., 92:388-396.

Kesner, R. P., 1980, An attribute analysis of memory: The role of the hippocampus, Physiol. Psychol., 8:183-197.

Kesner, R. P., Dixon, D. A., Pickett, D., and Berman, R. F., 1975, Experimental animal model of transient global amnesia: Role of the hippocampus, Neuropsychologia, 13:465-480.

Kinsbourne, M., and Wood, F., 1975, Short-term memory processes and the amnesic syndrome, in: "Short-term Memory Processes," D. Deutsch and J. A. Deutsch, eds., Academic Press, New York.

Kolb, B., and Whishaw, I. Q., 1980, "Fundamentals of Human Neuropsychology," W. H. Freeman and Company, San Francisco.

Milner, B., 1968, Preface: material-specific and generalized memory loss, Neuropsychologia, 6:175-179.

Mishkin, M., 1978, Memory in monkeys severely impaired by combined but not separate removal of amygdala and hippocampus, Nature, 273:297-298.

Nadel, L., and O'Keefe, J., 1974, The hippocampus in pieces and patches: an essay on modes of explanation in physiological psychology, in: "Essays on the Nervous System. A Festschrift for Professor J. Z. Young," R. Bellairs and E. G. Gray, eds., Clarendon Press, Oxford.

Nadel, L., O'Keefe, J., and Black, A., 1975, Slam on the brakes: a critique of Altman, Brunner, and Bayer's response-inhibition model of hippocampal function, Behav. Biol., 14:151-162.

O'Keefe, J., 1976, Place units in the hippocampus of the freely moving rat., Exp. Neurol., 51:78-109.

O'Keefe, J., 1979, A review of the hippocampal place cells, Prog. Neurobiol., 13:419-439.

O'Keefe, J., and Black, A. H., 1978, Single unit and lesion experiments on the sensory inputs to the hippocampal cognitive map, in: "Functions of the Septo-hippocampal System," Ciba Foundation Symposium 58, Elsevier, New York.

O'Keefe, J., and Conway, D. H., 1978, Hippocampal place units in the freely moving rat: why they fire where they fire, Exp. Brain Res., 31:573-590.

O'Keefe, J., and Dostrovsky, J., 1971, The hippocampus as a spatial map. Preliminary evidence from unit activity in the freely moving rat, Brain Res., 34:171-175.

O'Keefe, J., and Nadel, L., 1978, "The Hippocampus as a Cognitive Map," Oxford University Press, Oxford.

O'Keefe, J., and Nadel, L., 1979, Precis of O'Keefe and Nadel's The Hippocampus as a Cognitive Map, Behav. Brain Sci., 2 :487-533.

O'Keefe, J., Nadel, L., Keightley, S., and Kill, D., 1975, Fornix lesions selectively abolish place learning in the rat, Exp. Neurol., 48:152-166.

Olds, J., 1972, Learning and the hippocampus, Review of Canadian Biology, 31:215-238.

Olton, D. S., 1978a, Characteristics of spatial memory, in: "Cognitive Aspects of Animal Behavior," S. H. Hulse, H. Fowler, and W. K. Honig, eds., Lawrence Erlbaum, Hillsdale, N.J.

Olton, D. S., 1978b, The function of septo-hippocampal connections in spatially organized behavior, in: "Functions of the Septo-hippocampal System," Ciba Foundation Symposium 58, Elsevier, New York.

Olton, D. S., 1979, Mazes, maps, and memory, Amer. Psychol., 34: 583-596.

Olton, D. S., in press, Spatial abilities of animals: Behavioral and neuroanatomical analyses, in: "The Neural and Developmental Bases of Spatial Orientation," M. Potegal, ed., Academic Press, New York.

Olton, D. S., Becker, J. T., and Handelmann, G. E., 1979a, Hippocampus, space, and memory, Behav. Brain Sci., 2:313-322.

Olton, D. S., Becker, J. T., and Handelmann, G. E., 1979b, A re-examination of the role of hippocampus in working memory, Behav. Brain Sci., 2:353-359.

Olton, D. S., Becker, J. T., and Handelmann, G. E., 1980, Hippocampal function: Working memory or cognitive mapping? Physiol. Psychol., 8:239-246.

Olton, D. S., and Collison, C., 1979, Intramaze cues and "odor trails" fail to direct choice behavior on an elevated maze, Anim. Learn. and Behav., 7:221-223.

Olton, D. S., Collison, C., and Werz, M. A., 1977, Spatial memory and radial arm maze performance in rats, Learn. and Motiv., 8:289-314.

Olton, D. S., and Feustle, W., 1981, Hippocampal function and non-spatial memory, Exp. Brain Res., 41:380-389.

Olton, D. S., Handelmann, G. E., and Walker, J. A., 1981, Spatial memory and food searching strategies, in: "Foraging Behavior: Ecological, Ethological, and Psychological Approaches," A. C. Kamil and T. D. Sargent, eds., Garland STPM Press, New York.

Olton, D. S., and Papas, B. C., 1979, Spatial memory and hippocampal function, Neuropsychologia, 17:669-682.

Olton, D. S., and Samuelson, R. J., 1976, Remembrance of places passed: spatial memory in rats, J. Exp. Psychol.: Anim. Behav. Proc., 2:97-116.

Olton, D. S., Walker, J. A., and Gage, F. H., 1978, Hippocampal connections and spatial discrimination, Brain Res., 139: 295-308.

Olton, D. S., Walker, J. A., and Wolf, W. A., in press, A disconnection analysis of hippocampal function, Brain Res.

Rawlins, J. N. P., and Olton, D. S., 1981, The septo-hippocampal system and cognitive mapping. Submitted manuscript.

Schacter, D. L., and Tulving, E., in press, Memory, amnesia, and the episodic/semantic distinctions, in: "Expression of Knowledge," R. L. Isaacson and N. E. Spear, eds., Plenum Press, New York.

Sidman, M., Stoddard, L. T., and Mohr, J. P., 1968, Some additional quantitative observations of immediate memory in a patient with bilateral hippocampal lesions, Neuropsychologia, 6:245-254.

Suzuki, S., Augerinos, G., and Black, A. H., 1980, Stimulus control of spatial behavior on the eight arm maze in rats, Learn. Motiv., 11:1-18.

Terry, R. D., and Davies, P., 1980, Dementia of the Alzheimer type, Ann. Rev. Neurosci., 3:77-95.

Thomas, G. J., 1978, Delayed alternation in rat after pre- or post-commissural fornicotomy, J. Comp. Physiol. Psychol., 92:1128-1136.

Thomas, G. J., 1979, Comparison of effects of small lesions in posto-dorsal septum on spontaneous and re-run correction (contingently reinforced) alternation in rats, J. Comp. Physiol. Psychol., 93:685-694.

Thomas, G. J., Brito, G. N. O., and Stein, D. P., 1980, Medial septal nucleus and delayed alternation in rats, Physiol. Psychol., 8:467-472.

Thompson, R. F., Berger, T. W., Berry, S. D., Hoehler, F. K., Kettner, R. E., and Weisz, D. J., 1980, Hippocampal substrate of classical conditioning, Physiol. Psychol., 8:262-279.

Thompson, R. F., Berger, T. W., Cegavske, C. F., Patterson, M. M., Roemer, R. A., Teyler, T. J., and Young, R. A., 1976, The search for the engram, Amer. Psychol., 31:209-227.

Tulving, E., 1972, Episodic and semantic memory, in: "Organization of Memory," E. Tulving and W. D. Donaldson, eds., Academic Press, New York.

Walker, J. A., and Olton, D. S., 1979a, The role of response and reward in spatial memory, Learn. and Motiv., 10:73-84.

Walker, J. A., and Olton, D. S., 1979b, Spatial memory deficit following fimbria-fornix lesions. Independent of time for stimulus processing, Physiol. Behav., 23:11-15.

Walker, J. A., and Olton, D. S., 1981, Fimbria-fornix lesions impair spatial working memory but not cognitive mapping. Submitted manuscript.

Wallace, J. E., Krauter, E. E., and Campbell, B. A., 1980, Animal models of declining memory in the aged: Short-term and spatial memory in the aged rat, J. Gerontol., 35:355-363.

Watts, J., Stevens, R., and Robinson, C., 1981, Effects of scopolamine on radial arm maze performance in rats, Physiol. Behav., 26:845-851.

Winocur, G., 1980, The hippocampus and cue utilization, Physiol. Psychol., 8:280-288.

Winocur, G., and Olds, J., 1978, Effects of context manipulation on memory and reversal learning in rats with hippocampal lesions, J. Comp. Physiol. Psychol., 92:312-321.

ACKNOWLEDGEMENTS

This research was supported in part by Research Grant MH-24213 from the National Institute of Mental Health and by a Bio-medical Sciences Research Support Grant from the Johns Hopkins University to D.S.O. The author thanks M. Weigel for typing the manuscript.

NEURONAL SUBSTRATES OF LEARNING AND MEMORY: HIPPOCAMPUS AND OTHER STRUCTURES [1]

R.F. Thompson, T.W. Berger, S.D. Berry, G.A. Clark, R.N. Kettner, D.G. Lavond, M.D. Mauk, D.A. McCormick, P.R. Solomon, D.J. Weisz
Stanford University
Stanford, CA 94305

Current studies of the hippocampus in the context of learning and memory offer an embarrassment of riches. Neuronal activity shows clear and often striking relations to behavioral plasticity, both in terms of original learning and in terms of memory retrieval.

We have focussed on the hippocampal as one aspect of the neural basis of learning in a broader project concerned with identification, localization and analysis of the neuronal substrates of learning and memory in the mammalian brain (Thompson et al., 1976). A simple and well-characterized form of associative learning is used as a model system: classical conditioning of the rabbit nictitating membrane (NM) response, an aspect of eyelid conditioning. This preparation, developed by Gormezano (Gormezano et al., 1962) has a number of advantages for analysis of brain substrates of learning (Thompson et al., 1976; see also Disterhoft et al., 1977): the animal is motionless but not drugged or paralyzed, significant learning occurs within a single 2 hour training session, the air-puff UCS (as opposed to shock) does not give artifact, the learned response is very well characterized, under very good behavioral control (Gormezano, 1972), obeys the fundamental laws of classical or Pavlovian conditioning, learning vs. performance substrates can be distinguished at both behavioral and neuronal levels and the amplitude-time course of the behavioral response can be measured easily and precisly. Finally, the learned (eyelid) response has the same basic properties in humans.

The standard training paradigm is short delay conditioning: a paired trial of a tone CS (1 KHz, 85 db, 350 msec) and corneal airpuff UCS (210 g/ cm^2 source pressure, 100 msec) with the UCS overlapping the last 100 msec of the tone CS. Intertrial intervals are approximately 1 min. Control animals are given a random sequence of unpaired CS and UCS stimuli with an interstimulus interval of approximately 30 sec. Both paired conditioning and unpaired control animals thus receive the same number and kind of stimuli. More recently we have also used the trace paradigm where a period of no stimulation intervenes between CS offset and UCS onset (CS duration 250 msec, UCS duration 100 msec, CS-UCS onset interval 750 msec - trace interval of no stimulation thus being 500 msec). Animals with prior bilateral ablation of the hippocampus are unable to learn the trace CR (Weisz, Solomon and Thompson, 1980).

It is necessary to comment briefly on the nature of the conditioned response. Investigators typically record either extension of the NM, which is a largely passive consequence of eyeball retraction (Cegavske et al. 1976), or closure of the external eyelid. However, with standard NM training both become conditioned in a coordinated manner, together with some degree of contraction of the periorbital facial musculature (McCormick and Thompson, 1982). Both the NM and eyelid components of the CR develop initially at the time of onset of the UCS (corneal airpuff or periorbital shock) and gradually move forward in time as training continues. In a well-trained animal, the conditioned response has a latency somewhat less than 100 msec. (eyelid somewhat shorter than NM) Conditioning of the NM/or eyelid using corneal airpuff or periorbital shock does not develop in animals (or humans) if the CS-UCS interval is 50 msec or less. In terms of at least these properties, conventional eyelid and NM conditioning differ markedly from the very short latency eyelid response to glabellar tap in cat studied by Woody and associates (Brons and Woody, 1980). It will be of great interest to compare the neuronal substrates of these two types of behavioral plasticity, both of which involve the eyelid response.

In our initial studies of the hippocampus we discovered a rather extraordinary learning-induced neuronal response (Berger, Alger and Thompson, 1976; Berger and Thompson, 1977; Berger and Thompson, 1978a,b,c). In brief, neurons in CA3 and CA1 increase their activity very rapidly and form a "temporal model" of the learned behavioral response (see Figure 1). This hippocampal response does not develop in unpaired control animals. Furthermore, under a wide range of conditions that alter, impair or block the development of the hippocampal unit response, the unit reponse is an invariable and predictive concomitant of the development of the learned behavioral response.

In a series of studies, the generality and significance of the learning induced hippocampal response were explored using the short delay paradigm. In brief, the learning-induced hippocampal unit response develops in the same manner with a light CS

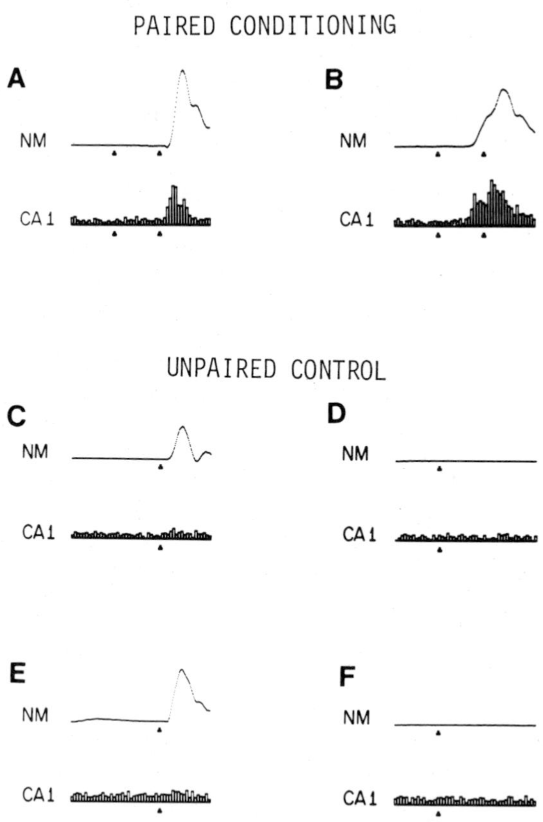

Fig. 1. Examples of eight-trial averaged behavioral NM responses and associated multiple-unit histograms of hippocampal activity for a conditioning (A, B) and a control (C-F) animal at the beginning and end of short delay training. Upper trace: Average nictitating membrane response for one block of eight trials. Lower trace: Hippocampal unit poststimulus histogram (15-msec time bins) for one block of eight trials. (A) First block of eight paired conditioning trials, Day 1. (B) Last block of eight paired conditioning trials, Day 1, after conditioning has occurred. (C) First block of eight unpaired UCS-alone trials, Day 1. (D) Last block of eight unpaired UCS-alone trials, Day 2. (E) First block of eight unpaired CS-alone trials, Day 1. (F) Last block of eight unpaired CS-alone trials, Day 2. Trace duration 750 msec, first cursor is tone onset, second is air puff onset. (From Berger & Thompson, 1978a).

as with a tone CS (Coates and Thompson, 1978), in approximately the same manner in classical conditioning of the cat NM (Patterson, Berger & Thompson, 1979) and in classical conditioning of the hindlimb flexor response in the rabbit (Thompson et al., 1980). In their pioneering studies, Olds and Segal reported increases in hippocampal unit activity in rats given combined classical and instrumental training with food reward (Olds et al., 1972, Segal, 1973). Best and Best (1976) report similar hippocampal unit increases with paired tone-shock in the rat. It is thus a very general phenomenon in simple learning paradigms.

A critically important issue concerns the extent to which the conditioned increase in hippocampal unit activity is related to the learning aspect of behavior. As noted above, in the trained animal, the hippocampal response seems very much like a motor response that correlates closely with behavioral performance. Can the learning vs. performance aspect of the hippocampal response be distinguished? Variation of the interstimulus interval (ISI) permits this distinction to be made (Hoehler & Thompson, 1980). Thus, in the 50 msec forward ISI, all stimuli are presented and in the same order as is the case for the 250 msec forward ISI condition which yields learning and the marked increase in hippocampal unit activity. Yet the 50 msec condition yields no learning and no conditioned increase in hippocampal unit activity, even though the animal gives robust reflex NM responses. The following additional points are worth noting as well. In unpublished work, we determined that the learning-induced hippocampal unit response develops in the ventral as well as the dorsal hippocampus and develops bilaterally, i.e. in both the left and right CA3-CA1 regions. We also found that in already trained animals, the hippocampal response is present in totally paralyzed, unanesthetized rabbits. This point is important because of the close similarity in the temporal forms of the hippocampal and behavioral responses, even though the hippocampal response precedes the measured behavioral response by about 40 msec (e.g., Berger, Laham and Thompson, 1980). Finally, analysis of the hippocampal unit response during extinction training (CS alone trials) showed that it began to extinguish earlier over trials than behavioral conditioned responses and predicted the occurrence of behavioral extinction (Berger and Thompson, 1981).

Results of all these studies can be summed up in the following rather simple statement: the growth of the hippocampal unit response is an invariable and strongly predictive concomitant of subsequent behavioral learning. If the hippocampal response does not develop, the animal will not learn. If it develops rapidly, the animal will learn rapidly. If it develops slowly, the animal will learn slowly. Further, the temporal form of the hippocampal response predicts the temporal form of the learned behavioral response. Another way of stating this is that the hippocampal response has all the properties of a relatively direct measure of the inferred processes of learning and memory retrieval in the brain.

The most direct way of testing this hypothesis is to manipulate variables that influence either hippocampal activity or learned behavior and determine the effect on the other. Note that this goes beyond simple correlaton - the prediction is: manipulations that systematically influence one dependent variable will have the same effect on the other. This is as strong a causal statement as can be made when two kinds of measures - in this case neural and behavioral - are compared. It does not necessarily mean that one directly causes the other but it does mean that the two are causally linked. Three such experiments are described below, one involving lesions, one involving a drug effect and one involving a behavioral manipulation.

Medial septal lesions have a profound influence on the activity of the hippocampus, essentially abolishing EEG theta activity and markedly altering unit activity. Small bilateral lesions of the medial septum markedly reduce the growth of the learning induced unit response in the CA1 field of the hippocampus and have an identical effect on the rate of acquisition of the learned response (Berry and Thompson, 1979).

The second experiment concerns the effects of morphine. In pilot studies we discovered that a dose of 5 mg/Kg of morphine given i.v. after animals had learned to a criterion of 8/9 CRs totally abolished the CR but had no effect on the UCR (Mauk et al., 1982). This, incidentally, illustrates one of the great advantages of the classical conditioning paradigm - the possibility of differentiation between the effects of a drug or other treatment on learning and on performance (see above). In this case, effects of morphine on the execution of the behavioral response, per se, can be excluded. The strong prediction here is that morphine will also abolish the learned increase in hippocampal unit activity. This is precisely what occurs (see Fig. 2). Effects of morphine on both the learned behavioral and hippocampal responses are immediately reversed by a low (0.1 mg/Kg) dose of naloxone. This suggests a specific receptor action, possibly on the mu receptors, which preferentially bind morphine and for which naloxone has its highest affinity.

This morphine effect provides a potentially very useful tool for identification of the neuronal circuitry that codes the learned response - the memory system. Thus, the fact that the unconditioned response is completely unaffected by morphine indicates that the reflex pathways that generate the unconditioned response are not a part of the essential neuronal plasticity coding memory.

Perhaps the most powerful test of the hypothesis would be a situation in which the learned behavioral response is given on only a part of the trials to a constant intensity stimulus. Signal detection provides such a paradigm. Rabbits are trained, overtrained and taken to threshold, using a white noise CS

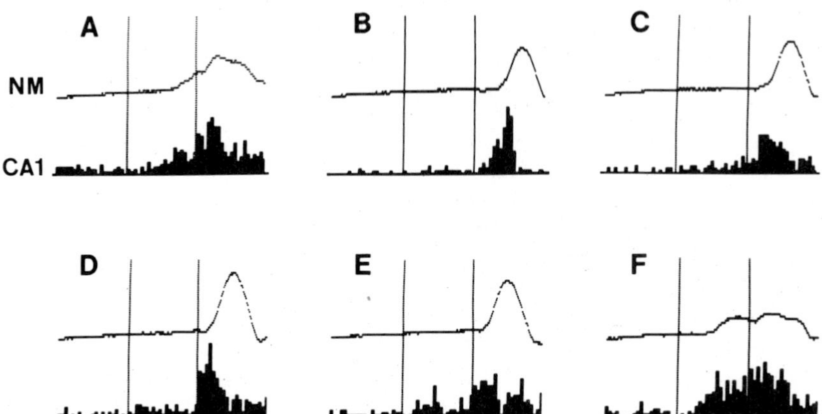

Fig. 2. Examples of eight-trial-averaged behavioral NM responses (upper trace) and associated multiple unit histograms of hippocampal activity (lower trace, 12 msec time bins) for a single animal. The early vertical line indicates tone onset, later line indicates airpuff onset. Total trace length equals 750 msec. (A) block of eight trials immediately preceding injection of morphine. Note the (conditioned) increase in hippocampal activity in the CS period (CS-UCS interval) which is completely absent immediately following injection of morphine (B). The unit increase begins to redevelop in later post morphine blocks; blocks 3-5 (C-E). Both the behavioral and unit conditioned responses recover fully following injection of naloxone (F). (From Mauk et al., 1981).

(Kettner et al., 1980). A Staircase procedure is used so each animal asymptotes at 50% detection (50% CRs) to a constant intensity threshold level CS. Interestingly, the behavioral detection response (NM extension) is dichotomous at threshold, being clearly present on detection trials and completely absent on non-detection trials. In this sense it is very similar to the all-or-none response typically used in human threshold studies.

In order to indicate behaviorally the detection of a threshold level stimulus, the organism must make use of learned responses. When an organism is detecting a constant stimulus at threshold, the learned response is activated on 50% of the trials. The neuronal circuitry that plays an essential role in this memory retrieval must be activated on behavioral detection trials and either not activated or not sufficiently activated on non-detection trials. Consequently, any neuronal regions or systems in the brain that do show dichotomous, or at least differential, activation by detected and non-detected stimuli are candidate substrates for the circuitry. Conversely, neurons and circuits

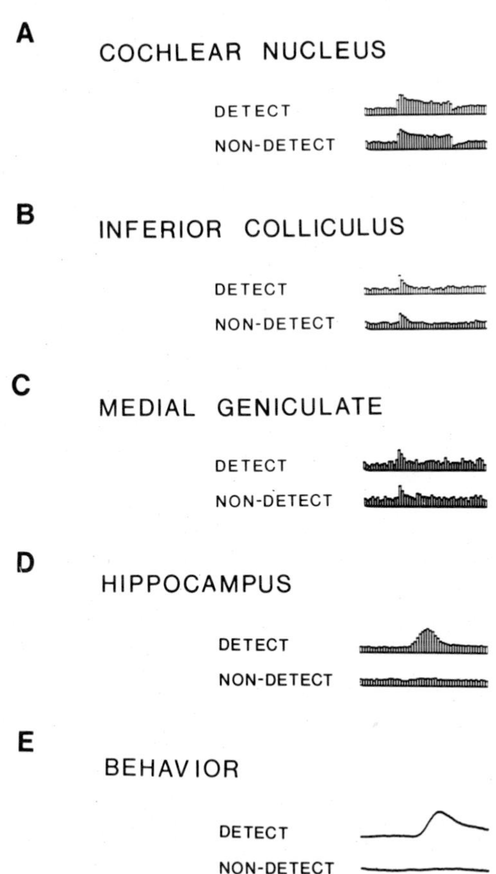

Fig. 3. Comparison of multiple-unit responses from auditory relay nuclei and hippocampus during detect vs. nondetect trials. A through D: Average poststimulus histograms (15-msec time bins) created by averaging from 200 to 300 trials (obtained from several testing sessions) for cochlear nucleus (A), inferior colliculus (B), medial geniculate (C), and hippocampus (D) on detect (upper histogram) vs. nondetect (lower histogram) trials. E: Average nictitating membrane response for detect (upper trace) vs. nondetect (lower trace) trials. Note the large difference between hippocampal response during detect vs. nondetect trials in comparison with difference in responses of the auditory relay nuclei. (From Thompson et al., 1980).

activated identically by detected and non-detected stimuli are not a part of the neuronal substrate of the memory circuitry.

Unit responses in the primary auditory relay nuclei - anteroventral cochlear nucleus, central nucleus of the inferior colliculus and the ventral division of the medial geniculate body - are substantial and identical on both behavioral detection and non-detection trials (see Figure 3). The auditory system reliably and identically detects the stimulus on all trials at behavioral threshold. Consequently, the primary auditory relay nuclei are not a part of the memory system.

In marked contrast, the learning-induced hippocampal unit response is present and well developed on detection trials and completely absent on nondetection trials (Fig. 3). It is actually possible to predict the occurrence of behavioral detection and non-detection responses with a probability very close to one from the occurrence of the learning-induced neuronal response in the hippocampus. All these data support the general hypothesis that unit activity in the hippocampus provides a relatively direct measure of processes of learning and memory retrieval in the brain.

Thanks to the anatomical organization of the hippocampus, it is possible to identify conclusively one category of cells using physiological techniques - the pyramidal neurons. To date we have focussed on pyramidal neurons sending axons out the fornix. A stimulating electrode is implanted in the fornix and recording microelectrodes in CA3. Pyramidal neurons are identified using antidromic (Berger and Thompson, 1978b) and collision methods (see Swanson, Teyler and Thompson, 1982). The primary criteria for antidromic response are short latency and very low variability of latency at threshold (no more than .1 msec). Collision, if positive, is conclusive. A spontaneous discharge of the soma-dendrites is used to trigger fornix stimulation with a variable delay. If the spike-stimulus interval is within the approximate period of the antidromic conduction time the ortho-and antidromic spikes will collide and no antidromic spike will occur (see Fuller and Schlag, 1976). Note, however, that a negative outcome - no collision - is not conclusive. Thus, a dendritic spike might occur and be recorded but not initiate an axonic spike.

Of 72 two pyramidal neurons identified by antidromic criteria, 79% showed a clear positive correlation with the learned response, i.e. generated a model of the learned behavior (Berger and Thompson, 1982). All cells that met the collision criteria showed this same positive correlation. As can be seem from examples shown in Figure 4, the correlation between the increased frequency of individual cell discharges and the amplitude-time course of the behavioral NM response is extraordinarily high. Identified pyramidal neurons recorded at the beginning of training show the development of this "temporal model" of the learned behavioral response over the first few trials of training, long before the learned behavioral response develops.

The marked learning-induced response of pyramidal neurons in CA3-CA1 of the hippocampus either develops there or is projected from elsewhere. Data to date argue that it develops within the hippocampus. The two major sources of afferents to the hippocampus

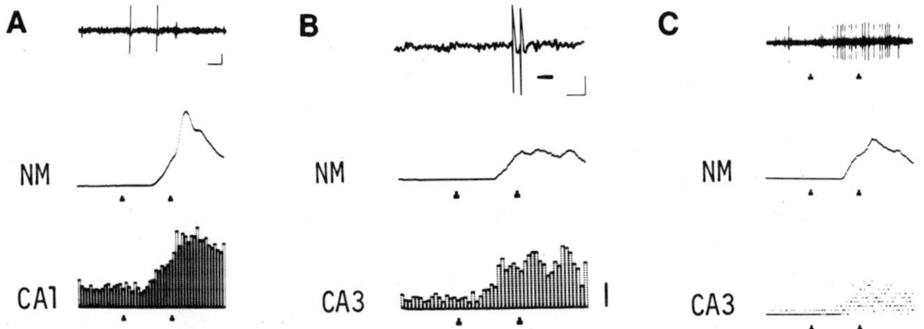

Fig. 4. Examples of learning-induced responses of identified pyramidal neurons in trained animals. Upper traces show individual raw unit records (A and B 100 msec duration; C one full trial of 750 msec duration). Middle traces show averaged NM responses and lower traces show histograms of pyramidal neurons for some blocks of trials, in all cases for at least 50 trials. (Berger & Thompson, 1978b; 1982).

are the medial septum and the entorhinal cortex. Unit responses in the medial septum show a pattern of response very different from the hippocampus (Berger and Thompson, 1978c). In brief, they exhibit evoked onset responses to both tone and airpuff in both paired and unpaired animals, which tend to decrease over the course of training. They show no sign of learning-dependent plasticity but instead could provide information to the hippocampus about the occurrence of stimuli. Unit activity in layers 2 and 3 of the entorhinal cortex shows a small within-trial pattern of increased activity from the early stages of training; however, this activity does not increase over the course of training (Berger, Clark and Thompson, 1980). Although the initial pattern of unit response in the hippocampus may be "projected" to it from entorhinal cortex, the growth in hippocampal unit activity over the course of training appears to develop within the hippocampus itself.

The "principal circuit" of the hippocampus is from entorhinal cortex to dentate granule cells via the perforant path, from granule cells to pyramidal neurons of CA3 via the mossy fiber pathway and from CA3 pyramidal cells to CA1 pyramidal cells via the Schaffer collaterals. In classical conditioning, the pyramidal neurons of CA3 and CA1 show an apparently identical learning-induced increase in response. Weisz describes current work on dentate granule cells (see his chapter). Although they show marked, learning-induced changes in activity, they do not develop a temporal model of the learned behavioral response. Consequently, the learning-induced response of the pyramidal neurons of CA1-CA3 cannot be accounted for by either of its two major afferent systems - medial septum or dentate gyrus.

The learning-induced response of pyramidal neurons in the hippocampus (and neurons in related structures such as the lateral septum) appears to be an instance of neurons possessing "learning" or "Hebb" synapses. By definition, such neurons must show altered output to constant input, or at the very least an output that does not simply relay the input but changes relative to it. The cells show a marked and patterned increase in response frequency that is induced by behavioral learning, is strongly predictive of behavioral learning, and cannot be accounted for by the inputs to them, so far as is known at present. Further, these cells do not respond at all to the tone CS and often do not respond to the airpuff UCS at the beginning of training.

Pyramidal neurons in the CA1-CA3 region of the hippocampus thus provide a very promising model for analysis of the cellular mechanisms underlying learning-induced plasticity. We are not suggesting that the hippocampus is the only place in the brain where learning-induced plasticity develops, rather that it is a very good model. In terms of known processes, the most likely candidate mechanism is long-term potentiation (LTP) - this possibility was explored in detail in a recent volume (Swanson, Teyler and Thompson, 1982). A number of clear parallels do exist between the learning-induced plasticity we have described and LTP: 1) both are exhibited by hippocampal pyramidal neurons, 2) only a small number of stimulations is necessary to establish both, 3) they both develop with a similar time-course, 4) the magnitude of increase in response is very similar for both, 5) both are dependent on particular temporal parameters - a specific range of stimulation densities, and 6) both persist for very long periods of time.

In sum, the hippocampus clearly plays a very important role in learning and memory, even in simple associative learning paradigms like eyelid conditioning. Over a wide range of conditions that influence the development, maintenance and extinction of the learned behavioral response in both the short-delay and trace paradigms, alteration of the learning-induced hippocampal response invariably precedes and accurately predicts subsequent alteration of the learned behavioral resopnse. The activity of CA3-CA1 pyramidal neurons appears to provide a relatively direct measure of the inferred processes of learning and memory.

Depending upon one's view of how the neuronal substrates of learning are organized in the brain, it may or may not be surprising that rabbits with prior bilateral ablation of the hippocampus can learn the short delay conditioned NM response (Solomon and Moore, 1975). An analysis of the effects of the CS-UCS interval on both hippocampal unit activity and behavioral learning, together with consideration of the lesion-behavior literature, led to the prediction that the hippocampus plays a critical role in the temporal aspects of learned behavior (Hoehler and Thompson, 1980, see also Solomon, 1979). More specifically, it was suggested that hippocampal lesions would severely impair learning of the trace conditioned response, where a period of no stimulation intervenes between CS offset and UCS onset. The outcome of such a lesion study was as expected - animals with bilateral ablation of hippocampus were unable to learn the trace CR (Weisz, Solomon and Thompson, 1980). When these same animals are then shifted to the short delay paradigm, they learn in a normal number of trials - the deficit is specific to the trace paradigm, which is perhaps the simplest task requiring "delayed" memory. It is similar in some ways to Olton's notion of working memory (Olton, et al., 1980). Other types of learning paradigms that place sufficient demands on the learning and memory system also reveal substantial impairments after hippocampal lesions. A particularly clear example is discrimination reversal (see chapters by Berger and Deadwyler).

Multiple unit recordings from the CA3-CA1 region of the hippocampus in the trace paradigm suggest that the "neural trace" may actually develop in the hippocampus (see Figure 5). Early in training, long before the behavioral CR develops, hippocampal activity builds up and persists over the entire trace period. As behavioral learning develops, this unit response coalesces into a predictive model of the learned behavioral response. It is important to emphasize that the "endpoint" learning-induced neuronal response in the hippocampus is essentially identical in both short delay and trace paradigms. The hippocampus invariably develops the neuronal response that predicts the occurrence of the learned behavioral response in animals that learn.

As noted above, rabbits with bilateral ablation of the hippocampus can learn the standard short-delay CR, as can neodecorticated animals (Oakley and Russell, 1972). In fact, rabbits with all brain tissue above the thalamus can do so (Enser, 1976), as can decerebrate cats (Norman et al., 1975). Although several alternative inferences are possible from these observations, perhaps the most straightforward is that there is an essential circuit in the midbrain-brainstem that serves to code the short delay CR. We have adopted this as a working hypothesis and are in process of exploring the roles of various structures and systems in the midbrain-brain stem that may serve as the loci of essential neuronal plasticity coding the short delay conditioned NM and eyelid responses. In recent work we feel we have succeeded in localizing this learning circuit, or at least an essential part of it, to the cerebellum (McCormick, et al., 1981).

Our initial approach to identification of this circuit was to map the entire brainstem in already trained animals by recording neural unit activity during paired training trials. In the course of this mapping we discovered a striking unit response in portions of the ipsilateral cerebellum. There is both stimulus evoked

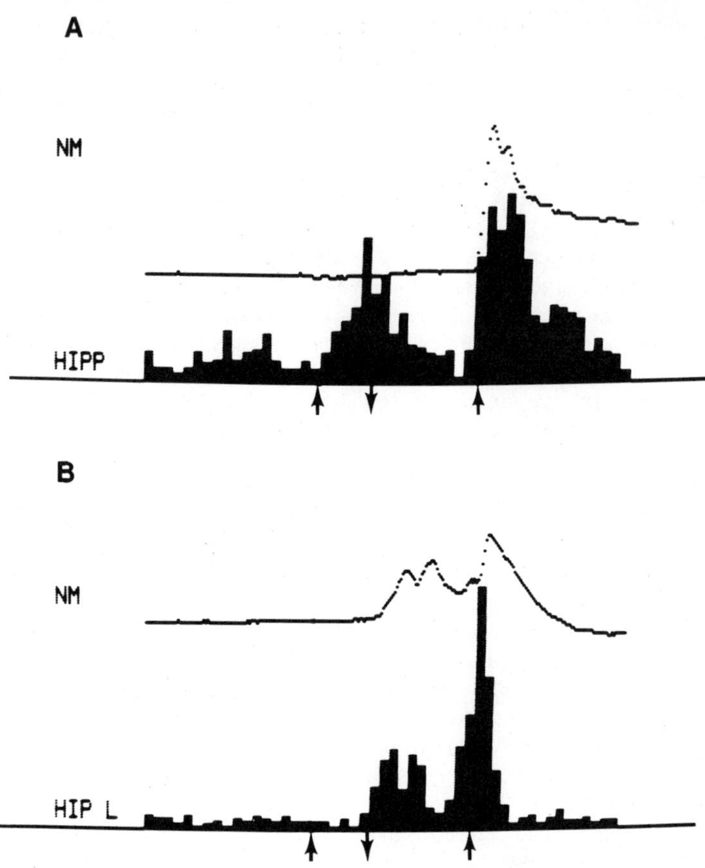

Fig. 5. Behavioral and hippocampal unit response in trace conditioning. A. An 8-trial block average taken early in training before behavioral NM conditioning has developed. Total sweep duration is 2250 msec, tone on at first upward arrow, tone off at downward arrow, air-puff on at second upward arrow. Upper trace, averaged NM response, lower trace, histogram of hippocampal (CA1) multi-unit activity. Each time bind is 45 msec. Note marked build-up and decay of hippocampal unit activity from tone on to air puff on. B. As in A. but taken after the animal has learned the behavioral conditioned response. Note that the hippocampal unit response has "coalesced" into a very good temporal model of the conditioned NM response.

activity and a model of the learned behavioral response. The latter closely resembles the learning induced response in the hippocampus.

We also completed two types of lesion studies in animals that were very well trained: ablation by aspiration of the ipsilateral lateral cerebellar hemisphere and more localized stereotaxic electrolytic lesions of the ipsilateral dentate nucleus. All animals in both studies learned in less than two days of training preoperatively and were all given one full day of overtraining and then subjected to lesion. After recovery, they were all given four full days of retraining.

In all ablation animals (five), large removal of the ipsilateral neocerebellum completely abolished the conditioned response (NM and eyelid) but had no effect at all on the unconditioned response. None of the animals showed any signs of relearning the original conditioned response. Lesions in all animals included at least the ansiform and paramedian lobes.

A total of six stereotaxic lesion animals have been run to date. Lesions localized to the dentate nucleus and vicinity produced complete abolition (n=2) or severe impairment (n=2) of the CR (NM and eyelid). Lesions that were dorsal and caudal to the dentate nucleus (n=2) had no effect at all on the CR. In two of the animals in which the CR was abolished or severely impaired there were no detectible motor symptoms.

At the end of the four full days of postoperative training to the eye ipsilateral to the cerebellar lesion, three animals who showed not a single CR in postoperative training - two with a large ablation and one with a localized stereotaxic lesion - were then given training to the contralateral eye. All three learned in a few trials and maintained a robust and consistent CR. Training was again shifted back to the original (ipsilteral) eye and none of the three animals showed any signs of conditioned responding.

We would like to suggest that the primary engram for short-delay classical conditioning of the NM and eyelid is localized within the ipsilateral cerebellum. The studies of Welker and associates showing an exquisitely detailed tactile projection to the lateral neocerebellar cortex suggest that the critical regions may be very localized (Shambes et al., 1978). Our results are consistent with this hypothesis. However, it is also possible that only a part of the engram, albeit an essential part, is in the cerebellum. In other current work, we have found complete abolition of the same CR with lesions in the ipsilateral pontine reticular formation (Lavond et al., 1981). However, the effective lesion site is at the lateral edge of the decussation of the superior cerebellar peduncle and may interrupt essential cerebellar efferents. Moore has found that ipsilateral lesions in a rather different region of the pons can also abolish the CR (Moore, personal communication).

The cerebellum has long been suggested as a possible locus for the coding of learned motor responses (e.g., Eccles et al., 1967; Marr, 1969). We know of no reason to suppose that the cerebellum has a special role for such movements as NM extension and eyelid closure. Consequently, we argue that the present result may hold for all simple learned responses involving discrete, striated muscle movements. Although cerebellar lesions have been reported to impair a variety of skilled movements in animals (e.g., Brooks, 1975), to our knowledge the present experimental results are the first to show that damage to the ipsilateral cerebellum can selectively abolish a simple learned response. This result is nicely consistent with our earlier suggestion that the engram for simple learned responses is some form of a "motor plan" (Thompson et al., 1980).

If the cerebellum is indeed the locus of the primary engram for simple learned responses, it seems very possible that higher brain structures may exert their modulatory influences on learning and memory by acting on the cerebellum. Thus, there is a pathway from hippocampus to cerebellum via the subiculum to cingulate gyrus to pontine nuclei (Berger et al., 1980; Berger, personal communication). Indeed, relations between hippocampus and cerebellum appear to be close and reciprocal insofar as learning is concerned. In current and preliminary observations we have seen the following (Clark et al., 1982): in trained animals showing the typical hippocampal response (recorded from the left CA1 region), a stereotaxic lesion of the cerebellar dentate nucleus ipsilateral to the trained NM (left eye) abolishes the learned response and the learning-induced hippocampal response in the CS period. When training is then given to the right NM, it learns rapidly and the learning-induced response in the left hippocampus returns. When training is shifted back to the left eye, the left NM shows no CRs but the right eye of course continues to do so and the hippocampal response is maintained. Perhaps the most parsimonious explanation of this effect is that the learning-induced plasticity that develops in the hippocampus requires some type of input or influence from the cerebellum to express itself. It is possible that our current results on the cerebellum may provide the key that has so long been sought in the analysis of the neuronal substrates of simple associative learning of striated muscle responses in the mammalian nervous system.

REFERENCES

Berger, T.W., Alger, B.E. and Thompson, R.F., 1976, Sci., 192:483
Berger, T.W. and Thompson, R.F., 1977, Sci., 197:587.
Berger, T.W. and Thompson, R.F., 1978(a) Brain Res., 145(2):323.
Berger, T.W. and Thompson, R.F., 1978(b) Nat.Acad.Sci., 75(3):1572.
Berger, T.W. and Thompson, R.F., 1978(c), Brain Res., 156:293.
Berger, T.W., Milner, T.A., Swanson, G.W., Lynch, G.A. and Thompson, R.F., 1980, Brain Res., 201:411 (1980).
Berger, T.W., Clark, G.A. and Thompson, R.F., 1980, Physiol. Psychol., 8(2): 155.
Berger, T.W., Laham R.I. and Thompson, R.F., 1980, Brain Res.,193:229
Berger, T.W. and Thompson, R.F., in press, 1981, Behav. Brain Res.
Berger, T.W. and Thompson, R.F., in preparation, 1982.

Berry, S.D. and Thompson, R.F., 1979, Sci., 205:209.
Best, M.R. and Best, P.R., 1976, Exp. Neurol., 51:546.
Brons, J.F. and Woody, C.D., 1980, J. Neurophysiol., 44:605.
Brooks, V.B., 1975, Can. J. Neurol. Sci., 2:265.
Cegavske, C.F., Thompson, R.F., Patterson, M.M. and Gormezano, I., 1976, J. comp. physiol. Psych., 90:411.
Clark, G.A., McCormick, D.A., Lavond, D.G. and Thompson, R.F., 1982, in preparation.
Coates, S.R. and Thompson, R.F., 1978, Neurosci. Abstr., 4:792
Disterhoft, J.F., Kwan, H.H. and Lo, W.D., 1977, Brain Res., 137:127
Eccles, J.C., Ito, M. and Szentagothai, J., 1967, Springer-Verlag, Berlin.
Enser, D., 1976, personal communication.
Fuller, J.H. and Schlage, J.D., 1976, Brain Res., 112:283.
Gormezano, I., Schneiderman, N., Deaux, E., and Fuentes, I., 1962, Sci., 138:33.
Gormezano, I., 1972, New York: Appleton-Century-Crofts.
Hoehler, F.K. and Thompson, R.F., 1980, J.comp.phys.Psych., 94:201.
Kettner, R.E., Shannon, R.V., Nguyen, T.M. Thompson, R.F., 1980, Percep. & Psychophys., 28(6):504.
Lavond, D.G., McCormick, D.A., Clark, G.A., Holmes, D.T. and Thompson, R.F., in press, 1981.
Marr, D., 1969, J. Physiol. (London), 202:437.
Mauk, M.D., Warren, J.T. and Thompson, R.F., in preparation, 1982.
McCormick, D.A., Lavond, D.G., Clark, G.A., Kettner, R.E., Rising, C.E. and Thompson, R.F., in press, 1981, Bull. Psychon. Soc.
McCormick, D.A. and Thompson, R.F., 1982, in preparation.
Norman, R., Buchwald, J. and Villablanca, J.,1975, Program Abstr., 5th Annual Meeting, Soc. for Neurosci., N.Y., Nov. 2-6.
Oakley, D.A. and Russell, I.S., 1972, Phys. & Behav., 8:915.
Olds, J., Disterhoft, J.F., Segal, M., Kornblith, C.L. and Hirsch, R., 1972, J. Neurophysiol., 35:202.
Olton, D.S., Becker, J.T., and Handelmann, G.E., 1980, Physiol. Psych., 8:239.
Patterson, M.M., Berger, T.W. and Thompson, R.F., 1979, Brain Res. 163:339.
Segal, M., 1973a, Brain Res., 64:281.
Segal, M., 1973b, J. Neurophysiol., 36:840.
Shambes, G.M., Gibson, J.M. and Welker W., 1978, Brain Behav. & Evol., 15:94.
Solomon, P.R. and Moore, J.W., 1975, J.comp.physiol.Psych., 89:1192.
Solomon, P.R., 1979, Psychol. Bull., 86:1272.
Swanson, L.J., Teyler T.J. and Thompson R.F., in press, 1982, Neurosci. Res. Prog. Bull.
Thompson, R.F., Berger, T.W., Cegavske, C.F., Patterson, M.M., Roemer, R.A., Teyler, T.J., and Young, R.A., 1976, Amer. Psychol. 31:209.
Thompson, R.F., Berger, T.W., Berry, S.D., Hoehler, F.K., Kettner, R.E. and Weisz, D.J., 1980, Physiol. Psychol., 8(2):262.
Weisz, D.J., Solomon, P.R. and Thompson, R.F., 1980, Bull. Psychon. Soc. Abstr., 193:244.

[1]Supported in part by National Science Foundation research grant BNS - 8106648.

ACTIVITY OF DENTATE GYRUS DURING NM CONDITIONING IN RABBIT

Donald J. Weisz - Dept. of Psychology, Yale University

Gregory A. Clark, Bo-yi Yang, and Richard F. Thompson
Dept. of Psychology, Stanford University

Paul R. Solomon - Dept. of Psychology, Williams College

SUMMARY

Two studies were conducted to characterize the role of dentate gyrus during classical conditioning of the rabbit nictitating membrane response. In the first study, dentate field potentials elicited by perforant path stimulation were recorded before and during training to test for changes in granule cell excitability. Results showed above-baseline increases in population spike amplitude over the course of training in paired but not unpaired animals. In a second study, the activity of identified single granule cells was recorded during conditioning to determine if they exhibited the same neuronal response patterns seen in hippocampal pyramidal cells and in entorhinal cortex. Unlike responses in these other areas, granule cell responses did not develop a model of the behavioral response; instead they were tied more to stimulus presentation, with many cells exhibiting stimulus-evoked theta-frequency bursting in paired but not in unpaired animals. Taken together these studies suggest an intimate involvement of the dentate gyrus in the associative process; however dentate's role appears to be different from that of other hippocampal regions.

INTRODUCTION

We have been involved in the tracing of neuronal responses through limbic system structures during classical conditioning of the nictitating membrane (NM) response in rabbit. In the initial study Berger and Thompson (1) found that, very early in the course of NM conditioning, hippocampal units greatly increased their firing rate in response to paired CS-US presentations. The conditioned unit response grew over training, preceded the conditioned behavior by approximately 30-35 msec, and developed a temporal model of the conditioned behavior. An analysis of the first few trials indicated that the conditioned hippocampal response was not present on the first trial but began to emerge as early as the second paired trial. The hippocampal conditioned response did not develop in unpaired control animals nor was it a sensory evoked response or a motor potential per se. More recently the hippocampal conditioned response (CR) was found to be exhibited by the principal cell type of hippocampus proper -- the pyramidal cells of CA3 and CA1 (2).

Subsequent investigations have focussed on the origin of the hippocampal CR. Two structures providing major input to the hippocampus have been examined. Berger and Thompson (3) reported that conditioned changes in hippocampus cannot be accounted for solely on the basis of activity in the medial septum. Multiple unit activity in the medial septum exhibited onset evoked responses to training stimuli in both paired experimental and unpaired control animals, but the responses decreased across trials in both groups. Multiple unit recordings from entorhinal cortex revealed a within-trial conditioned unit response that is similar (though not identical) to that in hippocampus (4). Over the course of training there was a significantly larger increase in the growth of the conditioned hippocampal unit response than of the conditioned entorhinal unit response.

These findings suggest that the marked learning-dependent growth in unit activity may occur within the hippocampus itself and that the hippocampus may do so by facilitating and enhancing a neuronal "model" of the behavioral response received from entorhinal cortex. Certainly, entorhino-hippocampal connections are capable of an extraordinary degree of physiological and anatomical plasticity including relatively permanent changes in synaptic efficacy. The most likely loci for the enhancement of the conditioned unit response observed in entorhinal are the perforant path synapses on the granule cells of dentate gyrus.

To begin to test this possibility, we conducted experiments in which we recorded electrophysiological activity from dentate gyrus during NM conditioning. In one study, we examined dentate field potentials elicited by perforant path stimulation to test for increases in granule cell excitability. If entorhino-dentate connections are in fact sites of learning-induced synaptic plasticity, responses elicited by perforant path stimulation should grow larger over the course of conditioning. In a second study we recorded responses of identified single granule cells during learning to determine whether these cells would also exhibit a "neuronal model" of the learned behavioral response, or whether their discharge patterns would suggest a functional role of a different nature.

METHODS

Surgical procedures

Male New Zealand White rabbits weighing 1.9 to 2.5 kg were used in these studies. Two types of implant procedures were used. For recording dentate field potentials, a recording electrode was chronically implanted in the dentate granule cell layer, while for isolated single unit recording, a base for a custom microdrive was implanted over dentate gyrus. For both groups, chronic stimulating electrodes were implanted in perforant path.

For the field potential experiment animals were anesthetized with halothane and mounted on a custom stereotaxic holder. Using stereotaxic coordinates in conjunction with electrophysiological recording, an insulated stainless steel recording electrode (3-5 u tip diameter, 40 u shaft exposed at tip) was implanted in the cell body layer of dentate granule cells (upper blade, left hemisphere). A pair of stainless steel stimulating electrodes (5-7 u tip diameter, 500 u exposed shaft, 1 mm tip separation) were implanted into the perforant path. Final placements of stimulating and recording electrodes were based on the shape and latency of elicited field potentials. Wires previously attached to the electrodes were connected to pins of a headstage which was mounted to the skull. A small nylon loop was sutured in the nictitating membrane for recording of behavioral responses during conditioning.

Surgical procedures for the single-unit study were essentially the same except, prior to cementing, the dentate recording electrode was withdrawn, and the base of the microdrive system was implanted over the dentate recording site.

Behavioral procedures

All animals were allowed at least one week of recovery prior to training. Prior to each training session, the animal was placed in a Plexiglas restraining box, and eyeclips inserted into the left eye to hold the lids open during training. A headgear containing first-stage FET amplifiers, a potentiometer for transduction of nictitating membrane (NM) movement, and an airpuff delivery nozzle was bolted to a chronically implanted stage on the animal's head. Both experimental (paired) and control (unpaired) animals received one day of adaptation to the experimental chamber followed by at least two days of training.

Experimental animals were trained in a classical conditioning paradigm in which a 1 kHz, 85dB, 350 msec tone conditioned stimulus (CS) was paired with a 100 msec airpuff unconditioned stimulus

(UCS). UCS onset (measured at cornea) followed CS onset by 250 msec, and the two stimuli co-terminated. Animals in this group received 117 trials per day consisting of 13 blocks of training, with one tone-alone and eight tone-airpuff paired trials constituting each block. The intertrial interval (ITI) ranged from 40 to 60 sec in pseudo-random fashion, with a mean of 60 sec.

Animals in the control group were given explicitly unpaired training. These animals received 208 trials consisting of 13 blocks of training, with eight tone-alone and eight airpuff-alone trials presented in pseudo-random order constituting each block. Thus experimental and control animals received virtually the same number of stimuli, but for control animals, the two stimuli never occurred together within a single trial. ITI's for the control group ranged from 20 to 40 sec, with a mean of 30 sec.

In the first experiment field potentials elicited by perforant path stimulation were recorded from the cell body layer of dentate gyrus before and during training to test for any changes in granule cell excitability. Just prior to the beginning of behavioral training, input-output curves were obtained by varying stimulus intensity. On the basis of the input-output curve, the stimulus intensity which elicited spikes approximately 30% of the reliable maximum was used to elicit 18 (in paired) or 16 (in unpaired) potentials immediately prior to the onset of behavioral conditioning. These procedures established a baseline against which any possible changes in excitability could be assessed. The stimulus intensity used to determine the baseline was used to elicit potentials during the training sessions.

During the course of conditioning, the perforant path was stimulated 225 msec after tone onset (25 msec prior to airpuff onset in the paired conditioning group). The 225 msec interval corresponds to a time at which conditioned changes in single and multiple unit activity have been demonstrated to occur in entorhinal cortex and in CA1 and CA3 regions of hippocampus. Field potentials were elicited during all trials in the paired conditioning group and during all tone-alone presentations in the unpaired group. Potentials were also elicited between trials when no tones or airpuffs were being presented.

During training sessions, elicited field potentials were amplified using battery-powered, solid-state FET amplifiers (gain = 500, filter cutoff points = 0.5 Hz and 10 KHz, input impedance = 60 Mohm). Amplified potentials were recorded on audio tape both directly and as frequency modulations of a carrier wave. During subsequent off-line analysis, field potentials were bandpass filtered (20Hz to 2KHz), digitized every 0.2 msec, and analyzed on a PDP-12 computer system using a program developed by the first author. This program scored each potential individually, and all averages were computed from measurements taken from the individual trials. The insert in Figure 1 shows the method used for measuring spike amplitude.

Procedures for the single unit study were similar, with the necessary modifications for single unit recording. At the start of each training session, etched microelectrodes (1-3 Mohm impedance at 1 KHz) were lowered to the granule cell layer of the upper blade of dentate gyrus and a unit was isolated. The field potential elicited by perforant path stimulation was used to help identify electrode recording position. Criteria for isolation were that the waveform of the unit was of constant amplitude (at least three times greater than the background) and of constant shape and duration. Once a unit was isolated, the perforant path was stimulated to test if the cell could be driven orthodromically. Responses to stimulation were considered to be monosynaptic if they occurred within or before the population spike recorded from the same electrode. Activation latencies were generally 4-6 msec.

The system for recording single units was similar to that described above. Generally the unit was amplified and stored on two tape channels in filtered (500-10,000 Hz) and unfiltered (0.5-10,000 Hz) form. EEG from the unfiltered preamplifier was collected, frequency modulated and stored on tape for later analysis.

The paired and unpaired paradigms used in the single cell experiment were identical to those described for the field potential study. After a cell had been isolated and characterized, animals received at least five blocks of training. At the end of each training session, the unit was tested to determine if it could still be driven. Animals were run for as many as six training sessions.

At the conclusion of the studies animals were anesthetized with pentobarbital, small lesions were made by passing current through the electrode tips, and intracardial perfusions of 0.9% saline followed by 10% formalin were performed. Standard histological procedures revealed that recording electrode tips were in or very near to the dentate granule cell layer and stimulating electrodes were in the perforant path for all animals reported here.

RESULTS

An NM extension of greater than 0.5 mm was considered to be a response and an NM response occurring during the 250 msec CS-US period was scored as a conditioned response (CR). For animals in the unpaired group, an NM response occurring within 250 msec after

CS onset was scored as a CR. For the first experiment all paired animals (n=7) acquired conditioned NM responding, and by the end of Day 2 animals were reponding with CR's on approximately 80 % of the trials. The mean number of trials to acquisition criterion (8 CR's out of 9 consecutive trials) occurred at the end of Block 2 on Day 2. Unpaired animals (n=7) exhibited NM responses to CS presentations on approximately 6 % of the trials.

Figure 1 depicts the results from the first experiment in which dentate population spikes were elicited between trials (top part of figure) and during tone presentations (bottom part). Individual amplitudes for each animal were scored as a percent of pretraining baseline which is indicated on the graphs by the dashed lines. As can be seen, spike amplitudes elicted in paired animals were larger than those elicited in unpaired animals, especially on Day 2. It should be noted that the major portion of the increase in spike amplitude occurred after animals met acquisition criterion. The only consistent change observed for unpaired animals was an increase in amplitude during the first half of Day 1 for potentials elicited during tone presentations. Initially there was a marked inhibition of population spikes which attenuated over blocks 2-7. Finally there was an inhibition of population spikes elicited during tone presentations for both paired and unpaired groups.

All of these observations were supported by statistical analysis. A 2x2x26 analysis of variance for repeated measures (paired-unpaired groups vs. during tone-no tone vs. blocks of training) was performed on spike amplitudes. While the Groups effect only approached significance (F=3.97, df=1,12, p<.10), the Groups x Blocks interaction was statistically significant (F=1.72, df=25,300, p<.05). The effect of Tone was significant (F=8.43, df=1,12, p<.05) as was the effect of Blocks (F=2.63, df=25,30, p<.05). In addition the Groups x Tone x Blocks interaction was significant (F=1.58, df=25,300, p<.05). Newman-Keuls tests revealed significant differences between paired and unpaired population spikes elicited during the tone (within-trial) on blocks 3,12, and 13 on Day 1 and on blocks 3,5,6,8, and 10-13 on Day 2. Significant paired and unpaired differences for spikes elicited between trials were found on blocks 4,5,6,11, and 12 on Day 1 and on blocks 4,5, and 7-13 on Day 2. The Day 2 pretraining baselines (not plotted) for paired animals was 97.1 % of the Day 1 baseline while the figure for unpaired animals was 109.6 %. The 12.5 % difference was not significant.

For the second experiment we recorded the activity of 27 presumed granule cells in 9 conditioning animals and of 15 granule

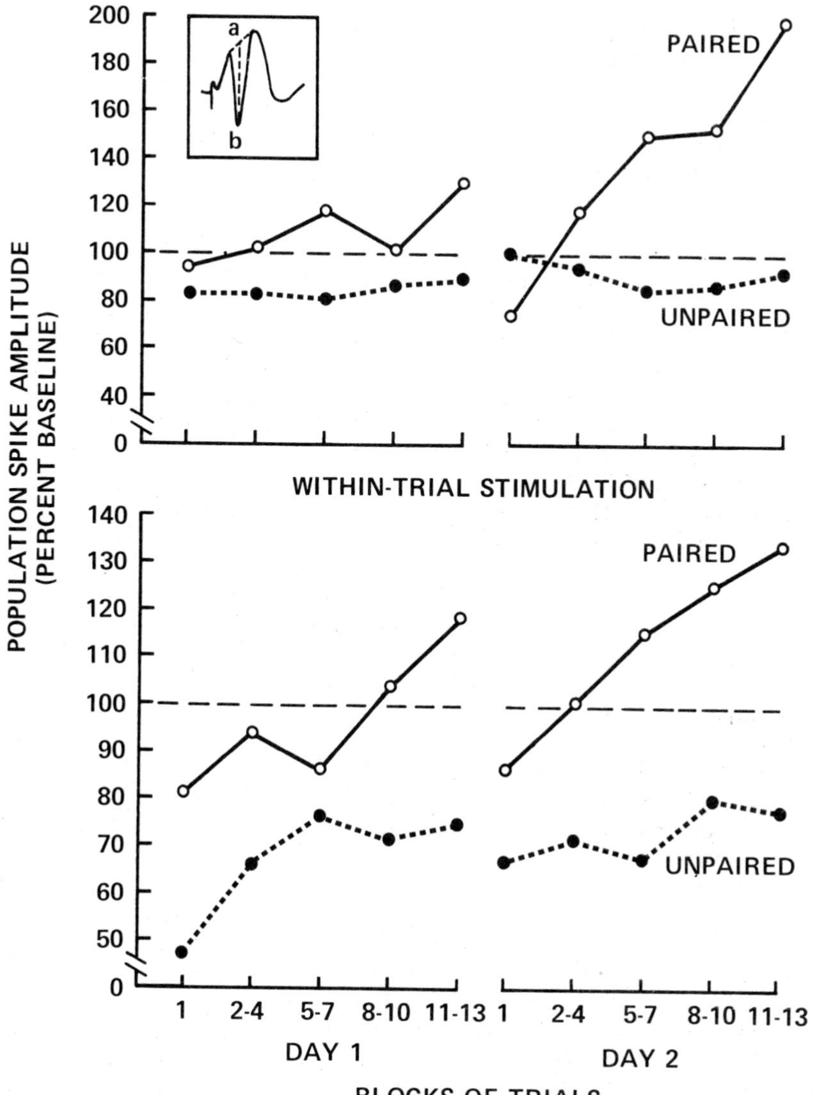

Fig. 1. Average amplitude of dentate granule cell population spikes is plotted as a function of conditioning trials. The baseline amplitude (set at 100 %) was determined by averaging the amplitudes of 16 (paired) or 18 (unpaired) spikes elicited immediately prior to the start of training on Day 1. The inset depicts the measurement used for the amplitude determination. The distance from a to b was measured as the spike amplitude.

cells in 6 unpaired control animals. Cells which could be activated within or before the monosynaptic population spike, were located at the granule cell layer (based on laminar profiles of elicited field potentials and on subsequent histology), and possessed spike widths of .15-.25 msec were considered to be granule cells. Almost all of these cells at times fired in synchrony with 4-8 Hz EEG activity as recorded at the electrode tip. The range of baseline firing rate for granule cells was 5.8-35.5/sec.

Marked differences appeared between paired and unpaired cell responses. The dominant response of paired cells in 8 of 9 animals was an increased firing rate beginning in the tone period and continuing through the air puff period. Although the latency varied across cells (30-100 msec), the increased firing appeared to be locked to the tone and within a cell the latency of the firing was stable. For approximately 1/2 of the cells the increased firing took the form of rhythmical bursting with an interburst interval of approximately 125 msec, which is in the range of theta. In general when the theta bursting pattern was exhibited by a cell, the EEG recorded at the tip displayed large amplitude theta.

There was a great deal of consistency for all granule cells recorded from a given animal. Figure 2A shows a cumulative post-stimulus histogram for a granule cell on trials 10-18 on Day 1. The animal showed no sign of behavioral conditioning at this point; however there was a rhythmical burst beginning in the tone period and lasting throughout the trial. Figure 2B depicts the average block response from the same granule cell later on Day 1 when behavioral conditioned responses first appeared, and Figure 2C shows the response from another granule cell from the same animal on trials 1-9 on Day 2. By Day 2 the animal had developed a well-conditioned NM response, but there was no obvious change in the granule cell firing pattern from the early Day 1 pattern. Overall, following the first 18 paired trials, there were no major changes in the cell response patterns (in either latency or amplitude) to the tone and air puff across cells within a given animal. Furthermore the response patterns in conditioning animals appeared as early as the first block of trials. For 5 conditioning animals presumed granule cells were held during the first training block of 9 trials. In all 5 cases the cells exhibited increased within-trial firing rates, and in some cases the within-trial responses grew over trials 10-18.

While there were no major changes across trials in the paired granule cell responses, there were major differences between the paired responses and the responses of unpaired granule cells. Figures 3A and 3C show representative stimulus histograms for an unpaired granule cell during block 1 of training on Day 1, and

Figures 3B and 3D show histograms for the same cell on block 5 of Day 1. The dominant response to tone-alone and air puff-alone presentations was inhibition during the first block of unpaired training. For most cells inhibition to the air puff remained throughout the first two days of unpaired training; however in

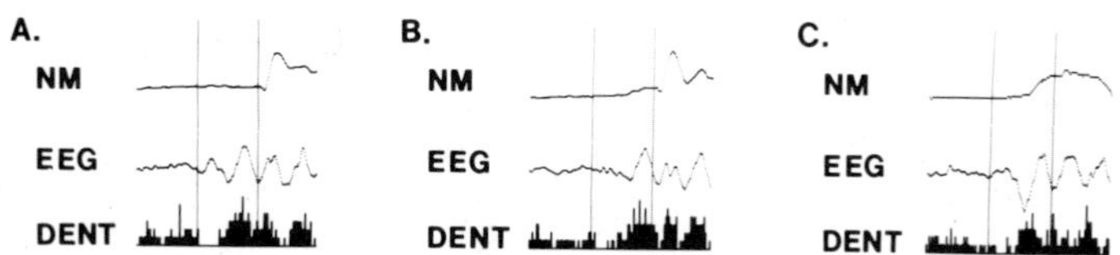

Fig. 2. Examples of eight-trial-averaged behavioral NM responses and associated single-unit histograms for a paired conditioning animal. Upper trace: Average nictitating membrane response for one block of eight trials. Middle trace: Average EEG for one block of trials. Lower trace: Granule cell histogram for one block of eight trials. (A) Second block of eight paired conditioning trials, Day 1, Cell 1. (B) Thirteenth block of eight paired conditioning trials, Day 1, Cell 1. (C) First block of eight paired conditioning trials, Day 2, Cell 2. First cursor indicates CS onset. Second cursor indicates UCS onset. Trace duration is 750 msec.

almost all cases inhibition to the tone decremented with further tone-alone presentations. In addition the spontaneous activity decreased in unpaired animals. This can be seen in Fig. 3 by examining the unit activity prior to CS delivery. There were no consistent EEG patterns elicited by unpaired tone and air puff presentations.

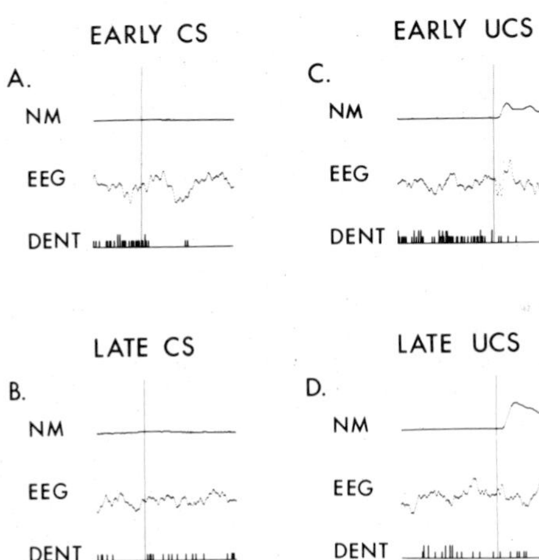

Fig. 3. Examples of eight-trial-averaged behavioral NM responses and associated EEG and single-unit histograms for an unpaired control animal. Upper trace: Average nictitating membrane response for one block of eight trials. Middle trace: Average EEG for one block of eight trials. Lower trace: Granule cell histogram for one block of eight trials. (A,C) First block of eight CS-alone (A) or UCS-alone (C) presentations, Day 1, Cell 1. (B,D) Fifth block of eight CS-alone (B) or UCS-alone (D) presentations, Day 1, Cell 1. Cursor indicates stimulus onset. Trace duration is 750 msec.

DISCUSSION

The primary finding of these experiments is that the excitability of dentate granule cells during tonal CS presentations is greater in animals receiving paired nictitating membrane (NM) conditioning than in animals receiving unpaired stimulus presentations. This result was demonstrated using recordings of monosynaptic population spikes elicited in dentate gyrus by electrical stimulation of the perforant path and by recordings of single dentate granule cells. Differences in excitability between paired and unpaired animals were seen within the first block of training. Using population spike recordings, we demonstrated that granule cell excitability during tone presentations and between trials increased after paired conditioning animals had acquired conditioned NM responding. Finally tone presentations in the context of unpaired training resulted in marked inhibition of granule cell excitability over the first four blocks of training.

The single cell response patterns observed in dentate during NM conditioning were qualitatively and quantitatively different from the responses previously reported for pyramidal cells in CA1 and CA3 of hippocampus (1,2). There were at least three major differences between the conditioned unit responses of pyramidal cells and of dentate granule cells. First, the granule cells responded at a fixed latency to the presentation of the tone throughout conditioning. In contrast pyramidal cell responses preceded the NM response by approximately 30-35 msec, and, as an animal acquired the conditioned NM response, the behavior and the pyramidal unit responses both moved closer to the tone onset. Second, the patterns of conditioned unit responses were different for the two types of cells. The firing patterns of pyramidal cells but not granule cells formed temporal models of the conditioned NM responses. Third, granule cells responded with inhibition to both tone and air puff presentations in unpaired control animals while pyramidal cells increased slightly their firing rates following air puff presentations and exhibited no change following tone presentations. The same three contrasts can be made between the granule cell responses and those previously observed for multiple units in entorhinal cortex.

These results strongly suggest that the dentate gyrus is not merely involved in passing information from entorhinal cortex to CA3 of hippocampus. Our results and those of Segal, Disterhoft, and Olds (5), Segal and Olds (6), and very recently of Rose and Lynch (7) suggest that dentate gyrus has a role during behavioral conditioning that is different from the roles of CA3 and CA1. Segal and colleagues (5,6) reported that rat dentate units showed increased firing to a tone that signalled food and decreased firing to one that preceded shock; whereas CA3 and CA1 units augmented their firing rates in both conditioning paradigms. Segal (8) found that dentate cells required fewer trials to develop conditioned unit responses than did CA3 cells and that dentate cells extinguished their conditioned responses first. Segal concluded that the dentate cells appeared to be responsible for both the acquisition and extinction of cells in CA3. Working with Lynch, Rose (7) reported differential firing patterns in rat of dentate granule cells and of CA3 pyramidal cells in both one-tone and two-tone conditioning tasks. During an appetitive task, granule cells exhibited high firing rates following CS presentation while pyramidal cells did not. The granule cell results of Rose and Lynch were very similar to the previously reported findings of Deadwyler and colleagues (9). Using a two-tone discrimination task, they reported that granule cells increased their firing rate following both CS+ and CS- presentations with a latency of 80 msec. While the increased firing persisted for more than 1 sec following CS+ presentations, it was short-lasting following the CS-.

The differences in firing patterns between granule cells and pyramidal cells observed in the present study should not obscure one important similarity between the conditioned responses of the two cell types. Both the field potential and single cell experiments revealed that as early as the first block, there were differences between paired and unpaired animals in the excitability of granule cells. Throughout training dentate single cells and population spikes responded to tone presentations with increased excitability while unpaired cells inhibited. Both approaches also showed that the greatest inhibition to the tone in unpaired animals occurred on the first block of training. The one major difference in the two sets of findings is that the field potential experiment revealed increased cell excitability during the last half of Day 2 while the single cell results failed to show this. One possible explanation is that more granule cells were recruited across training rather than any one cell gradually increasing its firing rate as the animal learned. More single cells need to be recorded early in training before conclusions can be made regarding this possibility.

The dentate population spike data are consistent with the hypothesis that long-term potentiation may underlie the neural plasticity induced in hippocampus by NM conditioning. Increased amplitudes over the course of paired training were observed for population spikes elicited both during CS presentation and between trials when no conditioning stimuli were presented. The demonstration of increased population spike amplitude between trials eliminates the possibility that the increased excitability only represents a CS-induced event. It is possible that conditioned unit responses in entorhinal cortex are relayed to dentate and that the perforant path-granule cell synapse is potentiated as a result of the repetitive entorhinal input. Of course, the results of the present study provide only preliminary support for this view and evidence needs to be gathered regarding synaptic events. For example, the effect of conditioning on the monosynaptic EPSP needs to be assessed. In conjunction the afferent fiber volley needs to be recorded to determine if there is a change in the number of axons being activated. Furthermore long-term effects of NM conditioning on granule cell excitability need to be studied. The finding that behavioral conditioning can enhance population spike amplitude is a first step in locating a hippocampal site of synaptic change which accompanies NM conditioning.

An alternative interpretation of the results of the present experiments is that the experimental and control procedures differentially affected the excitability of granule cells via an input other that from entorhinal cortex. Winson (10,11) has shown that behavioral state changes are reflected in altered excitability of dentate population spikes. During slow-wave sleep (SWS), spikes are significantly larger than those elicited during the still-alert state (SAL). He found that the enhancement of the spikes during SWS was dependent on an intact input from median raphe (MR). Furthermore prepulsing MR resulted in even larger perforant path elicited spikes. Winson could not enhance dentate population spikes elicited during SAL by prepulsing MR, and he hypothesized that there may be a tonic suppression of dentate during SAL possibly mediated by the noradrenergic input from locus coeruleus. Indeed intraventricular administration of 6-OHDA released the suppression during SAL (Note 1). Thus changes in the inputs from either MR or locus coeruleus (LC) as a result of NM conditioning could lead to changes in the excitability of the dentate granule cells. For example, a release of a suppressive influence by LC could account for the growth of the population spike on Day 2 of paired NM conditioning.

In approximately one-half of the paired animals phase-locked theta or rhythmical slow activity (RSA) was observed following CS presentation. This is in agreement with similar findings in cat (12) and in rat (13). Busaki and colleagues (13) noted that in their study phase-locked RSA coincided with the stage of conditioning when the CS acquired significance and, with continued training on the appetitive classical conditioning task, the phase-locked RSA was replaced by a short-latency evoked potential. Hippocampal EP′s previously were found by Deadwyler and associates (9) using an appetitive two-tone discrimination task in rat. In our aversive task no major changes in the EEG were seen over the course of conditioning; however several procedural differences, including electrode site, task, and type of recording electrode (monopolar vs. bipolar), could account for the discrepancy.

One final point concerns the inhibitory effect of tone presentations on granule cell excitability. The smallest spikes relative to a pretraining baseline were elicited early in unpaired training. While the inhibition attenuated over the first 6 blocks in unpaired animals, there remained throughout the rest of training a slight reduction in spike amplitude following tone presentations. Inhibition of dentate cells to sensory stimuli has been found previously. Vinogradova (14) reported that 30 % of the cells recorded in rabbit dentate gyrus exhibited inhibitory responses to stimulus presentations. The inhibitory responses were not specific to one sensory modality. In general habituation of dentate responses to sensory stimuli was not observed, although habituation of CA3 and CA1 responses occurred frequently. Mays and Best (15) found similar results using rat but only when animals were aroused from sleep by stimulus presentations. Lidsky and colleagues (16) further supported the importance of arousal state on hippocampal unit responses in rat. They found that many hippocampal cells reduced their firing rates in response to stimulus presentations when a stimulus aroused the animal from slow-wave sleep. While it appears that hippocampal cells in awake rats may not inhibit following sensory stimulation, Vinogradova's work and our work suggest that in rabbit dentate cells may show inhibition even when the animals are awake.

Note 1. J. Winson, 1981, presentation at Neuroscience Research Program, Boston.

REFERENCES

1. T. W. Berger and R. F. Thompson, 1978, Neuronal plasticity in the limbic system during classical conditioning of the rabbit nictitating membrane response. I. The hippocampus, Br. Res., 145:323.
2. T. W. Berger and R. F. Thompson, 1978, Identification of pyramidal cells as the critical elements in hippocampal neuronal plasticity during learning, PNAS, 75:1572.
3. T. W. Berger and R. F. Thompson, 1978, Neuronal plasticity in the limbic system during classical conditioning of the rabbit nictitating membrane. II. Septum and mammillary bodies, Br. Res., 156:293.
4. G. A. Clark, T. W. Berger, and R. F. Thompson, 1978, The role of entorhinal cortex during classical conditioning: Evidence for entorhinal-dentate facilitation, Neurosci. Abstr., 4:673.
5. M. Segal, J. F. Disterhoft, and J. Olds, 1972, Hippocampal unit activity during classical aversive and appetitive conditioning, Sci., 175:792.
6. M. Segal and J. Olds, 1973, Activity of units in the hippocampal circuit of the rat during differential classical

conditioning, J. comp. physiol. Psychol., 82: 195.
7. G. Rose, 1980, Physiological analysis of the hippocampus during behavior, Doctoral dissertation presented to University of California, Irvine.
8. M. Segal, 1973, Flow of conditioned responses in limbic telencephalic system of the rat, J. Neurophys., 36:840.
9. S. A. Deadwyler, M. West, and G. Lynch, 1979, Activity of dentate granule cells during learning: Differentiation of perforant path input, Br. Res., 169:29.
10. J. Winson, 1980, Influence of raphe nuclei on neuronal transmission from perforant pathway through dentate gyrus, J. Neurophysiol., 44:937.
11. J. Winson and C. Abzug, 1978, Dependence upon behavior of neuronal transmission from perforant pathway through entorhinal cortex, Br. Res., 147:422.
12. M. Radulovacki and W. R. Adey, 1965, The hippocampus and the orienting reflex, Exp. Neurol., 12:68.
13. G. Busaki, E. Grastyan, I. N. Tveritskaya and J. Czopf, 1979, Hippocampal evoked potentials and EEG changes during classical conditioning in the rat, Electroenceph. clin. Neurophysiol., 47:64.
14. O. S. Vinogradova, Functional organization of the limbic system in the process of registration of information: Facts and hypotheses. in: "The Hippocampus," R. L. Isaacson and K. H. Pribram, ed., Plenum Press, New York (1975).
15. L. E. Mays and P. J. Best, 1975, Hippocampal unit activity to tonal stimuli during arousal from sleep and in awake rats, Exp. Neur., 47:268.
16. T. I. Lidsky, M. S. Levine, and S. MacGregor, 1974, Hippocampal units during orienting and arousal in rabbits, Exp. Neur., 44:171.

A BIOPHYSICAL BASIS FOR MOLLUSCAN ASSOCIATIVE LEARNING

Daniel L. Alkon

Section on Neural Systems, Laboratory of Biophysics
National Institutes of Health at the
Marine Biological Laboratory
Woods Hole, Massachusetts 02543

The nudibranch mollusc *Hermissenda crassicornis* can be conditioned to change its normal positive phototactic behavior. This behavioral change is pairing specific (i.e. paired but not randomly associated light and rotation produce the change), stimulus specific, increases as a function of practice and is of long-duration (at least three to five days). The synaptic relations of identified neurons within the sensory pathways which mediate this behavior have been described in considerable detail at every stage of neural integration: sensory, interneuron, and motorneuron. With this knowledge of neural systems from input of environmental stimuli to output of animal movement, membrane changes of specific neurons were implicated as primary steps in a causal sequence responsible for the conditioning. In summary, repeated stimulus pairing results in short-term cumulative membrane depolarization (associated with elevated intracellular Ca^{++}) of the Type B photoreceptor. This cumulative depolarization results in long-term inactivation of an early voltage-dependent outward K^+ current. This inactivation causes enhanced depolarizing responses of the Type B cells and, sequentially, increased inhibition of ipsilateral Type A cells, ipsilateral hair cells, interneurons and motorneurons, and ultimately retarded phototaxis. This causal sequence is contrasted with those responsible for short-term behavioral changes such as reflex facilitation and sensitization.

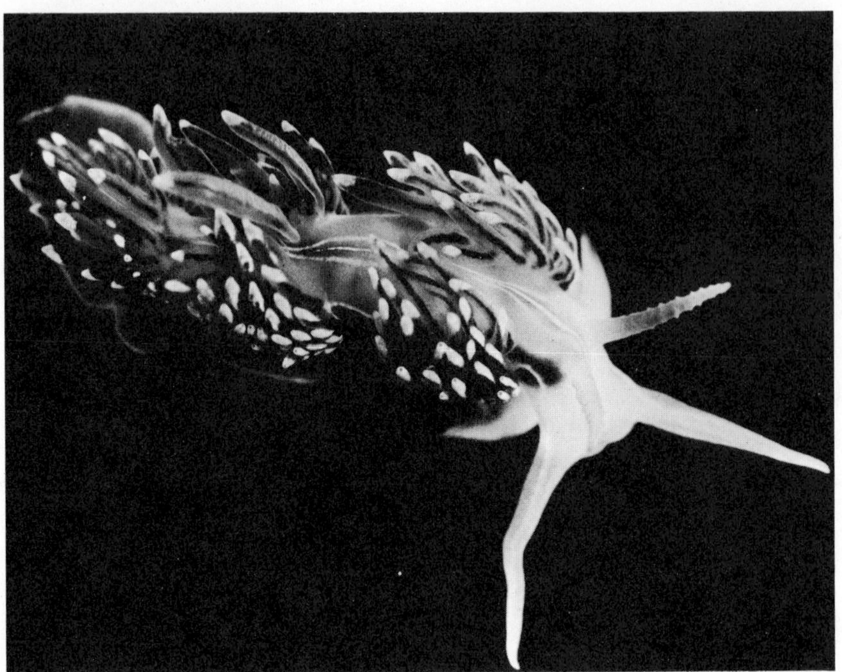

Figure 1. The nudibranch mollusc Hermissenda crassicornis. Note the small black spot (the right eye) at the base of the lower rhinophore. Length of the animal is ∿ 4 cm (Alkon, 1980).

There is no difficulty in generating a host of possible cellular mechanisms for associative learning. The challenge is determining which possibility actually functions in a natural context. We know of neuronal structural changes during an animal's growth and development, of increased number of sensitive receptors with presynaptic degeneration, of regeneration, facilitation, post-tetanic potentiation, habituation, etc. Which of these apply?

Ideally, to answer this question we should identify those neurons which cause clear-cut associative learning of a vertebrate species and analyze those biophysical and biochemical steps which are crucial to the behavioral transformation. Some of us interested in this problem have turned to invertebrates, which often have relatively few neurons, accessible to intracellular recording techniques. With these preparations, however, new questions arise. Is the behavioral change of interest really associative learning as defined for vertebrates? If so, do diverse invertebrate and vertebrate

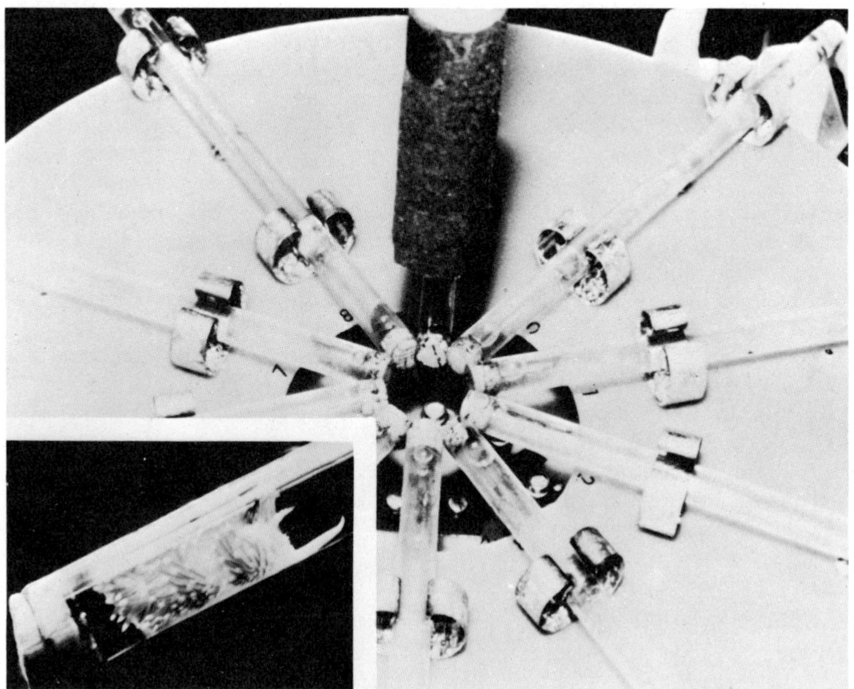

Figure 2. Training and testing apparatus. The response latencies to enter a light spot projected onto the center of the turntable by an overhead illuminator were recorded automatically when the Hermissenda moved toward the light source (direction of the arrows) and interrupted the light between illuminator and photocells (arrowhead).

(Inset) Hermissenda were subjected to different behavioral treatments consisting of light and rotation while confined to the end of glass tubes filled with seawater (Crow and Alkon, 1978).

species share common cellular mechanisms for this learning? Finally, the demonstration of a causal sequence from transduction of environmental stimuli through neural integration and motor output, although greatly simplified, remains formidable, even for the more elementary nervous systems of such invertebrates as gastropod molluscs.

It has been possible to produce, for the nudibranch mollusc, *Hermissenda crassicornis* (Fig. 1), a behavioral change which shares many of the features of vertebrate associative learning (Alkon, 1974a; Crow and Alkon, 1978; Lederhendler et al., 1980; Crow and Offenbach, 1980; Farley and Alkon, 1981). When light is repeatedly paired with rotation the animal's normal positive response to light is markedly reduced (Figs. 2, 3). This behavioral change is truly associative since it is not produced by randomized light and rotation (i.e. light and rotation stimuli which occur with no fixed temporal relation) as well as a number of other control training procedures. The behavioral change is specific in that responses to stimuli other than light (e.g. food, darkness, and gravity) are not changed by the associative training. Finally, it is of long duration (at least three to five days) depending on the number of repetitions of temporally associated light and rotation to which the animal was exposed. A teleologic description of this learning might be one of aversive conditioning. The aversive quality of rotation, which is a noxious stimulus, may be considered to be *associated* with the previously neutral or positive stimulus, light.

To arrive at cellular principles of associative learning for *Hermissenda* we first determined, with some completeness, genetically specified, i.e. invariant neural systems which process information within and between the visual and statocyst pathways which mediate the associated stimuli, light and rotation. We established, by electrophysiologic and morphologic criteria, those neurons and the synaptic relations between them which were reproducible from animal to animal (Alkon and Fuortes, 1972; Alkon, 1973a, b; 1974; Alkon et al., 1978; Akaike and Alkon, 1980). For example, each of three Type B photoreceptors in each eye are mutually inhibitory (Fig. 4) and also inhibit optic ganglion cells, but Type B photoreceptors also inhibit Type A photoreceptors (of which there are two in each eye) which do not have synaptic interactions with each other. Type A photoreceptors excite a specific ipsilateral hair cell (there are twelve hair cells in each statocyst). Type B photoreceptors also inhibit some as well as excite other ipsilateral interneurons (Fig. 5) within the cerebropleural ganglion. Caudal (but not cephalic) hair cells inhibit photoreceptors which undergo a prolonged excitatory rebound following this inhibition (Fig. 6). The synaptic interactions of many other neural elements, including interneurons and motorneurons are now well known (Fig. 7). For example, Dr. Yasumasa Goh and I have recently established that the medial Type A photoreceptor excites interneurons which ultimately excite a pedal ganglion motorneuron. This motorneuron responds to light focused on the animal's eyes and excitation (by intracellular current injection) of this motorneuron causes movement of a behaving animal. Thus it has now become possible to describe for Hermissenda input-output relations mediating visual and gravitational stimuli from sensory receptors to motorneurons to muscular responses.

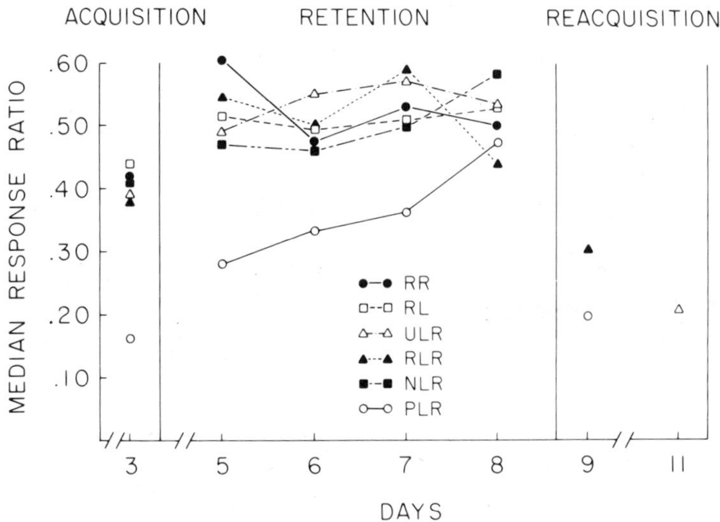

Figure 3. Median response ratios for acquisition, retention and reacquisition of a long-term behavioral change of Hermissenda in response to a light stimulus [random rotation (●), random light (□), unpaired light and rotation (△), random light and rotation (▲), nothing (■), and paired light and rotation (○)]. The response ratio in the form of 1-A/(A+B) compared the latency during the test (A) with the baseline response latency (B). Group data consists of two independent replications for all control groups and three independent replications for the experimental group (Crow and Alkon, 1978).

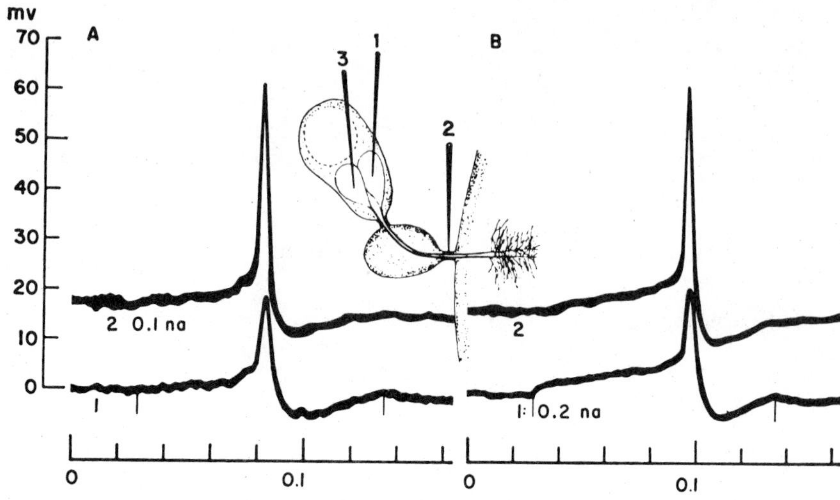

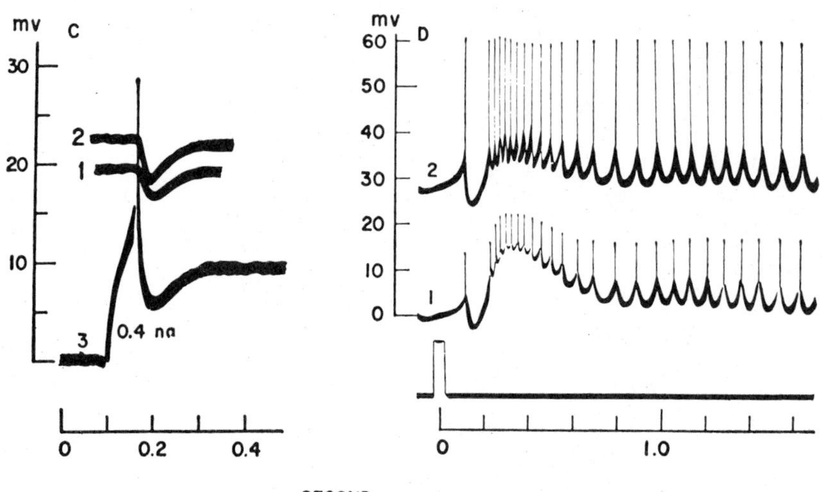

Figure 4. Responses recorded from soma and axon of same cell. The distance between the two electrodes was 80-100 μm. A) Responses to a step of depolarizing current through axonal electrode. B) Responses to a step of current through the soma electrode. In either case the spike is larger and earlier in the axon. C) Two electrodes were inserted, respectively, in the soma and axon of one receptor and a third electrode was inserted in the soma of a second receptor. A step of depolarizing current through this third electrode evokes a spike in one receptor and

(Fig. 4, continued) a hyperpolarizing synaptic potential in the other. The synaptic potential is larger and has shorter time to peak in the axon. D) Responses to a flash of light. The generator potential is larger at the soma (lower trace) while the spikes are larger at the axon. Downgoing bars in (A) and (B) indicate timing of current steps (Alkon and Fuortes, 1972).

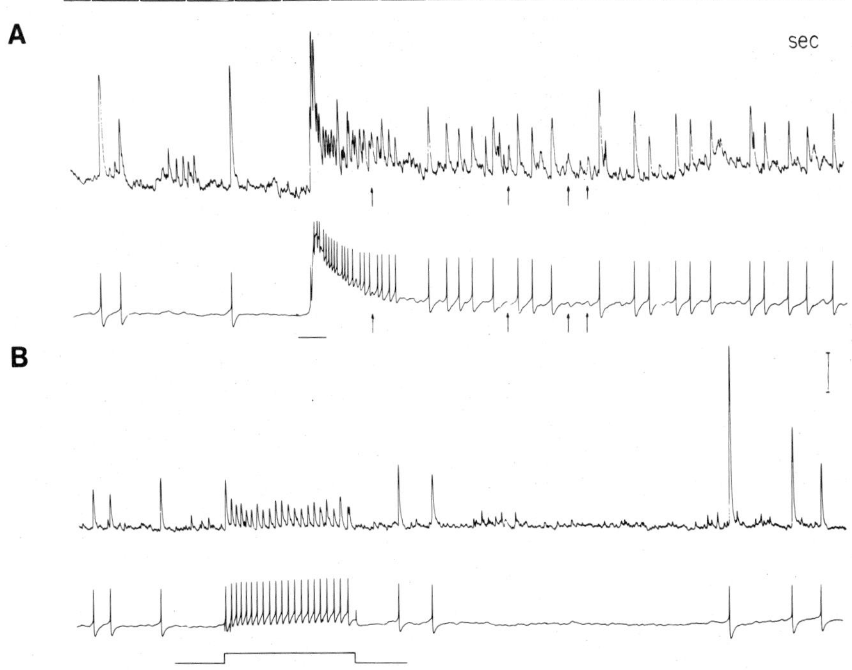

Figure 5. EPSP's recorded from a second-order visual neuron associated with each impulse of a Type B photoreceptor. Upper trace: CPG neuron; this neuron was hyperpolarized -40 mV from the resting level by injection of current (-2.1 nA). Lower traces: recording from Type B photoreceptor. A: responses to light as indicated by horizontal bar (intensity: -3.0). B: responses to depolarizing current step (0.22 nA) applied to the Type B cell, as indicated in the lowest trace. Arrows indicate IPSP's in the Type B cell and corresponding small EPSP's in CPG neuron. Voltage calibration: 5 mV for upper traces, 10 mV for lower traces (Akaike and Alkon, 1980).

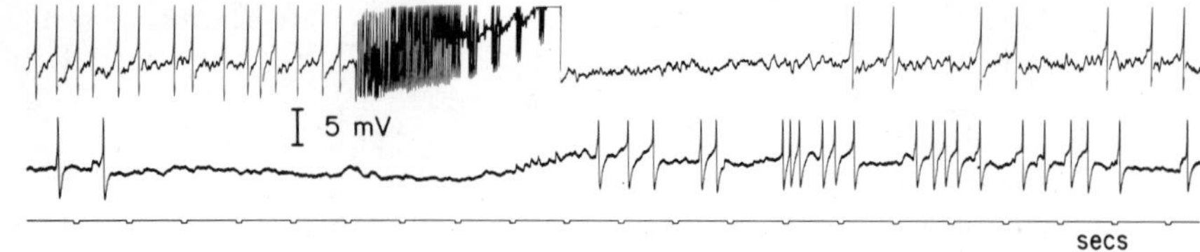

Figure 6. Depolarization of Type B photoreceptor (lower record) follows impulse train of ipsilateral caudal hair cell (upper record). A positive current pulse (+0.5 nA) injected into hair cell elicits increased firing of hair cell and slight inhibition of Type B cell. After high frequency firing, hair cell remains slightly hyperpolarized and without impulse activity while Type B cells show increased EPSP's and prolonged depolarization (Tabata and Alkon, in preparation).

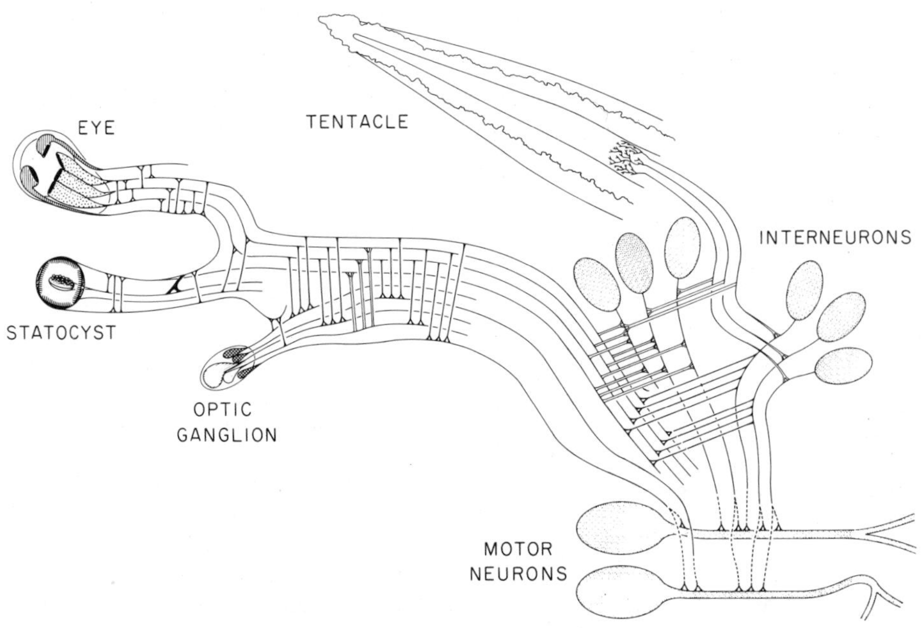

Figure 7. Schematic summary (partial) of ipsilateral neural interactions within and between the visual, statocyst and chemosensory pathways. Branches perpendicular to lines (representing axons) indicate inhibitory synapses. Double branch lines perpendicular to axonal lines indicate excitatory synapses. Dash lines indicate synaptic interactions presently under study. No contralateral ipsilateral interactions (which have been investigated) are included (Alkon, 1980).

With intracellular microelectrodes we then measured within these neural systems changes which occurred during and persisted after associative training (Alkon, 1975, 1976b; Crow and Alkon, 1978, 1980; West et al., 1981; Farley and Alkon, 1981; Lederhendler and Alkon, in preparation). A number of neuronal changes within identified neurons were limited to associatively trained animals. It was then possible to construct a causal sequence beginning with a specific cell type, Type B, and continuing through Type A, hair cell, interneurons and ultimately motorneurons. This causal sequence will now be briefly described.

Because of several convergence points, i.e. sites of synaptic interaction between the statocyst and visual pathways, there is, during acquisition, synaptic enhancement of a light-induced depolarization of the Type B photoreceptor when light and rotation are temporally associated (Alkon, 1979). Due to the specificity of the synaptic organization, this enhancement only occurs when caudal (not cephalic) hair cells are excited (Alkon, 1980; Farley and Alkon, 1980). A kind of regenerative or positive feedback mechanism (Alkon, 1979) contributes to the progressive depolarization of the Type B cell during acquisition of the associative learning behavior. Light-induced depolarization enhances synaptic depolarization, which in turn enhances the light-induced depolarization, and so forth (Fig. 8). With each successive trial, residual depolarization potentiates and adds to depolarization following the next stimulus pair. When light is repeatedly paired with rotation, membrane depolarization progressively increases, i.e. it accumulates (Alkon, 1980). We have measured this accumulation by recording from Type B cells during and after associative training (Fig. 9). How does cumulative membrane depolarization in turn cause a very long-lasting change which can account for the animal's decreased positive phototactic behavior? There was another change in the Type B membrane which accompanies and then outlasts cumulative depolarization. This change was first manifest to us a few years ago as an increased input resistance of the Type B soma membrane, i.e. Type B cells with impulse-generating zone and synaptic interactions removed by axotomy show an increased input resistance (Fig. 10) on days following associative training but not control procedures (Crow and Alkon, 1980; West et al., 1981). An increased input resistance at least in part explains (see below) an enhanced depolarizing response (Fig. 11) of the Type B cell after light (Crow and Alkon, 1980; West et al., 1981) also recorded from associatively trained but not control animals. Enhanced Type B depolarization and higher impulse frequency during and following a light step will cause greater inhibition of the Type A cell, the hair cell, ipsilateral interneurons and the motorneurons which control the animal's movement toward light. Thus ultimately enhanced Type B depolarization is expressed as a decreased positive phototaxis.

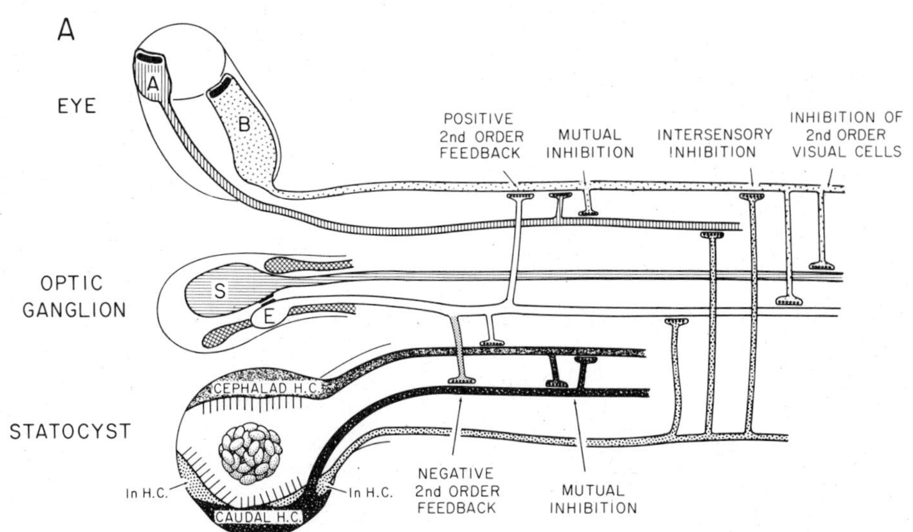

Figure 8A. Neural system (schematic and partial diagram) responsive to light and rotation. Each eye has two Type A and three Type B photoreceptors; each optic ganglion has thirteen second-order visual neurons; each statocyst has twelve hair cells. The neural interactions (intersection of vertical and horizontal processes) identified to be reproducible from preparation to preparation are based on intracellular recordings from hundreds of pre- and post-synaptic neuron pairs. Abbreviations: IN HC, hair cell $\sim 45^{0}$ lateral to caudal north-south equatorial pole or statocyst; S, silent optic ganglion cell, electrically coupled to E cell; E, optic ganglion cell, pre-synaptic source of EPSP's in Type B photoreceptors. The E second-order visual neuron causes EPSP's in Type B photoreceptors and cephalad hair cells and simultaneous inhibitory post-synaptic potentials (IPSP's) in caudal hair cells (Alkon, 1979).

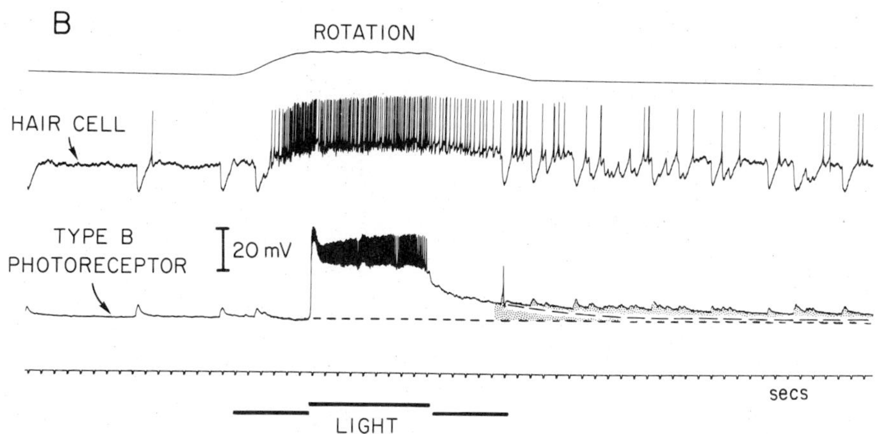

Figure 8B. Intracellular recordings (simultaneous) from caudal hair cell and Type B photoreceptor show increase of EPSP's (Type B cell, lower record) and simultaneous IPSP's (caudal hair cell, upper record) after light paired with rotation. The LLD after stimulus pairing is greater than that after light alone (line of long dashes). The line of short dashes indicates level of resting membrane potential. The lowest trace indicates light duration; top trace, angular velocity of turntable (effecting 1.2 g) (Alkon, 1979).

These changes of Type B properties, observed one and two days following the last days of associative training could be due, it was hypothesized (Crow and Alkon, 1980; West et al., 1981) to long-term reduction of voltage-dependent K^+ currents across the Type B photoreceptor membrane. With voltage clamp techniques (Fig. 12) two such currents were determined (Shoukimas and Alkon, 1980) for this membrane (in the absence of light): an early, rapidly inactivating voltage-dependent K^+ current (I_A) and a late slowly inactivating voltage-dependent K^+ current (I_B). It has been possible to separate these currents pharmacologically: I_A is blocked by 10 mM 4-aminopyridine and I_B by tetraethylammonium ion (Shoukimas and Alkon, in preparation).

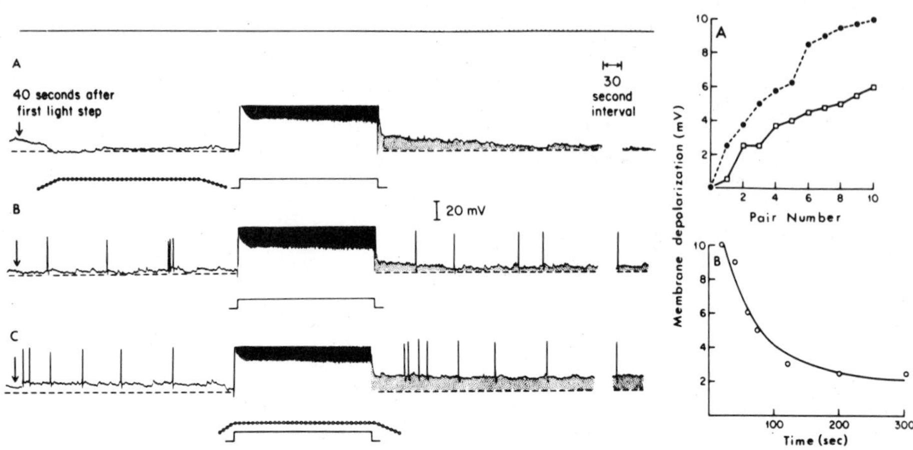

Figure 9. (Left) Intracellular voltage recordings of Hermissenda neurons during and after light and rotation stimuli. (A) Responses of a Type B photoreceptor to the second of two succeeding 20-second light steps (with a 90-second interval intervening). The cell's initial resting potential, preceding the first of the two light steps in (A), (B), and (C), is indicated by the dashed lines. Depolarization above the resting level after the second of the two light steps is indicated by shaded areas. (A) Light steps ($\sim 10^4$ ergs$\cdot$cm$^{-2}\cdot$sec^{-1}) alternating with rotation (caudal orientation) generating $\sim$ 1.0 g. The end of the rotation stimulus preceded each light step by 10 seconds. (B) Light steps alone. (C) Light steps paired with rotation. By 60 seconds after the first and second light steps, paired stimuli cause the greatest depolarization and unpaired stimuli the least. The minimal depolarization was in part attributable to the hyperpolarizing effect of rotation. Depolarization after the second presentation of paired stimuli was greater than that after the first. (Right) (A) Increase of Type B membrane depolarization with repetition of the stimulus pairs. Membrane potential was measured instantaneously 20 seconds (filled circles) and 60 seconds (open squares) after successive presentations of light steps paired with rotation. (B) Decrease of Type B membrane depolarization after repeated presentation of stimulus pairs as described in (A) (Alkon, 1980).

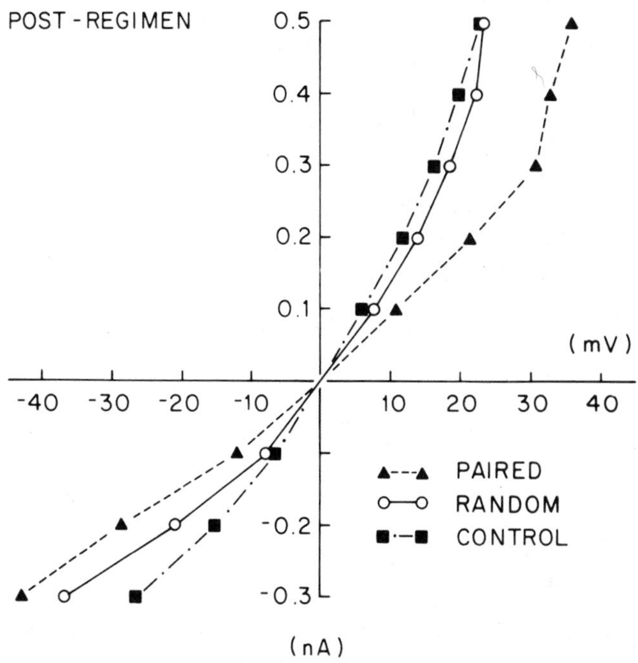

Figure 10. Current-voltage relations of Type B photoreceptors. Post-regimen values were obtained by measuring the steady-state voltage changes produced by current pulses through an intracellular microelectrode. The Paired cells showed significantly greater voltage changes particularly for positive pulses. This difference of Paired cells (as compared to Random and Control cells) was greater for the Post- as compared to the Pre- regimen values (West et al., in press).

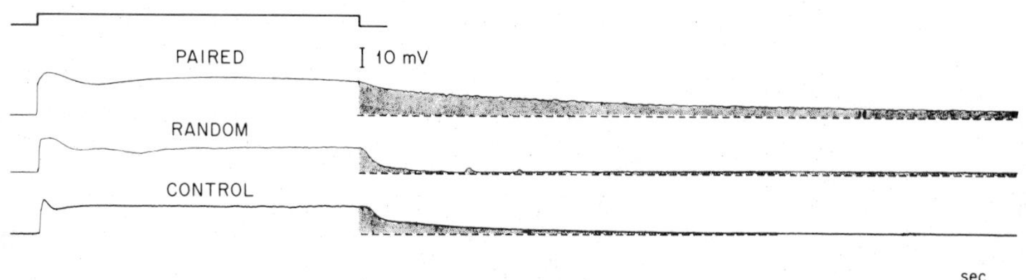

Figure 11A. Responses to first light step of Type B photoreceptors from Paired, Random and Control groups. Shaded areas indicate LLD (long-lasting depolarization) following the light step (monitored by top trace). Note that the Paired LLD is clearly larger than Random and Control.

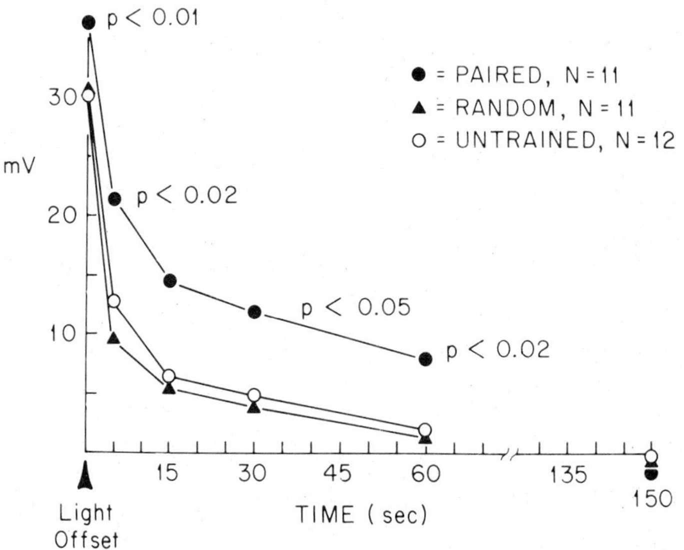

Figure 11B. LLD responses of Type B photoreceptors. Values taken from actual voltage recordings at pre-chosen time points (0, 5, 15, 30, 60 sec) following the first light step. Note that the Paired LLD values are significantly greater than Random and Control, using a 2-tail Mann-Whitney U-test (West et al., in press).

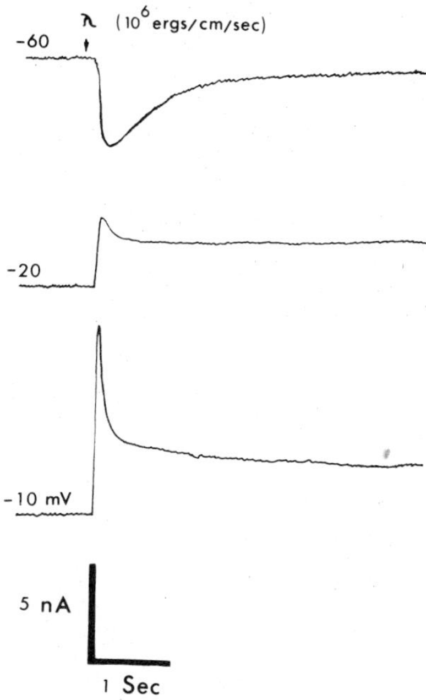

Figure 12. Voltage-clamp recordings from Type B photoreceptor. Top current recording shows inward Na^+ current during a light step whose onset is indicated by arrow. Middle and bottom current recordings are of outward K^+ currents (elicited in the dark by positive command pulses from -60 to -20 and from -60 to -10 mV), onsets also indicated by arrow (Shoukimas and Alkon, in preparation).

To test the hypothesis of a reduced I_A and/or I_B, axotomized Type B cells, using a blind procedure were isolated from paired, random or control animals and voltage-clamped with two microelectrodes inserted in the soma one and two days following the third day of training. The peak amplitude of I_A but not I_B in response to positive voltage command pulses was significantly reduced only for the paired cells (Fig. 13). Similarly a measure of the rate of inactivation of I_A provided by a twin pulse ratio was significantly increased only for the Type B cells isolated from associatively trained animals. These changes of I_A then were truly a result of pairing light with rotation rather than an effect of phototransduction itself. This separation of phototransduction effects and conditioning effects on I_A and I_B was further demonstrated by an additional experiment (Fig. 13). I_A peak amplitude was unchanged by simultaneous presentation of a light step whereas I_B was markedly reduced. The conditioning procedure, however, unlike light, does change I_A but leaves I_B unaltered. A reduced I_A for paired animals will result in greater depolarization during the in-

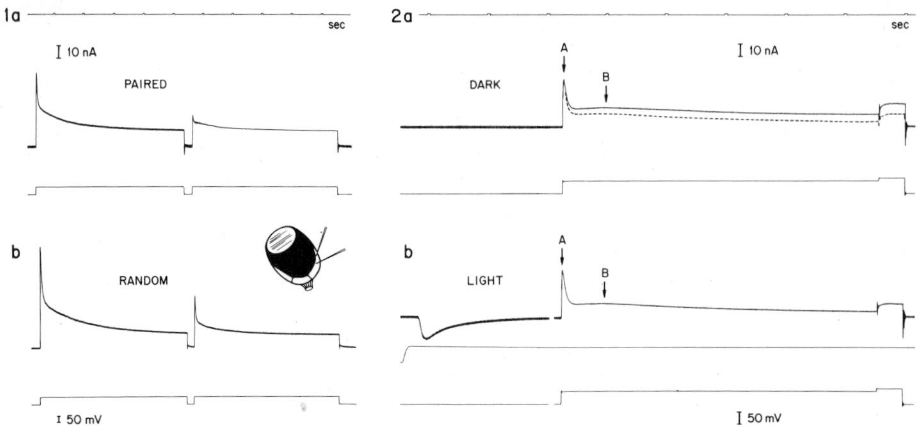

Figure 13. Outward K^+ currents of Type B cell. 1a, b: Outward currents elicited by command pulses to 0 mV. Initial peaks are the early rapidly inactivating K^+ currents (I_A). Late outward K^+ currents (I_B) not obvious in these records reach maximum values at approximately 1.0 sec after the onset of the command pulse. Note that I_A Paired is smaller than for I_A Random for both first and second command pulses. Note also that the ration of I_A Paired for second pulse to I_A for first pulse is smaller for Paired than for Random. Cartoon depicts impalement of medial Type B cell with two microelectrodes.

2a, b: Outward currents elicited by command pulses to -10 mV in darkness (a) and during light (b). Breaks in current trace of (b) is 10 sec until approximate steady-state current during light was achieved. Note that I_A is unchanged by light while I_B is significantly reduced when measured 1.0 sec after the command pulse to -10 mV and in response to a second command pulse to 0 mV 30 µsec after the first pulse. Dashed line in (a) represents superimposed current record of (b) to show differences. I_A is known to be entirely inactivated during the second command pulse (Alkon et al., in press).

itial phase of the Type B light response. This initial depolarization results from a light-induced transient inward Na^+ current (Alkon, 1979). The initial depolarization, if larger for the paired animals, will trigger a larger light-induced voltate-dependent Ca^{++} current which, because of its slow inactivation (Alkon, 1979) will be associated with a larger and more prolonged depolarizing response of the Type B cell during and following a light step. In summary, I_A, a specific membrane current intrinsic to the Type B cell soma, is charged by conditioning and this change is such that it can explain a number of other neuronal changes (see above) which can account for or control the animal's learning behavior.

What is the underlying biochemistry of this primary membrane change? We have some clues. Within eyes isolated from conditioned animals a low molecular weight protein band showed increased phosphorylation when compared to eyes from control (i.e. trained with randomized light and rotation or naive) animals (Neary et al., 1981). Injection of the catalytic subunit of protein kinase, which catalyzed phosphorylation, produced an increased input resistance and enhanced depolarizing response to light in isolated Type B somata (Acosta-Urquidi et al., 1981). These results suggest that the reduction of I_A across the Type B membrane is related to a change of phosphorylation within this cell. Intracellular injection of the catalytic subunit of cyclic-AMP-dependent protein kinase (which catalyzed phosphorylation) reduced I_B (the slow voltage-dependent outward K^+ current) which was also reduced by light. The kinase injection did not affect I_A which changed during associative learning. This raised the possibility that a Ca^{++}-calmodulin-dependent protein kinase might catalyze phosphorylation which is responsible for I_A and its modification during learning. Such a possibility was given further support by recent experiments which have implicated intracellular Ca^{++} in long-term changes of I_A (Alkon et al., in preparation). When light is repeatedly presented to isolated Type B cells during a command pulse to -10 mV (from a holding level of -60 mV) I_A in response to subsequent commands to -60 mV in the absence of light remains smaller for several minutes. This effect is not produced by repeated presentations of light alone nor command pulses alone, nor light alternating with command pulses. The effect of pairing under these conditions is to produce a voltage-dependent light-induced flow of Ca^{++} into the cell (Alkon, 1979). Thus, this inward Ca^{++} current apparently reduces I_A. Consistent with this interpretation was another finding that I_A is enhanced when extracellular Ca^{++} is negligible and reduced for many minutes following intracellular injection of Ca^{++} into the cell (Alkon et al., in preparation). Thus, during associative training, repeated pairing of depolarizing steps with light-induced Ca^{++} currents may raise intracellular Ca^{++} levels which in turn activate a Ca^{++}-calmodulin-dependent protein kinase. A change of phosphorylation catalyzed by this kinase could then cause a long-term reduction of I_A.

What are some possible implications of our findings with Hermissenda? The first implication is that the associative learning occurs via pre-existing converging sensory pathways. These pathways don't grow or develop during the learning but instead define the potential for learning. The "plasticity" if you will, already resides, dormant within the neural systems of Hermissenda. The incredible specificity of this learning potential was illustrated by the opposite effects of stimulus pairing for the caudal orientation (with the animal's head toward the center of rotation) vs. the cephalic orientation. The synaptic organization is such (Fig. 14) that stimulus pairing only causes enhanced depolarization

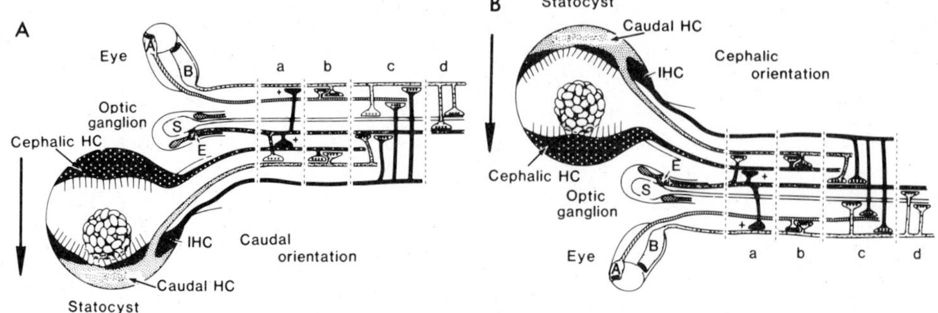

Figure 14. Schematic diagram of interactions between Hermissenda visual and statocyst systems. The neural interactions (intersection of vertical and horizontal processes) identified to be reproducible, from preparation to preparation, are based on intracellular recordings from hundreds of pre- and post-synaptic neuron pairs as well as light and electron microscopic studies. (A) Caudal orientation. When caudal hair cells are depolarized by rotation (as they are for the caudal orientation) their inhibition of the E optic ganglion cell increases. Following inhibition by these hair cells as well as inhibition by the ipsilateral Type B photoreceptor, the E cell undergoes rebound depolarization. During this depolarization the E cell increases its synaptic excitation of the Type B cell. The E cell is also responsible for synaptic inhibition of the caudal hair cell. During rebound depolarization of the E cell, the inhibition of the Type B cell by the caudal hair cell is also increasingly inhibited. The resultant of these synaptic effects is increased synaptic excitation of the Type B cell after rotation (for caudal orientation) alone and after light alone, but particularly after light paired with rotation. This is so because during stimulus pairing (for the caudal orientation), the caudal hair cell (or cells) depolarized both in response to rotation and because of decreased inhibition from the E cell, which is now inhibited both by the caudal hair cells and the Type B photoreceptors. (B) Cephalic orientation. When cephalic hair cells are depolarized by rotation, the resultant synaptic effect is slight inhibition after stimulus pairing. The arrow indicates direction of the centrifugal force vector produced by rotation. The darkened vertical processes with plus signs represent the only excitatory synaptic interactions within this network (Farley and Alkon, 1980).

and cumulative depolarization of the Type B cell for a caudal orientation. The function of this pre-existing convergence of sensory pathways predicts opposite behavioral effects which were in fact confirmed (Farley and Alkon, 1980). Animals trained with stimulus pairing in the caudal orientation should and do move to a light less readily. Animals trained in the cephalic orientation should and do move to a light source more readily. That this convergence between the visual and statocyst pathways occurs at the level of the sensory receptors (as well as interneurons) reflects the necessity of a relatively small number of neurons to fulfill multiple information processing functions. With more evolved species the very much greater number of neurons allows more specialized function for individual neurons. Phototransduction, for example, is performed by retinal rods and cones and intermodal sensory convergence occurs, with few exceptions, within more central neuronal structures of vertebrate species (Alkon, 1976b). Similarly, the biophysical changes which were observed to occur within Hermissenda photoreceptors are more likely to occur at points of convergence within more central neuronal structures of vertebrate species. The substitution of multiplicity of neuronal function for specialization may also require, for the Hermissenda photoreceptors, unique biophysical features (e.g. I_A) which are usually reserved for vertebrate neurons which are not primary sensory receptors.

A second implication concerns the possible generality of our findings thus far. Voltage-dependent K^+ currents are not uncommon in neurobiology. Prolonged inactivation, lasting many seconds is not uncommon. To me it is quite reasonable that accumulated depolarization associated with elevated levels of intracellular Ca^{++} can result from specific stimulus patterns in many nervous systems, including our own, and that prolonged inactivation of voltage-dependent K^+ currents, lasting many days, follows this accumulated depolarization. A cellular mechanism for associative learning is provided, therefore, by this accumulated depolarization and resulting K^+ current change. It may not be able to account entirely for the learning even of Hermissenda -- it may not be the only mechanism operating. But it is a functional means of long-term storage of information concerning the association of stimuli within a neuronal membrane and it is a mechanism which is eminently possible in many other more highly evolved nervous systems.

A number of other phenomena in neurobiology involve inactivation of K^+ channels. The importance of this inactivation, however, as a cellular mechanism, how it arises and how it affects subsequent information processing differs enormously when one is discussing associative learning for Hermissenda, visual transduction, dishabituation, or the propagation of an action potential. For associative learning, where pairing specificity and stimulus specificity are essential, accumulated depolarization arises from stimulation of precise pre-existing synaptic networks leading to K^+ current inactivation. For dishabituation, a transient K^+ inactivation has been studied at an *Aplysia* cell body but not at the synapse where sensitization is believed to occur. The proposed K^+ inactivation of dishabituation has been thought to begin with a neurochemical event at the synapse which somehow becomes manifest at the cell body (Klein and Kandel, 1980). Unlike the long-lasting K^+ inactivation of associative learning this reduced K^+ conductance can apparently arise in response to serotonin or pre-synaptic facilitation with no preceding membrane depolarization. A neurohumor-induced change of conductance is well suited to the more generalized, nonspecific nature of sensitization or dishabituation in contrast to the precise long-term storage of information concerning stimulus relationships necessary for associative learning. Many strong stimuli mediated by many different neural pathways will arouse or sensitize an animal thereby raising responsiveness to a host of stimuli and stimulus combinations. A means for producing such diffuse effects is provided by the release of a hormonal messenger into an organism's circulation. This again is in contrast to restricted information flow within a well-ordered neural network such as we have found occurs for the associative learning of *Hermissenda*.

Thus, differences of behavioral phenomena such as conditioning, sensory adaptation, and arousal are paralleled by differences of causal cellular mechanisms. Such parallelism points to the improbability of one cellular mechanism, e.g. for sensory adaptation, explaining several other behavioral phenomena, e.g. associative learning. The data available thus far indicate quite the contrary -- namely, *there is no unified basis for behavioral changes*. What seems much more likely is a multiplicity of mechanisms. This is not to say, however, that there can't be some shared features within these mechanisms -- just as there are undoubtedly some shared features of learning changes and those of developmental and regeneration changes. The sequence of biophysical and biochemical steps which precedes these changes is almost certainly not shared. Stimulation of single pre-synaptic terminals with the correct magnitude and frequency of current injection will cause post-tetanic potentiation, facilitation, or habituation. For the associative learning of *Hermissenda* we have seen that paired stimulation of converging sensory pathways results in cumulative depolarization and elevation of intracellular Ca^{++}. This in turn causes (possibly by inducing changes of protein phosphorylation) long-lasting inactivation of a voltage-dependent K^+ current which ultimately affects the entire neural pathway as it responds to subsequent light stimuli. Synaptic facilitation also involves elevation of intracellular Ca^{++} (cf. Zucker, in this volume), yet how it arises and its biophysical consequences are quite distinct from those for associative learning of *Hermissenda*.

Another implication of the biophysical steps we have found for associative learning of *Hermissenda* concerns what have been taken for granted as the necessary sites of neural changes which cause learning. For decades it has been assumed that learning must occur at synapses. Unlike the short-lived electrophysiologic changes of habituation which have been studied at spinal reflex synapses, the crayfish neuromuscular junction, the frog neuromuscular junction, and the *Aplysia* sensory-motor cell synapse, the long-lasting current changes I have described here for associative learning of *Hermissenda* occur at the cell body. The inactivation of K^+ currents of *Hermissenda* specifically results from paired stimulation of the synaptic networks, but this inactivation is not tied to specific neurotransmitters or neurotransmission itself. If our findings have meaning for other species, sites of learning may include a variety of membrane loci including somata, dendrites, axons, axonal branches and synapses.

In closing, I would like to briefly address the issue of causality. All of the participants in the symposium are interested in identifying those neuronal changes which cause the learning behavior demonstrated for our experimental animals. Theoretically, to demonstrate causality one needs a fairly complete knowledge of the neural circuitry to describe the flow of information through the nervous system to finally produce behavior. For none of these preparations is the neural circuitry completely understood -- although some are better understood than others. So we must approximate cellular location of changes which cause learning. We can do this by (1) correlation of behavioral with electrophysiologic change, (2) establishing changes which are intrinsic to neurons which are isolated physically and electrically from all other neurons, (3) sampling neurons at sensory, integrative and motor stations which are sufficiently representative to provide some input-output description of the nervous system, (4) making lesions at specific sites within the nervous system to assess the functional importance of neurons and neuron groups.

Ultimately, a neuronal change can be said to cause learning if it can be shown that this change (1) occurs as a direct consequence of the training paradigm (e.g. paired stimuli), (2) persists following training in the absence of further input from other neurons, and (3) produces a behavioral change which in some way expresses or reveals what has been learned (e.g. that one stimulus is "associated" with another stimulus as manifest by similarities of behavioral responses elicited by each stimulus following training). We know that the Type B photoreceptor changes satisfy the first two conditions. We know also that light, *after* repeated pairing with rotation, elicits a greatly diminished overall movement of the animal, just as rotation prior to pairing diminishes overall movement. What remains is to show that the Type B changes actually produce the behavioral changes. Ideally, with intracellular electrodes within Type B photoreceptors of fully behaving animals, the appropriate neuronal changes effected by current injected into the Type B cells would bring about the predicted behavioral changes. In lieu of this ideal experiment, which has never been fully accomplished with any form of learning for any preparation, we use the approximations of causality mentioned above (correlation, isolation, sampling, and lesions) to construct a model which corresponds to our observations. As the model becomes increasingly unique, our confidence in the causal role of neuronal changes is increased. We know that the changes of Type B impulse activity produced by training will cause changes of the Type A cells, interneurons and motorneurons which actually cause turning in response to light. We don't yet know how good the quantitative fit of the predicted effect of these neural changes is to the observed behavioral changes.

A quantitative description of neural changes which cause behavioral change must include ensembles of neurons. We have localized, for instance, primary neuronal changes during associative learning of *Hermissenda* which are intrinsic to isolated Type B cells -- but these changes are only meaningful when considered within the context of the Type B cells' interrelationships with many other neurons within the nervous system. These relationships then also lead us to sites of learning although they are secondary sites which ultimately may not require biochemical transformations which primary membrane changes almost certainly do.

REFERENCES

Acosta-Urquidi, J., Alkon, D.L., Olds, J., Neary, J.T., Zebley, E., and Kuzma, G., 1981, Intracellular protein kinase injection simulates biophysical effects of associative learning on *Hermissenda* photoreceptors. *Soc. Neurosci.* 7:944.

Akaike, T., and Alkon, D.L., 1980, Sensory convergence on central visual neurons in *Hermissenda*, *J. Neurophysiol.*, 44:501.

Alkon, D.L., 1973a, Intersensory interactions in *Hermissenda*, *J. Gen. Physiol.*, 62:185.

Alkon, D.L., 1973b, Neural organization of a molluscan visual system, *J. Gen. Physiol.*, 61:444.

Alkon, D.L., 1974a, Associative training of *Hermissenda*, *J. Gen. Physiol.*, 64:70.

Alkon, D.L., 1974b, Sensory interactions in the nudibranch mollusc *Hermissenda crassicornis*, *Fed. Proc.*, 33:1083.

Alkon, D.L., 1975, Neural correlates of associative training in *Hermissenda*, *J. Gen. Physiol.*, 65:46.

Alkon, D.L., 1976a, Neural modification by paired sensory stimuli, J. Gen. Physiol., 68:341.

Alkon, D.L., 1976b, The economy of photoreceptor function in a primitive nervous system, in "Neural Principles in Vision", F. Zettler and R. Weiler, eds., Springer-Verlag, New York, pp. 410-426.

Alkon, D.L., 1979, Voltage-dependent calcium and potassium ion conductances: A contingency mechanism for an associative learning model, Science 205:810.

Alkon, D.L., 1980a, Cellular analysis of a gastropod (Hermissenda crassicornis) model of associative learning, Biol. Bull., 159:505.

Alkon, D.L., 1980b, Membrane depolarization accumulates during acquisition of an associative behavioral change, Science 210:1375.

Alkon, D.L., Akaike, T., and Harrigan, J.F., 1978, Interaction of chemosensory, visual and statocyst pathways in Hermissenda. J. Gen. Physiol., 71:177.

Alkon, D.L. and Fuortes, M.G.F., 1972, Responses of photoreceptors in Hermissenda, J. Gen. Physiol., 60:631.

Alkon, D.L., Lederhendler, I., and Shoukimas, J.J., 1982, Primary changes of membrane currents during associative learning, Science, in press.

Crow, T.J. and Alkon, D.L., 1978, Retention of an associative behavioral change in Hermissenda, Science 201:1239.

Crow, T.J. and Alkon, D.L., 1980, Associative behavioral modification in Hermissenda: Cellular correlates, Science 209:412.

Crow, T. and Offenbach, N., 1979, Response specificity following behavioral training in the nudibranch mollusk Hermissenda crassicornis, Biol. Bull., 157:364.

Farley, J. and Alkon, D.L., 1980, Neural organization predicts stimulus specificity for a retained associative behavioral change, Science 210:1373.

Farley, J. and Alkon, D.L., 1981, Associative neural and behavioral change in Hermissenda: Consequences of nervous system orientation for light- and pairing-specificity, Soc. Neurosci., 7: 352.

Klein, M. and Kandel, E.R., 1980, Mechanism of calcium current modulation underlying presynaptic facilitation and behavioral sensitization in Aplysia, Proc. Nat. Acad. Sci. USA, 77:6912.

Lederhendler, I.I., Barnes, E.S., and Alkon, D.L., 1980, Complex responses to light of the nudibranch Hermissenda crassicornis. Behav. Neural Biol., 28:218.

Neary, J.T., Crow, T., and Alkon, D.L., 1981, Change in a specific phosphoprotein band following associative learning in Hermissenda. Nature 293:658.

Shoukimas, J.J. and Alkon, D.L., 1980, Voltage-dependent, early outward current in a photoreceptor of Hermissenda crassicornis. Soc. Neurosci., 6:17.

West, A., Barnes, E., and Alkon, D.L., 1981, Primary neuronal changes are retained after associative learning, Biophys. J., 33:93a.

West, A., Barnes, E., and Alkon, D.L., 1982, Primary neuronal changes during retention of associatively learned behavior, *J. Neurophysiol.*, in press.

Zucker, R.S., 1982, Processes underlying one form of synaptic plasticity: facilitation, in, "Conditioning: representations of involved neural function", C. Woody, ed., Plenum Pub. Corp., New York, in press.

A POSTSYNAPTIC MECHANISM UNDERLYING LONG-LASTING CHANGES IN THE EXCITABILITY OF PYRAMIDAL TRACT NEURONES IN THE ANAESTHETIZED CAT

Lynn J. Bindman, O.C.J. Lippond and Alex R. Milne

The Department of Physiology
University College London
London, WC1E 6BT, England

SUMMARY

1. Changes in the excitability of pyramidal tract (PT) neurones that last for hours can be induced by altering their firing rates for brief periods, in cats that are anaesthetized and paralyzed.

2. Long-lasting increases in excitability can be induced by trains of antidromic conditioning shocks (e.g. 100Hz, 0.2 ms width, train duration 6 sec to 10 min). In this experimental situation the site of the underlying change could be pre- or postsynaptic. However, we have evidence that a postsynaptic mechanism exists, shown in the following way. Synaptic transmission was blocked by the application of $MgCl_2$ solution to the pial surface. Antidromic conditioning trains were then given to the PT at the medulla; an increase in the excitability of PT cells resulted, and persisted undiminished, for up to 3 hours (ref. 1). This observation needs to be taken into account when considering the cellular basis of conditioning and learning.

3. Long-lasting decreases in excitability of PT neurones were produced by stimulation of the contralateral PT when synaptic transmission was not impaired by the application of Mg (1). The decreases in excitability persisted without decrement for more than 1 hour. Conditioning stimuli given to the contralateral tract affect cells whose axons run in the ipsilateral tract via synapses alone, either via axon collaterals or more circuitous pathways. The site of the underlying change in this case may be pre or postsynaptic; it could be due to a prolonged decrease in excitability of PT cells, or to a prolonged increase in excitability of inhibitory interneurones.

INTRODUCTION

Persistent changes in the firing rate of cortical neurones can be elicited in anaesthetized animals by a variety of experimental procedures that briefly alter the firing rate of the cell.[1] It is not known if the underlying mechanisms are presynaptic, postsynaptic or both. In the experiments reported here we investigated the possibility of a postsynaptic contribution to long term changes in cortical neuronal excitability. We found evidence for a postsynaptic mechanism in PT cells of the cat, initiated by repetitive, antidromic firing.

METHODS

Experiments were performed on 124 cats, anaesthetized with urethane (1.5/Kg body weight). This anaesthetic was used because it kept the cats fully anaesthetized at a steady level for at least 20 hr, and because cortical excitability remained stable. Gallamine triethiodide (i.v.) was used to abolish evoked muscle twitches; the cats were ventilated to maintain a constant end-expiratory PCO_2. Arterial BP was measured continuously.

Structures in the neck were dissected to expose both medullary pyramidal tracts. A hole (ca. 2 cm dia) was made in the skull to expose part of the precruciate and much of the parietal cortex. The dura mater was removed, and a watertight cup was cemented to the skull. Non-polarizable electrodes for delivery of test shocks were placed on the pial surface of the cortex; a recording electrode was inserted into the primary somatosensory cortex. All the electrodes were fixed rigidly to the inner wall of the cup. The cup was filled with NaCl (9g/l), then sealed at the top, and was connected by a side arm to a reservoir. The animal was rotated into a supine position. The dura over the medullary pyramids was removed, and recording and stimulating electrodes were placed on the ventral surface (see diagram inset into Fig. 2). Electrodes were arranged so that the same axons were stimulated by the PT conditioning shocks as by the cortical test shocks (shown by occlusion). The fluid in the reservoir was adjusted to the level of the exposed medullary surface. The cavity was then filled with a gel of agar in NaCl. The cortex could be irrigated with $MgCl_2$ via the reservoir, cup and an outlet tube.

The effect of Mg on the cortex was monitored by examining the waves in the PT response to cortical stimulation, spike activity and the contralateral forepaw evoked response in the cortex. A 1M solution was needed to block synaptic transmission throughout the depth of the sensorimotor cortex. Controls for the effects of osmolarity were carried out. Further details are given in refs. 1 & 4.

RESULTS

Experiments in which synaptic transmission was blocked by Mg. A $MgCl_2$ solution was applied to the pial surface to block synaptic transmission throughout the depth of the somatosensory and motor cortex. The completeness of the block was judged by the abolition of unitary firing and cortical evoked responses. Sub-maximal test shocks (T) were applied at 1 per 2 sec to the pial surface to excite PT cells. The mass axonal response was recorded on the ventral surface of the ipsilateral medullary pyramid. Averages of 32 responses (inset of Fig. 1) were measured successively for a control period of at least an hour. Conditioning shocks (C) were applied via separate, caudal electrodes at the pyramid; collision between impulses evoked by T and C shocks showed that the same population of cells was excited in each case. Following a conditioning train, the axonal mass response to the T shock was increased (Fig. 1). In 11 cats, 13 statistically significant increases were found, that were maintained undiminished for 1h to 3h. No decreases were obtained.

Experiments without synaptic block by Mg. Prolonged increases in excitability of PT cells were also obtained in the absence of Mg following antidromic C stimulation. In this case synaptic activity and/or antidromic activity could be responsible. Fig. 2 shows (●) the increased ipsilateral response to T produced after ipsilateral C stimulation. The responses to the same T shocks, recorded from cells that were not excited antidromically, because their axons travel in the contralateral pyramidal tract, show (■) no significant increase in the hour following the C train.

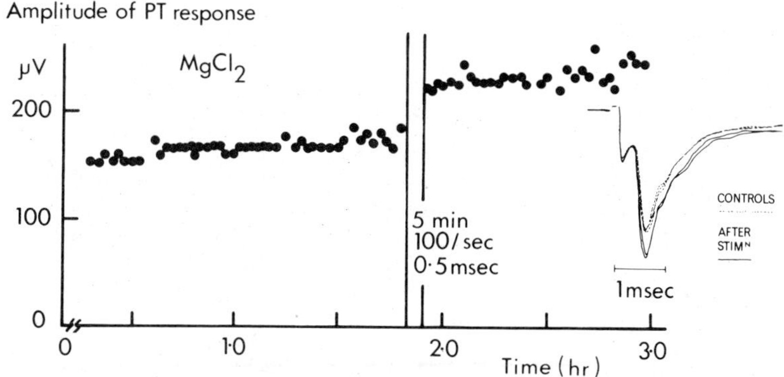

Fig. 1. Long-lasting increase in presence of 1M $MgCl_2$. For methods see ref 1. Cats were anaesthetized with ethyl carbamate which maintains a stable level of anaesthesia for hours.

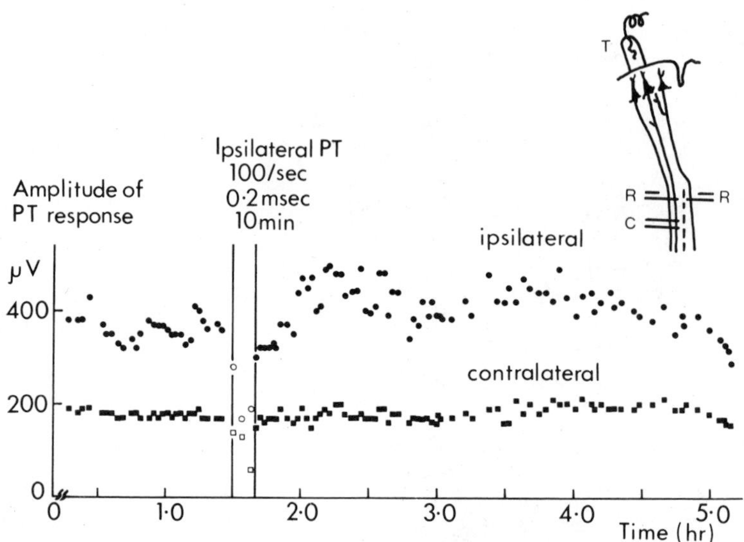

Fig. 2. Long-lasting increase without added Mg.

In 7 cats in which C shocks were given to the ipsilateral PT to excite cells antidromically, 10 statistically significant non-decrementing increases were obtained, plus 1 transient increase of 35 min. Three further conditioning periods produced a decrease in excitability and 3 were without effect.

The increase in the axonal mass response was not due to effects of the C train on the axons. When the T shock was applied to the sub-cortical white matter, no increase in the axonal mass response was found following C stimulation, in 8 out of 8 experiments.

Long-lasting decreases, but no increases in excitability were found when PT cells were affected via synapses alone during PT stimulation. The C shocks were applied to the contralateral pyramid and the response to the T shocks in the ipsilateral pyramid was recorded. Twenty-three non-decrementing decreases were obtained in 18 cats; 2 decreases of 10 to 20 min were also found.

Table 1. Summary of results showing After-Effect of PT Stimulation on the Excitability of a Population of Pyramidal-Tract Cells.‡

Stimulation	Number of cats	Effect	Number of experiments
Antidromic activation via ipsilateral tract when synaptic transmission blocked by Mg.	15	Long-lasting increase△	13
		Long-lasting decrease	0
		No change*	4
Antidromic plus synaptic inputs via ipsilateral tract, in the absence of additional Mg.	7	Long-lasting increase□	10
		transient increase	1
		Long-lasting decrease	3
		No change	3
Synaptic inputs alone via contralateral tract, in the absence of additional Mg.	18	Long-lasting increase	0
		Long-lasting decrease	23
		transient decrease	2

Mean increase in amplitude of PT response, as % of control:
△when synaptic transmission blocked by Mg 17.46% S.E. 2.31%
□in absence of additional Mg 8.6% S.E. 2.12%

*In 2 of these experiments occlusion was not obtained and in the other 2 experiments supramaximal test shocks were used.
‡All increases and decreases significant at $p < 0.001$ (t test)

DISCUSSION

A postsynaptic mechanism has been implicated in the production of long-lasting increases in neuronal excitability both in the hippocampus[5] and in the motor cortex[9]; the post-synaptic change was induced in each case by way of normal synaptic pathways onto the neurones.

We have shown that a postsynaptic mechanism is involved in PT cells after they have been excited antidromically. In the anaesthetized, paralyzed cat, a persisting increase in the excitability of a population of PT cells can be observed following trains of conditioning stimuli applied to the ipsilateral pyramidal tract[1,2]. In some of these experiments, the PT cells could have been excited synaptically as well as antidromically, either via recurrent collaterals to the PT cell population or by other pathways. However, in other of our experiments synaptic transmission was blocked, and the neurones were excited during the conditioning train only by antidromic impulses. The change in this situation must be of postsynaptic origin.

What cellular events might be involved in the production of postsynaptic increases in excitability when synaptic transmission is blocked? Three possibilities are as follows. First, a modulator chemical could be released from the presynaptic endings during the conditioning train, which acts to increase postsynaptic excitability for at least several hours. It would be necessary for its release to be unaffected by a concentration of Mg that abolishes all spontaneous firing of cortical cells, and synaptically evoked potentials[4]. There is no evidence at present that such a modulator exists; moreover Woody, Swartz & Gruen[10] have shown that a combination of depolarization produced by iontophoretically-applied acetylcholine (ACh) and an increased rate of spike discharge is sufficient to elicit a persistent increase in input resistance in cortical neurones. The increase in input resistance is usually associated with an increase in excitability of the cells.

Second, it may be that in our experiments where synaptic transmission was blocked by added Mg, the presynaptic terminals of axon collaterals were nevertheless releasing transmitter during the conditioning train. Together with the increase in firing rate initiated by antidromic excitation of the axons, a postsynaptic change might be induced as in the experiments of Woody et al[10]. Indeed it has been shown that iontophoretically applied Mg ions reduce postsynaptic excitability in the cortex[7]; it could be argued that the block of synaptic transmission by Mg in our experiments resulted from a postsynaptic action of Mg.

We have now made direct measurements of ACh released from the cortex at the same time as electrical recordings of the direct cortical response (a post-synaptic potential evoked in the superficial layers of the cortex by weak electrical stimulation of the cortical surface). Topically applied Mg reduced the amount of ACh released from the cortex. At a concentration of Mg that abolished the postsynaptic electrical response, the amount of ACh released following stimulation was indistinguishable from the background control levels of ACh, in any one experiment. Nevertheless, measurements pooled from several experiments indicated that a small, significant increment in ACh release could be observed as a result of stimulation, even when the postsynaptic electrical response was abolished (Bindman & West, unpublished observations). If this evoked ACh release in the presence of Mg is consequent upon presynaptic impulses, we cannot exclude the second possibility, namely that transmitter plus cell discharge induced the after-effects.

The data of Table 1 show that a persisting increase can be produced more reliably in the presence of Mg than without it; a comparison of the magnitude of the after-effects shows that the mean increase in the presence of Mg is significantly greater than without synaptic block. We think therefore that it is not likely that the release of transmitter is a causative factor in our experiments using antidromic conditioning stimuli.

A third possibility to consider is that the repetitive antidromic firing of PT cells at high frequency is the determinant. Woody, Swartz & Gruen were not able to elicit persisting changes in input resistance in cortical neurones by current-induced firing of cells in the absence of added transmitter[10]. In the 17 control neurones they examined, the lower limit of discharge frequency during current-induced firing was 3Hz; it is not clear from their paper what was the upper limit of firing rate, produced by 10 msec depolarizing pulses applied at 10 Hz. It may well have been considerably lower than the 100, 200 or 300 Hz we used to stimulate PT axons.

The question arises as to what are the normal rates of firing of PT cells <u>in vivo</u>. Evarts[6] has reported that in monkeys carrying out learned movements, mean rates of firing were in the range of 80 to 100/s at the start of the learned task. Individual interspike intervals in PT cells can be much higher than these mean values, even in the cat.

In our experiments carried out in the absence of additional Mg, we were usually able to elicit either a prolonged decrease[3] or a prolonged increase in excitability (see Table 1). Prolonged increases were never seen when synaptic inputs alone were activated, which presumably reflects a predominance of inhibitory interneurones excited via the contralateral PT. The prolonged increases were produced by ipsilateral PT stimulation, when cells could have been excited synaptically or antidromically, or both. In the latter situation, prolonged decreases were obtained in a few experiments. The proportion of excitatory and inhibitory effects is different from that found by Tzebelikos & Woody[8]. Following antidromic excitation of PT cells, they found 9 persistent increases in excitability and 14 persistent decreases; following synaptic but not antidromic excitation, they observed 21 persistent increases and 6 persistent decreases in excitability. The experimental situation was different from ours in that a) low frequency (1-6 Hz) stimulation of the pes pedunculi was used, and b) no anaesthetic was employed. In our animals the anaesthetic may have altered the balance of excitatory and inhibitory effects.

Finally, we must admit that antidromic activation of PT cells would not occur in the normal life of a cat. However we have shown that long-lasting changes of excitability can be induced in neurones by an experimental method that excludes synaptic transmission, and considerably reduces transmitter release at synapses. We suggest that the consequences of high-frequency firing of the postsynaptic cell should be taken into account in addition to synaptic events when considering the cellular mechanisms underlying information storage in the cortex.

REFERENCES

1. Bindman, L.J., Lippold, O.C.J. & Milne, A.R. (1979). Prolonged changes in excitability of pyramidal tract neurones in the cat: a post-synaptic mechanism. J. Physiol., 286, 457-477.
2. Bindman, L.J., Lippold, O.C.J. & Milne, A.R. (1976). Long-lasting changes of post-synaptic origin in the excitability of pyramidal tract neurones. J. Physiol., 258, 71-72P.
3. Bindman, L.J., Lippold, O.C.J. & Milne, A.R. (1976). Prolonged decreases in excitability of pyramidal tract neurones. J. Physiol., 263, 141-142P.
4. Bindman, L.J. & Milne, A.R. (1977). The reversible blocking action of topically applied magnesium solutions on neuronal activity in the cerebral cortex of the anaesthetized rat. J. Physiol., 269, 34P.
5. Bliss, T.V.P. & Lømo, T. (1973). Long-lasting potentiation of synaptic transmission in the dentate area of the anaesthetized rabbit following stimulation of the perforant path. J. Physiol., 232, 331-356.
6. Evarts, E.V. (1965) Relation of discharge frequency to conduction velocity in pyramidal tract neurons. J. Neurophysiol., 28, 216-228
7. Sömjen, G.G. & Kato, G. (1968) Effects of magnesium and calcium on neurons in the central nervous system. Brain Res., 9, 161-164
8. Tzebelikos, E. & Woody, C.D. (1979) Intracellularly studied excitability changes in coronal-pericruciate neurons following low frequency stimulation of the corticobulbar tract. Brain Res. Bull., 4, 635-641.
9. Woody, C.D. & Black-Cleworth, P. (1973) Differences in excitability of cortical neurones as a function of motor projection in conditioned cats. J. Neurophysiol., 36, 1104-1116.
10. Woody, C.D., Swartz, B.E. & Gruen, E. (1978) Effects of acetylcholine and cyclic GMP on input resistance of cortical neurones in awake cats. Brain Res., 158, 373-395.

DIRECT MEASUREMENTS OF cAMP EFFECTS ON MEMBRANE CONDUCTANCE, INTRACELLULAR Ca^{2+} AND pH IN MOLLUSCAN NEURONS

John A. Connor
Philip E. Hockberger

University of Illinois, Urbana, IL
Bell Telephone Laboratories, Murray Hill, NJ

SUMMARY

We have investigated the effects of cAMP on membrane conductances, internal Ca^{2+} levels, and internal pH in 14 identifiable giant neurons of *Archidoris monteryensis*. Injecting cAMP in amounts which should have elevated the internal concentration by 50-200 µM (ignoring possible breakdown) had a strong excitatory effect on all the neurons tested, forcing them into repetitive firing or into a burst generating mode. Heavier doses resulted in a large, reversible depolarization. The membrane mechanism underlying the excitation was a long lasting conductance increase to Na^+ which was induced specifically by cAMP. The pH changes which resulted from cAMP injection were not as stereotyped as the membrane conductance change. The most commonly observed response was a transient acidification which persisted for 10 to 20 minutes following an injection. In some neurons, however, a transient alkalinization occurred. Both responses were within the range of .05 to .1 pH unit change and were graded with the size of the injection. Addition of the phosphodiesterase inhibitor IBMX to the bath before injection of cAMP caused a significant prolongation of both the current and pH responses. Multiwavelength absorbance measurements of the indicator dye, arsenazo III, were used to probe for changes induced by cAMP in resting [Ca^{2+}] or in the characteristics of Ca influx or regulation during electrical activity. We were unable to detect significant changes in any of the above parameters.

INTRODUCTION

The role of cyclic adenosine - 3′:5′ - monophosphate (cAMP) as a second messenger for regulating intracellular processes is widely recognized and a number of findings have implicated its involvement in such things as neural plasticity. There exist, however, relatively few studies which have attempted to measure specific membrane or cytoplasmic changes mediated by the agent under *in vivo* conditions in neurons. In molluscs where most of the *in vivo* work has been done, the effects of cAMP on various identifiable neurons have proven to be quite variable. The compound, or any of several analogs, has an inhibitory action on cell R15 of *Aplysia* (the parabolic burster), apparently causing an increase in membrane potassium conductance (Treistman and Levitan, 1976; Drake and Treistman, 1980). In other neurons from *Aplysia* the effect is excitatory, e.g. the neurosecretory "bag cells" showing an enhancement of a triggered firing pattern with cAMP injection (Kaczmarek and Strumasasser, 1981) while other identifiable neurons are brought from their normally quiescent state into firing by application of the phosphodiesterase inhibitor IBMX (Treistman and Drake, 1979). Pellmar (1981) has reported the induction of a calcium influx following cAMP injection into *Aplysia* cells in two identified clusters of neurons (LB & RB). Both excitatory and inhibitory effects have been reported in neurons from other molluscs as well (Liberman, *et al*., 1975; Treistman and Levitan, 1976; Gillette et al., 1981). Studies on the sensory neuron, R11, from *Aplysia* have indicated a direct role of cAMP in membrane mechanisms underlying behavioral sensitization (Brunelli, et al., 1976; Klein and Kandel, 1978).

This diversity of effects of cAMP, a widely utilized messenger substance, should probably not be surprising given the varied functional characteristics of neurons. It does require, though, that a large population of neurons be examined before general features of the action of this substance can be deduced. In the present study we have examined the effects of elevated cAMP concentrations on membrane conductances, internal Ca^{2+} levels and internal pH in a population of 14 reidentifiable giant neurons located in the various ganglia of the brain of *Archidoris monteryensis*, a marine gastropod.

EXPERIMENTAL METHODS

Experiments were performed on the population of reidentifiable giant neurons of *Archidoris monteryensis* shown diagrammatically in Figure 1. Cell body diameters generally ranged from 300-600 μm. Isolated single ganglia (i.e., pleural, pedal) were used in the recording apparatus with the exception that the cerebral ganglia were left connected to their respective pleural neighbor when the cerebral giants were studied. Standard experimental saline was; 490 mM NaCl, 8mM KCl, 20 mM $MgCl_2$, 30 mM $MgSO_4$, 10 mM CaCl, 5mM $C_6H_{12}O_6$, 10 mM MOPS buffer at pH 7.6. Ganglia were stored in this medium at 9°C until used and were quite stable with regard to their cAMP responses for periods of 1 to 2 days after removal from healthy specimens. In a number of cases the same neuron was examined on two consecutive days. Trypsin was routinely used in the removal of connective tissue and separation of ganglia. In about 10% of the experiments no enzyme treatment was employed. All experiments were carried out at 12°C.

Voltage clamp and dye absorbance experiments have been described elsewhere (Connor, 1979; Ahmed and Connor, 1979, 1980). Recessed tip pH electrodes were fabricated by Thomas' procedure (Thomas, 1978). Electrodes having slopes of 54 to 57 mV and tip diameters of 1 to 2 µm were used for the measurements reported.

cAMP (crystalline free acid, Sigma Chemical, St. Louis, MO) was injected either iontophoretically or by pressure. Pressure injections were calibrated by injecting a mixture of cAMP and arsenazo III, measuring the resulting transneuron absorbance

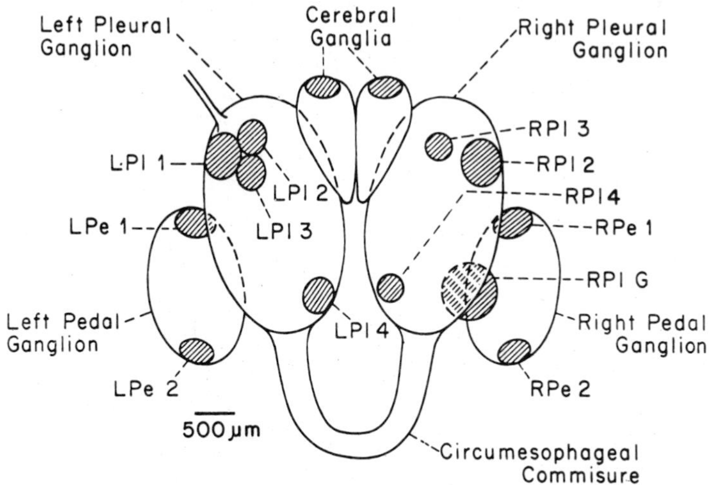

Figure 1: Diagram of Archidoris brain showing usual location and the designation of the 14 giant neurons used in these experiments. White cells are LPL 2 and LPL 3. Calibration bar is appropriate for cells of a large specimen (70 gr.).

change at 570 nm, and calculating the injected amount from this absorbance change and the known extinction coefficient for the dye. (c.f. Ahmed, Kragie & Connor, 1980). Injected amounts of cAMP are reported as "equivalent" concentrations, # moles injected/neuron volume. This measure overestimates the actual concentration change because hydrolysis of cAMP is not taken into account. In several experiments the pH of the injection solution was adjusted over the range 7.0 to 7.9 to check for pH changes resulting directly from the pH of the injected substance. Normally the pH of the injected solutions was 7.2 - 7.3. Absorbance was simultaneously monitored at 700nm, a wavelength at which dye absorbance is very small, in order to detect possible movement artifacts during injection or excessive volume changes.

RESULTS

Figure 2 illustrates an experiment in which three separate injections of cAMP were given to neuron RPl 3. Membrane voltage (V_m) is shown in the top trace while transneuron absorbance at 580 and 700 nm and the difference of these absorbances is shown in the lower 3 traces. Prior to the first injection the repetitive firing characteristics of the neuron were tested by applying a 1nA step of depolarizing current (far left, top trace). The cell responded with a steady train of action potentials at 3 per sec (tonic discharge). This cell was normally quiescent, or nearly so. The cell began firing spontaneously within a few seconds of the start of cAMP injection and continued firing throughout the course of the injection and for several minutes afterward. Injection periods are marked by the horizontal bars located between the 580 and 700 nm absorbance traces. Entry of cAMP/arsenazo into the cell is most clearly shown in the 580-700 nm trace where the absorbance increases as long as the mixture is entering the cell and reaches a plateau as the rate drops to zero.

The second and third injections also produced periods of spontaneous firing with the third injection producing a period of "slow-burst" discharge instead of tonic repetitive firing (see also Heyer and Lux, 1976). An interval of such slow-burst discharge is shown at expanded time and voltage scales in the lower part of the figure. The type of slow-burst discharge we have observed in this set of neurons is different from burst activity in the widely studied R-15 of *Aplysia* in that growing oscillations always precede spike activity, and there are substantially fewer spikes per slow-burst.

The response of the cell to constant current stimulation (1nA) was tested following the first and third injections after the cell had ceased to be spontaneously active. During the first of these tests the cell fired a slowly adapting spike train similar to that observed before injection, whereas it gave slow-burst discharge during the second test (see right hand portion of record). We have examined a total of 131 neurons in the present series of experiments and have divided the population according to the firing pattern developed after the injection of cAMP. Ninety-eight neurons (N_1) developed tonic discharge only while 33 (N_2) showed a tonic discharge followed by a slow-burst pattern, either spontaneously or in response to constant current injection. Thus, injection of cAMP either induced spontaneous firing or increased the spontaneous firing rate in all the neurons. The group N_2 was comprised mostly but not exclusively, of neurons, LPl 1, LPl 4, and RPl 4. While we have not succeeded in determining an exact correspondence between cAMP dose and the type of firing pattern developed, it has become clear that larger doses are required to elicit bursting rather than simple tonic firing even in neurons LP1 1, 4 and RP1 4. Controls for non-specific effects have been tested by injecting 5′AMP, arsenazo

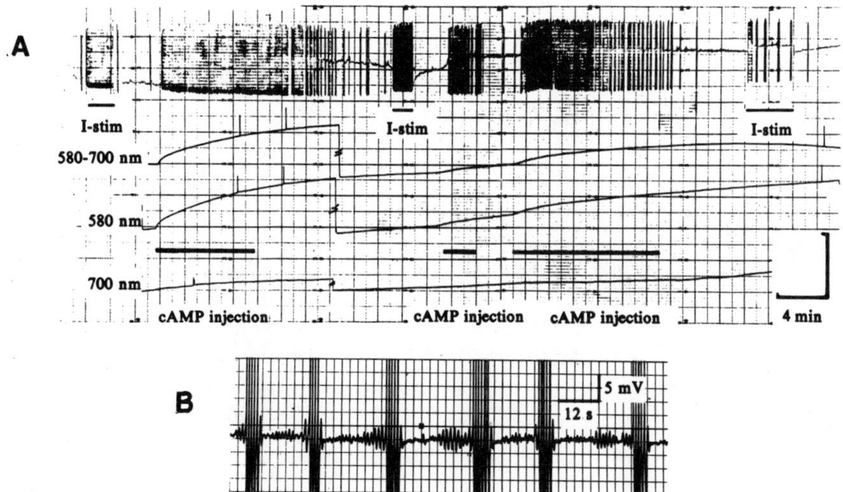

Figure 2A: Effects of cAMP on neural firing pattern. Membrane voltage (V_m) is shown in the top trace. Neuron absorbance at the wavelengths and wavelength pair indicated is shown in the lower three traces. Arsenazo III was injected along with the cAMP so that absorbance increases as the injection proceeds. Periods during which cAMP was injected are indicated by the heavy horizontal bars between the 580 & 700 nm traces. Baselines are reset after the first injection. 2B: High gain record of "slow burst" activity recorded after heavy cAMP injection. Action potentials are severely distorted by the low frequency response of the chart recorder.

III, and 350 mM KCl. None of these controls had an appreciable effect on cell excitability or pH (see below) when injected volumes were up to ten-fold greater than those used in the cAMP injections.

In order to investigate the basis of the increased excitability, cAMP injections were made while the cell was held under voltage clamp. This allows changes in net membrane current to be measured and also eliminates internal [Ca^{2+}] and pH changes which occur during periods of spike activity (cf. Ahmed and Connor, 1979, 1980). The experiments of Figures 3 and 4 were run with V_m clamped at -40 mV (near the normal resting potential) and with an intracellular pH electrode in place.

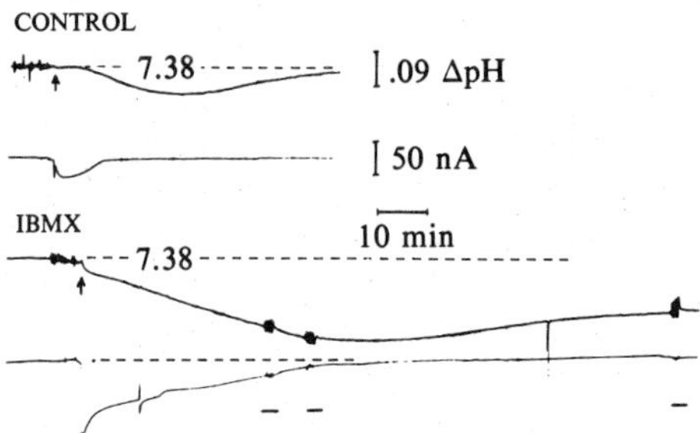

Figure 3: Internal pH (upper traces) and membrane current (lower traces) under voltage clamp following a pressure injection of cAMP. Arrows indicate when pressure pulse was applied. A: control. B: after exposure to 1mM IBMX. Short horizontal bars denote normal saline washes. The concentration equivalent of total injected cAMP was .8 mM in A and 1.7 mM in B. Cell: RPe 1.

Figure 3A illustrates one of two types of membrane current-internal pH response to cAMP injection. There is a rapidly developing net inward current which persists for several minutes and would drive the cell into repetitive firing if it were not held in voltage clamp. This current is more than large enough to account for repetitive firing like that shown in Figure 2. In the record of Figure 3A as in most, there is a reversible acidification following cAMP injection, characterized by a rapid and a slow phase. At present we regard the more rapid phase as an artifact which arises from a pH mismatch of injection fluid (7.2) and cytoplasmic pH (usually 7.3-7.4). The cellular response, the slower phase, does not develop until long after the injection period; in many cases the injection electrode had been removed from the neuron before this phase of the response got underway. Both the inward current and the pH response magnitudes were graded with injection size. In all the records obtained, the current response developed before the pH change with most of the pH change occurring during the recovery phase of the current or after the current had returned nearly to baseline.

Although the magnitudes of both the current and pH responses were graded with injection size, a considerable degree of variation existed in some cases between responses elicited by approximately equivalent injections into the same neuron. For example repeated doses which varied by no more than $\pm$20% (as estimated from $\Delta A_{570-690}$) often gave rise to inward currents which varied by as much as 50%. Generally there was a progressive increase. Due to these variatons we have been unable to derive a standard dose-response curve for either the current or pH.

Figure 3B illustrates behavior of the same neuron as in Fig. 3A when a comparable cAMP injection was preceded by a 20 min exposure to the phosphodiesterase (PDE) inhibitor IBMX (10^{-3} M). Under these conditions both current and pH responses are prolonged with pH recovery facilitated following several normal saline washes. It should be noted that the maximum internal pH change is considerably larger, in IBMX not so much because the rate of change is greater but because the acidification continues at a steady rate for a far longer time in the presence of IBMX. We assume that this type of result reflects the condition of a prolonged elevation in internal [cAMP]; its hydrolysis having been blocked, the injected cAMP is able to modulate the processes responsible for the pH change for a longer period of time. This observation would also seem to rule out the possibility that a significant portion of the pH change simply reflects the breakdown of cAMP since this rate should be greatly retarded by the PDE inhibitor IBMX.

Figure 4 illustrates the behavior often found in the two white pigmented giant neurons of the left pleural ganglion and on occasion in the twelve orange pigmented cells. The injection of cAMP produced a net inward current, but gave rise to an initial alkalinization which may or may not be followed by an acidification. It can be seen that the time relationship between the two parameters, current and pH, is similar in both categories of cell. None of the effects shown in Figures 3 and 4 was seen if like amounts of buffered 5′ AMP, arsenazo III, 5′AMP + 350 mM KCl were injected instead of cAMP.

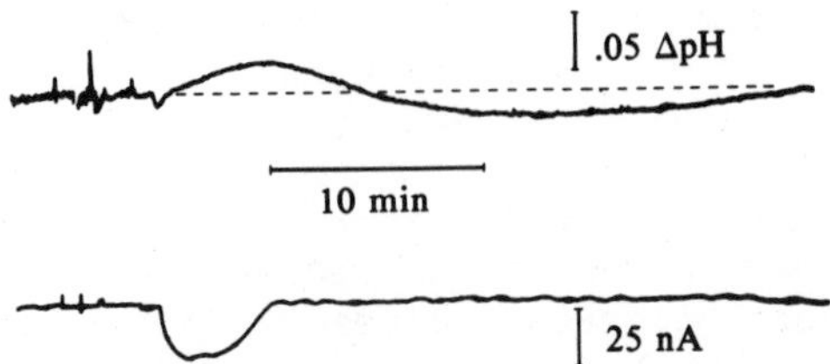

Figure 4: Internal pH (upper traces) and membrane current (lower traces) under voltage clamp following a pressure injection (arrow) of cAMP. Injected concentration equivalent of cAMP was 3.5 mM. Cell: RPe 1.

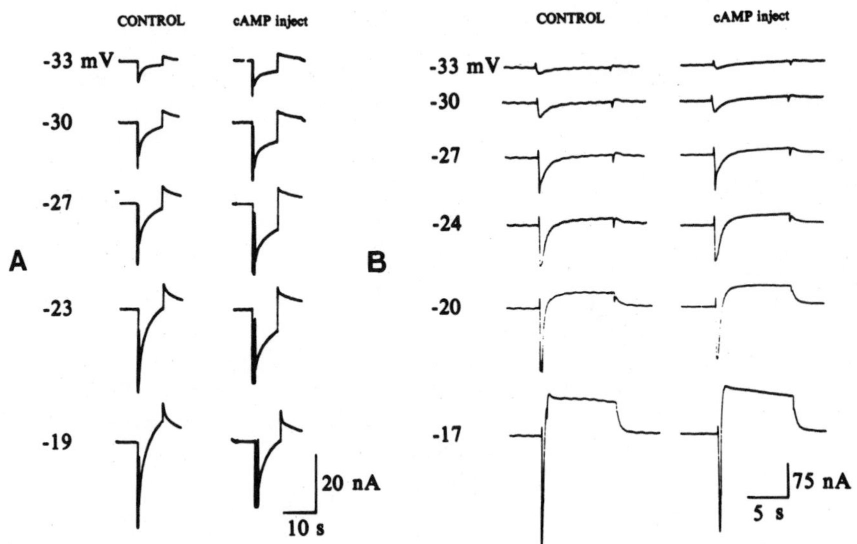

Figure 5: Voltage clamp currents illustrating the two general categories of conductance behavior. A: Negative slope resistance displayed under control conditions (left column). Injection of cAMP increases net inward current (right column). B: Cell without NSR (left column) showing small increase in outward current following injection (right column).

Removal of Na from the external bathing medium (replacement with either Tris-methane or tetramethylammonium) reversibly abolished the inward current. On the other hand where Ca was replaced by Mg we were unable to detect significant changes in inward current induced by cAMP. However, the responses were generally variable enough under control conditions to make it impossible to rule out a minor contribution of calcium current to the total. The pH changes persisted in the zero Na runs, and we would conclude though that the membrane current responses and the pH changes were not coupled.

The effects of cAMP on membrane currents activated by step voltage clamps are complex and variable in detail. The clearest, most consistent effects were observed in spontaneously firing cells where the current-voltage (I-V) curves showed a negative slope resistance (NSR) region for long clamp pulses; that is, for small positive voltage steps (5 to 20 mV) from the resting potential, membrane current was inward instead of outward. Voltage clamp records of this type are shown in Figure 5A (left column) and the corresponding I-V curves in Figure 6A. In these cells the effect of cAMP was always to increase the net inward current during small clamp steps. This step response current was measured relative to the prestep current baseline, which was not necessarily zero I_m for -40mV holding potentials. The step response increase was greatest during the period of steady inward current flow (c.f. Figures 3 and 4) but in many cases persisted for several minutes after the steady current had decayed. The records of Figure 5A (right column) were taken from one such cell. Ion substitution and pharmacological studies have been carried out and indicate that the inward current induced by cAMP, both the steady current and the increase during voltage clamp pulses is carried by Na^+.

About 50% of the total neuron population tested did not show a slow NSR; rather, the membrane current quickly became outward following a voltage step, as illustrated in Figure 5B and 6B. In these cells the net effect of cAMP was to increase the outward current, Figure 5B (right column). We have not been able to sort out the more basic changes in current underlying this net effect as yet. That is, even in cells where the total I_m records are like those of Figure 5B, one can demonstrate the presence of a rather constant inward current (c.f. Connor, 1979) which is simply of smaller size than the outward current carried by other channels. We have tentatively concluded that the characteristics of both inward and outward current carrying channels may be altered as a result of cAMP injection and where outward current dominates the slow voltage clamp records, any effect on inward current is masked.

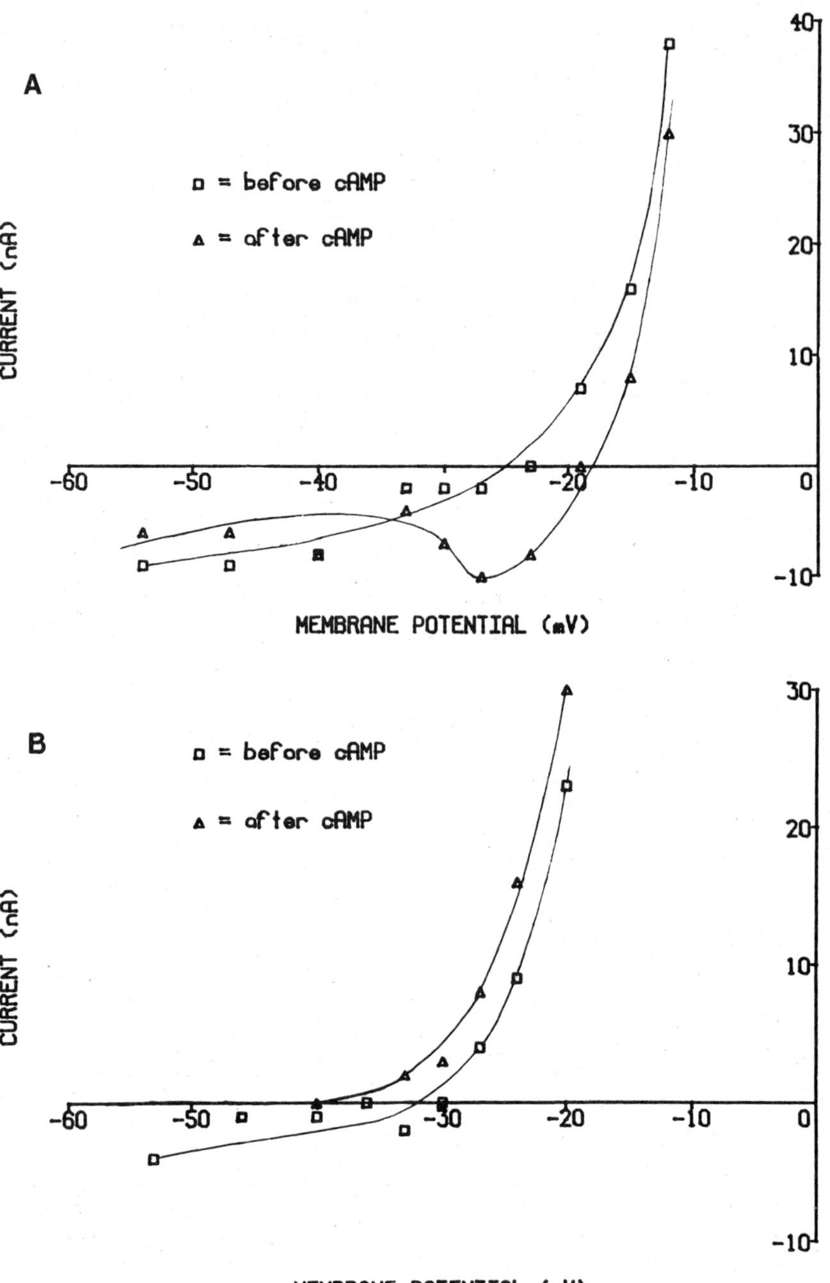

Figure 6: I-V relations constructed from the data of Figure 5 reading membrane current at the end of the voltage clamp pulses.

We found that the 4 pedal ganglion neurons studied almost invariably showed a NSR while LP1 4, RP1 4, and LP1 1 generally did not. The remaining neurons were observed to fall into either category an appreciable fraction of the time. Since the effect of cAMP seemed to be a strengthening of either type of characteristic (NSR or non-NSR) rather than a conversion from one characteristic to another, it appears unlikely that the nucleotide is directly involved in establishing the variability seen in the individual neurons. It should be noted that the cells which were capable of displaying a slow-burst firing mode were characterized by a non-NSR I-V relation.

Using the indicator arsenazo III, we have looked for changes in $[Ca^{2+}]_i$ and Ca influx which might be brought about by increased $[cAMP]_i$. It seemed reasonable to expect such changes given the extensive literature linking these two important second messengers in a variety of cells. Figure 7 illustrates the sensitivity of the arsenazo III detection for changes in internal $[Ca^{2+}]$. In Figure 7A membrane voltage was held at -60 mV for several minutes to establish an absorbance baseline and then stepped to -40 mV. These voltages are in the range of normal resting potentials for _Archidoris_ neurons and at least 10 mV more negative than the action potential threshold. There is a clear absorbance increase at 660 nm, the wavelength at which the difference spectrum for the Ca-arsenzao complex is maximum _in situ_, indicating a rise in $[Ca^{2+}]_i$. If one assumes that the change in $[Ca^{2+}]$ is uniform within the cell, the signal represents approximately a 150 nM change in $[Ca^{2+}]$. The initial concentration is partially restored over several minutes after V_m is returned to -60 mV. We often noted only partial recovery of the absorbance signal following small changes of $[Ca^{2+}]$ in both single wavelength measurements, as shown in the figure, or with dual wavelength measurements (660 - 690 nm). We are uncertain what this latter observation may mean. The second record of Figure 7A shows a larger ΔA associated with a voltage step to -33 mV. In this case there is nearly complete recovery following return of the voltage to -60 mV. We were not able to demonstrate subthreshold Ca influx in all the neurons of our population. Figure 7B shows the absorbance increase recorded from LPe 2 when external [Ca] was increased from 10 to 30 mM, while Figure 7C illustrates the small decrease in ΔA when this same cell was exposed to nominally Ca-free saline. Different neurons showed differing abilities to regulate $[Ca]_i$ in the face of changes in extracellular [Ca]. Some neurons showed almost no increase in Ca_i^{2+} with 10 to 20 min exposures to high external [Ca].

The injection of cAMP, while it produced an indicator absorbance decrease at 660 nm, also caused a larger absorbance decrease at 610 nm, a wavelength where dye absorbance is predominantly pH sensitive because of the binding and debinding

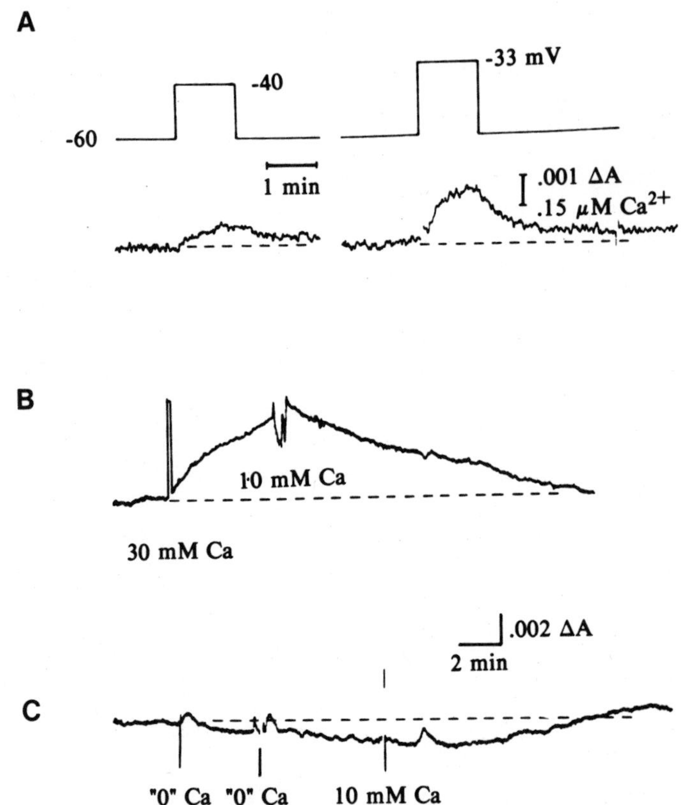

Figure 7: A - Voltage (upper) and absorbance (lower) records showing the increase of Ca^{2+} during subthreshold voltage changes. Single wavelength absorbance (λ = 660 nm) shown. The absorbance trace was given a downward offset between the two pulses. B - Absorbance changes resulting from a transient change of [Ca] in external saline from 10 to 30 mM. Solution changes are indicated by arrows and are accompanied by large transient offsets in the optical trace. C: Absorbance decrease resulting from exposure to nominally Ca-free saline. Two bath exchanges of "0" Ca were given.

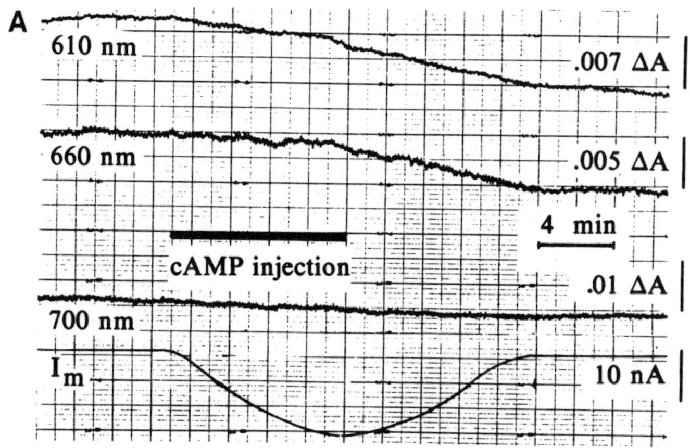

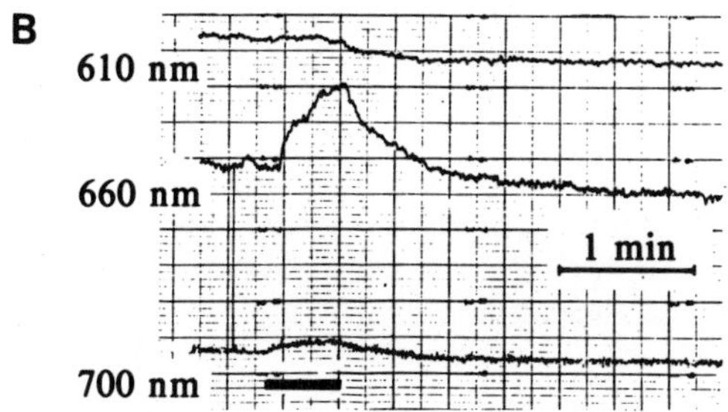

Figure 8: A - Triple wavelength measurements of arsenazo III absorbance changes (upper traces) during and after iontophoretic injection of cAMP. Injection period indicated by horizontal bar. Simultaneous membrane current under voltage clamp has been plotted in the bottom trace. The optical density of arsenzo is small at 700 nm and the 700 nm signal is included as a control for light scattering and incident beam intensity changes. B: Records at the same 3 wavelengths taken during (horizontal bar) and after a train of spikes elicited by current stimulation. Period of spike activity indicated by horizontal bar. Spike frequency approximately 0.5/s. Calibrations same as Part A.

of Mg. Figure 8 illustrates a record typical of data from a total of 35 neurons. Iontophoretic injection of cAMP was employed for these measurements making the delivery time longer than for the pressure injections of Figures 3 and 4 and the dose somewhat smaller. It can be seen that during the period when inward current is maximally activated there is relatively little change in either the 660 or 610 nm absorbance signal indicating either that $[Ca^{2+}]$ and pH are both constant or that both are

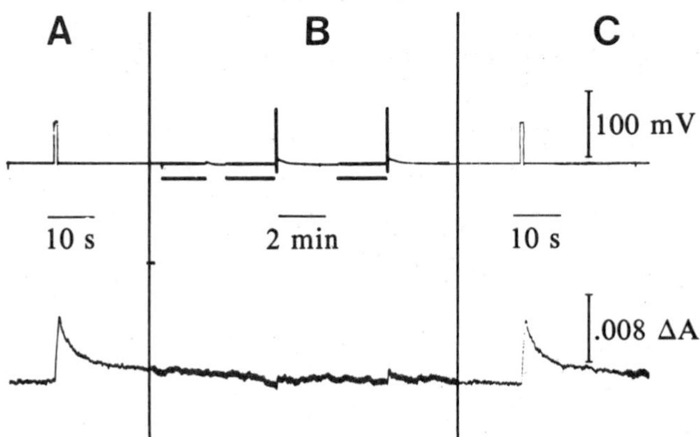

Figure 9: A and C - Arsenzo III absorbance changes at 660 nm (lower trace) generated by identical voltage clamp pulses (upper trace) before and after iontophoretic injections of cAMP. The two records are nearly identical indicating no change in Ca^{2+} influx or regulation characteristics. B: Absorbance and voltage records during cAMP injection. Bars underlining the voltage trace indicate 3 periods of iontophoretic injection. Following each injection period voltage clamp was discontinued. The 2nd and 3rd injections were followed by a burst of action potentials. Record B is contiguous with A while two additional injections were interposed between the end of record B and the start of record C.

changing in exactly a manner to produce a null (e.g., $[Ca^{2+}]$ is increasing and pH decreasing or the converse). However, this possibility is unlikely since independent pH measurements made with glass electrodes show that pH is nearly constant during like iontophoretic injection periods. The "delayed" pH decrease discussed in connection with Figure 3 occurred in this neuron also and is indicated by the delayed decrease in dye absorbance at 610 and 660 nM.

Figure 9 shows arsenazo response data for voltage clamp pulses before and after iontophoretic injections of cAMP. The pulses (shown in 9A and C) were of 1 sec duration to +25 mV and the Ca influx generated a sizeable absorbance changed (λ = 660 nm). It can be seen that the magnitude of the absorbance change as well as the recovery time course are nearly the same before and after the injections. Part B illustrates the dye absorbance during a period when 3 separate injections were given (horizontal bars under the voltage trace). Following each injection the voltage clamp loop was opened allowing voltage to vary freely. A brief period of spike activity and depolarization followed the 2nd and 3rd injections, illustrating the usual excitatory effect of cAMP. The dye absorbance remains relatively constant throughout the injection period with small transient increases occurring during the spike activity.

DISCUSSION

The results presented here have demonstrated that raising cytoplasmic levels of cAMP in a defined set of neurons leads to the generation of a steady inward sodium current, complicated changes in voltage dependent conductances, and the modulation of cellular processes involved in H^+ generation or pumping. This is the first example of which we are aware where cAMP has been shown to affect membrane sodium conductance, most other preparations showing effects on potassium or calcium conductances. Our data indicate that the conductance changes are not directly related to the pH changes since (1) a pH response occurs in sodium free media where there is no inward current, and (2) since the normal inward current response has been noted to occur in conjuction with either an acidification or alkalinization (c.f. Figure 3,4). At present we have no data to suggest what processes in particular are causing the pH changes. We have noted that the generally observed acidificaiton does not seem to be a simple reflection of cAMP breakdown since the pH changes become much larger when PDE activity is inhibited (c.f. figure 4). The buffering power of these neurons for H^+ is considerable, i.e. in the neighborhood of 10-20 mEq/unit pH (Ahmed and Connor, 1980; see also Thomas, 1976); therefore a pH change of 0.1 unit reflects a rather large change in total H^+ evolution. The data of Figure 3 might also serve as a cautionary note, in that, where PDE inhibitors or non-hydrolysible analogs of cAMP are employed, there are quite probably significant pH changes occuring in the cytoplasm.

Most of the results shown here have been for relatively large injected amounts of cAMP (0.1 - 1.0 mM) in order that a robust effect on conductance or pH might be illustrated. Changes in physiological activity, such as spontaneous firing rates, were detectible with much smaller injections. For example the 0.8 mM injected quantity of Figure 3A produced an inward current change of approximately 30 nA, whereas 1 to 2 nA of steady inward current is sufficient in most cases to drive a quiescent neuron into repetitive firing (see Figure 2). We are unable to relate injected amounts of cAMP to actual concentration changes in the cytoplasm because the rate at which the compound is broken down is unknown. We suspect however that the time course of [cAMP] elevation is directly mirrored by the time course of the inward membrane current due to the persisitence of this current when PDE activity has been inhibited - e.g. by IBMX in Figure 3 or when slowly hydrolyzed analogs such as dibutyryl-cAMP are injected (unpublished data). If this is true then most of the cAMP injected, even by the large pressure pulses illustrated here, is broken down within 5 to 10 minutes.

As illustrated in Figures 8 and 9 there is very little effect of cAMP injection on internal free calcium concentrations under the experimental conditions used. While this result can mean either that there are truly no direct effects on Ca^{2+} regulation or transport systems, or that the measurement system is not sufficiently sensitive, it should be noted that increased [cAMP] will have a large effect on internal calcium levels under more physiological conditions (given some of the observations presented here and elsewhere). That is, the steady sodium current induced by cAMP, if large enough, will cause a neuron to fire action potentials, each of which briefly opens voltage dependent calcium channels in the cell membrane and allows Ca influx. This phenomenon has been extensively studied (c.f. Hagiware, 1973), and in molluscan giant neurons the incremental changes in [Ca^{2+}] have been followed using the Ca-luminescent protein, aequorin, as well as arsenazo III (c.f. Stinnarke and Tauc, 1973; Chang, Gelperin, and Johnson, 1974; Gorman and Thomas, 1978; Ahmed and Connor, 1979). Even if the sodium current induced by cAMP is insufficient to cause action potential discharge but only subthreshold depolarization, data such as that shown in Figure 7 would indicate that one would expect Ca increases in some neurons.

ACKNOWLEDGEMENTS

That part of the work performed at the University of Illinois was supported by NIH grants NS15186 and 2T32GM07143.

BIBLIOGRAPHY

1. Ahmed, Z., and Connor, J. A. (1979). "Measurement of Calcium Influx under Voltage Clamp in Molluscan Neurons using the Metallochromic Dye Arsenazo III." J. Physiol. 286, 61-82.

2. Ahmed, Z., and Connor, J. A. (1980). "Intracellular pH Changes Induced by Calcium Influx During Electrical Activity in Molluscan Neurons." J. Gen. Physiol. 75, 403-426

3. Ahmed, Z., Kragie, L., and Connor, J. A. (1980). "Stoichiometry and Apparent Dissociation Constant of the Calcium-Arsenazo III Reaction under Physiological Conditions." Biophys. J. 32, 907-920.

4. Brunelli, M., Castellucci, V., and Kandel, E. R. (1976). "Synaptic Facilitation and Behavioral Sensitization in Aplysia: Possible Role of Serotonin and Cyclic AMP." Science 194, 1178-1181.

5. Chang, J., Gelperin, A., and Johnson, F. (1974). "Intracellularly Injected Aequorin Detects Transmembrane Calcium Flux During Action Potentials in an Identified Neuron from the Terrestrial Slug, Limax Maximus." Brain Res. 77, 431-442.

6. Connor, J. A. (1979). "Calcium Current in Molluscan Neurons: Measurement under Conditions which Maximize its Visibility." J. Physiol. 286, 41-60.

7. Drake, P., and Treistman, S., (1980). "Alteration of Neuronal Activity in Response to Cyclic Nucleotide Agents in Aplysia." J. Neurobiology 11, 471-482.

8. Gillette, R., Gillette, M., and Davis, W. J. (1982). "cAMP Activates Command Function in a Feeding Neuron of Pleurobranchia." J. Comp. Physiol. B (in press).

9. Gorman, A. L. F. and Thomas, M. V. (1978). "Changes in the Intracellular Concentration of Free Calcium Ions in a Pace-Maker Neurone, Measured with the Metallochromic Indicator Dye Arsenazo III." J. Physiol 275, 357-376.

10. Hagiwara, S. (1973). "Ca Spike." Advan. in Biophys. 4, 71-102.

11. Heyer, C. and Lux, H. D. (1976). "Properties of a Facilitating Calcium Current in Pacemaker Neurones of the Snail, Helix pomatia." J. Physiol. 262, 319-348.

12. Klein, M., and Kandel, E. R., (1978). "Presynaptic Modulation of Voltage-Dependent Ca^{+2} Current: Mechanism for Behavioral Sensitization in Aplysia Californica." PNAS (USA) 75, 3512-3516.

13. Kaczmarek, L. K., and Strumwasser, F. (1981). "The Expression of long-lasting Afterdischarge by Isolated *Aplysia* Bag Cell Neurons." *J. Neuroscience* 1, 626-634.

14. Liberman, Y. A., Minima, S. and Golubtsov, K., (1975). "The Study of Metabolic Synapse. I. Effect of Intracellular Microinjection of 3′, 5′-AMP." *Biofizika* 20, 451-456.

15. Pellmar, T. (1981). "Ionic Mechanism of a Voltage-Dependent Current Elicited by Cyclic AMP." *Cell Mol. Neurobiol.* 1, 87-97.

16. Stinnakre, J., and Tauc, L. (1973). "Calcium Influx in Active *Aplysia* Neurons Detected by Injected Aequorin." *Nature New Biol.* 242, 113-115.

17. Thomas, R. C. (1976). "The Effect of Carbon Dioxide on the Intracellular pH and Buffering Power of Snail Neurones." *J. Physiol.* 255, 715-735.

18. Thomas, R. C. (1978). "Ion Sensitive Intracellular Microelectrodes." Academic Press, London.

19. Treistman, S., and Levitan, I. (1976). "Alteration of Electrical Activity in Molluscan Neurones by Cyclic Nucleotides and Peptide Factors." *Nature* 261. 62-64.

20. Treistman, S., and Drake, P. (1979). "The Effects of Cyclic Nucleotide Agents on Neurons in *Aplysia*." *Brain Research* 168, 643-647.

CELLULAR BASIS OF OPERANT-CONDITIONING OF LEG POSITION

Graham Hoyle

Department of Biology
University of Oregon
Eugene, Oregon

SUMMARY

Leg position learning is accomplished rapidly and successfully by insect thoracic ganglia in operant-conditioning paradigms using either negative or positive reinforcements. This opens up the possibility of analysis of the cellular mechanisms underlying learning and retention because the neurons are relatively few in number, identifiable and repeatedly addressable. Starting with positions controlled by single identified motorneurons we find that these are changed in relation to reinforcement either by very long-lasting frequency shifts or by adjustment of the strength and repetition interval of spontaneously-occurring plateau movements, depending on the paradigm. Postural change is accomplished by altered resistance of a motorneuron, specifically associated with potassium conductance. The resistance range is from 3-10 MΩ, with associated mean frequency range of 5-30 Hz. Only goal-related inputs lead to postural shifts, by way of association of reinforcement with efference or afference memory.

CAPABILITIES OF POSTURAL LEARNING BY INSECTS

A variety of tethered insects (Horridge, 1962; Hoyle, 1965; Eisenstein, 1972; Tosney & Hoyle, 1977) and some crustaceans (Hoyle, 1976) learn to alter the position of a single joint when this is coupled to a reinforcement. Negative reinforcement in the form of aversive electric shocks has been used most commonly, but natural ones such as loud noises are also very effective (Hoyle, 1980). The average time taken to learn avoidance is much less than that taken to learn a reward in the form of food brought mechanically to the mouth, or desirable temperature regulated by a heat lamp. The difficulty of the task is proportional to the extent of displacement from the preferred, or most frequently-occupied position. It is also proportional to the narrowness of the limits by which the position is defined, i.e. the angular position within which the reinforcement occurs. Extension is more difficult than flexion, which is the natural defense posture. Animals seldom learn a highly extended position that is sufficient to generate a strong resistance reflex if this is the initial task, but they do learn it quickly if first trained to a more moderate one in the same direction.

Some 'smart' individuals learn simpler aversive tasks with a single trial: the 'dullest' require many trials. The learning of a position in which aversive stimuli are avoided is lost without savings if reinforcement is omitted even a single time. This is not the case in food reward learning. If the insect finds a position in which food comes automatically to its mouth, this position is not held indefinitely so that food is available continually. Instead, the desired position is adopted for a few minutes only, once or twice every hour. This type of movement is termed a plateau movement (PM) from its appearance on a chart record of position. Such movements are made randomly in untrained animals, but very infrequently and with a wide range of plateau (position) levels. In training in the presence of the reward the insect first makes PMs more frequently, then 'experiments' with the plateau position until the correct one has been found. This is then repeated and accompanied by steady feeding.

Warmth may be used either as a simple reward, with a distant heat source for an animal placed in a cold room, or as a combined reward/punishment by placing the heat source so close to the insect it will be cooked if left on (Hoyle, 1979, 1980). Since the insect has control over the heat by adopting the coupled posture only periodically, it can in principle learn to thermoregulate. In practice locusts learn both constant heat reward and thermoregulation very quickly and very efficiently. No individual has yet died in our laboratory as a result of failing to learn heat regulation, even when the minimum safe period was as little as 5 minutes.

The learning is quickly changed not only in the same positional direction, but also in the reverse one, provided there is no break in the reinforcement regime, merely a shift from one position to another. Position as such is not a necessary variable. The insect learns equally quickly to adjust the antagonist motorneuron outputs, whose mean frequencies are the principal determinants of position, when these are coupled to the reinforcement rather than angular position (Hoyle, 1966). In these experiments the leg is held fixed or even cut off and the motor output recorded. These experiments proved that the insect can use a memory of the central nervous efference copy, the efference memory (Hoyle, 1982) of its fluctuating output, to adjust subsequent motor output, in relation to the reinforcement.

Two basic mechanisms are available for postural adjustment and used either singly or co-operatively. The insect is able to alter basic tonus (BT) by mechanisms which are not understood, that are neurally-controlled but not driven by conventional neuromuscular excitation. However, this is limited to weak adjustments. Stronger ones required altering the mean frequency of discharge in specific tonic motorneurons (MNs).

What makes the above results especially significant to the cellular neurophysiologist is that, as Horridge (1962) first discovered with flexion to avoid electric shock, the insects learn the task faster, and with far fewer errors, when the head has been cut off. The learning changes are taking place within the single ganglion that contains the MN cell bodies (Eisenstein & Cohen, 1965). The third thoracic ganglion of locusts proved to be amenable to intracellular studies that were greatly facilitated by the introduction of intracellular dye techniques at about this time. In less than a decade a majority of the MNs had been mapped (Hoyle, 1975) and a start had been made on locating and examining the antecedent interneurons (Burrows & Siegler, 1978). The principal muscle involved in adjusting the position of the entire leg is the anterior adductor of the coxa (AAdC), which turned out to be innervated by a single excitatory MN (Fig. 1)

The Location of the Cellular Change is in the Motorneuron

A computer-controlled electric shock paradigm developed by Tosney and Hoyle (1977) permitted automatic entrainment of AAdC, or

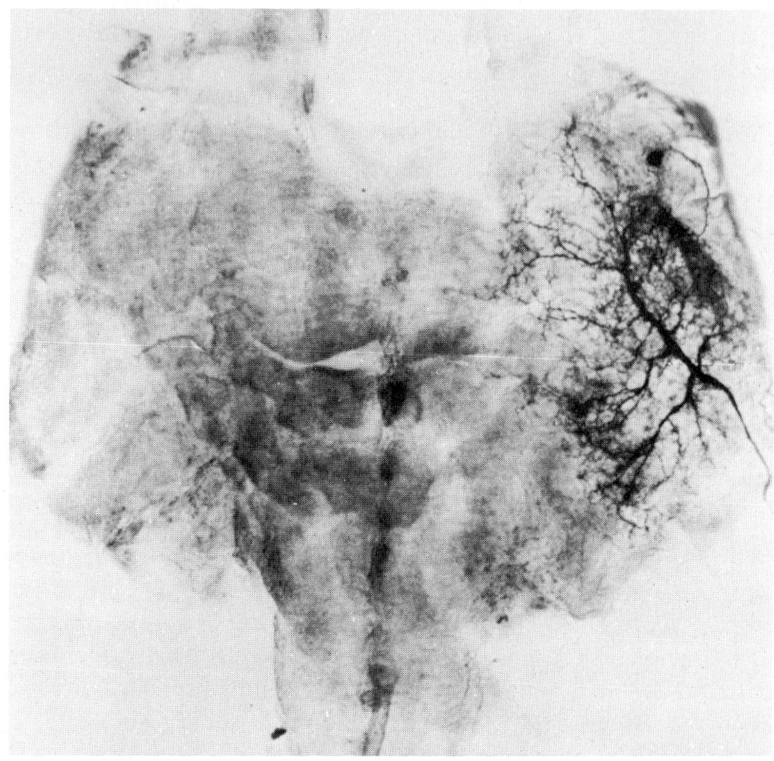

Fig. 1. Cobalt fill (intensified) of AAdC motorneuron, the sole excitor of the coxal adductor muscle used to raise the whole leg in electric shock avoidance. From Hoyle, 1980.

indeed any other tonic MN. It may be used to either increase (up-training mode) or decrease (down-training mode) mean frequency. Once trained, the frequency remains at the new level for up to a few hours without, and indefinitely with, continued reinforcement. This can then be used to train the neuron under conditions that permit intracellular and ganglion manipulation. The natural output is highly erratic, with large fluctuations in interval between successive inputs, though the mean is fairly steady. Following training the mean alters and also becomes quite steady, especially in up-training (Fig. 2). Intracellular recording revealed that sort-term fluctuations are due to the erratic occurrence of single large EPSPs and IPSPs onto the MN. When this input was blocked by infusion into the ganglion of high Mg^{++}/low Ca^{++} saline the discharge became extremely regular, but without any significant change in the mean in many cells (Fig. 3). This meant that the MN has intrinsic pacemaker capability.

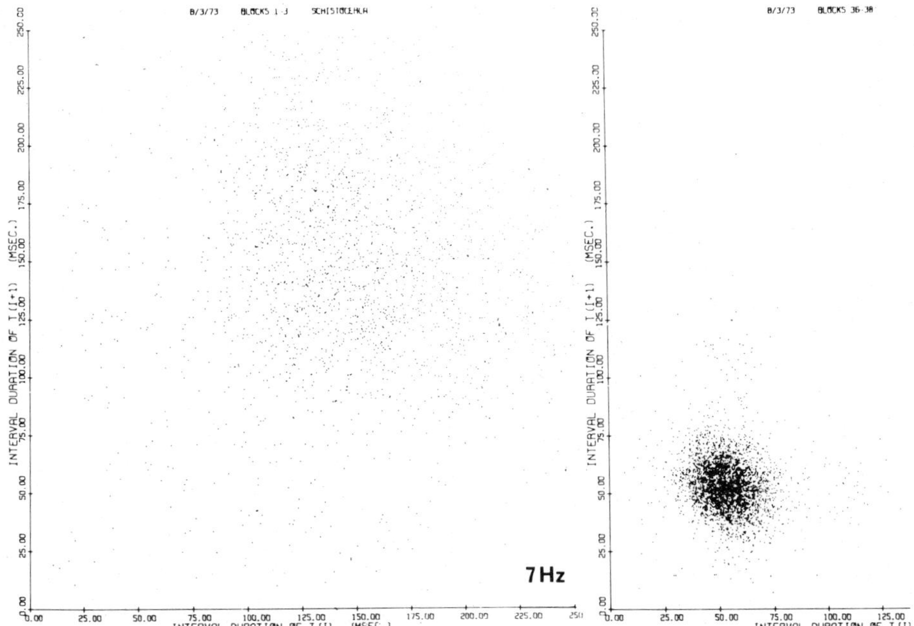

Fig. 2. Left: computer plot of T + 1 against T intervals of naive preparation firing at 7 Hz.
Right: computer plot of T + 1 against T intervals of naive preparation firing for a similar time following a single period of computer-controlled up-training. From Hoyle, 1982.

When the pacemaker rate was determined, first before training, then after, it was found to have shifted stably to a value equal to the new mean frequency. Therefore, either the learning change occurs within the MN itself, or is transferred to it: in the final event it is embodied within the cell in such a way as to alter its pacemaking.

Nature of the Cellular Event

We then set out to determine the nature of the cellular event(s) underlying the pacemaker shift, and also to try to locate any antecedent interneuron that might be bringing it about. From the MN frequency records we knew that when the critical event is triggered it follows an exponential time-course, being substantially complete in about 3 s. An interneuron was located by Dr. Malcolm Burrows (1978), that

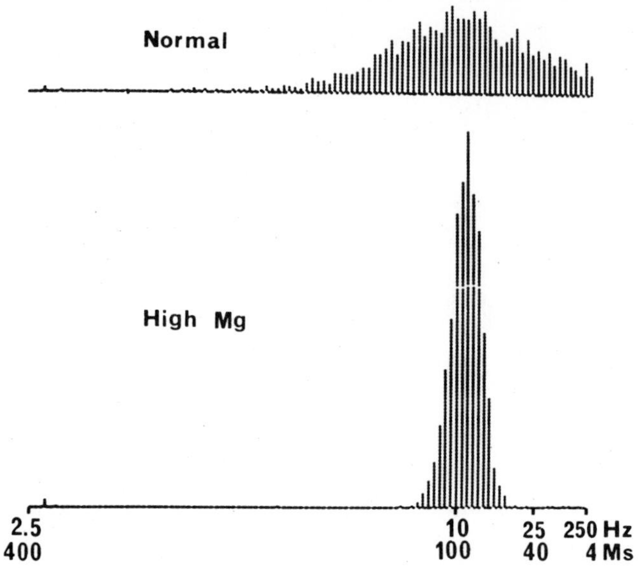

Fig. 3. Pacemaker aspect of AAdC. Above: graphics computer record of distribution of intervals between succeeding impulses with the ganglion bathed in normal saline. Below: same after infusion of high Mg^{++}/low Ca^{++} saline into the ganglion (under its sheath) until all synaptic activity onto the neuron was blocked. From Woollacott & Hoyle, 1977.

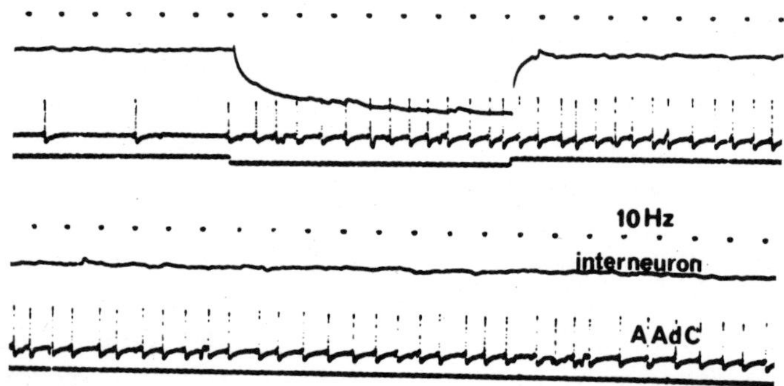

Fig. 4. Non-spiking interneuron that leads to relatively long-lasting change in frequency of AAdC MN following a brief hyperpolarization. Courtesy of Dr. M. Burrows, unpublished.

can bring about a long-lasting change in AAdC frequency (Fig. 4). This is a non-spiking interneuron and it is especially interesting that this cell is effective by being briefly hyperpolarized: there is no change when it is hyperpolarized. However, the change it produces is abrupt compared with the exponential one with a time-constant of 1.2 s (Fig. 5) seen in learning, and not nearly as long-lasting as the learning event. The critical cell(s) has (have) yet to be discovered.

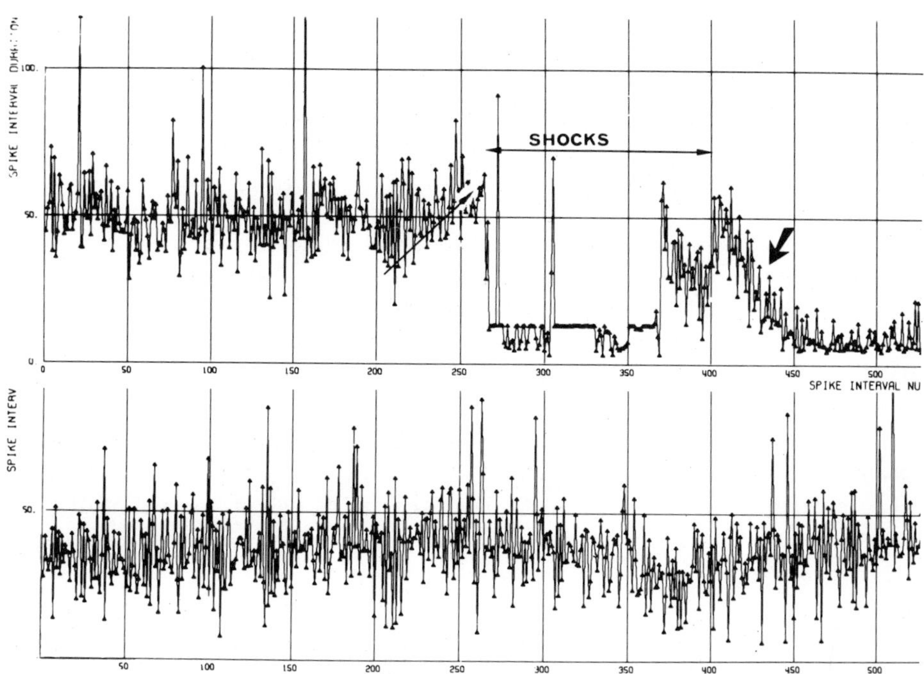

Fig. 5. Above: time-course of frequency change, indicated by heavy arrow, occurring as a result of aversive shocks delivered by computer that were correlated with statistically significant increments in frequency. Spike interval duration (ordinate), plotted by computer, as a function of spike interval number. Up-training was applied starting at the small arrow. Initial mean frequency 20 Hz.
Below: sample of intervals taken during stable period at the new higher mean frequency, which was 28 Hz.
Plotted by Dr. James Sidey from taped data of Tosney & Hoyle, 1977.

Unfortunately it has turned out to be a very frustrating (and ulcerating) event to track. With each stage in manipulation -- opening the thorax, setting up the ganglion, infusion of saline, penetration of the ganglion with a microelectrode, and determining the resistance of the cell by passing various strengths of constant-current pulses into it -- the learning ability was impaired. Nevertheless, we have obtained values for resistance in both before- and after-training only, resistance testing, and with also continuous pulsing (Fig. 6). These were the least successful in up- and down-learning. We did these tests with double-barreled soma electrodes, but have so far failed to obtain satisfactory voltage clamping.

However, the results were all both consistent and surprising. During up-training the resistance increased and during down-training it decreased. The mean slope was 0.50 M Ω /Hz. The resistances of naive animals having different mean frequencies naturally fall on a slope that is not greatly different, 0.33 M Ω /Hz.

There is a major change in the soma action potential shape during training (Fig. 7). At low frequencies (5-15 Hz) there is a very large, slow undershoot of 5-6 mV, though the spike remnant is a mere 5-7 mV. The change is progressively greater with further increase in frequency, until the undershoot entirely disappears at about 30 Hz (Fig. 8).

Conversely, the undershoot is small or absent in cells discharging naturally at a high frequency (30-40 Hz), but it appears in association with training. The undershoot of a slowly-firing cell is immediately lost following intracellular injection of TEA or extracellular permeation with γ-amino pyridine.

The change is therefore due to altered gK, and this could be the final event determining the altered pacemaking. It acts simply by the effect of gK on E_M, following the Nernst relation. The pacemaker frequency is directly proportional to the difference between $E_{M(A)}$, the resting potential in the axon near the impulse initiation zone (IIZ), and $E_{M(IIZ)}$ which is lower. IIZ is located within the ganglion, fairly close to both the main dendritic field and the soma. Any change in gK of either the soma, the dendrites, or both, alters $E_{M(IIZ)}$. Current flows from the axon through IIZ in proportion to the local difference in E_M which in turn determines the frequency.

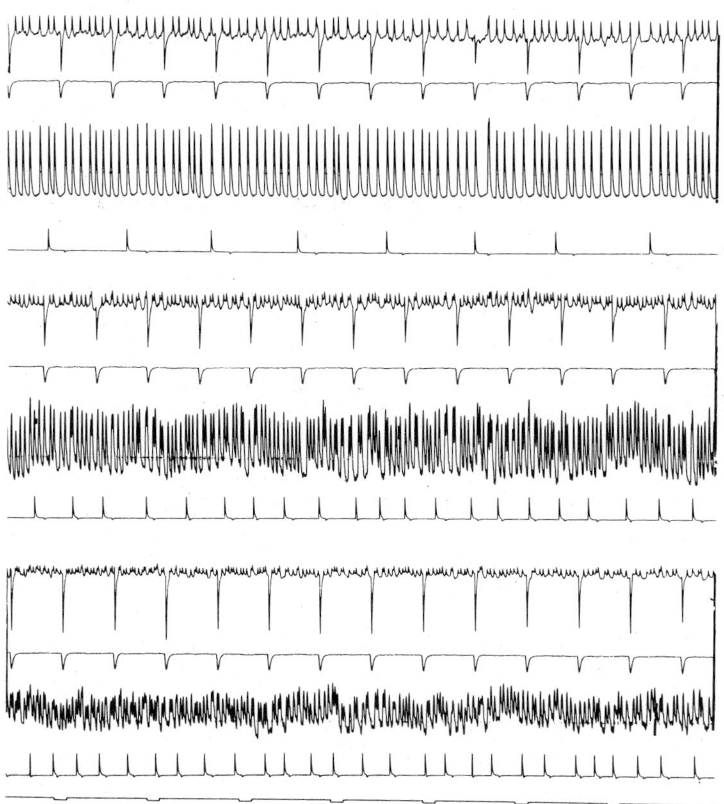

Fig. 6. Intracellular recordings from the AAdC soma (top traces), with continuous constant-current pulses (current monitored on middle traces). Lower traces are intracellular recordings from AAdC muscle cell.
TOP: Naive preparation
MIDDLE: After first session of up-training
BOTTOM: After second session of up-training
Note increasing resistance and changed shape of intracellular MN action potentials (see Figs. 7 & 8).
From Hoyle, 1982.

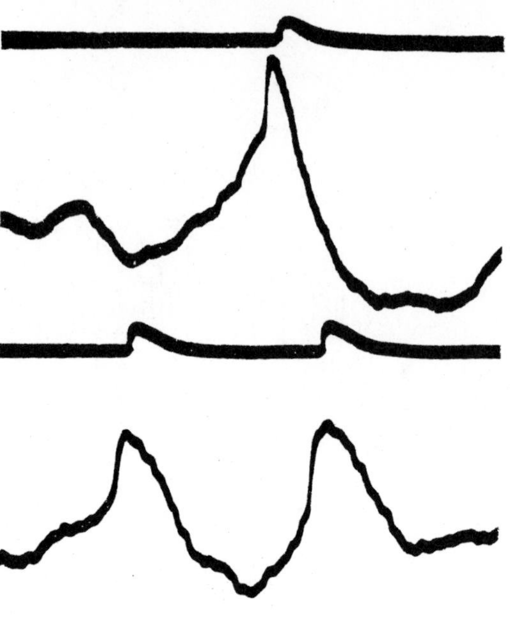

Fig. 7.
Change in shape of soma-recorded AAdC MN spike associated with training.
Above: naive preparation
Below: following up-training
Top traces are EJPs recorded from AAdC muscle cell.
Note small increase, due to facilitation, at higher frequency. From Wollacott & Holye, unpublished.

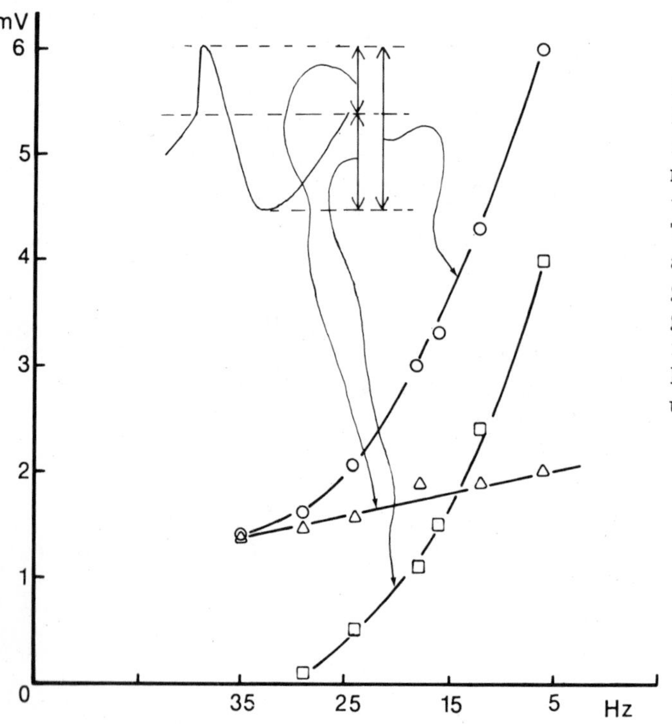

Fig. 8.
Relationship of soma spike parameters to mean frequency as altered by training. The changes are attributed to progressively reduced gK and associated increased resistance. From G. Hoyle, unpublished data.

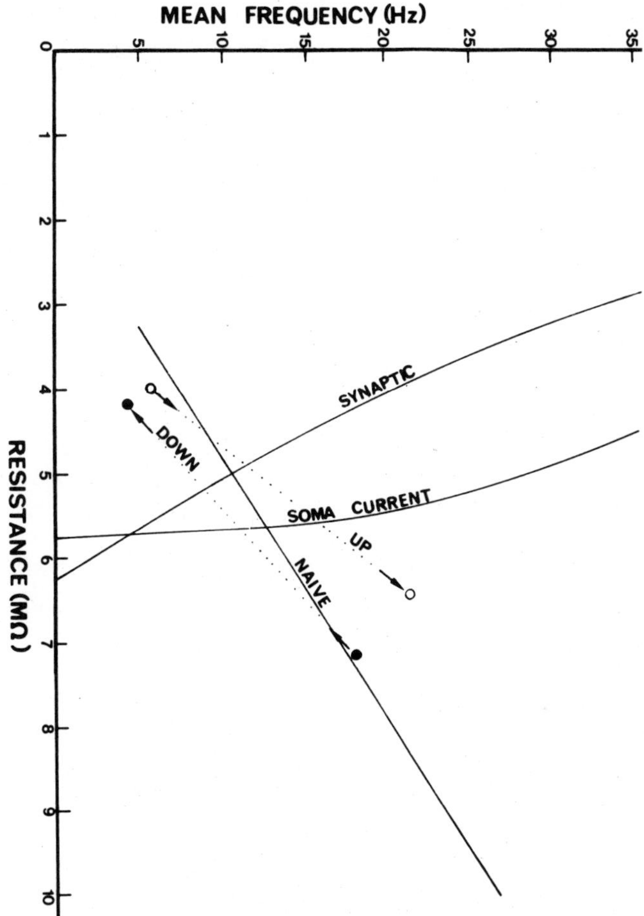

Fig. 9. Mean frequency/resistance relation in AAdC MN in: naive preparation having different natural frequencies (solid line with positive slope), and up-trained and down-trained preparations (averages indicated by dotted lines). The slightly curved lines with negative slopes show the frequency/resistance relations when frequency was changed by excitatory or inhibitory synaptic inputs, and by passing current into the soma, respectively. From unpublished data of M. Woollacott & G. Hoyle.

Lack of Influence of Normal Synaptic Inputs on Learning

It was a relatively easy experiment to cause falls in mean frequency by electrically driving inhibitory inputs to the MN and coupling the falls in mean frequency to the shocks automatically. But such correlations, although followed by brief reflex rises in frequency never led to long-term up-learning changes. Likewise, when similar aversive shocks were correlated with electrically-driven excitatory inputs there was no down-learning. The same shock-derived inputs to the cell must have been operating as those that do lead to stable learning and the same positional afference memory or efference memory systems also, so why didn't they work? The only possible difference lies within the MN. In natural operant-conditioned learning the animal makes its own trials. These could be initiated by unique interneurons not accessible to our electrically-driven inputs, or they may be occurring as spontaneous 'trial' events within the MN. In either case a molecular mechanism located in the MN is involved, that adjusts the long-term control of gK.

Cellular Mechanisms in other Learning Paradigms

A similar mechanism to that observed in the AAdC MN can in principle explain postural learning in any MN. We are preparing to test events in other identified MNs of locust, especially the slow extensor SETi, and the slow levator and depressor tarsi. The feeding behavior learning could be achieved in part by adjusting the resistance of the MN until the regular neural inputs causing PMs produce the appropriate tension. But we are not able to examine the mechanism because this paradigm no longer works after making the necessary dissection.

'Homeostatic' Model of the Learning Events

It is the gK regulating mechanism that is 'hit' by the various goal-related inputs that can bring about stable postural change. This mechanism must be part of the genome read-out that regulates the K conductance channels normally.

A model scheme of the events known to be involved, together with hypothetical ones associated with causing them to change in learning paradigms, is presented in Fig. 10. To initiate this, as in all operant-conditioning, a 'spontaneous' change must be initiated independently within the nervous system. The consequences of the change, altered motor output, are stored for a short time as

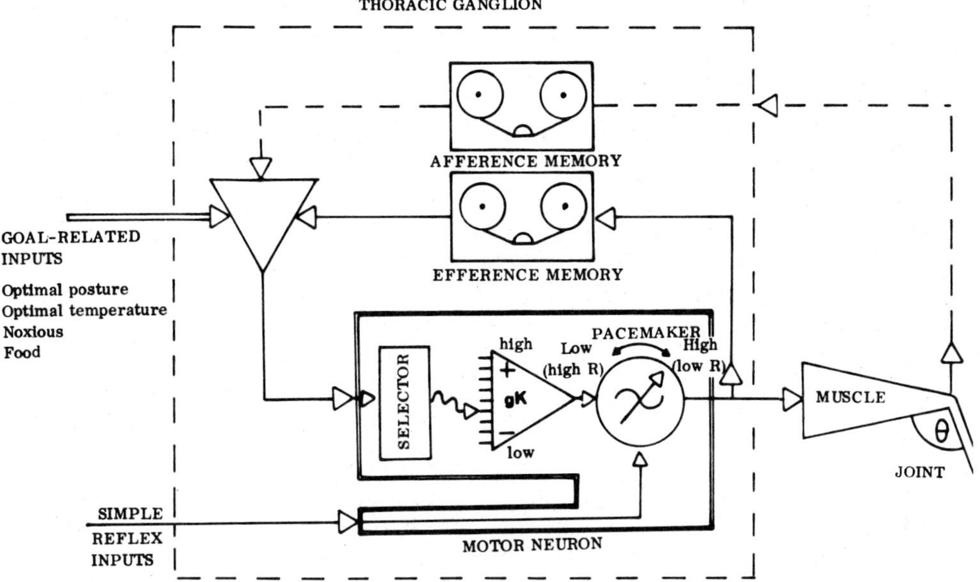

Fig. 10. Model of learning system and mechanism. The MN is symbolized by the double-walled outline: it receives two significantly different inputs, ones associated with ordinary reflex actions (below), the other associated with goal-related events (above). Only the latter can bring about a learned change. There is an association region (open triangle) within the ganglion where goal-related inputs interact with memory of recent efference (efference memory), which is entirely within the ganglion, or recent proprioceptive input occurring as a consequence of the motor output (afference memory). Input to the MN from this region initiates a long-term change in its gK which causes associated resistance and membrane potential change. These alter the pacemaker frequency, and therefore motor output and posture. From Hoyle, 1982.

efference memory, and also, when behavior occurs, as afference memory of the associated changes in proprioceptive input. Either can promote the cellular learning change that is manifested as altered gK.

If these mechanisms smack of the anciently-conceived regulatory devices termed homeostasis, that is hardly surprising. All learning is a form of automatic adaptation, using the plastic capabilities of the nervous system to relate behavior to the environment. If the posture as genetically-determined is inappropriate, as it will be as the animal ages, especially with gonadal maturation, it is altered, not just reflexly on a short term basis, but by a much more satisfactory long-term one of altered MN gK. Perhaps it is regulation of gene expression that shifts; certainly it is a natural built-in capability. The organism apparently also has a built-in mechanism for testing the appropriateness of its basic motor outputs because these are shifted slightly from time to time. All organisms fidget, none more so than locusts. If the altered output leads to improved goal-related inputs the trend is perpetuated and may be further accentuated. If it leads to an aversive input, either the opposite trend is generated or the 'experiment' automatically annuls itself.

When an investigator sets up an operant-conditioning paradigm he merely provides another disturbance of the natural equilibrium for the organism to adjust to. Perhaps this is not a true form of 'learning', any more than is classical conditioning, but at least we know that we are dealing with a form of nerve cell plasticity that underlies long-term change. A stable shift in gK is the simplest cellular event that could underlie learning in any neuron. It will be worth while examining this aspect of neurons in any learning situations in which the neurons involved can be located and tested.

ACKNOWLEDGMENT

This research was supported by National Science Foundation Research Grant No. BNS 0075-463 to G. Hoyle.

REFERENCES

Burrows, M., and Siegler, M.V.S., 1978. Graded synaptic transmission between local interneurones and motor neurones in the metathoracic ganglion of the locust. J. Physiol., 285: 231-255.

Eisenstein, E.M., 1972. Learning and memory in isolated insect ganglia. Adv. Insect Physiol., 9: 111-181.

Eisenstein, E.M., and Cohen, M.J., 1965. Learning in an isolated prothoracic insect ganglion. Anim. Behav., 13: 104-108.

Horridge, G. A., 1962. Learning leg position by the ventral nerve cord of headless insects. Proc. Roy. Soc. Lond. B., 157: 33-52.

Hoyle, G., Neurophysiological studies on 'learning' in headless insects. in: "Physiology of Insect Central Nervous Systems". J. Treherne, ed., Academic Press, London & N. Y. (1965).

Hoyle, G., 1966. An isolated ganglion-nerve-muscle preparation. J. Exp. Biol., 44: 413-429.

Hoyle, G., 1975. Identified neurons and the future of neuroethology. J. Exp. Zool., 194: 51-74.

Hoyle, G., 1976. Learning of leg position by the ghost crab Ocypode ceratophthalma. Behavioral Biol., 18: 147-163.

Hoyle, G., 1979. Mechanisms of simple motor learning. Trends in Neurosci., 2: 153-159.

Hoyle, G., 1980a. Learning, using natural reinforcements, in insect preparations that permit cellular neuronal analysis. J. Neurobiol., 11: 323-354.

Hoyle, G., Neural mechanisms. in: "Insect Biology in the Future". M. Locke and D. S. Smith, eds., Academic Press, London & N. Y. (1980b).

Hoyle, G., The role of pacemaker activity in learning. in: "Cellular Pacemakers". D. O. Carpenter, ed., Wiley, N. Y. (1982).

Tosney, T., and Hoyle, G., 1977. Computer-controlled learning in a simple system. Proc. Roy. Soc. Lond. B., 195: 365-393.

Woollacott, M., and Hoyle, G., 1977. Neural events underlying learning: changes in pacemaker. Proc. Roy. Soc. Lond. B., 195: 395-415.

SYNAPTIC PLASTICITY UNDERLYING THE CEREBELLAR MOTOR LEARNING INVESTIGATED IN RABBIT'S FLOCCULUS

Masao Ito

Department of Physiology, Faculty of Medicine
University of Tokyo, 7-3-1 Hongo, Bunkyoku
Tokyo 113, Japan

SUMMARY

An old concept that the cerebellum is equipped with capabilities of motor learning has been substantiated by recent theoretical exploration of neuronal network models of the cerebellum and by experimental investigation of adaptive motor phenomena which involve the cerebellum. The cerebellar flocculus is inserted into the oculomotor system as a sidepath of the vestibulo-ocular reflex (VOR) arc, and it also receives visual information. It has thus been hypothesized that the flocculus is the site of adaptive modification of the VOR which takes place under visual-vestibular interaction. This flocculus hypothesis of the VOR control has been supported by lesion experiments and by recording impulse signals from flocculus Purkinje cells. Marr-Albus' modifiable neuronal network model of the cerebellum predicts that this flocculus action is effected through plastic modifiability of synaptic transmission from granule cells to Purkinje cells in the flocculus cortex. The prediction has been substatiated by recent demonstration of a long-lasting depression at granule cell-Purkinje cell synapses after conjunctive stimulation of visual and vestibular inputs to the flocculus.

INTRODUCTION

The possibility that the cerebellum is equipped with learning capabilities has been pointed out by classic experiments of Flourens (1842) and Luciani (18 91). However, this interesting aspect of cerebellar functions has been left out for a long time because of lack of experimental evidence. In recent years, new light has been shed to this problem from two lines of approach. First, on the basis of ample experimental data of neuronal circuitry structures of the cerebellum (Eccles, Ito and Szentágothai, 1967), possible learning mechanisms of the cerebellum has been explored by theorists. Marr (1969) and Albus (1971) built a theoretical model of the cerebellum equipped with learning capabilities. Second, several concrete examples of adaptive motor phenomena have been shown to imply a simple form of cerebellar learning. The adaptive modification of the vestibulo-ocular reflex (VOR) which takes place under visual-vestibular interaction is one of these examples. This adaptive modification of the VOR was demonstrated by Gonshor and Melvill-Jones (19 76a, b) and was related to the possible learning capabiliti of the cerebellar flocculus which has been conceived from a neuronal circuitry analysis (Ito, 1970, 1972, 1974). Thus, the flocculus has provided an advantageous material for investigaying mechanisms of cerebellar learning with Marr-Albus model as a guide. This presentation outlines recent outcome from investigations of rabbit's flocculus conducted in my laboratory.

MARR-ALBUS MODEL OF THE CEREBELLUM

The cerebellar cortex receives two distinctively different inputs, mossy fibers and climbing fibers. Marr (1969) postulated that mossy fibers provide major inputs to the cerebellar cortex which are eventually converted to Purkinje cell outputs, while climbing fibers carry "instruction" signals which have an acton of reorganizing the relationship between mossy fiber inputs and Purkinje cell outputs (Fig. 1). This arrangement enables us to construct a learning machine like a Simple Perceptron (Albus, 1971). Marr's (1969) model of the cerebellum is based on a plasticity assumption that the transmission efficacy of a parallel fiber synapse mediating mossy fiber signals to a Purkinje cell is modified when impulses of this parallel fiber attain at the Purkinje cell dendrite with impulses of a climbing fiber (Fig. 1). Marr (1969) suggested that this heterosynaptic interaction from a climbing fiber to a parallel fiber enhances the the transmission efficacy, but Albus (1971) preferred the opposite, i.e., a depression instead of enhancement for some practical reasons.

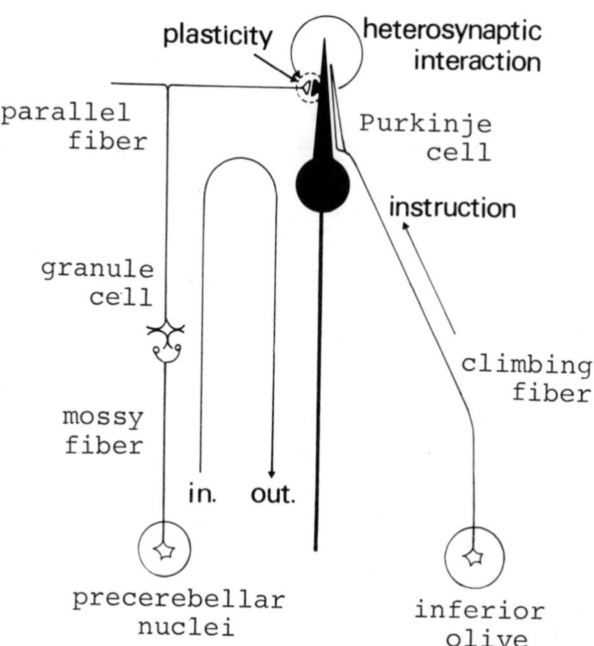

Fig. 1 Diagrammatical illustration of Marr-Albus Model. Inhibitory neuron is filled in black.

FLOCCULUS HYPOTHESIS OF THE VOR CONTROL

As the flocculus receives primary vestibular fibers as a mossy fiber input and in turn project to relay cells of the VOR, it is incorporated into the oculomotor system as a sidepath to the major VOR arc (Fig. 2). The flocculus also receives climbing fibers which convey visual signals. From these structural aspects, it has been hypothesized that the flocculus adaptively controls the VOR by referring to retinal error signals (Ito, 1970, 1972, 1974). Since retinal error signals imply "instruction' concering the performance of the VOR, the hypothesis is in good accordance with Marr-Albus model of the cerebellum; retinal error signals conveyed by climbing fibers would modify parallel fiber-Purkinje cell synapses in the flocculus and thereby alter the signal transfer characteristics of the flocculus sidepath, which eventually would lead to adaptive modification of the VOR.

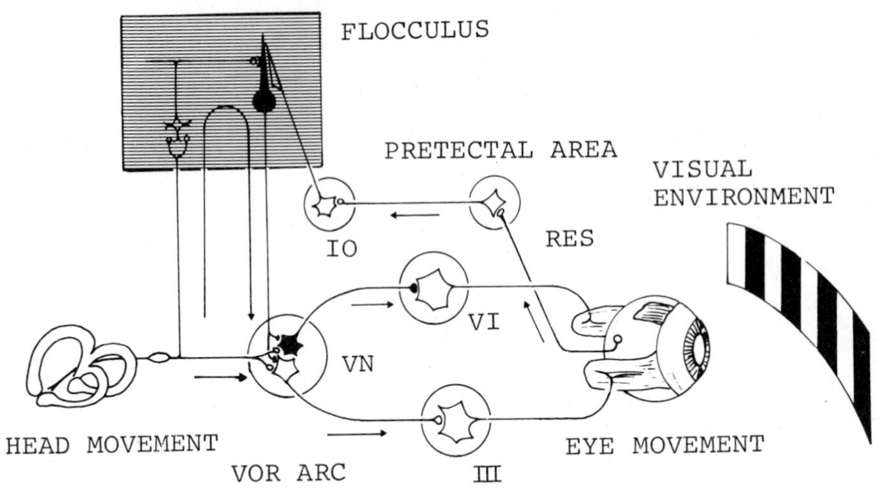

Fig. 2 Connections of the flocculus with the horizontal VOR. RES, retinal error signals. IO, inferior olive. VN, vestibular nuclei.

SUPPORT FOR THE FLOCCULUS HYPOTHESIS FROM LESION EXPERIMENTS

The adaptability of the VOR can be tested either by using prism goggles (Gonshor and Melvill-Jones, 1976a, b) or X2 spectacle glasses (Miles, Braitman and Dow, 1980), or by moving visual fields in various combinations with head rotation (Ito, Shiida, Yagi and Yamamoto, 1974). The VOR adaptability so tested was abolished by ablation of the flocculus (Ito et al. 1974) or of the vestibulocerebellum including the flocculus (Robinson, 1976). Similar results were obtained with chemical destruction of the flocculus by local injection of kainic acid (Ito, Jastreboff and Miyashita, 1981) which , differing from ablation of the flocculus, does not cause retrograde degeneration of the inferior olive neurons (Ito, Jastreboff and Miyashita, 1980). Destruction of the dorsal cap of the inferior olive which mediates visual climbing fiber pathway to the flocculus also abolished the VOR adaptability (Ito and Miyashita, 1975; Haddad, Demer and Robinson, 1980). Death of olivary neurons induces a depression of inhibitory action of Purkinje cells on VOR relay cells (Dufossé, Ito and Miyashita, 1978), but this complication can be avoided by interrupting visual climbing fiber pathway prior to the dorsal cap, without involving dorsal cap neurons in lesions, which still abolishes the VOR adaptability (Ito and Miyashita, 1975).

SUPPORT FOR THE FLOCCULUS HYPOTHESIS FROM RECORDING OF PURKINJE CELL IMPULSES

In rabbits, it was demonstrated that responsiveness of flocculus Purkinje cells to vestibular mossy fiber inputs during head rotation altered in parallel with the VOR adaptation (Dufossé, Ito, Jastreboff and Miyashita, 1978). The change occurred in the direction which accords with the flocculus hypothesis that it is causal to the VOR adaptation. In monkeys, however, changes observed in Purkinje cell responsiveness to vestibular stimuli were in the opposite direction to the theoretical prediction, and therefore were regarded as secondary effects of VOR adaptation (Miles et al. 1980). This seemingly conflicting data in monkeys, however, should be interpreted with caution, because direct connection from sampled Purkinje cells to relay cells of the horizontal VOR was not tested in monkeys. Rabbit's flocculus is now divided into five longitudinal zones, only one of which is connected to relay cells of the horizontal VOR. Microzonal structures have not yet been dissected in monkey's flocculus, and there is no solid basis for assuming that flocculus Purkinje cells responding in connection with horizontal gaze velocity, as tested by Miles et al. (1980), have a direct connection with horizontal VOR relay cells. For this reason, it is difficult to interprete the monkey data immediately for or against the flocculus hypothesis.

DEMONSTRATION OF THE PLASTICITY AT PARALLEL FIBER-PURKINJE CELL SYNAPSES

A more direct test of Marr-Albus' plasticity assumption has recently been performed by substituting electric pulse stimulation of a vestibular nerve and the inferior olive in high decerebrate rabbits for natural vestibular and visual stimulation in alert rabbits (Ito, Sakurai and Tongroach, 1981a, b). In this experiment, Purkinje cells were sampled from the rostral flocculus and identified by their characteristic responses to stimulation of the contralateral inferior olive. Basket cells were also sampled and identified by absence of olivary responses and also by their location in the molecular layer adjacent to identified Purkinje cells. Single pulse stimulation of a vestibular nerve, either ipsilateral or contralateral, at a rate of 2/sec excited Purkinje cells with a latency of 3-6 msec. This early excitation represents activation through vestibular mossy fibers, granule cells and their axons (Fig. 2). Similar excitation was common also among putative basket cells.

Conjunctive stimulation of a vestibular nerve at 20/sec and the inferior olive at 4/sec, for 25 sec per trial, effectively depressed the early excitation of Purkinje cells by that nerve, without an associated change in spontaneous discharge. The depression recovered in about ten minutes, but it was followed by the onset of a slow depression lasting for an hour (Fig. 3). No such depression occurred in the early excitation by the vestibular nerve not involved in the conjunctive stimulation. Therefore, the depression is a specific effect of conjunctive stimulation. No depression was detected in early excitation of putative basket cells from either vestibular nerve, nor in the inhibition or rebound facilitation in Purkinje cells following the early excitation. Vestibular nerve-evoked field potentials in the granular layer and white matter of the flocculus were not affected. These responses represent impulse transmission in mossy fibers and cortical networks except for the parallel fiber-Purkinje cell synapses. It can be concluded that the depression occurs specifically at parallel fiber-Purkinje cell synapses activated simulatenously with climbing fiber-Purkinje cell synapses, in the manner postulated by Albus (1971).

INVOLVEMENT OF TRANSMITTER-SENSITIVITY OF PURKINJE CELL DENDRITES

Iontophoretic application of glutamate,i.e., the putative neurotransmitter of parallel fibers (Sandoval and Cotman, 1978; Hacket, Hou and Cochran, 1979), in conjunction with 4/sec olivary stimulation was found to depress very effectively the glutamate sensitivity of Purninje cells; aspartate sensitivity was depressed to a much lesse degree. The depression diminished in about ten minutes, but this recovery was followed by a slow depression lasting for an hour. This observation suggests that subsynaptic chemosensitivity of Purkinje cells to the putative neurotransmitter of parallel fibers is involved in the depression observed after conjunctive stimulation of a vestibular nerve and the inferior olive.

POSSIBLE MECHANISMS OF THE PLASTICITY AT PARALLEL FIBER-PURKINJE CELL SYNAPSES

There are two possibilties to be tested by a further experiments. First, since climbing fiber activation of Purkinje cells appears to involve a voltage-dependent increase of calcium permeability of the dendritic membrane (Llinás and Sugimori, 1980), Ekerot

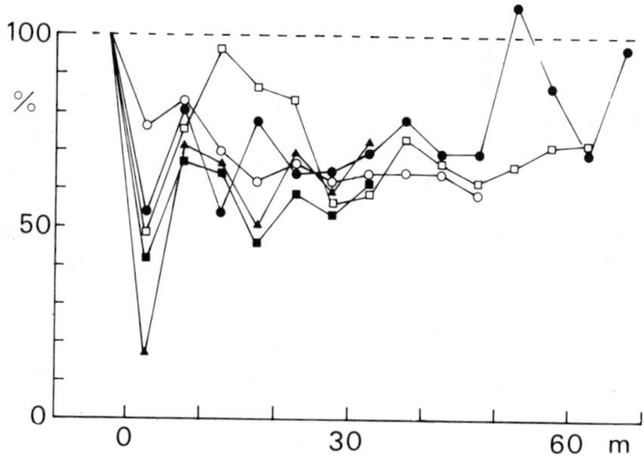

Fig. 3 Recovery time course after conjunctive vestibular-olivary stimulation. Ordinate, values of the firing index of Purkinje cells of rabbit's flocculus activated by electric supramaximal stimulation of a vestibular nerve at 2/sec. The plotted values of firing index are normalized by control values before conjunctive stimulation which happened at the zero time (Ito, Sakurai and Tongroach, 1981b).

and Oscarsson (1981) suggested than an increased intradendritic calcium concentration affects subsynaptic receptors of Purkinje cell dendrites, just as intracellular calcium is supposed to desensitize acetylcholine receptors in muscle endplates (Miledi, 1980). Second, climbing fibers may liberate a chemical substance(s) which reacts with subsynaptic receptor molecules at parallel fiber neurotransmitter, thereby rendering the receptors insensitive to the parallel fiber neurotransmitter. An analogous phenomenon has been reported in cerebral cortical cells (Renaud, Blume, Pittman, Lamour and Tan, 1980), that application of thyrotropin-releasing hormon causes a reduction in glutamate sensitivity without affecting aspartate sensitivity. These two possible ways for climbing fiber impulses to affect a parallel fiber-Purkinje cell synapse are diagrammatically illustrated in Fig. 4.

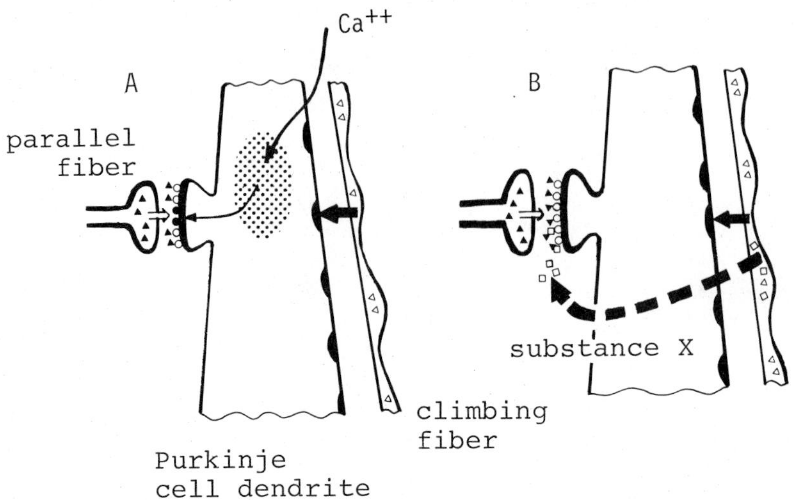

Fig. 4 Diagrammatical illustration for the two possible mechanisms of the heterosynaptic intercation between a climbing fiber and a parallel fiber-Purkinje cell synapse.

COMMENT

Results from neuronal circuitry analyses, eye movement studies, and recording from flocculus Purkinje cells all support the flocculus hypothesis of the vestibulo-ocular reflex control, even though there is still much to do for eliminating seeming conflicts among experimental data on different animals and under different experimental conditions. The flocculus hypothesis conforms to Marr-Albus model of the cerebellum. The long lasting depression at parallel fiber-Purkinje cell synapses and associated change in glutamate sensitivity further provide a strong support for Marr-Albus model. However, it is not yet clear whether the recovery of the depression involves a still slower process analogous to a permanent memory. To pursuit a long-termed time course of the depression and to investigate its molecular mechanisms are important tasks of future experiments.

REFERENCES

Albus, J.S. (1971) A thoery of cerebellar function. Math. Biosci. 10, 25-61.

Dufossé, M., Ito, M. and Miyashita, Y. (1978) Diminution and reversal of eye movements induced by local stimulation of rabbit cerebellar flocculus after partial destruction of the inferior olive. Exp. Brain Res. 33, 139-141.

Dufossé, M., Ito, M., Jastreboff, P.J. and Miyashita, Y. (1978) A neuronal correlate in rabbit's cerebellum to adaptive modification of the vestibulo-ocular reflex. Brain Res. 150, 511-616.

Eccles, J.C., Ito, M. and Szentágothai, J. (1967) The Cerebellum as a Neuronal Machine. New York, Heidelberg: Springer.

Ekerot, C.-F. and Oscarsson, O. (1981) Prolonged depolarization elicited in Purkinje cell dendrites by climbing fibre impulses in the cat. J. Physiol. 318, 207-221.

Flourens, P. (1842) Recherches experimentales sur les propriétés et les fonctions du système nerveux dans les animaux vertébrés. Paris: Bailliere.

Gonshor, A. and Melvill-Jones, G. (1976a) Short-term adaptive changes in the human vestibulo-ocular reflex arc. J. Physiol. 265, 361-379.

Gonshor, A. and Melvill-Jones, G. (1976b) Extreme vestibulo-ocular adaptation induced by prolonged optical reversal of vision. J. Physiol. 256, 381-414.

Hacket, J.T., Hou, S.-M. and Cochran, S.L. (1979) Glutamate and synaptic depolarization of Purkinje cells evoked by parallel fibers and by climbing fibers. Brain Res. 170, 377-380.

Haddad, G.M., Demer, J.L. and Robinson, D.A. (1980) The effect of lesions of the dorsal cap of the inferior olive on the vestibulo-ocular and optokinetic system of the cats. Brain Res. 185, 265-275.

Ito, M. (1970) Neurophysiological aspects of the cerebellar motor control system. Int. J. Neurol. 7, 162-176.

Ito, M. (1972) Neural design of the cerebellar motor control system. Brain Res. 40, 81-84.

Ito, M. (1974) The control mechanisms of cerebellar motor system. In The Neurosciences, Third Study Program, ed. F.O. Schmitt, F.G. Worden, 293-303.

Ito, M. and Miyashita, Y. (1975) The effects of chronic destruction of inferior olive upon visual modification of the horizontal vestibulo-ocular reflex of rabbits. Proc. Jpn Acad. 51, 716-760.

Ito, M., Jastreboff, P.J. and Miyashita, Y. (1980) Retrograde influence of surgical and chemical flocculectomy upon dorsal cap neurons of the inferior olive. Neurosci. Lett. 20, 45-48.

Ito, M., Sakurai, M. and Tongroach, P.(1981a) Evidence for modifiability of parallel fiber-Purkinje cell synapses. In Advances in Physiological Sciences 2,97-105. Oxford: Pergamon.
Ito, M., Shiida, T., Yagi, N. and Yamamoto, M. (1974) The cerebellar modification of rabbit's horizontal vestibulo-ocular reflex induced by sustained head rotation combined with visual stimulation. Proc. Jpn Acad. 50, 85-89.
Llinás, R. and Sugimori, M. (1980) Electrophysiological properties of in intro Purkinje cell dendrites in mammalian cerebellar slices. J. Physiol. 305, 197-213.
Luciani, L. (1891) Il Cerevelletto: Nuovi Studi di Fisiologia normale e pathologica. Flourens: Le Monnier.
Marr, D. (1969) A theory of cerebellar cortex. J. Physiol. 202, 437-470.
Miledi, R. (1980) Intracellular calcium and desensitization of acetylcholine receptors. Proc. Roy. Soc. B 209, 447-452.
Miles, F.A., Braitman, D.J. and Dow, B.M. (1980) Long-term adaptive changes in primate vestibuloocular reflex. IV. Electrophysiological observations in flocculus of adpated monkeys. J. Neurphysiol. 43, 1477-1493.
Renaud, L.P., Blume, H.W., Pittman, Q.J., Lamour, Y. and Tan, A.T. (1979) Thyrotropin-releasing hormone selectively depressed glutamate excitation of cerebral cortical neurons. Science N.Y. 205, 1275-1277.
Robinson, D.A. (1976) Adaptive gain control of vestibulo-ocular reflex by the cerebellum. J. Neurophysiol. 39, 954-969.
Sandoval, M.E. and Cotman, C.W. (1978) Evaluation of glutamate as a neurotransmitter of cerebellar parallel fibers. Neurosci. 3, 199-206.

CLASSICAL CONDITIONING MEDIATED BY THE RED NUCLEUS IN THE CAT

Nakaakira Tsukahara

Department of Biophysical Engineering
Faculty of Engineering Science
Osaka University, Toyonaka, Osaka and
National Institute for Physiological Sciences
Okazaki, Japan

SUMMARY

We have attempted to develop a behavioral and neuronal model for the study of classical conditioning using the corticorubrospinal system. A conditioned stimulus (CS) was applied to the cerebral peduncle (CP) in cats which had lesions that interrrupted the corticofugal fibers caudal to the red nucleus. The unconditioned stimulus (US) was an electric shock to the skin of the forelimb that produced flexion of the limb. After pairing of the CS and US in close temporal association, an initially ineffective stimulus to the cerebral peduncle was found to give rise to flexion of the elbow. Extinction of this conditioned response could be achieved by applying the CS alone, or by reversing the sequence of the stimuli (US-CS:backward pairing). The US when used alone did not produce an increase in the effectiveness of the CS, and pairing a fixed CS with a US at random intervals did not produce any increase in performance in response to the CS. In these respects, the observed behavioral modification has the features of associative conditioning.

Because both the threshold for and strength of elbow flexion induced by stimulation of the nucleus interpositus of the cerebellum were identical in experimental and control animals, it is unlikely that the interpositorubrospinal system is the neuronal site of behavioral change. Instead, since the conditioned response is most probably mediated the corticorubrospinal system, it is likely that a modification of the corticorubral synapses underlies the change in behavior. Extracellular recording from red nucleus cells in unanesthetized cats has shown that stimulation of the CP induces a greater degree of excitation in the red nucleus in animals that have undergone conditioning than control animals. (The control group contained cats which had received no training, or those which had received backwardly paired stimulation, or random CS-US pairing).

INTRODUCTION

Recent studies (Tsukahara et al., 1975; Murakami et al., 1977; Tsukahara and Fujito, 1976; Tsukahara et al., 1981; Fujito et al., 1981) have shown that sprouting of the corticorubral synapses occurs after neonatal as well as adult lesions and after cross-innervation of peripheral flexor and extensor nerves and the newly-formed symapses are physiologically effective. The latter is particularly important, because this finding suggests that sprouting occurs in intact central neurons and that it might therefore be involved in naturally occurring adaptive behavior such as learning.

In order to test this idea, we have attempted to reconstruct the learning behavior using the corticorubral synapses as the modifiable elements of the network for the learning behavior. Classical conditioning was used in this experiment as the learning behavior, since there is already evidence that midbrain structures are important for classically conditioned avoidance responses. Furthermore, it has been established that rubral lesions abolished a conditioned forelimb flexion responses where a tone was used as the conditioned stimulus (CS) and an electric shock to the forelimb nerves as the unconditioned stimulus (US) (Smith, 1970). An attempt was made to simplify this paradigm by limiting both the afferent pathway involved and the conditioned behavior mediated by the red nucleus. This was done by applying the CS to the corticorubral fibers as they pass through the cerebral peduncle (CP). The CS is delivered in the form of electric pulses in a preparation in which the cerebral corticofugal outflow is largely restricted to the corticorubrospinal pathway by section of the cerebral peduncle caudal to the red nucleus. In this preparation we have found that after paired conditioning (by stimulating the CP as the CS and applying electric shocks to the skin of the forelimb as the US in close temporal association) initially ineffective stimuli to the corticorubral fibers give rise to forelimb flexion; this has never been observed after random control, after CS alone, after US alone, or after backward pairing of the two stimuli. In this article, details of this experiment and cellular correlates of conditioning by analyzing unit activities of the red nucleus in unanesthetized conditioned cats will be presented.

METHODS

During conditioning, the animals were given 120 periods of training per day with CS-US paired trials; once every five trials, the CS was presented alone. The intertrial interval was fixed at 30 sec. The CS was a train of five pulses each with a duration of 0.1 msec and was presented at intervals of 2 msec. In order to avoid electrode polarization, the polarity of the pulse was automatically reversed after every train of pulses. The US was an electric pulse with a duration of 10 msec; this was preceded by the CS some 60 to 200 msec earlier (but most often 100 msec). CS-US pairing of 120 trials, at intervals of 30 sec, constituted the training session on any given day. The ratio of positive responses in 24 such trials, without the US, provided the score of performance for that day.

Control procedures consisted of (1) presentation of the CS alone; (2) the US alone; (3) backward pairing of the stimuli; (4) random presentations; the animals received the CS and US in the same session in random sequence; the CS was presented at regular intervals of 30 sec, but the US was presented randomly anywhere from 0 to 30 sec after the onset of the CS. This random US stimulus was achieved by controlling the stimulator by a microcomputer in which random numbers had been stored in memory.

A potentiometer was attached to the elbow joint. The output of this potentiometer was connected to an amplifier and the amplified signals were recorded by a penrecorder and also were recorded through the analogdigital converter to the microcomputer for processing. The resolution of the movement at the elbow joint was 0.05°. Teflon-coated needles were inserted into the biceps and triceps brachii muscles of the right arm for electromyographic (EMG) recording. The electromyograms were amplified and displayed on the pen recorder simultaneously with the associated elbow movements. The electromyogram was also displayed on an oscilloscope and photographed.

Current intensity for the CS was selected in the following way. First, the stimulus intensity required to evoke elbow flexion was determined; next, the proportion of positive response (out of a total of 20 trials) was estimated; then this was defined as the "score of performance" for that current intensity. A positive response was defined as a flexion at the elbow joint of more than 0.05°, which was the maximum resolution of our recording system for elbow movements. The "score of performance" increased as the CS stimulus intensity was increased. A current intensity that produced a 50% "score of performance" was accepted as "50% current" and the average for this 50% current (during four consecutive pretraining days) was determined. Seventy-five percent of this 50% current intensity was used during the subsequent training session for the CS.

RESULTS

ESTABLISHMENT AND TIME COURSE OF CONDITIONING

We have found that after paired conditioning (by stimulating the CP as the CS and applying electric shocks to the skin of the forelimb as the US in close temporal association) initially

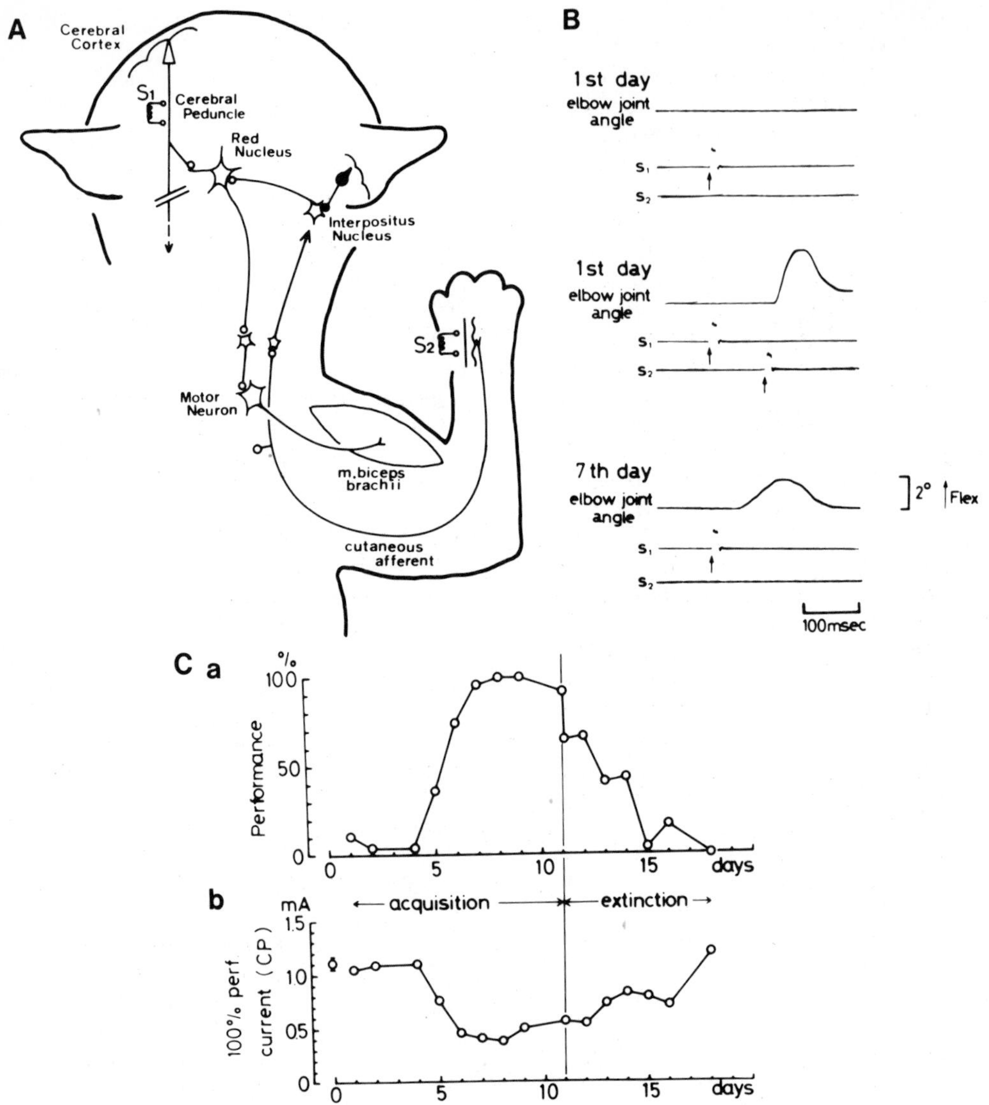

Fig. 1 Associative conditioning mediated by the red nucleus in the cat. A: Arrangement of the experimental set-up. S1, conditioned stimulus (CS), S2, unconditioned stimulus (US). B: Specimen record of elbow flexion (uppermost traces) on 1st day and 7th day after conditioning. Upward arrows of middle and lowermost traces indicate the onset of the timulus. S1, CS., S2, US. C: Change in performance (Ca) and change of minimum current for eliciting 100% correct performance (100% performance current) (Cb) during forward and backward pairing (Ordinates). Abscissa; day after onset of training, CS-US interval of 100 msec. After eleventh day, stimulus sequence was reversed as US-CS with interval of 900 msec. (modified from Tsukahara et al., 1981).

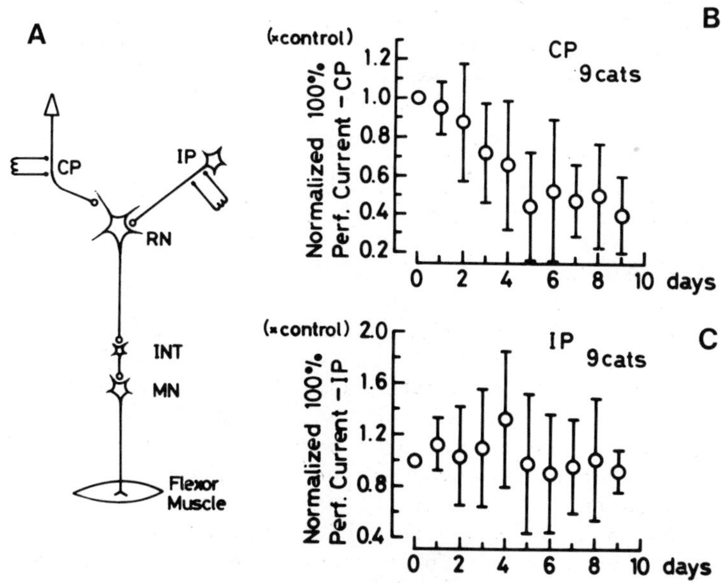

Fig. 2 Primary site of conditioned changes
A: CP, cerebral peduncle, IP, interpositus necleus of the cerebellum, RN, red nucleus, INT, interneurons interpolated in the rubrospinal system, MN, flexor motoneurons. B: Current intensity of CP stimulation for producing 100% performance to CS. C: Current intensity producing 100% performance by stimulation of IP with the same train of pulses and in the same cats as used in B. The data from nine cats are illustrated. Ordinates for B & C: Normalized 100% performance current; abscissa, day after onset of conditioning of CS to CP and US to the skin of the forearm.

ineffective stimuli to corticorubral fibers gives rise to forelimb flexion; this has never been observed in control experiments. Typical changes of the responses to CS illustrated in Fig. 1B show an example of elbow flexion on the 1st and 7th days after CS-US paired conditioning. On the 1st day of training, the CS alone produced no response, whereas the US by itself produced an elbow flexion. After CS-US pairing for 7 days, the CS alone produced a flexion at the same stimulus intensity as was used before. Fig. 1C shows an example of the time course in the change of "score of performance" after training. The score of performance as defined by the probability of positive responses with a fixed CS stimulus intensity increased gradually until it reached a plateau after about 7 days. With extinction (produced by reversing the sequence of the stimuli, i.e., US-CS), the score of performance, the minimum current intensity required to produce 100% of the score of performance progressively decreased. Furthermore, the degree of the observed elbow flexion also increased.

PRIMARY SITE OF THE CONDITIONAL CHANGE

The pathway mediating the conditioned response in this experimental paradigm is considered to be relatively simple in view of the fact that (a) corticofugal fibers were surgically eliminated just caudal to the red nucleus and (b) CS electrodes were implanted within the cerebral peduncle which contains cortico-rubral fibers that are presynaptic to the cells in the red nucleus. The shortest latency of electrical activity elictied in the biceps muscle in response to CS 8 msec, which accords well with the shortest time required for the transmission of impulses along the corticorubrospinal pathway.

The neuronal changes that occur after conditioning do not appear to involve any detectable alteration in neuronal elements caudal to the red nucleus, since the efficacy of transmission along the interposito-rubrospinal pathway does not change (Fig. 2), whereas there is a remarkable increase of a transmission efficacy in the corticorubrospinal system. This suggests that the primary site of the conditioned change is to be found in the transmission of the corticorubral synapses. This is exactly the site of the modifiable synapses as described previously.

CELLULAR CORRELATES OF CONDITIONING

Units were recorded using either glass or tungsten micro-electrodes. Red nucleus (RN) cells were identified by orthodromic activation from the nucleus interpositus (IP) of the cerebellum, and also by histological verification of the microelectrode tracks after experiments.

Fig. 3 shows a comparison of the firing probability of RN neurons to the CS (with the same number and intensity of stimuli as applied for behavioral experiments) before and after the

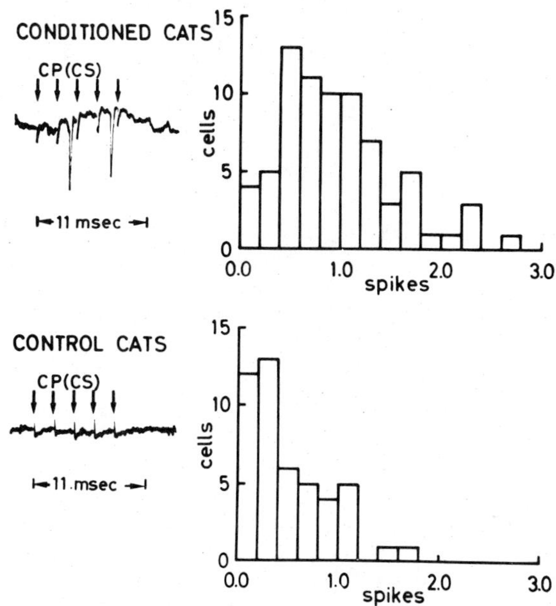

Fig. 3 Modification of rubral unit activity during conditioning. Mean number of spikes during five pulses of CP stimuli (during 11 msec from the onset of the stimuli) from 74 RN units of conditioned cats (upper histogram) and from 47 RN units of control (random, non-stimulated and extincted cats) (lower histogram) in abscissa and number of cells in ordinate. Specimen RN units in conditioned cats (upper left) and record of no spike response in control cats are illustrated. Downward arrows mark the CP stimuli.(modified from Oda et al., unpublished).

establishment of conditioning. The firing probability increased in some RN neurons after conditioning. This result is consistent with the conclusion reached from the above-mentioned behavioral experiment that transmission along the cortico-rubrospinal pathway increases after conditioning, although there is no change in transmission efficacy in the interposito-rubrospinal system. This is taken to support the idea that the primary site of change is to be found in transmission at the corticorubral synapses. However, some investigators might raise a question as to whether stimulation of the interposito-rubrospinal and corticorubrospinal pathways activate common RN neurons in this experimental condition. This possibility has been tested experimentally, using recording from inidividual RN neurons. Out of 90 RN cells, 63 RN cells were activated by both CP and IP stimuli used in the behavioral experiments. These data show that the majority of RN neurons are in fact excited by both the corticorubral CS stimuli and the interpositorubral stimuli.

The latency of electrical activity recorded in the biceps muscle in response to a CS was 8 msec, which accords well with the shortest time which would be needed for the transmission of impulses along the corticorubrospinal pathway to the muscle. This is calculated in the following way: (1) 1 msec, for conduction from the CP to the red nucleus and the onset of corticorubral EPSPs (Tsukahara and Kosaka, 1968); (2) 2 msec, from the onset of the corticorubral EPSPs to the initiation of impulses in the neurons of the red nucleus, assuming that the neurons are excited during the rising phase of the corticorubral EPSPs, which have a mean time-to-peak of 3.6 msec (Tsukahara et al., 1975); (3) 2 msec, from the onset of spike initiation in the neurons of the red nucleus to the onset of EPSPs in the forelimb motoneurons (Illert et al., 1976); (4) 3 msec, from the onset of EPSPs in the motoneurons to the initiation of electrical activity in the biceps muscle. This total of 8 msec is considered to be the shortest possible time.

In this article, some attempts to correlate the plasticity of the mammalian red nucleus with learning behavior have been presented. The strategy proposed here: to identify neuronal plasticity in the neuronal network first, then to pursue behavioral correlates of this neuronal plasticity (i.e. a "bottom-up" approach) appears to be a valid and useful way to obtain insight into the mechanisms underlying learning, and promises to yield further information in the future.

REFERENCES

Fujito, Y., Tsukahara, N., Oda, Y., and Yoshida, M., 1981, Formation of functional synapses in the adult feline red nucleus from the cerebrum following cross-innvervation of forelimb flexor and extensor nerves. II. Analysis of newly-appeared postsynaptic potentials. Exp. Brain Res. (in press).

Illert, M., Lundberg, A., and Tanaka, R., 1976, Integration in descending motor pathways controlling the forelimb in the cat.a. Convergence on neurones mediating disynaptic corticomotoneuronal excitation. Exp. Brain Res. 26:521.

Murakami, F., Tsukahara, N., and Fujito, Y., 1977, Analysis of unitary EPSPs mediated by the newly-formed cortico-rubral synapses after lesion of the nucleus interpositus of the cerebellum. Exp. Brain Res. 30: 233.

Oda, Y., Kuwa, K., Miyasaka, S., and Tsukahara, N. Modification of rubral unit activities during classical conditioning of the cat. (in preparation).

Smith, A. M., 1970, The Effects of rubral lesions and stimulation on conditioned forelimb flexion responses in the cat. Physiol. Behav. 5: 1121.

Tsukahara, N., and Fujito, Y., 1976, Physiological evidence of formation of new synapses from cerebrum in the red nucleus following cross-union of forelimb nerves. Brain Res. 106:184.

Tsukahara, N., and Kosaka, K., 1968, The mode of cerebral excitation of red nucleus neurons. Exp. Brain Res. 5:102.

Tsukahara, N., Hultborn, H., Murakami, F., and Fujito, Y., 1975, Electrophysiological study of formation of new synapses and collateral sprouting in red nucleus neurons after partial denervation. J. Neurophysiol. 38:1359.

Tsukahara, N., Oda, Y., and Notsu, T., 1981, Classical conditioning mediated by the red nucleus in the cat. J. Neurosci., 1: 72.

Tsukahara, N., Fujito, Y., Oda, Y., and Maeda, J. Formation of functional synapses in adult red nucleus from the cerebrum following cross-innervation of forelimb flexor and extensor nerves. I. Appearance of new synaptic potentials Ex. Brain Res. (in press).

NEUROPHYSIOLOGIC CORRELATES OF LATENT FACILITATION

C.D. Woody

Departments of Anatomy and Psychiatry
UCLA Medical Center
Los Angeles, CA 90024

SUMMARY

Classical conditioning is now recognized to represent a combination of several different underlying phenomena. Some of these phenomena may be produced nonassociatively in the course of conditioning. These are not simply epiphenomena of conditioning, but, as recent studies indicate, each may contribute significantly to major facets of conditioning itself. The present report concerns neurophysiologic correlates of latent facilitation. Latent facilitation of subsequently learned motor responses is thought to occur nonassociatively following repeated presentations of a US. In cats, latent facilitation of an eyeblink response is paralleled by the development of increased excitability in neurons of the motor cortex and in facial motoneurons projecting to the musculature involved with blinking. This facilitation may result, in part, from activation of cholinergic pathways to the pyramidal cells of the motor cortex.

INTRODUCTION

Behaviorally, it has long been recognized that repeated presentation of a stimulus used later as a US in classical conditioning may inhibit the development of subsequent conditioning (Kimble and Dufort, 1956; Leonard et al, 1972; MacDonald, 1946). Nonetheless, it appears that some facilitatory effects of presenting the US may also occur. In the literature these effects are either termed pseudoconditioning (Kimble, 1961; Kimble et al, 1955), reflex dominance (Ukhtomsky, 1911; Ukhtomsky, 1927), or simply facilitation (Graham-Brown and Sherrington, 1912; Bindman and Lippold,

1981). In cats, as a result of repeated presentations of glabella tap US, one can observe both a facilitation of the rate of acquisition of subsequent eyeblink conditioning (Matsumura and Woody, 1982) and increases in the excitability of neurons of the motor cortex that last sufficiently long to contribute to this behavioral phenomenon (Brons and Woody, 1980). A series of experiments, the results of which are described below, lead one to the conclusion that this facilitation may result, in part, from activation of cholinergic pathways to the pyramidal cells of the motor cortex. Additional changes occur subcortically at the level of involved motoneurons (Jordan et al, 1976; Matsumura and Woody, 1982).

METHODS

Details of the methods used in these studies have been described elsewhere (Woody and Black Cleworth, 1973; Woody et al, 1978). Four different approaches were taken. The first was to apply cholinergic agents and putative second messengers iontophoretically to study their effects on intracellularly recorded neurons of the motor cortex of awake cats (Woody et al, 1978; Swartz and Woody, 1979). The agents used were acetylcholine, extracellularly, and cyclic GMP, intracellularly. Second, the effects on neural excitability of both orthodromic and antidromic activation of pyramidal cells were evaluated by stimulating the pyramidal tract at the level of the facial nucleus (Tzebelikos and Woody, 1979). Third, the excitability of neurons of the motor cortex to intracellularly applied currents was measured directly in cats given serial presentations of tap US in the absence of any presentations of CS (Brons and Woody, 1980). These measures of excitability were then compared with measurements in animals given presentations of CS alone or paired presentations of CS and US. (The latter resulted in eyeblink conditioning.) Fourth, the behavioral consequences of serial presentations of the tap US were evaluated on rates of subsequently acquired conditioned blinking (see Matsumura and Woody, 1982).

RESULTS

1. Long-lasting Increases in Membrane Resistance of Cells Given Applications of Acetylcholine Plus Current-Induced Cell Discharge

Iontophoretic applications of acetylcholine (ACh) were made extracellularly for 30 seconds while recording intracellularly from neurons of the motor cortex. From 1/3 to 1/2 of the cells tested showed a transient increase in membrane resistance (Rm) following application of ACh. Pooled data from one such group of cells are shown in Fig. 1. In part B a transient increase in acetylcholine can be seen, reaching a peak approximately 2 minutes after cessation of iontophoresis. In the remaining cells no increase in Rm was seen. Most cells showing an increase in Rm following application of ACh

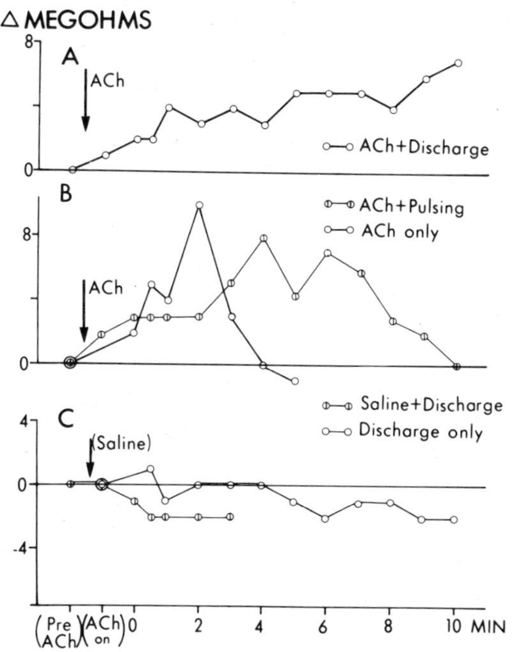

Figure 1. Average changes in membrane resistance in cells given: A) iontophoresis of ACh plus depolarizing current sufficient to repeatedly discharge the cell (ACh plus discharge); B) iontophoresis of ACh alone (ACh only) and iontophoresis of ACh plus depolarizing current insufficient to repeatedly discharge the cell (ACh plus pulsing); A and B are data from cells that responded with some increase in input resistance; C) iontophoresis of saline plus current-induced discharge (saline plus discharge) and injection of depolarizing current sufficient to produce repeated discharge (discharge only). Ordinate shows mean differences in resistance (Rm) in megohms from initial value, the latter set to zero. Abscissa: pre ACh - before administration of ACh; ACh on - during iontophoresis of acetylcholine; 0 - immediately after cessation of iontophoresis of ACh; remaining numbers - time in minutes after cessation of ACh. Rm determined by Frank-Fuortes method, except for ACh-plus-pulsing where Rm was determined by bridge balance (from Woody et al, 1976b).

also showed an increased rate of discharge (cf Krnjevic et al 1971; Woody et al 1978).

When iontophoresis of acetylcholine was performed while repeatedly discharging the cell with depolarizing current pulses, the increases in input resistance were maintained throughout the period of recording. (Again, about half of the cells tested did not respond to acetylcholine, i.e., had no increase in resistance following application of ACh). Figure 1A shows the persistent increase in Rm in data averaged from 12 cells responding to acetylcholine plus depolarization-induced discharge.

Control studies were performed in which (1) the effects of depolarization-induced discharge alone were studied and (2) iontophoresis of saline rather than acetylcholine was combined with depolarization-induced discharge. The results are shown in Fig. 1C. Increases in resistance were significant ($p<.05$, Chi Sq.) in comparison with these controls.

Fig. 2 shows the effect on the resistance of a single

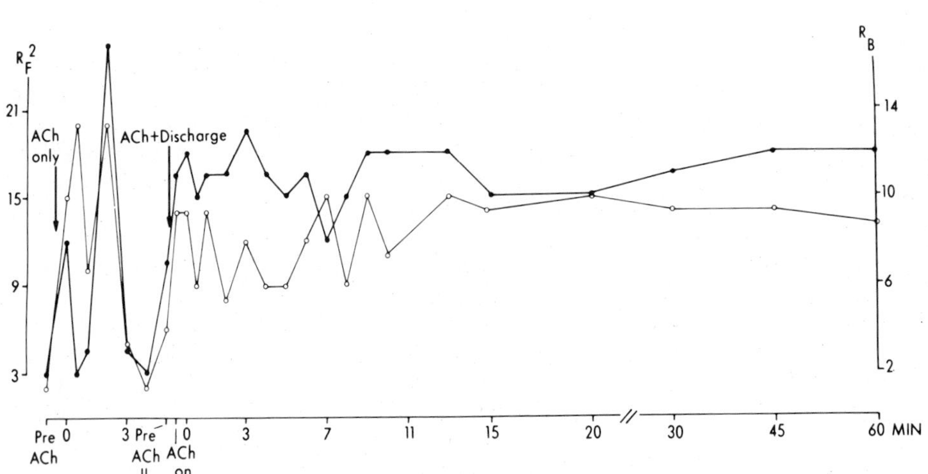

Figure 2. Changes in membrane resistance in a cell given acetylcholine without current-induced discharge (ACh only) followed by acetylcholine plus current-induced discharge (ACh plus discharge). Abscissa and ordinate as in Fig. 1. Determination of resistance by Frank Fuortes method ($R_F 2$), open circle,and by bridge balance (R_B), filled circles (from Woody et al, 1976b).

neuron of giving first ACh alone and then ACh plus depolarization-induced cell discharge. As can be seen ACh alone produced a transient increase in resistance whereas ACh plus depolarization-induced discharge produced an increase in resistance which lasted for one hour (at which time the cell was lost).

Attempts were made to determine whether the persistent increases

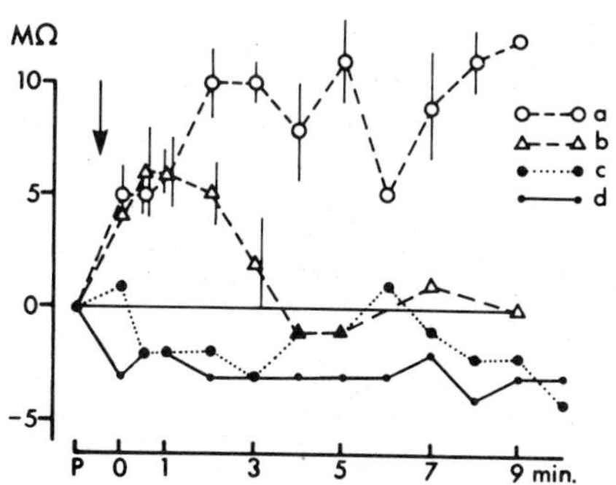

Figure 3. Average changes in input resistance (Rm) in different groups of neurons following (arrow) intracellular iontophoresis of cyclic GMP (cGMP) or control iontophoresis of 5′ GMP in awake cats: (a) neurons responding to cGMP plus current-induced discharge with increased Rm, (b) neurons responding to cGMP alone with increased Rm, (c) neurons given 5′ GMP, and (d) neurons which failed to respond to cGMP with increased Rm. Vertical bars show standard errors of means that are significantly increased above control values. Ordinate shows resistance in megohms determined by method of Frank and Fuortes. Abscissa: p = before iontophoresis of cGMP; remaining values as in Fig. 2 (from Woody et al 1978).

in Rm depended on repetitive discharge of the cells or on injection of the depolarizing current. Results from 23 neurons in which iontophoresis of ACh was paired with injection of depolarizing current pulses insufficient in magnitude to discharge the cell repeatedly are shown in Fig. 1B. As can be seen, the increase in resistance was prolonged beyond its normal point of termination but failed to persist throughout the period of recording.

2. Effects of Cyclic GMP

Effects on resistance of injecting cyclic GMP intracellularly were essentially similar to those of applying acetylcholine extracellularly. One-third to one-half of cells given cGMP responded with an increase in resistance. When cGMP was administered alone, the increase was transient, reaching a peak between 30 sec and 2 minutes after cessation of the iontophoresis and returning to baseline 3 to 5 minutes after cessation. When cGMP was applied together with depolarizing current sufficient to produce repeated spike discharge, a persistent increase in resistance resulted. These effects are illustrated in Fig. 3 for 24 neurons given cGMP plus current-induced discharge and 13 neurons given cGMP alone.

In addition to the cells which failed to respond to cGMP with an increase in Rm (part d of Fig. 3, N=39), an additional group of 41 neurons were given 5′ GMP as a control. As can be seen in Fig. 3, these neurons also failed to respond with an increase in Rm. In the group of cells given 5′ GMP, nineteen were given depolarizing current sufficient to produce repeated spike discharge during application of the nucleotide. The absence of an increase in Rm in this group was similar to that in the other group of 22 neurons in which the depolarizing current given during application of 5′ GMP was insufficient to produce repeated spike discharge. In the former group only one cell showed an increase in Rm and it was transient; in the latter group only one cell showed an increase in Rm and it was persistent.

3. Effects of Sequential Application of ACh and cGMP

Further studies (Swartz and Woody, 1979) were done in which the effects of sequential application of acetylcholine and cyclic GMP were investigated in single neurons. In these cases ACh was first applied extracellularly, then atropine was applied to block the muscarinic effects of ACh, and then ACh was given again. Finally, after these procedures were completed, cGMP was applied intracellularly to determine if the resistance could be increased. The results of these studies showed that of 15 cells responding initially to ACh with an increase in Rm, 14 failed to respond to a second administration of ACh after extracellular iontophoresis of atropine. All 13 of the cells that could be held for a lengthy period responded with a further increase in membrane resistance to subsequent

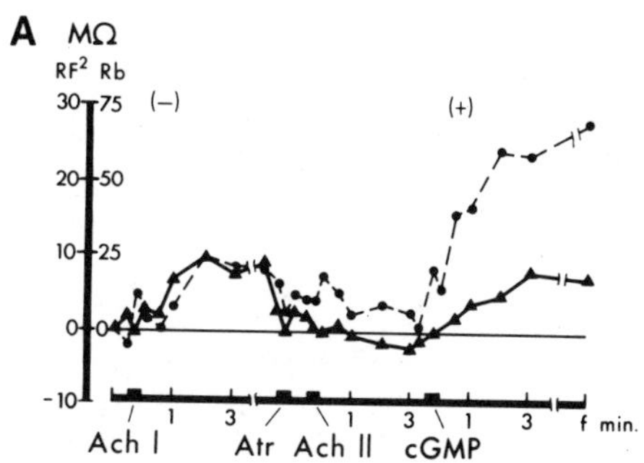

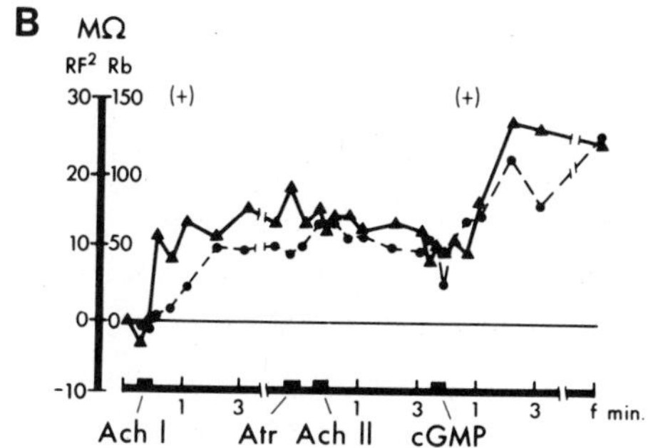

Figure 4. Changes in input resistance in cells which received extracellular iontophoresis of acetylcholine (ACh I), followed by extracellular iontophoresis of atropine (ATR), another extracellular iontophoresis of acetylcholine (ACh II), and then intracellular iontophoresis of cGMP. A. Average data from cells which did not receive current-induced spike discharge (-) during ACh I but did receive current-induced discharge (+) during cGMP. B. Average data from cells which received current-induced discharge during ACh I and cGMP. The ordinate shows changes in resistance (Rm) in megohms, determined by the method of Frank and Fuortes (RF^2, solid lines) and by the bridge balance method (RB, broken lines). Initial values of Rm were set to zero and subsequent values normalized to changes about this value to construct averages. Scales of RF2 are on the left; scales of RB are on the right. Time course of changes in resistance is shown in minutes; f is the final value before losing the cell. The 20 sec iontophoretic period is shown by thickened horizontal bars on the abscissa scales (from Swartz and Woody, 1979).

TABLE 1*

SUMMARY OF ELECTROPHYSIOLOGICAL CHARACTERISTICS

	Number of Cells	AP(mV)	MP(mV)	Firing Rate (spike/sec) Before Activation	After Activation
Antidromically activated cells	13	40 ± 7	52 ± 10	9 ± 3	10 ± 3
Orthodromically activated cells	14	47 ± 12	46 ± 11	12 ± 4	13 ± 5

SUMMARY OF CHANGES IN INPUT RESISTANCE AND SPONTANEOUS FIRING RATE

	A. Input Resistance			B. Spontaneous Discharge	
	Increase	Decrease	No Definite Change	Increase	Decrease
Antidromically activated cells	1	8	4	6	7
Orthodromically activated cells	9	3	2	8	6
	(Difference between antidromically and orthodromically activated cells significant at $p<0.05$, Fisher test.)			(Difference between antidromically and orthodromically activated cells not significant.)	

*(From Tzebelikos and Woody, 1979)

iontophoresis of cGMP. (Two of the 15 cells could not be held long enough to apply cGMP).

Cells given ACh without associated current-induced discharge showed a transient response to ACh; then, when subsequently given cGMP with current-induced discharge, they showed a persistent increase in input resistance. This can be seen in Fig. 4A. Cells given ACh plus current-induced discharge showed a persistent increase in Rm that was not abolished by administration of atropine. Thereafter, when given cGMP plus current-induced discharge, an even higher increase in resistance was observed. this increase also persisted for as long as the cells could be held (Fig. 4B).

4. Effects of Orthodromic and Antidromic Stimulation of Pyramidal Cells.

Effects of stimulating the pyramidal tract were studied in 27 neurons of the motor cortex. Of these, 13 were activated antidromically by PT stimulation and 14 were activated orthodromically (Table 1). Most antidromically activated cells showed a decrease in input resistance and excitability whereas most cells activated orthodromically showed an increase in input resistance and excitability. Interestingly, there was no change in rates of spontaneous discharge associated with the changes in Rm. This mirrored the effects on neuronal excitability found in relation to the behavioral experiments described in the next section. Examples of the changes of excitability following antidromic and orthodromic stimulation are shown in Fig. 5.

5. Effects of US Alone on Neural Excitability at the Motor Cortex

The excitability of cortical neurons to intracellularly injected currents was compared among animals given serial presentations of US alone, those given CS only, and another group given combined CS and US. The method used to determine the excitability of the neurons to injected current is illustrated in Fig. 6. The results (Fig. 7) showed an increased excitability in neurons projecting polysynaptically to the muscles involved with the UR and CR in cats given serial presentations of US but not so pronounced an increase in excitability as in cats given presentations of both CS and US. Further studies showed that the effects of serial presentations of the US were transient, lasting approximately four weeks. (The changes induced by associative presentation of CS and US were persistent.)

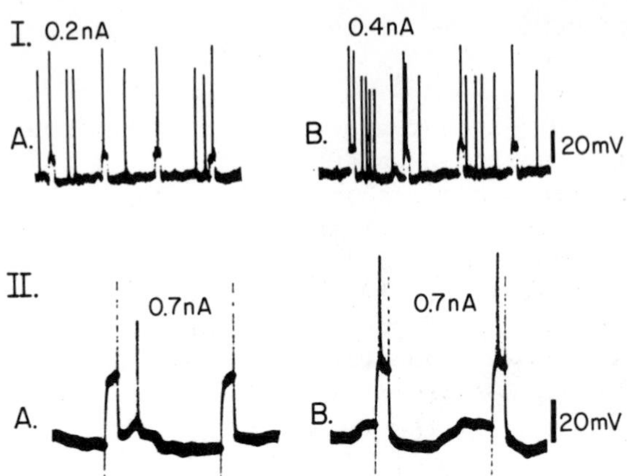

Figure 5. Changes in neural excitability following (I) antidromic activation and (II) orthodromic activation of cortical neurons: (A) prior to activation, (B) subsequent to activation. In I double the current was required for spike elicitation following activation. In II, the same current which failed to produce discharge prior to activation succeeded in producing repetitive discharge thereafter. The upward going rectangles are 10 msec depolarizing current pulses, values as indicated (from Tzebelikos and Woody, 1979).

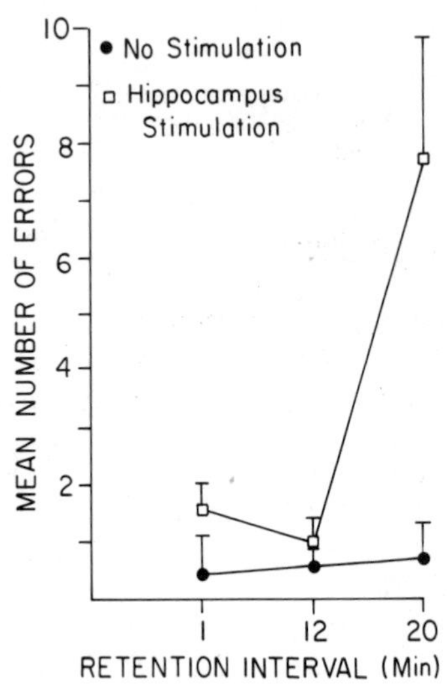

Figure 6. Examples of effects of different levels of intracellularly injected pulse currents on spike activity: a. 0.5 nA hyperpolarization; b. 2.0 nA depolarization; c. 5.0 nA depolarization. Pulses have their onset 6 msec before the end of the sweep. The pulses were 10 msec in duration and were given at rates of 10 Hz. Each trace is 3 superimposed sweeps (from Woody, 1977).

The time course of the changes following nonassociative presentations of the US approximated the time course of the behavioral effects of latent facilitation. Behavioral studies showed that the facilitation of rates of acquisition of conditioning was absent in animals tested four weeks after serial presentations of US (Matsumura and Woody, 1982). The conditioned behavioral response can be elicited over a year after association of these stimuli. Conditioning did not develop to presentations of US only.

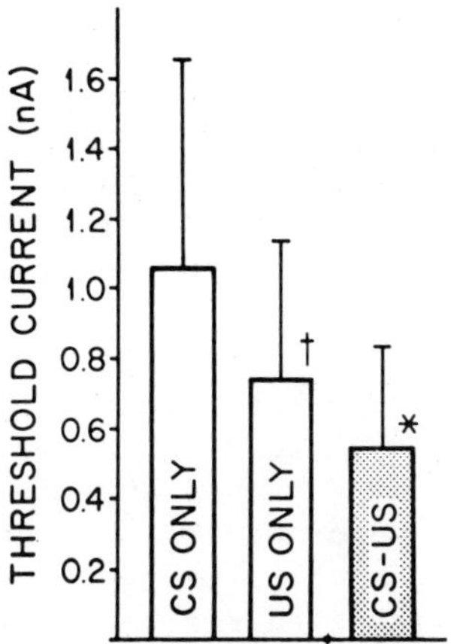

Figure 7. Mean (± SD) threshold currents (in nanoamps) required to discharge cells projecting to both eyeblink (orbicularis oculi) and nosetwitch (levator oris) muscles in cats given serial presentations of CS only versus cats given serial presentations of US only. Less current was required in the latter ($P<0.10$); significantly less current ($P<0.05$) was required in cats given paired CS/US presentations. All data were obtained within 4 weeks of stimulus presentations. (from Brons and Woody, 1980).

DISCUSSION

Latent facilitation of facial movements can arise from repeated presentations of an unconditioned stimulus (e.g. glabella tap) and last for periods of approximately four weeks. We suggest that the type of latent facilitation studied herein is induced, in part, by cholinergically mediated discharge of cortical pyramidal cells projecting polysynaptically to the musculature involved in performing the unconditioned response to the US. In order for conditioning to develop at the behavioral level, it is necessary to have a CS associated with presentation of the US. These associations appear 1) to transform the excitability changes induced by the US from transient changes into persistent changes (Brons and Woody, 1980) and 2) to produce critical associative changes in other neurons that are needed for the development of discriminative conditioning (Woody et al, 1976a). When both changes occur there results performance of a behavioral response to the CS.

Still other neural changes occur during classical conditioning, notably those supporting latent inhibition (or habituatory adaptation) and sensory preconditioning. The former are relatable to a decreased excitability of cortical neurons to weak, extracellularly applied current and decreased rates of spontaneous neuronal discharge (Brons and Woody, 1978). The latter are relatable to an increased excitability of cortical neurons to weak extracellular current and to increased rates of spontaneous firing (Buchhalter et al, 1978). Still other important changes occur, for example those in the hippocampus, thalamus, and cingulate cortex, and they are described elsewhere in this volume. Finally, in the course of presenting the CS and US, neural changes related to presynaptic facilitation and presynaptic inhibition may be expected to occur. Their manifestations appear to be obscured by the other effects of conditioning described herein.

Activation of cholinergic pathways to cells of the motor cortex may be involved in the development of latent facilitation. Aceylcholine (or cyclic GMP) produced increases in resistance that persisted when depolarizing currents sufficient to repeatedly discharge neurons of the motor cortex were applied. Orthodromic (trans-synaptic) activation of cells of the motor cortex by PT stimulation resulted in an increased resistance and excitability comparable to that found with administration of ACh. Antidromic activation did not. This latter finding was in agreement with the observation that current-induced discharge alone failed to produce an increase in resistance without application of ACh. Much stronger stimulation of the pyramidal tract (Bindman et al, 1979) may produce long term increases in the excitability of cortical PT cells by the combination of (orthodromic) cholinergic synaptic discharge with the elicitation of multiple spikes due to antidromic activation. PT cells are thought to receive cholinergic inputs

(Krnjevic and Phillis, 1963; Crawford and Curtis, 1966; Woody and Gruen, 1980) and are thought to mediate changes in the motor cortex supporting Pavlovian eyeblink conditioning with an auditory CS with an auditory CS (Sakai and Woody, 1980). PT stimulation is known to serve as a satisfactory US for producing classical conditioning (O´Brien et al, 1977).

A combination of ACh, depolarization, and an increased rate of discharge appears to be necessary for the increases in resistance to last for more than a few minutes. Repetitive cell discharge per se is not responsible for the persistent increase in Rm since increases in firing rate produced in control experiments in which ACh was not given (Fig. 1C) failed to produce increases in Rm. Depolarizing current itself is also not responsible for the persistent increase in Rm. Pulse depolarizations insufficient to repeatedly discharge cells given ACh resulted in a prolonged incease in Rm but not in a persistent increase. The ranges of current used in the studies shown in Fig. 1B overlapped those shown in Fig. 1A in which ACh plus current-induced discharge resulted in a persistent resistance increase. In the experiments with cGMP, ranges of currents delivered in cells with transiently increased Rm overlapped those in the cells with persistently increased Rm. Thus, the level of current per se also failed to be the decisive factor leading to a persistent increase in Rm.

Increases in firing rate produced as a consequence of administration of ACh or cGMP ranged between 13 and 87% of the increases in firing rate in cells given ACh (or cGMP) plus current-induced discharge, yet only the latter resulted in a persistent increase in Rm. In O´Brien and colleagues´ experiments, PT stimulation had to produce spiking in the studied unit for conditioning to occur. This, again, points to the need for cell activation beyond that arising from simple cholinergic transmission for changes of this type to develop. Besides ACh, the critical variable controlling the production of a persistent increase in Rm may be narrowed to two possibilities. The first would be the combination of depolarization and an increased rate of discharge as above. The second, an increasingly promising possibility, is that of spike entrainment, i.e., doublets or triplets of spike discharges encroaching on refractory periods during the injection of depolarizing current. (It should be noted that the possibilities are by no means mutually exclusive.)

Once formed after the combination of cholinergic synaptic transmission with repetitive, current-induced postsynaptic discharge, the increases in resistance are resistant to disruption. Atropine does not interfere with the changes in resistance once they are established, nor does it interfere with whether or not the increases in resistance to cyclic GMP persist. The resistance to disruption may be useful in mediating latent facilitation of motor performance over periods as long as four weeks.

ACKNOWLEDGEMENT

I acknowledge with pleasure the collaboration of John Brons, Ehud Gruen, and other colleagues (see references) in these studies. The research was supported by BNS 78-24146, HD-05958, and AFOSR #81-0179.

REFERENCES

Bindman, L.J., Lippold, C.J., and Milne, A.R., 1979, Prolonged changes in excitability of pyramidal tract neurones in the cat: post-synaptic mechanism. J. Physiol. 28:457

Bindman, L. and Lippold, O., 1981, "The Neurophysiology of the Cerebral Cortex," E. Arnold: London

Brons, J. and Woody, C.D., 1978, Decreases in excitability of cortical neurons to extracellularly delivered current after eyeblink conditioning, extinction, and presentation of US alone, Soc. Neurosci. Abs. 4:255

Brons, J.F. and Woody, C.D., 1980, Long-term changes in excitability of cortical neurons after Pavlovian conditioning and extinction, J. Neurophysiol. 44:605

Buchhalter, J.R., Brons, J., and Woody, C., 1978, Changes in cortical neuronal excitability after presentations of a compound auditory stimulus. Brain Res. 156:162

Crawford, J.M. and Curtis, D.R., 1966, Pharmacological studies on feline Betz cells, J. Physiol. (Lon) 186:121

Graham-Brown, T. and Sherrington, C.S., 1912, On the instability of a cortical point. Proc. Roy. Soc. B. 85:250

Jordan, S.E., Jordan, J., Brozek,G., and Woody, C.D., 1976, Intracellular recordings of antidromically identified facial motoneurons and unidentified brain stem interneurons of awake, blink conditioned cats, Physiologist 19:245

Kimble, G.A., 1961, "Hilgard and Marquis' Conditioning and Learning," Appleton-Century-Crofts: New York (Second Edition)

Kimble, G.A., Mann, L.I., and Dufort, R.H., 1955, Classical and instrumental eyelid conditioning. J. exp. Psychol. 49:407

Kimble, G.A. and Dufort, R.H., 1956, The associative factor in eyelid conditioning. J. exp. Psychol. 52:386

Krnjevic, K. and Phillis, J.W., 1963, Acetylcholine-sensitive cells in the cerebral cortex, J. Physiol. (Lon) 166:296

Krnjevic, K., Pumain, R., and Renaud, L., 1971, The mechanism of excitation by acetylcholine in the cerebral cortex, J. Physiol. (Lon.) 215:247

Leonard, D.W., Fischbein, L.C., and Monteau, J.E., 1972, The effects of interpolated US alone (USa) presentations on classical nictitating membrane conditioning in rabbit (Oryctolagus cuniculus), Conditional Reflex 7:107

MacDonald, A., 1946, The effects of adaptation to the unconditioned stimulus upon formation of conditioned avoidance responses, J. exp. Psychol. 36:1

Matsumura, M. and Woody, C.D., 1982, Excitability changes of facial motoneurons of cats after acquisition of conditioned and unconditioned facial motor responses. In: "Conditioning: Representation of Involved Neural Function," C.D. Woody, ed., Plenum: New York

O Brien, J.H., Wilder, M.B., and Stevens, C.D., 1977, Conditioning of cortical neurons in cat with antidromic activation as the unconditioned stimulus, J. Comp. Physiol. Psychol. 91:918

Sakai, H. and Woody, C. D., 1980, Identification of auditory responsive cells in coronal-pericruciate cortex of awake cats, J. Neurophysiol., 44:223

Swartz, B. and Woody, C., 1979, Correlated effects of acetylcholine and cyclic guanosine monophosphate on membrane properties of mannalian necortical neurons, J. Neurobiol. 10:465

Tzebelikos, E. and Woody, C.D., 1979, Intracellularly studied excitability changes in coronal-pericruciate neurons following low frequency stimulation of the corticobulbar tract. Br. Res. Bull. 4:635

Ukhtomsky, A., 1911, "On the Dependence of Cortical Motor Reactions upon Central Associated Influences," (Russian), Moscow

Ukhtomsky, A.A., 1927, Concerning the condition of excitation in dominance, Psychol. Abstr. 1:2388

Woody, C.D., Vassilevsky, N.N., Engel, J., Jr., 1970, Conditioned eye blink: unit activity at coronal-precruciate cortex of the cat, J. Neurophysiol. 33:851

Woody, C.D. and Engel, J., Jr., 1972, Changes in unit activity and thresholds to electric microstimulation at coronal pericruciate cortex of cat with classical conditioning of different facial movements. J. Neurophysiol. 35:230

Woody, C.D. and Black-Cleworth, P.A., 1973, Differences in the excitability of cortical neurons as a function of motor projection in conditioned cats, J. Neurophysiol. 36:1104

Woody, C.D., Yarowsky, P., Owens, J., Black-Cleworth, P., and Crow, T., 1974, Effect of lesions of coronal motor areas on acquisition of conditioned eye blink in the cat, J. Neurophysiol. 37:385

Woody, C.D., Knispel, J.D., Crow, T.J., and Black-Cleworth, P.A., 1976a, Activity and excitability to electrical current of cortical auditory receptive neurons of awake cats as affected by stimulus association, J. Neurophysiol. 30:1045

Woody, C.D., Carpenter, D.O., Gruen, E., Knispel, J.D., Crow, T.W., Black-Cleworth, P., 1976b, Persistent increases in membrane resistance of neurons in cat motor cortex, AFRRI SR76:1

Woody, C.D., 1977, Changes in activity and excitability of cortical auditory receptive units of the cat as a function of different behavioral states, Ann. N.Y. Acad. Sci. 290:180

Woody, C.D. and Gruen, E., 1980, Effects of cyclic nucleotides on morphologically identified cortical neurons of cats, Proc. Intl. Un. Physiol. Sci. 14:789

Woody, C.D., Swartz, B.E. and Gruen, E., 1978, Effects of acetylcholine and cyclic GMP on input resistance of cortical neurons in awake cats, Brain Res. 158:373

The following article came to my attention while the manuscript was in press, and is of sufficient significance to warrant insertion: Kopytova, F.V., Mednikova, Yu. S., and Rusinova, E.V. Analog of a conditioned reflex of sensomotor cortical units following microinjection of acetylcholine. Neurosci. Behav. Physiol. 11: 213-220, 1981.

PROCESSES UNDERLYING ONE FORM OF SYNAPTIC PLASTICITY: FACILITATION

Robert S. Zucker

Physiology-Anatomy Department
University of California
Berkeley, CA 94720

SUMMARY

Facilitation is one of the most prevalent forms of synaptic plasticity, and is often invoked as a quality which is important in the nervous system's ability to generate adaptive behavior. The squid giant synapse provides an excellent opportunity to explore the biophysical mechanism of synaptic facilitation. Previous studies showed that facilitation is not due to changes in presynaptic action potentials or after-potentials. Evidence summarized here indicates that facilitation is also not a consequence of presynaptic calcium channel properties, nor is it a reflection of growing increments in presynaptic calcium concentration with repeated activity. Moreover, arsenazo III absorbance microspectrophotometry has revealed a residual calcium following presynaptic activity, and injection of calcium presynaptically facilitates spike-evoked transmitter release. A non-linear relation between calcium and transmitter release is demonstrated, and this plus a mathematical model of diffusive calcium movements within the presynaptic terminal account for both the time course of transmitter release and the magnitude and decay of facilitation following an action potential.

INTRODUCTION

Significance of Facilitation

Synapses, and especially chemically transmitting synapses, do not transmit information in a static fashion. Instead, the efficacy with which a presynaptic action potential influences the firing of the postsynaptic neuron is often a strong function of the level of preceding presynaptic activity. One of the most prominent forms of short-term synaptic plasticity at many synapses is synaptic facilitation, or homosynaptic facilitation, which refers to the enhancement of the strength of synaptic transmission following activity in the presynaptic neuron. Ever since this phenomenon was first described by Feng in 1940, it has attracted the attention of neurobiologists and psychologists. In the last four decades, hundreds of the former have concentrated on its mechanism and integrative function, while since the nineteenth century dozens of the latter have speculated on its role in adaptive behaviors such as conditioned reflexes and higher forms of learning (Ramon y Cajal, 1894; Freud, 1954; Hebb, 1958; Young, 1964; Deutsch, 1971; Rosenzweig et al., 1972; Thompson et al., 1972; Eccles, 1973; Mark, 1974). Recently, a special form of heterosynaptic facilitation, involving the presynaptic facilitatory effect of one pathway upon the efficacy of transmission in another pathway, has been implicated in behavioral sensitization, a simple form of learning sharing some of the characteristics of conditioning (Klein et al., 1981).

Hypothetical Mechanisms of Synaptic Facilitation

In every synapse in which a quantal analysis has been performed, facilitation has been found to be due to an increase in the amount of transmitter released by a nerve impulse (reviewed in Zucker, 1973). Two hypotheses about the mechanism for this presynaptic process enjoyed considerable popularity until recently: 1) the pre-spike hypothesis, which states that more transmitter is released by larger or broader presynaptic action potentials, and 2) the after-potential hypothesis, which proposes that facilitation is a consequence of long-lasting after-potentials in nerve terminals. However, in every synapse at which these hypotheses have been critically tested they have been shown to be false (Zucker, 1974*a*,*c*; Zucker and Lara-Estrella, 1979). The most elegant demonstration that facilitation can occur in the absence of changes in presynaptic action potential and resting potential is the study by Charlton and Bittner (1978*a*,*b*) on the squid giant synapse, where they observed directly with presynaptic intracellular recording from the nerve terminal the electrical events occurring during synaptic facilitation.

Two other hypotheses of the mechanism of facilitation have received more attention recently: 1) the calcium channel hypothesis, which assumes that facilitation is a property of calcium channels, such that they admit more calcium ions to successive depolarizations or repeated identical action potentials, and 2) the residual calcium hypothesis, which supposes that facilitation arises from the action of residual presynaptic intracellular calcium remaining after presynaptic electrical activity.

Both these hypotheses have received some positive experimental support. Measurements of calcium influx into neurons, using the nonlinear calcium-sensitive photoprotein aequorin, suggested that the calcium channels do themselves facilitate (Stinnakre and Tauc, 1973; Eckert et al., 1977; Lux and Heyer, 1977; Stinnakre, 1977). However, measurements of calcium influx using voltage-clamp recording of calcium current or the linear calcium-sensitive dye arsenazo III indicate that calcium channels do not facilitate (Akaike et al., 1978; Tillotson & Horn, 1978; Connor, 1979; Ahmed and Connor, 1979; Smith and Zucker, 1980; Gorman and Thomas, 1980). Unfortunately, none of these studies was performed on presynaptic membrane calcium channels, but rather on molluscan cell body membranes.

The idea that residual presynaptic calcium is responsible for synaptic facilitation was propounded by Katz and Miledi (1965). Several lines of evidence support this hypothesis: 1) Action potentials occurring in a calcium-free medium not only fail to release transmitter, but they also fail to facilitate subsequent transmitter release to later action potentials occurring after restoration of external calcium (Katz and Miledi, 1968). 2) Treatments believed to increase presynaptic calcium concentration, such as exposure to metabolic inhibitors (Alnaes and Rahamimoff, 1975) or fusion with calcium-containing liposomes (Rahamimoff et al., 1978) sometimes increase spike-evoked transmitter release. 3) Exposure to low calcium medium, which may reduce presynaptic calcium during spike activity, reduces the post-tetanic increase in miniature EPSP freauency, which also is thought to arise from residual calcium (Erulkar and Rahamimoff, 1978). Two sub-hypotheses have been been proposed to explain how residual calcium may lead to facilitation: 1) If there is a nonlinear relation between internal calcium and transmitter release, as suggested by a nonlinear relation between external calcium and release (Dodge and Rahamimoff, 1967), then residual calcium will shift the release vs. calcium system to a steeper part of the operating curve. Now a given increment of presynaptic calcium due to the constant influx in an action potential will be more effective in enhancing release, while the same nonlinearity will minimize the effectiveness of residual calcium on spontaneous release rate (Katz and Miledi, 1968; Miledi and Thies, 1971). I call this the nonlinear release version of the residual calcium hypothesis. 2) Alternatively, the calcium entering during an action potential may act at one locus to phasically release transmitter, while residual calcium may act at a different locus to condition subsequent phasic releases and cause facilitation (Balnave and Gage, 1974). I call this the two-site version of the residual calcium hypothesis.

The remainder of this report will focus on two issues: First, I shall summarize experimental results collected at the Marine Biological Laboratory with the collaboration of Drs. Milton Charlton and Stephen Smith, which support a role for presynaptic residual calcium in generating synaptic facilitation at the giant synapse in the stellate ganglion of the squid. The full details of this work have been presented elsewhere (Charlton et al., 1981). Second, I shall present a theoretical model, developed in collaboration with Dr. Norman Stockbridge, of how the internal diffusion of residual calcium away from the plasma membrane can account for the magnitude and kinetics of facilitation at this synapse. Details of this model may be found in Dr. Stockbridge's Ph.D. dissertation (Stockbridge, 1981).

EXPERIMENTAL SUPPORT FOR THE RESIDUAL CALCIUM HYPOTHESIS

Presynaptic Calcium Currents Do Not Facilitate to Repeated Depolarizations

Before proceeding to a test of the residual calcium hypothesis, we explored the possibility that the calcium channels at the presynaptic terminal of the squid giant synapse exhibit intrinsic facilitatory properties. To do this, we used the three-electrode voltage clamp configuration of Adrian et al. (1970) to record the local membrane currents through the end of the presynaptic terminal. Sodium and potassium currents were blocked with external tetrodotoxin and 3,4-diaminopyridine and with presynaptic iontophoresis of tetraethylammonium. Paired brief depolarizing pulses were delivered to the presynaptic terminal and adjusted to evoke subthreshold facilitating EPSPs in the postsynaptic giant axon. Fig. 1A shows the currents recorded during depolarizing pulses. These currents include brief capacitance transients due to the charge and discharge of the presynaptic membrane during the onset and offset of the depolarizations, a large inward calcium current turning on during each pulse, and a superimposed smaller leak current due to the resting potassium and chloride permeability of the membrane. The current trace in Fig. 1B shows the leak and capacitance currents with inverted polarity during two hyperpolarizing pulses of equal magnitude. In Fig. 1C, leak and capacitance currents are also shown alone during depolarizing pulses in low-calcium sea water containing the calcium channel blocker cadmium. Comparison of Figs. 1A-C shows that the inward calcium current that turns on during each depolarization is identical, although the second pulse releases nearly twice as much transmitter as the first. The perfectly linear parts of the capacitance and leak currents can be removed by averaging equal numbers of responses to depolarizing and hyperpolarizing pulses (Fig. 1D), and again the calcium currents appear constant. There was no suggestion of calcium channel facilitation in nine similar experiments, except that in one instance when a very brief (less than 1 msec) interval separated pulses, we observed that the calcium current activated slightly faster during the second pulse. This interval is unphysiological in that it is less than the absolute refractory period, and when longer intervals of over 1 msec were used, no such effect was observed, while facilitation of transmitter release was substantial. Apparently, this effect represents a small priming of activation of calcium channels, probably due to the calcium channels not having returned to their resting state, although they were fully closed. It

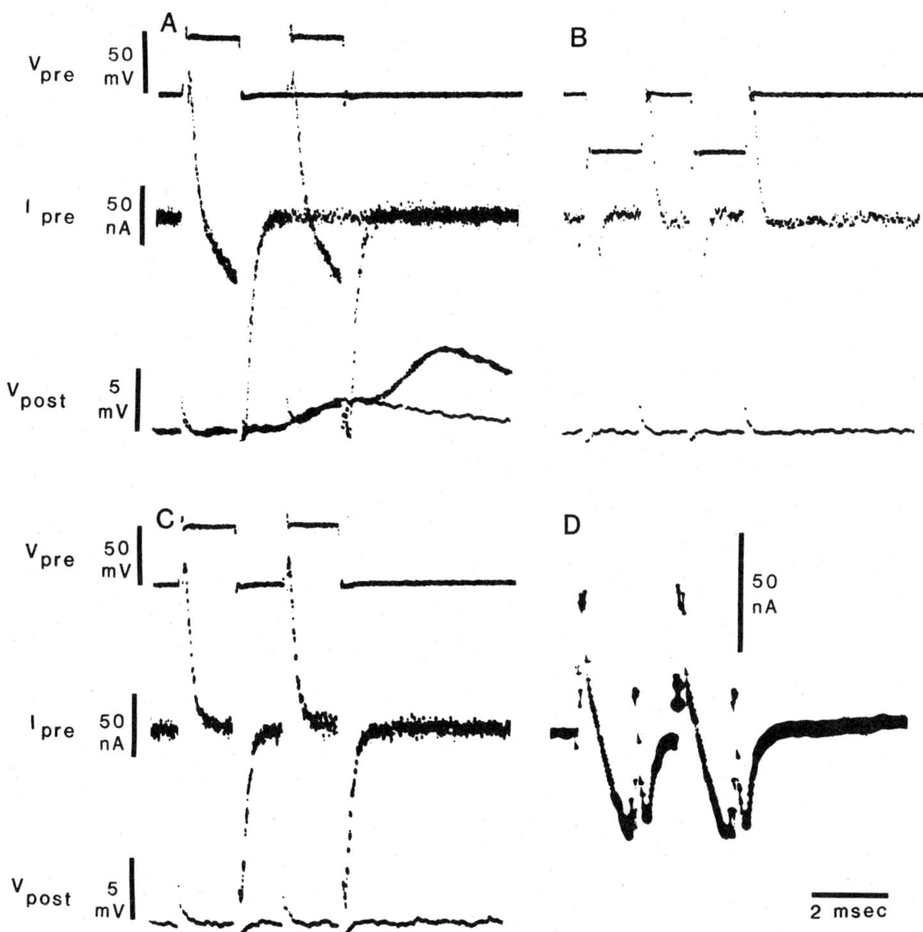

Fig. 1. Non-facilitating calcium currents in the presynaptic terminal. A: Superimposed records of presynaptic calcium, leak, and capacitance currents and postsyaptic potentials to both single and paired paired presynaptic depolarizations. B: Presynaptic leak and capacitance currents to paired hyperpolarizations. C: Presynaptic leak and capacitance currents after blocking calcium current with 1 m*M* cadmium in sea water with only 1 m*M* calcium. D: Presynaptic calcium current, obtained by averaging currents to 8 paired equal and opposite pulses as in A and B. Abbreviations: V_{pre}, presynaptic voltage-clamped potential; I_{pre}, presynaptic membrane current; V_{post}, postsynaptic potential.

is likely that under normal circumstances, facilitation of calcium channels is not involved in synaptic facilitation.

There is a Nonlinear Relation Between Calcium Influx and Synaptic Transmission

It is well known that elevating depolarization amplitude to about 0 mV absolute membrane potential increases both the amplitude of the presynaptic calcium current and the postsynaptic response (Llinas et al., 1981*a*,*b*). Facilitation, in contrast, apparently increases synaptic transmission without any concurrent increase in calcium influx. According to the nonlinear release version of the residual calcium hypothesis, this could arise from a nonlinear relation between internal calcium and transmitter release. We explored this possibility by measuring the relationship between presynaptic calcium current and transmitter release to brief depolarizing pulses of different amplitude. In three preparations, we plotted peak amplitude of presynaptic calcium current vs. peak amplitude of EPSP (after Martin correction), or peak amplitude of calcium current vs. initial slope of EPSP (which is a better measure of synaptic conductance change), or the area of the calcium current during a depolarization, including the tail current following the pulse, vs. EPSP area. In all cases, the data fit a power-law relationship such that when plotted on log-log co-ordinates, most points fall nearly on a straight line with slope of about 2. Two examples of this sort of plot of presynaptic calcium current area vs. EPSP area are shown in Fig. 2. This is a milder nonlinearity than that reported for some synapses (e.g., Dodge and Rahamimoff, 1965), but a steeper one that that reported for others (e.g., Zucker, 1974*b*). However, it is close to that expected from the relation between external calcium and transmitter release at the squid giant synapse (Katz anf Miledi, 1970; Lester, 1970).

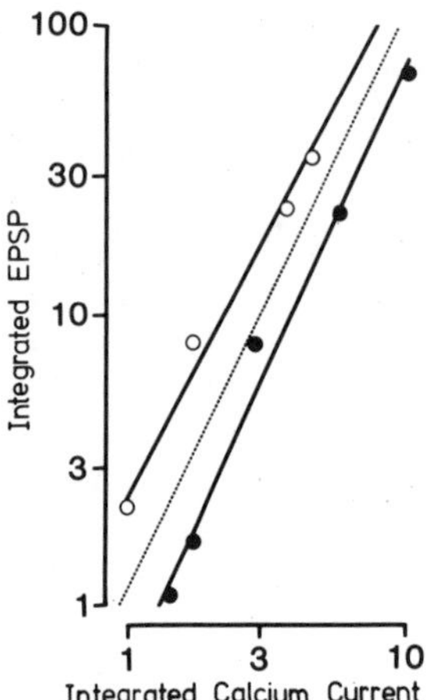

Fig. 2. Relation between transmitter release, measured as EPSP area, and integral of presynaptic calcium current, plotted on logarithmic co-ordinates. Data are from two synapses; units are arbitrary. Dotted line represents a power of 2.

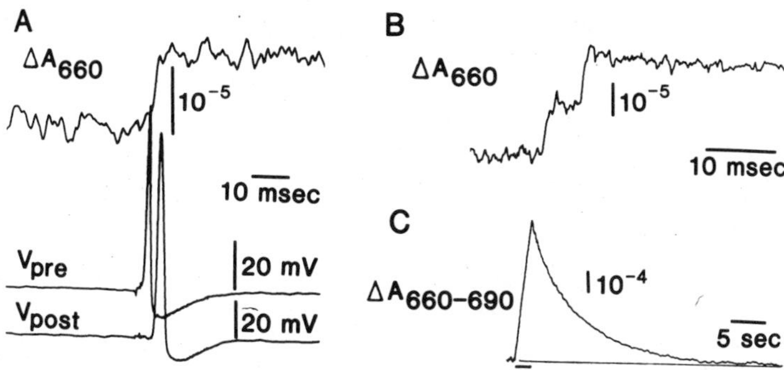

Fig. 3. Absorbance changes at 660 nm (ΔA_{660}) in 3 presynaptic terminals filled with about 0.25 m*M* arsenazo III. A: calcium concentration change and postsynaptic response accompanying one presynaptic action potential. B: Presynaptic calcium concentration transients accompanying paired action potentials. C: Presynaptic calcium concentration change elicited by a 33 Hz train of impulses for the duration of the open bar. Here differential absorbance change at 660 and 690 nm is displayed. Absorbance records are averages of 64 responses in A and 16 in B and C. ΔA of 10^{-5} corresponds roughly to a calcium concentration change of 50 n*M*.

Intracellular Calcium Changes to Repeated Action Potentials Are Constant and Long-Lasting

The above results show that calcium currents do not facilitate during spike-like depolarizations evoking facilitating EPSPs, but do not exclude the possibility that the presynaptic intracellular calcium concentration increments accompanying successive action potentials may facilitate, due for example to a saturation of internal calcium buffers. We measured intracellular calcium concentration changes during electrical activity by filling the presynaptic terminal with the calcium-sensitive dye arsenazo III and recording absorbance changes at several wavelengths of light passing through the terminal with a microspectrophotometer. Low levels of arsenazo III were used, so that the dye interfered very little with normal presynaptic calcium regulation, as indicated by the normal level of suprathreshold synaptic transmission characteristic of this synapse when it is activated in normal calcium medium and by full-size action potentials. Fig. 3A shows a typical presynaptic calcium signal from a giant nerve terminal during a presynaptic action potential, which elicits a suprathreshold postsynaptic spike. The intracellular calcium rises rapidly during the falling phase of the presynaptic spike, when most of the calcium enters the terminal (Llinas et al., 1981*b*), and the calcium level remains high for several seconds following the action potential. When two presynaptic action potentials are elicited in close succession, the EPSPs display a net depression, due to depletion of transmitter stores at high release levels in normal calcium medium with full-size action potentials. Nevertheless, facilitation still occurs normally, although it is masked by depression (Kusano and Landau, 1975; Charlton and Bittner, 1978a). Fig. 3B shows that the calcium increment caused by the second action potential evoking synaptic facilitation is identical to the calcium signal accompanying the first action potential. Finally, trains of presynaptic action potentials elicit a linearly rising absorbance change in the arsenazo-filled terminal, again indicating that facilitation of transmitter release occurs in the absence of any facilitation of transient changes in presynaptic calcium concentration (Fig. 3C). The records of Fig. 3 also show that there is indeed a residual calcium in the nerve terminal which persists long after presynaptic activity has ended (see also Miledi and Parker, 1981).

Injecting Calcium Presynaptically Facilitates Transmission

Until now no evidence has been adduced at any synapse that an increase in presynaptic calcium facilitates spike-evoked transmitter release without affecting the action potential. To test this possibility, we injected calcium by inter-barrel micro-iontophoresis into the presynaptic terminal and observed very little effect on spike-evoked release. It occurred to us that injection of calcium from one point is likely to influence only a small part of the giant synapse, which is about 1 mm long. We modified the experiment by working in a low-calcium medium to block transmission from most of the terminal and by restoring transmission locally with a focal extracellular calcium pipette near the same part of the terminal into which we were injecting calcium. Now only the part of the synapse we could

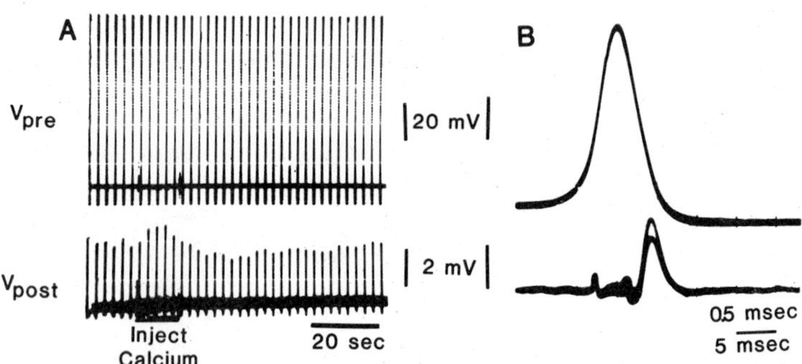

Fig. 4. Effect of presynaptic calcium injection on spike-evoked transmitter release. A: The presynaptic axon was stimulated every 3 seconds, and calcium was injected during the horizontal bar. B: Superimposed presynaptic action potentials and EPSPs in response to one stimulus before and one during presynaptic calcium injection.

influence intracellularly was transmitting in response to action potentials, and we regularly found that elevating intracellular calcium enough to increase the miniature EPSP frequency and elicit a noisy small postsynaptic depolarization (Miledi, 1973) invariably also facilitated spike-evoked release without having any effect whatever on the presynaptic action potential (Fig. 4). Apparently residual calcium exists and can cause facilitation.

THEORETICAL MODEL OF SYNAPTIC FACILITATION DUE TO PRESYNAPTIC DIFFUSION OF RESIDUAL CALCIUM

The above results suggest strongly that synaptic facilitation is due to some action of residual calcium on the release process, and that changes in the presynaptic action potential, resting potential, calcium channels, and size of calcium concentration increments are not involved. However, two important questions remain: 1) How can residual calcium persist for so long (many seconds) in the terminal, while transmitter release decays in a millisecond or two following a presynaptic spike and facilitation decays within a few tens of milliseconds? 2) Can the nonlinear release version of the residual calcium hypothesis explain the kinetic properties of release and facilitation, or must a two-site version be invoked?

With regard to the first question, it must be realized that our measure of residual calcium, using arsenazo III, detects free calcium anywhere in the cytoplasm in the last 3/4 mm of the presynaptic terminal. However, only the calcium ions in the immediate vicinity of transmitter release sites, immediately beneath the presynaptic plasma membrane, can influence transmitter release to an action potential. Facilitation is a short-lived process that is maximal immediately following an action potential. In contrast to post-tetanic potentiation, facilitation does not develop slowly, and cannot be due to changes in transmitter metabolism or to mobilization of stores. Thus, the residual calcium we detect with arsenazo anywhere in the terminal is not the same calcium that can influence transmission and facilitation. What we need is a measurement of the calcium level just beneath the membrane at transmitter release sites. This is not available.

Indeed, from earlier studies of the movement of calcium within cells (Smith and Zucker, 1980 and references therein), we expect that calcium entering a cell through surface membrane channels will rapidly diffuse into the interior of the cell after the channels close, quickly diluting the submembrane calcium concentration, but still being detected by arsenazo. Thus, calcium at release sites ought to decline much more rapidly than the arsenazo signal, which only reports the removal of free calcium from cytoplasm as a whole. Diffusion is just the sort of higher order process postulated in 1968 by Katz and Miledi to remove calcium rapidly from the presynaptic transmitter release sites.

To reconcile the arsenazo data with the characteristics of transmitter release and facilitation, I have used a computational model of calcium diffusion within a cell, originally developed for spherical symmetry by Thompson (1976) and Smith (1978). More recently, I have collaborated with Dr. Norman Stockbridge, who developed a similar model with cylindrical geometry (Stockbridge, 1981). The latter model presumes that calcium ions enter a cylindrical process at the surface, and then diffuse inward. The model includes binding to fixed cytoplasmic sites to account for the slow diffusion of calcium in cytoplasm. Calcium is removed from the system by a surface membrane calcium transport system, and a resting inward calcium current is included to yield a non-zero calcium level in steady state. The parameters of the system are adjusted to accord with physiological measurements of the relevant processes. Thus it is assumed that 1/40 of cytoplasmic calcium remains free while the remaining 97.5% is rapidly bound. This is similar to measurements of the rapid binding of calcium by cytoplasm (Brinley et al., 1977, 1978; Baker and Schlaepfer, 1978). A surface pump rate of 2×10^{-4} cm/sec was selected. This is within the range reported by Blaustein (1976) and DiPolo (1976). A surface leak of 2 f$\underline{M}$/cm^2.sec was selected, to yield a resting intracellular calcium concentration of 10 n$\underline{M}$ (DiPolo et al., 1976). The calcium influx during an action potential was represented as 25 p$\underline{M}$/cm^2.sec for 1 msec, as measured under voltage clamp for spike-like depolarizations by us and Llinas et al. (1981$\underline{a}$). The squid giant presynaptic terminal was represented as an infinitely long circular cylinder having a 0.025 mm radius. These parameters were used to drive the diffusion equation in cylindrical co-ordinates, and the equation was solved numerically for the spatial distribution of intracellular calcium as a function of time during and following one or more presynaptic action potentials.

Fig. 5 shows the behavior of this model in reponse to one or two spikes. In part A, the calcium concentration was integrated throughout the volume of the terminal, to yield an average cytoplasmic concentration as a function of time during and after a single action potential. This corresponds to the arsenazo measurement of intracellular calcium. It may be seen that the model predicts rather well the rate of removal of calcium from cytoplasm detected by arsenazo. The predicted peak in spatially averaged calcium concentration reached during an impulse is slightly lower than we estimate from our arsenazo calibrations (Fig. 3), but we must emphasize that the arsenazo calibration is extremely rough, due to uncertainties in path length, stray light, intracellular arsenazo concentration, and chemical factors affecting the calcium-arsenazo reaction. The rate of calcium removal is set largely by the rate of the calcium extrusion pump, and is nearly unaffected by other parameters.

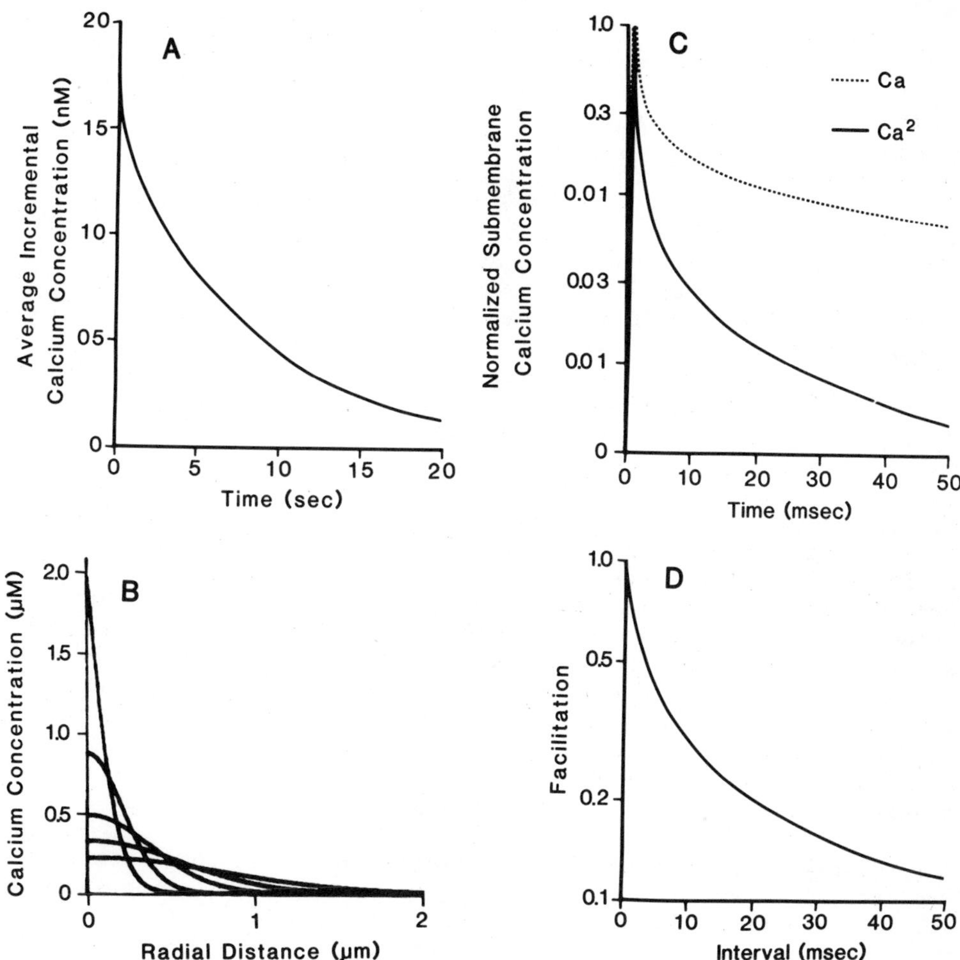

Fig. 5. Predictions of a diffusion model of calcium movements in the presynaptic terminal. A: Average increase in calcium concentration during and after an action potential at time 0. B: Presynaptic calcium concentration vs. distance from the membrane at (from the top) 0, 1, 4, 9, and 19 msec after the end of the action potential. C: Logarithm of submembrane calcium concentration, and its square, during and after a single spike, expressed as a fraction of the peak value at the end of the spike. 1.0 on the ordinate corresponds to 2.21 μM calcium and its square. D: Predicted logarithm of facilitation for two spikes separated by the interval shown on the abscissa. Facilitation is the fractional increase of the second EPSP compared to the first.

However, it is not this average calcium that triggers the release of neurotransmitter, but rather the calcium concentration just underneath the membrane. The calcium entering at the membrane surface diffuses rapidly into the interior of the terminal, so that the initially sharp gradient of calcium at the surface is almost entirely dissipated after about 10 msec (Fig. 5B). Fig. 5C shows the calcium concentration in the 10 nm thick shell just below the plasma membrane as a function of time during and after a nerve impulse (1 synaptic vesicle has a radius of about 25 nm). The submembrane calcium falls to about 50% in 1.5 msec. Since transmitter release depends on the square of the submembrane calcium concentration (see above), it seems more relevant to compare the time course of the square of the predicted submembrane calcium concentration to the time course of the release of transmitter. The latter can be estimated to be about as fast as the rate of decline of postsynaptic current under voltage clamp following a presynaptic action potential. This synaptic current declines with a half time of about 1 msec. The turn-off of transmitter release is probably the rate limiting factor in determining this decay rate, because when transmitter release is artificially shut off almost instantaneously by suddenly stepping the presynaptic membrane potential to the calcium equilibrium potential after a 1 msec moderate depolarization, the postsynaptic current is shortened to less than that following a regular impulse or depolarization (R. Llinas, S. Simon, and M. Sugimori, personal communication). Thus, the decline of the postsynaptic current probably is similar in time course to the decline in transmitter release. From Fig. 5C, it is also similar to the decline of the square in submembrane calcium concentration predicted by the diffusion model.

Finally, Stockbridge and I have used this model to predict the magnitude and time course of synaptic facilitation following a single impulse. We have driven the model with two action potentials separated by various intervals, and estimated the peak submembrane calcium concentration reached by the second peak. If we suppose the amount of transmitter released by a nerve impulse is related to the square of this calcium concentration, then we may predict the facilitation of the second EPSP (expressed as the fractional increase in EPSP size with respect to the first EPSP) by plotting the fractional increase of the peak squared submembrane calcium concentration reached during the second spike with respect to that reached during the first. This prediction is shown in Fig. 5D. Noting the semi-logarithmic co-ordinates, the curve may be described as showing a peak facilitation of about 100%, with a prominent early decline lasting about 10 msec and a slower and smaller component lasting a few tens of milliseconds. This is almost exactly how facilitation actually behaves at the squid giant synapse (Charlton and Bittner, 1978a).

CONCLUSIONS

From this and earlier work, we may conclude that synaptic facilitation is not caused primarily by changes in the presynaptic action potential, membrane potential, calcium channels, or calcium buffering. Rather, synaptic facilitation may be accounted for quantitatively as a consequence of a residual presynaptic calcium following nerve activity, operating on a nonlinear dependence of transmitter release on calcium to amplify the effect of a constant calcium influx accompanying nerve impulses. A final proof of this hypothesis must await the development of techniques to measure directly and selectively the submembrane calcium concentration following nerve activity, and to manipulate submembrane calcium accurately so as to measure precisely the dependence of transmitter release on submembrane calcium. Until then, the nonlinear release version of the residual calcium hypothesis will remain only our best hypothesis for the mechanism of this fascinating and ubiquitous form of synaptic plasticity.

ACKNOWLEDGEMENTS

I am indebted to Dr. Norman Stockbridge for his efforts in modifying his computer program and generating the predictions of Fig. 5. I also thank Dr. Rodolfo Llinas for sharing his unpublished results with me. The author's research is supported by NIH Grant NS 15114.

REFERENCES

Adrian, R. H., Chandler, W. K., and Hodgkin, A. L., 1970, Voltage clamp experiments in striated muscle fibres, J. Physiol., Lond., 208:607.

Ahmed, Z., and Connor, J. A., 1979, Measurement of calcium influx under voltage clamp in molluscan neurones using the metallochrome dye arsenazo III, J. Physiol., Lond., 286:61.

Akaike, N., Lee, K. S., and Brown, A. M., 1978, The calcium current of Helix neuron, J. gen. Physiol., 71:509.

Alnaes, A., and Rahamimoff, R., 1975, On the role of mitochondria in transmitter release from motor nerve terminals, J. Physiol., Lond., 248:285.

Baker, P. F., and Schlaepfer, W. W., 1978, Uptake and binding of calcium by axoplasm isolated from giant axons of Loligo and Myxicola, J. Physiol., Lond., 276:103.

Balnave, R. J., and Gage, P. W., 1974, On facilitation of transmitter release at the toad neuromuscular junction, J. Physiol., Lond., 239:657.

Blaustein, M. P., 1976, The ins and outs of calcium transport in squid axons: internal and external ion activation of calcium efflux, *Fedn. Proc.*, 35:2574.

Brinley, F. J., Jr., Tiffert, T., and Scarpa, A., 1978, Mitochondria and other calcium buffers of squid axon studied *in situ*, *J. gen. Physiol.*, 72:101.

Brinley, F. J., Jr., Tiffert, T., Scarpa, A., and Mullins, L. J., 1977, Intracellular calcium buffering capacity in isolated squid axons, *J. gen. Physiol.*, 70:355.

Charlton, M. P., and Bittner, G. D., 1978*a*, Facilitation of transmitter release at squid synapses, *J. gen. Physiol.*, 72:471.

Charlton, M. P., and Bittner, G. D., 1978*b*, Presynaptic potentials and facilitation of transmitter release in the squid giant synapse, *J. gen. Physiol.*, 72:487.

Charlton, M. P., Smith, S. J., and Zucker, R. S., 1981, Role of presynaptic calcium ions and channels in synaptic facilitation and depression at the squid giant synapse, *J. Physiol.*, in press.

Connor, J. A., 1979, Calcium current in molluscan neurones: measurement under conditions which maximize its visibility, *J. Physiol., Lond.*, 286:41.

Deutsch, J. A., 1971, The cholinergic synapse and the site of memory, *Science, N.Y.*, 174:788.

DiPolo, R., 1976, The influence of nucleotides on calcium fluxes, *Fedn. Proc.*, 35:2579.

DiPolo, R., Requena, J., Brinley, F. J., Jr., Mullins, L. J., Scarpa, A., and Tiffert, T., 1976, Ionized calcium concentrations in squid axons, *J. gen. Physiol.*, 67:433.

Dodge, F. A., Jr., and Rahamimoff, R., 1967, Co-operative action of calcium ions in transmitter release at the neuromuscular junction, *J. Physiol., Lond.*, 193:419.

Eccles, J. C., 1973, ''The Understanding of the Brain,'' McGraw-Hill, New York.

Eckert, R., Tillotson, D., and Ridgway, E. G., 1977, Voltage-dependent facilitation of Ca^{2+} entry in voltage-clamped, aequorin-injected molluscan neurons, *Proc. natn. Acad. Sci. U. S. A.*, 74:1748.

Erulkar, S. D., and Rahamimoff, R., 1978, The role of calcium ions in tetanic and post-tetanic increase of miniature end-plate potential frequency, *J. Physiol., Lond.*, 278:501.

Feng, T. P., 1940, Studies on the neuromuscular junction. XVIII. The local potentials around N-M junctions induced by single and multiple volleys, *Chin. J. Physiol.*, 15:367.

Freud, S., Project for a scientific psychology, *in*: ''The Origins of Psycho-Analysis. Letters to Wilhelm Fliess, Drafts and Notes: 1887-1902,'' M. Bonaparte, A. Freud, and E. Kris, eds., E. Mosbacher and J. Strachey, trs., Basic Books, New York.

Gorman, A. L. F., and Thomas, M. V., 1980, Intracellular calcium accumulation during depolarization in a molluscan neurone, *J. Physiol., Lond.*, 308:259.

Hebb, D. O., 1958, ''A Textbook of Psychology'', Saunders, Philadelphia.

Katz, B., and Miledi, R., 1965, The effect of calcium on acetylcholine release from motor nerve terminals, _Proc. Roy. Soc. Lond. B_, 161:496.

Katz, B., and Miledi, R., 1968, The role of calcium in neuromuscular facilitation, _J. Physiol., Lond._, 195:481.

Katz, B., and Miledi, R., 1970, Further study of the role of calcium in synaptic transmission, _J. Physiol., Lond._, 207:789.

Klein, M., Shapiro, E., and Kandel, E. R., 1980, Synaptic plasticity and the modulation of the Ca^{2+} current, _J. exp. Biol._, 89:117.

Kusano, K., and Landau, E. M., 1975, Depression and recovery of transmission at the squid giant synapse, _J. Physiol., Lond._, 245:13.

Lester, H. A., 1970, Transmitter release by presynaptic impulses in the squid stellate ganglion, _Nature, Lond._, 227:493.

Llinas, R., Steinberg, I. Z., and Walton, K., 1981_a_, Presynaptic calcium currents in squid giant synapse, _Biophys. J._, 33:289.

Llinas, R., Steinberg, I. Z., and Walton, K., 1981_b_, Relationship between presynaptic calcium current and postsynaptic potential in squid giant synapse, _Biophys. J._, 33:323.

Lux, H. D., and Heyer, C. B., 1977, An aequorin study of a facilitating calcium current in bursting pacemaker neurons of _Helix_, _Neuroscience_, 2:585.

Mark, R. F., 1974, ''Memory and Nerve Cell Connections,'' Oxford Univ., Oxford.

Miledi, R., 1973, Transmitter release induced by injection of calcium ions into nerve terminals, _Proc. Roy. Soc. Lond. B_, 183:421.

Miledi, R., and Parker, I., 1981, Calcium transients recorded with arsenazo III in the presynaptic terminal of the squid giant synapse, _Proc. Roy. Soc. Lond. B_, 212:197.

Miledi, R., and Thies, R., 1971, Tetanic and post-tetanic rise in frequency of miniature end-plate potentials in low-calcium solutions, _J. Physiol., Lond._, 212:245.

Rahamimoff, R., Meiri, H., Erulkar, S. D., and Barenholz, Y., 1978, Changes in transmitter release induced by ion-containing liposomes, _Proc. natn. Acad. Sci. U. S. A._, 75:5214.

Ramon y Cajal, S., 1894, La fine structure des centres nerveux, _Proc. Roy. Soc. Lond. B_, 55:444.

Rosenzweig, M. R., Bennett, E. L., and Diamond, M. C., 1972, Chemical and anatomical plasticity of brain: replications and extensions, _in_: ''Macromolecules and Behavior'', 2nd edn., J. Gaito, ed., Appleton-Century-Crofts, New York.

Smith, S. J., 1978, The mechanism of bursting pacemaker activity in neurons of the mollusc _Tritonia diomedia_, Ph.D. Dissertation, Univ. Washington, Seattle.

Smith, S. J., and Zucker, R. S., 1980, Aequorin response facilitation and intracellular calcium accumulation in molluscan neurones, _J. Physiol., Lond._, 300:167.

Stinnakre, J., 1977, Calcium movements across synaptic membranes and the release of transmitter, _in_: ''Synapses'', G. A. Cottrell and P. N. R. Usherwood, eds., Academic, New York.

Stinnakre, J., and Tauc, L., 1973, Calcium influx in active *Aplysia* neurones detected by injected aequorin, *Nature, New Biol.*, 242:113.

Stockbridge, N., 1981, Possible roles of calmodulin and diffusion in the release of transmitter from the neuromuscular junction of the frog, Ph.D. Dissertation, Duke Univ., Durham.

Thompson, R. F., Patterson, M. M., and Teyler, T. J., 1972, The neurophysiology of learning, *Psychol. Rev.*, 23:73.

Thompson, S. H., Membrane currents underlying bursting in molluscan pacemaker neurons, Ph.D. Dissertation, Univ. Washington, Seattle.

Tillotson, D., and Horn, R., 1978, Inactivation without facilitation of calcium conductance in caesium-loaded neurones of *Aplysia*, *Nature, Lond.*, 273:312.

Young, J. Z., 1964, ''A Model of the Brain'', Oxford Univ., Oxford.

Zucker, R. S., 1973, Changes in the statistics of transmitter release during facilitation, *J. Physiol., Lond.*, 229:787.

Zucker, R. S., 1974*a*, Crayfish neuromuscular facilitation activated by constant presynaptic action potentials and depolarizing pulses, *J. Physiol., Lond.*, 241:69.

Zucker, R. S., 1974*b*, Characteristics of crayfish neuromuscular facilitation and their calcium dependence, *J. Physiol., Lond.*, 241:91.

Zucker, R. S., 1974*c*, Excitability changes in crayfish motor neurone terminals, *J. Physiol., Lond.*, 241:111.

Zucker, R. S., and Lara-Estrella, L. O., 1979, Is synaptic facilitation caused by presynaptic spike broadening?, *Nature, Lond.*, 278:57.

ACTIVITY OF NEURONS IN AREA 4 AND IN AREA 5 OF MONKEY DURING OPERANT CONDITIONING OF A FLEXION MOVEMENT

Y. Burnod, B. Maton, and J. Calvet

INSERMU 3 CNRS
Hopital Salpetriere, 47 Bd Hopital
Paris, France

SUMMARY

Present data concern changes of neuronal activity in Area 4 and Area 5 of macaca Speciosa, during shaping of a self initiated flexion movement of the elbow without sensory cues. Two behavioral changes occur during this period and are quantified: increase in the frequency of movements and change in the shape (amplitude, muscular contraction of biceps and triceps). The authors propose a model to quantify neuronal patterns whose changes are compared with the changes in behavior. Two sets of neurons are described, one more active with the flexion movement, the other active with the taking of the reward by the ipsilateral arm; there is an important spatial overlap between them. Neurons active both with conditioned movement and taking of the reward can show an enhancement of their activity when the first series of movements appear. An increase in the regularity of the conditioned movement corresponds to a balance between the two sets described. Cells whose activity is maximal with the conditioned movement show changes parallel with performance. During the sessions in which there is an increase in the accuracy of the movement, some cells show an increase in activity at the onset of the flexion movement.

INTRODUCTION

The main topic of this study is to understand how learning of a new movement may be due to changes in the nervous system provoked by a temporal linkage between this movement and a reward. Monkeys can learn very precise movement of the arm. Neuronal activity of the different parts of the nervous system that may command and control this class of movement has been studied in naive monkeys and has been more precisely quantified in overtrained monkeys. For example, in Area 4 of the cerebral crotex , neurons discharge prior to muscle activity and their frequency is predictive of muscular contraction (EVARTS), and neurons in Area 5 discharge prior to arm projection and manipulation (MOUNTCASTLE et al.). Two points may be evaluated by recording electrical activity of neurons in these area during the first stage of operant conditioning, when repetition of a movement that fits a-priori criteria appears: 1) the possible temporal patterns of neuronal activity during the behavioral events of this period, i.e., conditioned movement and reward-related movement. 2) a cinoarusib between changes in neuronal activity and changes in behavior that occur during one conditioning session. Present data concern neuronal activity in Area 4 and 5 of the cerebral cortex of *Macaca Speciosa* during conditioning sessions of a self initiated flexion of the elbow.

METHODS

A monkey was placed in a primate chair; the right forearm was attached to a horizontal support which could retotate around a vertical axis corresponding to that of the elbow. The only possible movements of the right arm were flexions around this axis in an horizontal plane and were described by one parameter, angle of the arm, with a starting position "A". The flexion had to be performed against a constant load from a fixed position "A" to an arrival position "B"; "B" was any position within a sector determined by the conditioning program, without external signal or cue. A screen prevented the monkey from seeing the rotating arm. The EMGs of the surface of the biceps and triceps brachii was recorded and appeared in form of impulsions, the frequency of which was proportional to the surface of the rectified EMG. The reward was a piece of fruit given automatically on a tray in front of the free left arm. Movement of the left arm was controlled by photoelectric cells indicating when the monkey grasped the reward in the tray. A window in the skull allowed the penetration of microelectrodes from the arcuate to the intraparietal sulcus of the left hemisphere. Two microdrives allowed parallel but independent penetration of two platinum microelectrodes, one in area 4, the other in area 5. Two restricted parts of Area 4 and 5 were studied: that of Area 4 in the zone of the arm and that of Area 5 was located in the same lateral plane. The position of each recorded cell was measured relative to the four extreme penetrations which were histologically identified. This identification allowed the reconstruction of the position of each recorded neuron.

CONDITIONING PROGRAM-BEHAVIOR

Reward related movements of the left arm are stereotyped sequences triggered by the sight of the pece of fruit: extension of the arm, grasping of the fruit, flexion to the mouth; this sequence exists before conditioning and does not change during conditioning. Before conditioning the monkey performs few movements of the right arm. At the beginning the angular zone of arrival is broad. There is an increase of the frequency of reward due to an increase of the frequency of flexion movements. This increase is observed during several consecutive sessions. During the following sessions the angular zone of arrival is decreased. There is no increase in the frequency of flexion movements but an increase in the frequency of reward due to an increase in the proportion of flexion movements that fit the conditioning criteria. There is at the same time an increase in the temporal regularity of movements. When the frequency of reward does not increase more, the center of the angular zone of arrival is changed. There are new periods during which the frequency of reward increases due also to an increase in the proportion of flexion movements that fit the criteria. During a two hours session, the frequency of reward does not show a regular increase due to pauses, fatigue or satiety. However there are periods of about 15 minutes during which the frequency of reward increases in an obvious way. These periods are chosen to compare the changes in cell activity with the changes in behavior.

QUANTIFICATION OF CELLULAR ACTIVITY

Unitary discharges were studied only when they were well defined by both their amplitude and shape. Their frequency was determined every 20 msec by means of triggers and counters. A model is proposed to represent cellular activity by trapezoids (Fig. 1): constant levels separated by linear increases or decreases. Starting, ending position and amplitude of slopes are automatically determined by the least sqare method. The model is computed on means triggered by behavioral events (onset of movement, grasping of the reward) and cellular events (levels of neuronal activity, levels of IEMG). Four parameters of the model quantify the cell activity: lower (AB) and higher (AR+AB) level, latency of the onset (D) of increase, and latency of the higher level. These parameters allow a quantitative comparison of the cell activity between different events. When events correspond to different thresholds of the same variable, the model allows us to establish during each period the quantitative relationship between mechanical parameters of the movement (amplitude, velocity, acceleration) and cell activity. When the increase AR is significant at $p=.001$ the activity of the cell is said to be tied to the event. To get a good idea of how the model behaves when applied to the cell activities studied here, the ratio of standard deviation/ mean value is of the order of magnitude of 0.1. A relative increase of 1.1 is significant at .001 with 16 degrees of freedom.

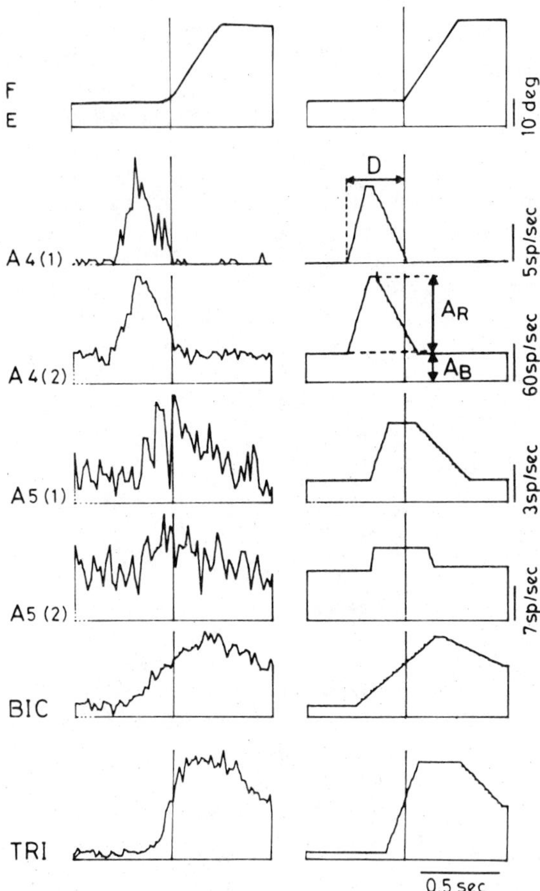

Fig. 1 Quantitative analysis of neuronal activities
Left: histograms of density of neuronal discharges and of the IEMG synchronized at the onset of successive movements (vertical line). Upper to lower: amplitude of the flexion movement (F, flexion; E, extension) A4(1) unitary activity in Area 4. A4(2) corresponding multi-unit activity. Same conventions for Area 5(A5). BIG and TRI: integrated EMG of biceps and triceps brachii.
Right: models of activities shown at left (see text). D measures the latency of the cell, AB the background activity, AR the increase at the onset of the movement.

SETS OF NEURONS

Before examining the time course during one training session, it is necessary to define the sets of cells observed in the explored regions in relation to the behavioral events: flexion movement of the contralateral arm and taking of the reward. Approximately 360 cells were recorded in each of the two zones in Area 4, the discharge of 209 neurons was studied in association with the flexion movement of the elbow (Fig. 1). Figure 2 shows the distribution of the latencies. There was a maximum between 160 and 80 msec prior to the onset of the movement. In Area 5, the discharge of 180 neurons was studied in association with the flexion movement (Fig. 1). Figure 2 shows that many neurons of Area 5 were active before the onset of the movement but there was no clear maximum in the distribution. Furthermore the increase of activity and the latency were more variable for successive movements than in Area 4. In the two areas these neurons were also active when the arm was moved by an external torque.

Another set of neurons contained neurons that were active when the monkey caught the reward with ipsilateral arm during one of the three phases: extension of the arm to the tray, grasping of the fruit or flexion to the mouth. Figure 6(left) shows two such neurons, one in area 4 and the other in area 5. 54 neurons in Area 4 and 96 in Area 5 were in this set. These cells were active with passive movements of the ipsilateral arm.

A third set of neurons was the intersection of the two sets described above. Neurons of this set are active during the flexion movement with the contralateral arm and during one of the phases of the taking of the reward with the ipsilateral arm (Fig. 3 for Area 5, Fig. 4 for Area 4). These cells are active during flexion movement without a reward (Fig. 4) and when the monkeys takes a fruit independently of a flexion movement. The model shows that the activity of some neurons is more important for movement with the ipsilateral than with the contralateral arm. Different combinations of timing and amplitude are observed. 46 neurons in Area 4 and 61 neurons in Area 5 are in this set. Neurons of Area 4 that are active bilaterally seem more frequent in the anterior part of this area. These neurons are driven by passive movements of the two arms. At the beginning of training there are two sets of neurons in each area that are active during the conditioned movement and during the taking of the reward. There is a spatial overlap between these two set, and some neurons are thus active two times when a movement is rewarded.

NEURONAL ACTIVITY DURING TRAINING SESSIONS

During the duration of each training session two neurons, one in Area 4 and the other in Area 5, were recorded simultaneously and analyzed in relation to the flexion movement. This was done during ninety training sessions with three monkeys, therefore giving ninety pairs of cells studied over periods from 30 minutes to 2 hours.

For neurons in Area 4 and Area 5 whose maximal activity occurs in relationship with the flexion movement, changes in cell activity and changes in behavior (frequency and shape of the flexion movement) are parallel. There is a good correlation between cell activity and performance. The same observations that are done on flexion movement can be done for these neuronal activities. During a conditioning session, when a movement is rewarded, the probability of repeating this movement increases; the probability of firing of these neurons increases in the same way. However because of the cell variability, the parallel changes of movement and cell activity become precise when the mean value of cell activity is computed from 5 to 20 successive movements. For neurons whose activity is not maximal at the onset of the movement, other types of changes can be observed.

a) The increase in the frequency of reward is due to an increase in the frequency of movements. After a period of isolated flexion movements, a series of repetitive movements occurs. The two periods are compared in Figure 5 for a neuron of Area 4 which is active before the onset of the movement and before the grasping of the reward. When the frequency of the movement is low, the two times of activity of the cell have a similar amplitude. But, since the first movement of the series, there is a strong enhancement of the activity of the cell during the taking of the reward; there is an addition of the two activities of the neuron.

b) The increase in the frequency of reward corresponds to an increase in the regularity of the intervals between movements. For cells whose activity is maximal with the taking of the reward (Fig. 6, left), it is possible to study the coupling between this maximal activity and the following flexion movement (Fig. 6, right). The mean values are synchronized to the end of the maximal activity of the neuron of Area 5 and for the flexion movement the results of two periods A and B are superimposed: A (dashed line) before and B after an increase in the frequency of reward. The probability that a flexion movement occurs in the next 100 msec after the cell activity has increased strongly. There is an increase of the temporal relationship between maximal cell activity and the onset of the next flexion movement. Regularity in the performance of the movement corresponds then to a balance between cell activity linked with flexion of the right arm and, in the same cortical area, cell activity linked with taking of the reward. There is a temporal overlap of the activities of these two sets at the onset of the movement. For cells whose activity is tied to the onset of the flexion movement but is not maximal at this time, it is interesting to notice that in period A the temporal

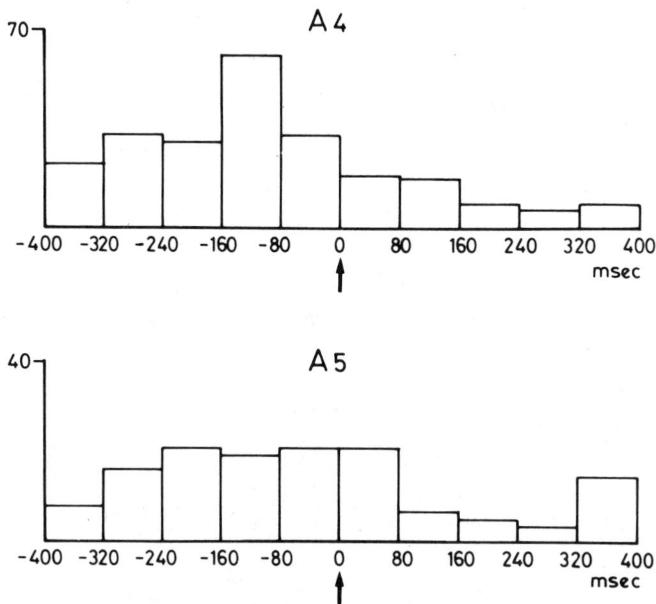

Fig. 2 Latency histogram of all the recorded neurons in Area 4 (upper) and in Area 5 (lower) active at the onset of the movement (arrow). Latency is parameter D of the model.

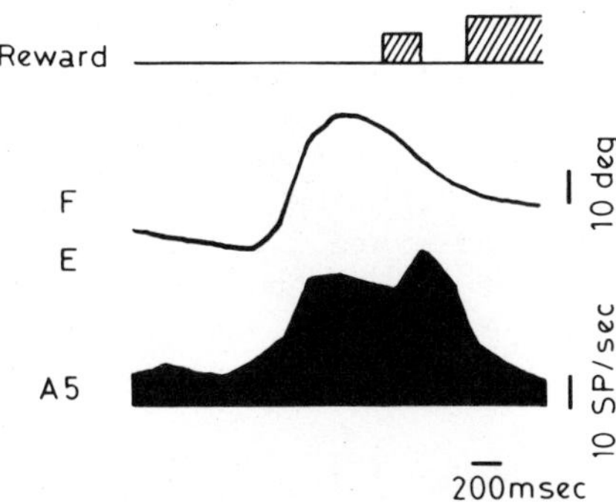

Fig. 3 Activity of a neuron of Area 5 with movement and reward. The two signals on the first line (REWARD) indicate the rotation of the tray that delivers fruit and the grasping of the fruit (thicker). Histogram synchronized on the rotation of the tray. Same conventions as for Fig. 1.

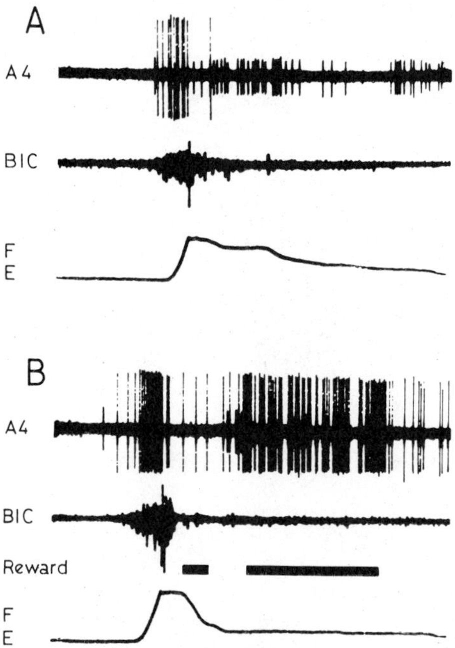

Fig. 4 Activity of a neuron of Area 4 active with the conditioned movement and the taking of the reward. A movement without a reward; B movement with a reward. Traces show discharges of the neuron of Area 4, IEMG of the biceps and amplitude of the flexion. Same conventions as for Fig. 1 and Fig. 3. The discharges of another neuron in the vicinity are recognizable.

regularity of this maximal activity can be higher than the regularity of the flexion movement, as demonstrated by interval histogram (Fig. 7). In period B the distribution of intervals between movements become more regular and the maximum of this distribution can be the same as for the cell.

c) Increase in the frequency of reward due to an increase in the precision of the movement. There is not change in the frequency of the flexion movement but an increase in the frequency of reward. Figure 8 represents the activity of a neuron of Area 5 during such a session. This neuron is active before the onset of the flexion movement as seen when the means are triggered by the onset of the movement. However, this activity is not the maximal activity of the cell as seen when the means are triggered by the highest level of cell activity. During the whole period when there is an increase in the frequency of reward, there is a constant increase in the activity of the cell at the onset of the flexion movement, and this activity reaches the maximum level at the end of the period. Parallel analysis of the mean parameters of the movement shows that this increase is not due to a change in the shape of the movement (the same analysis was done on velocity, acceleration, IEMG of biceps and triceps).

d) The frequency of reward increases after a change of the center of the sector of arrival. The adaptation of the monkey to a change in the center of the arrival sector is faster than the preceding learnings. As can be demonstrated by changing the starting position, the monkey learns the amplitude of the movement and not the absolute final position. The patterns of EMG of biceps and triceps show a co-contraction of the two muscles; the activity of the biceps increases in parallel with the amplitude of the movement. For cells active at the onset of the movement, but which are more active at other times (for example during the taking of the reward), it is possible to see an increase in activity at the onset of movement during the period of adaptation to the new sector (Fig. 9). This increase is similar to the increase shown in Figure 8; it is not parallel with the increase in the amplitude of the movement.

e) The relationship between cell activity and reward is as follows. In general, when a reward occurs just after an important activity of a neuron, there is not a short term enhancement of activity just after the reward. Two sets of cells show short term changes. For cells which have their maximal activity with the flexion movement, the probability of repetition of this activity increases (like for the flexion movement). For cells active both with movement and reward. There can be an enhancement during the second activity (Fig. 5).

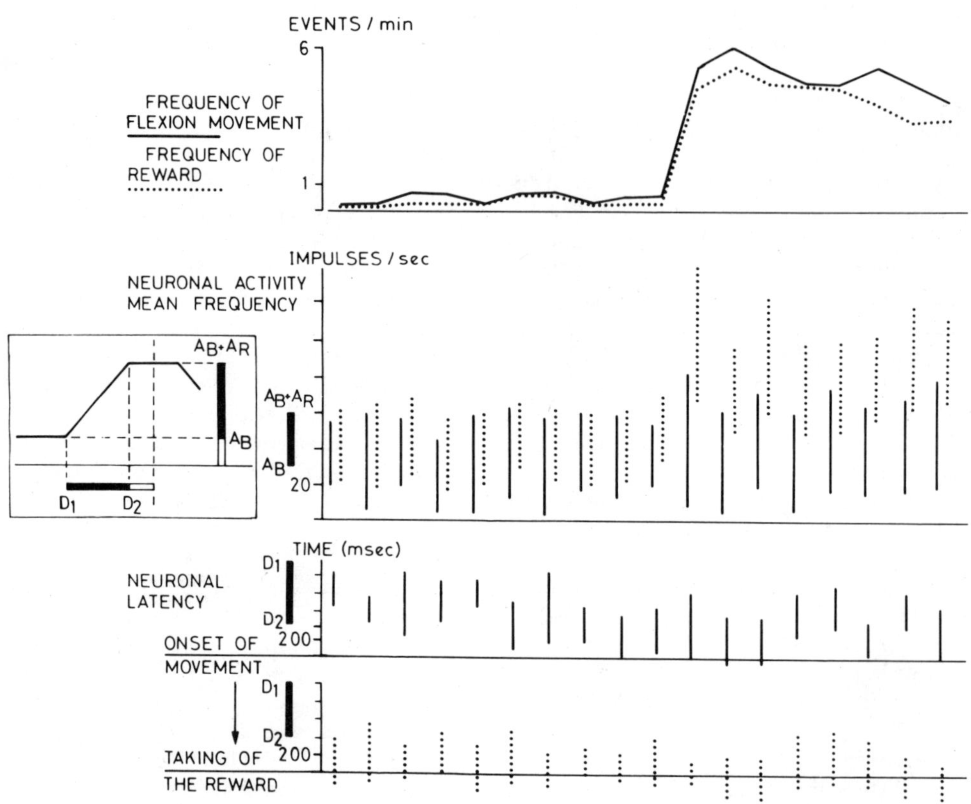

Fig. 5 Changes in the activity of a neuron in Area 4 during a session when the frequency of movement increases. Each of the three diagrams represents the results of successive periods of analysis during half an hour of a conditioning session.
Upper diagram: frequency of movement and frequency of reward.
Middle: each vertical double bar represents the increase of discharge frequency at the onset of the flexion movement (continuous bar) and at the grasping of the fruit (dotted bar); each double bar is the result of one period of analysis of 1 min. Lower and upper limit of each bar represents the two parameters AR and AR+AB computed by the model as shown at left.
Lower diagram: latency of the cell's activity with respect to the onset of the flexion movement (continuous bar) and to the grasping of the fruit (dotted bar). Each bar represents the two parameters D1 and D2 of the model as shown at left.

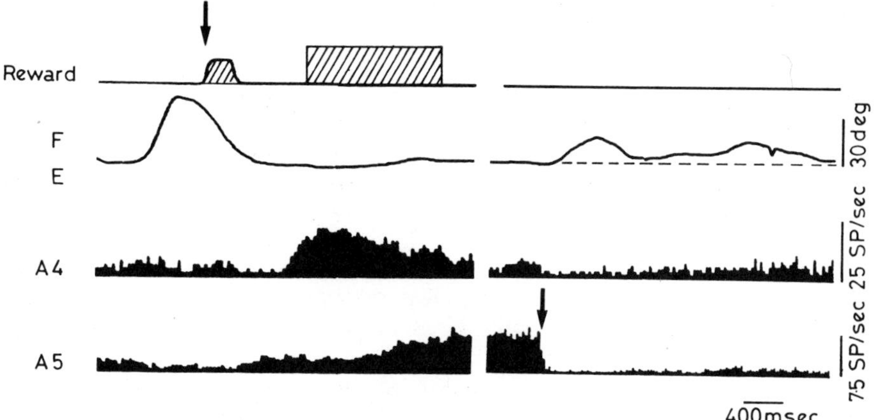

Fig. 6 Nex movement after a reward.
Left: the histograms are synchronized on the reward (arrow). Same conventions as for Fig. 1 and Fig. 3.
Right: histograms of the same cells synchronized on the end of activity of the cell in Area 5 (arrow). The mean value for the movement represents the superimposition of two periods before (dashed line) and after (continuous line) an increase in the frequency of reward.

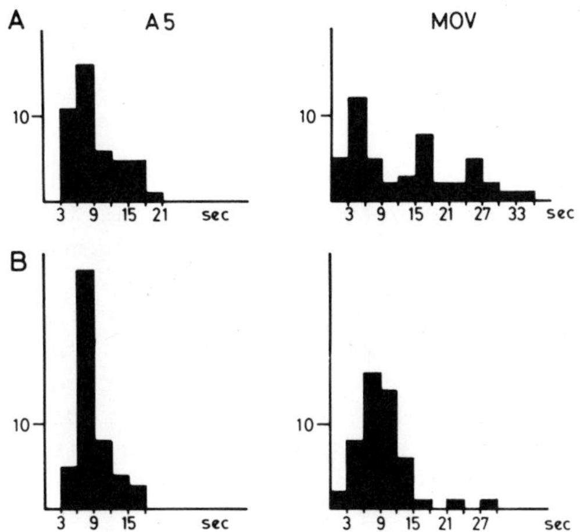

Fig. 7 Changes in the distribution of intervals between maximal activities of a neuron of Area 5 (left) and intervals between movements (right). A and B are two periods before and after an increase in the frequency of reward.

DISCUSSION

The training used to study the cellular activities in relation to behavior is achieved by successive adaptations, being rapidly performed. This rapidity limits both the number of cells that can be studied for each stage and the precision of the analysis of their functional and anatomical characteristics. It is also difficult to obtain a reversibility of the behavioral changes observed.

Before training, cell activities are similar to those described in naive monkeys (e.g., PHILLIPS and PORTER for Area 4, SAKATA et al. for Area 5). Since the beginning of training most of the cells recorded in this study can be classified following the criteria used by other authors for overtrained animals (see for example EVARTS for Area 4, MACKAY et al., BIOULAC and LAMARRE for Area 5). The cells of Area 5 active in association with the taking of the reward can be compared to arm projection and manipulation cells described by MOUNTCASTLE et al. However, the activities of the cells recorded in this study present a larger variability than cells studied by the authors mentioned above, even for successive movements that present similar kinematic characteristics. The histograms of latency are more widely distributed and shifted toward early latencies, mainly for Area 5. That may be explained in part by the differences in the paradigm (self initiated movement as opposed to movement triggered by a stimulus). Area 4 and Area 5 have direct and precise anatomical connections (JONES et al.) and timing of cell activities are overlapping; however, activity in Area 4 is more constant and more time locked with movement. Changes parallel with the movement are more frequent in Area 4, changes at the onset of the movement more frequent in Area 5. The changes described occur in time intervals (15 minutes) of sufficient size to establish new couplings by rewarding cell activities selectively (FETZ and BAKER, SCHMIDT et al.).

The enhancement of activity by reward is not observed in very neuron contingently active before a reward but is seen for cells which are linked both with the conditioned movement and the reward related movements. It is coherent with the fact that it is easier to obtain operant conditioning by successive differentiation of a natural movement (e.g., taking of the reward); the probability of occurrence of the natural movement is transferred to the conditioned movement. The differentiation from the taking of the reward to the flexion movement of the right elbow can occur via cells which are active in the two situations. Repetition of the conditioned movement corresponds to a direct loop that reactivates the movement at its end. Repetition occurs even if one movement is not rewarded. The enhancement of the activity of a subset of neurons of this loop by the taking of the reward may explain the increased probability of activation of the loop.

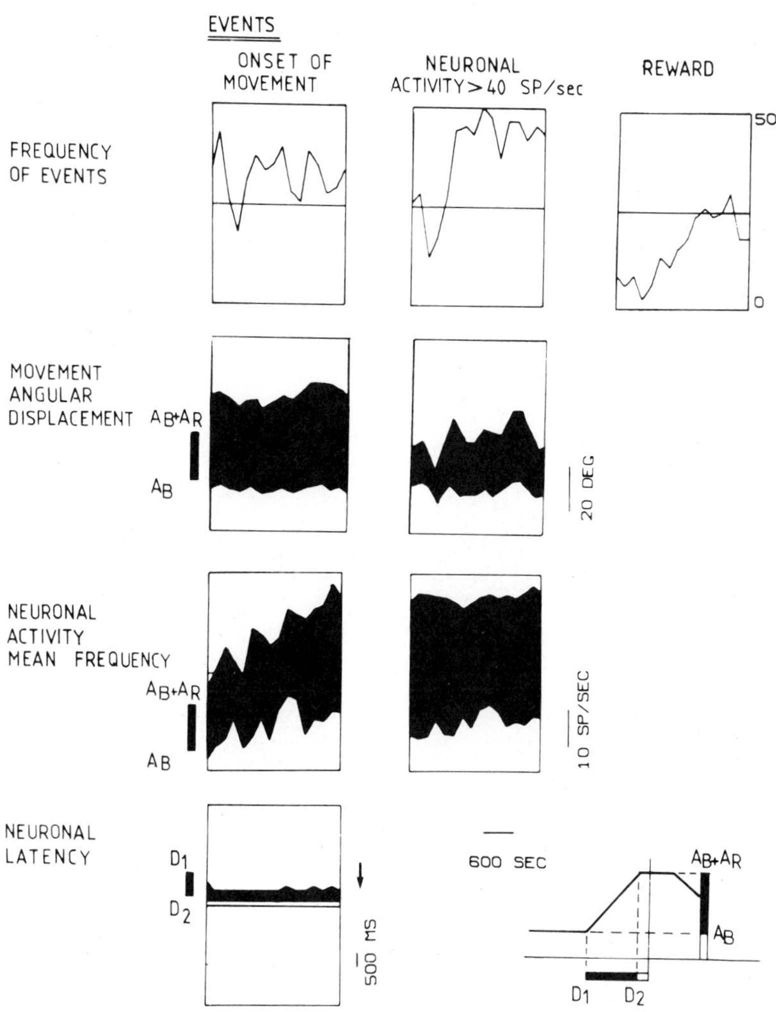

Fig. 8 Changes in activity of a neuron of Area 5 during a conditioning session. Each diagram represents the changes of one parameter during the whole session, with synchronization either by the onsets of flexion (left column) or by the maximal activities of the neuron (middle column). Diagrams use the same convention as in Fig. 5. The bars are jointive and appear in a continuous black surface. Upper to lower row: frequency of events, amplitude of angular displacement, neuronal activity and neuronal latency.

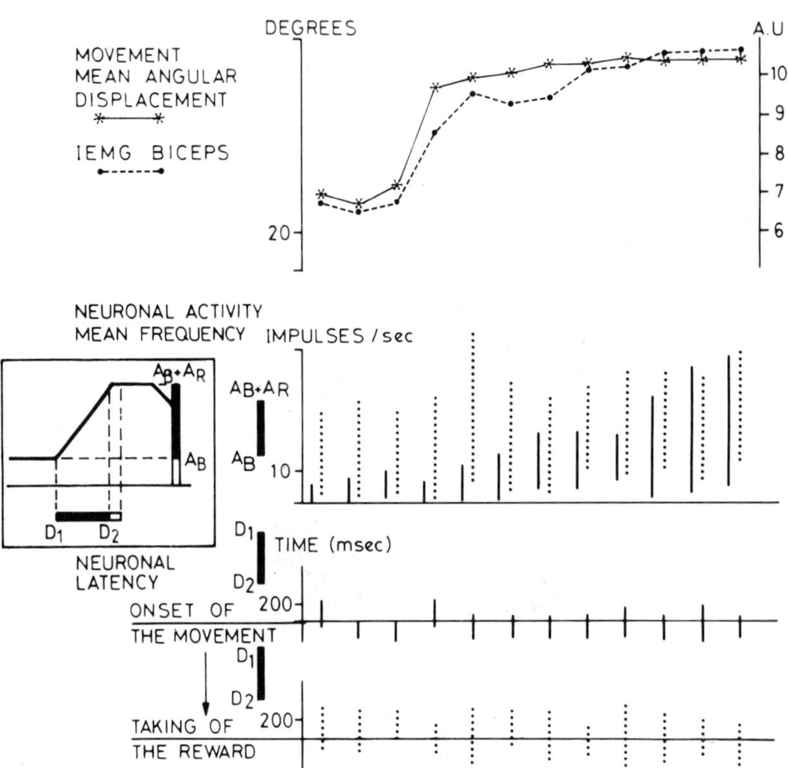

Fig. 9 Changes of the conditioned movement and the activity of a neuron of Area 4 after a change in the position of the sector of arrival.
Upper diagram: amplitude of the flexion and IEMG of the biceps during the period of adaptation.
Middle diagram: changes in cell activity at the onset of the movement and at the grasping of the fruit. Same conventions as in Fig. 5.
Lower diagram: latency of cell activity with respect to the onset of the flexion movement and with respect to the grasping of the fruit. Same conventions as in Fig. 5.

The behavioral regularity that occurs during learning corresponds to a balance between the activity of cells linked with the flexion of the right arm and the activity of cells linked with the taking of the reward by the left arm. This balance may be interpreted by the presence of reciprocal excitatory connnections and inhibitory ones that become stronger when the activity of one of the two subsets is above the threshold corresponding to the movement controlled by this subset.

During classical conditioning, a number of studies have shown that cells connected to the UR show an increase in activity when the CS is given after pairing with the US (cf. OLDS et al.). In Area 4 almost all cells connected to a movement of flexion-extension have their discharges modified by the occurrence of the stimulus indicating the direction of the movement to be performed (EVARTS). A part of the results presented here may be interpreted as an anticipation, at the onset of the movement, of the maximal cell activities. (With the model proposed, an anticipation does not appear as a shift in latency but as an increase of preexisting activity at the onset of the movement.) This anticipated activity can play a role in the control of the movement. The mechanism of this control is still unclear; it is not known if these cells are tuned for afferent inputs that could signal the proper movement.

REFERENCES

Y. Bioulac and Y. Lamarre, 1979, Activity of postcentral cortical neurons of the monkey during conditioned movements of a deafferented limb, Brain Res., 172:427.

E.V. Evarts, 1966, Pyramidal tract activity associated with a conditioned hand movement in the monkey, J. Neurophysiol., 29:1011.

E.V. Evarts, 1974, Gating of motor cortex reflexes by prior instruction, Brain Res., 74:479.

E. Fetz and M.A. Baker, 1973, Operantly conditioned patterns of precentral unit activity and correlated response in adjacent cells and contralateral muscles, J. Neurophysiol. 36:179.

E.G. Jones, J.D. Coulder, and S.H.C. Hendry, 1978, Intracortical connectivity of architectonic fields in the somatic sensory, motor and parietal cortex of monkeys, J. Comp. Neur. 181:291.

W.A. MacKay, M.C. Kwan, J.T. Murphy, and Y.C. Wong, 1978, Responses to active and passive wrist rotation in Area 5 of awake monkeys, Neuroscience Letters 10:235.

V.B. Mountcastle, J.C. Lynch, A. Georgopoulos, H. Sakata, and C. Acuna, 1975, Posterior parietal association cortex of the monkey:command functions for operations within extrapersonal space, J. Neurophysiol. 38(4):871.

J. Olds, J.F. Disterhoft, M. Segal, C.L. Kornblith, and R. Hirsch, 1972, Learning centers of rat brain mapped by measuring letencies of conditioned unit responses, J. Neurophysiol. 35:202.

C.G. Phillips and R. Porter, 1977, "Corticospinal neurons: their role in movement", Academic Press, London.

H. Sakata, Y. Takaska, A. Karasawak, and H. Shubitani, 1973, Somatosensory properties of neurons in the superior parietal cortex (Area 5) of the rhesus monkey, Brain Res. 64:85.

E.M. Schmidt, J.S. MacIntosch, L. Durelli, and J. Bak, 1978, Fine control of operantly conditioned firing patterns of percentral neurons, Exp. Neurology 61:340.

ROLE OF MOTOR CORTEX CELLS IN CONTROL OF OPERANTLY CONDITIONED MUSCLE ACTIVITY

Eberhard E. Fetz

Department of Physiology & Biophysics
and Regional Primate Research Center
University of Washington
Seattle, Wash.

INTRODUCTION

In the primate, precentral motor cortex plays an important role in both the learning and execution of voluntary limb movements, particularly those involving discrete patterns of muscle activity. A better understanding of the neural mechanisms underlying voluntary movements seems a prerequisite to the eventual goal of understanding the neural mechanisms of operant conditioning per se, i.e., how the occurrence of a reinforcing stimulus changes the probability of an operant response. The role of motor cortex cells in voluntary control of limb muscles has been elucidated recently by studies of neural activity in behaving animals, operantly conditioned to perform relevant motor responses. The functional relations between cortical cells and limb muscles are particularly well elucidated by experiments that test for constraints in their interactions.

The degree to which voluntary muscle responses can be differentiated appears to have definite limits. While different limb muscles may be activated in various combinations during voluntary movements, different motoneurons within a muscle cannot be activated so independently: their relative recruitment order is to a large extent fixed by inherent physiological constraints. The existence of comparable constraints in relative activation of motor cortex cells and motor units would be of some consequence to any final explanation of voluntary movement. This question is addressed by observations of cell and muscle activity during operantly conditioned response patterns.

This chapter reviews experimental evidence from a variety of studies in humans and monkeys that suggest differences in the degree to which activity of motor units and motor cortex cells may be independently controlled.

CONSTRAINTS IN RELATIVE RECRUITMENT ORDER

Motor Units

Initial experiments on the voluntary control of single motor units in human muscles had suggested a remarkable ability to recruit different motor units independently. For example, Harrison & Mortensen (1962) found that a human subject with auditory feedback could activate any one of six motor units in tibialis anterior independently of the others. These motor units were recruited at low force levels and "slight changes of the foot or leg were sometimes effective" in their isolation. Similar observations were reported by Basmajian (1973), who asked human subjects to fire different motor units in hand muscles at will. Under isometric conditions, however, in which limb movements are eliminated, the relative recruitment order of different motor units is more difficult to reverse. Whether or not two motor units can be activated independently depends on their critical firing level—i.e., the level of muscle force at which the unit normally begins to fire. Under isometric conditions, awake human subjects found it difficult to change the relative recruitment order of motor units whose critical firing levels differed appreciably (Henneman et al., 1976). Although the lower threshold unit could variably be activated in isolation, it was not possible to discharge the higher threshold unit without coactivating the lower threshold unit.

These apparently discrepant reports may be explained in part by the observation that when the subject is free to move, the motor unit recording electrode may be repositioned in the muscle and may therefore be isolating different motor units at different times and may record different waveforms for the same motor unit (Thomas et al., 1978). The regular recruitment order of motor units under controlled isometric conditions has been confirmed in a number of different laboratories (Henneman et al., 1976; Milner-Brown et al., 1973; Tanji & Kato, 1973; Thomas et al., 1978). However, there remains some evidence that the recruitment order observed during slower movements may be reversed during quick, rapid responses (Hanerz, 1973). Nevertheless, when recruitment was systematically related to peak ballistic force, Desmedt & Godaux (1976) found the same recruitment order for ballistic and slow contractions. It seems, therefore, that on balance the experimental evidence indicates a limit in the degree to which motor units of a muscle can be independently controlled.

Motor Cortex Cells

Just as motor unit discharge can be studied as an operant response, so can activity of cells in precentral motor cortex. Experiments in which single motor cortex neurons were operantly reinforced indicate that

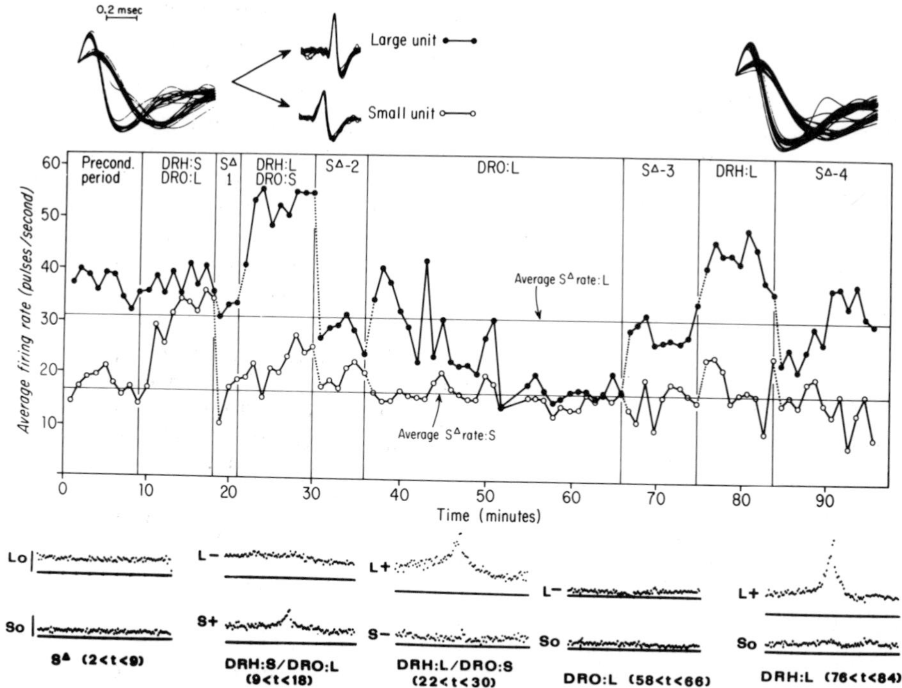

Fig. 1. Operant conditioning of a pair of adjacent motor cortex cells related to knee movement. Insets at top illustrate action potentials of large (L) and small (S) units, whose firing rates are plotted in 1-min intervals. During "Operant level" and SΔ periods, the reinforcement and meter feedback were turned off. During the "DRH:S/DRO:L" period, high rates of the small unit and simultaneous suppression of the large unit were reinforced; the reverse contingency was in effect during "DRH:L/DRO:S." During DRO:L, suppression of activity in the large unit was reinforced with no contingency on the small unit. Response averages (bottom) show time histograms of large and small unit rates for 2-sec periods aligned around feeder discharge; these were compiled during the time interval indicated in parentheses. Vertical bars calibrate 50/sec firing rate. (Fetz & Baker, 1973.)

conditioned monkeys could voluntarily activate virtually any motor cortex cell (Fetz & Baker, 1973; Schmidt et al., 1977; Wyler et al., 1975, 1980). In contrast to motor units of a muscle, adjacent motor cortex cells that were associated with a given movement could often be independently controlled. Figure 1 illustrates a pair of precentral cells that were consistently coactivated with active flexion of the knee and were both driven by passive extension of the knee. To test whether the monkey could activate the cells independently, we presented a differential schedule rewarding the monkey for increasing the firing rate of one cell and simultaneously reducing the activity of the other. As shown in Fig. 1, the monkey readily increased the activity of either cell without increasing the firing rate of the other. Moreover, the animal could also suppress cell firing as well as increase it. Similar results were obtained with other pairs of precentral cells, suggesting that the activation of motor cortex cells associated with a given joint may be more flexible than the recruitment of motor units of a given muscle. However, since the muscles to which these cells may have been linked remain unknown, the dissociation of adjacent motor cortex cells may be more analogous to the dissociation of adjacent muscles.

In studies rewarding the activity of motor cortex cells, the monkeys often performed some limb movement in association with the operant bursts of cell activity (Fetz, 1974; Schmidt et al., 1977; Wyler & Burchiel, 1978). These associated movements often became quite specific and sometimes dropped out as bursts of the same unit continued to be reinforced. Some precentral cells were activated in operant bursts with no associated movements or muscle activity (Fetz & Baker, 1973; Fetz & Finocchio, 1975).

Recruitment of Motor Cortex Cells Vs. Muscles

To test the relation of single motor cortex cells to specific forearm muscles directly, we operantly reinforced various patterns of isometric activity (Fetz & Finocchio, 1975). Figure 2 illustrates a representative precentral neuron that was consistently coactivated with the biceps muscle and with a wrist flexor under several different behavioral conditions. Isolated activation of biceps muscle produced clear coactivation of the cell (Fig. 2C), and operant reinforcement of unit activity with no contingency on the muscles produced coactivation of biceps, as well as wrist muscles (Fig. 2E). As might be expected, this unit was also coactivated with biceps during active elbow flexion. Yet, when the unit-biceps coactivation was directly tested by operantly rewarding its dissociation, the monkey activated the unit without coactivating any muscles (Fig. 2F). This degree of flexibility was revealed only when it was specifically tested. All the motor cortex cells that were similarly tested could be readily activated without coactivating any of the muscles that had been previously associated with the cell.

The reverse dissociation—muscle activation in the absence of motor cortex cell activity--was not so readily achieved. Figure 2G illustrates the response patterns obtained with this schedule; although the monkey increased the relative amount of biceps activity, this was still accompanied by some activity in the unit. It remains possible that the inability to suppress the cortical cell activity did not reflect a physiological constraint, but rather was due simply to behavioral causes. This last schedule was presented after the monkey had worked many hours on other schedules, so the fact that he did not achieve greater unit suppression may be attributable to satiation or fatigue.

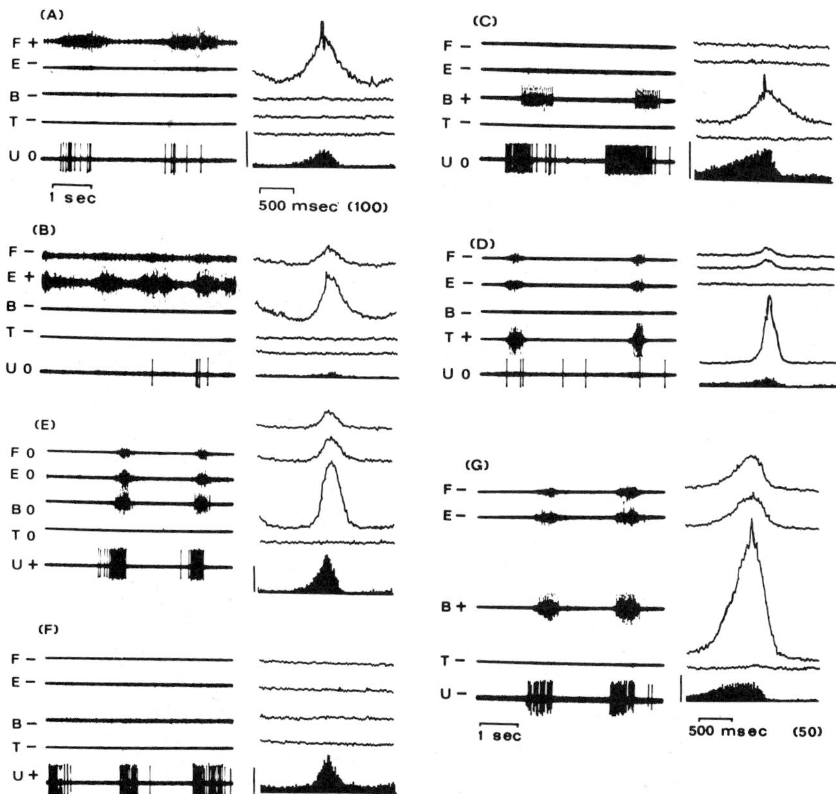

Fig. 2. Operantly conditioned response patterns of precentral cell and four contralateral forearm muscles. Response trials at left illustrate successive reinforced activity patterns and response averages at right show profile of reinforced responses. These isometric responses were performed with the elbow angle fixed at 90° and the wrist at 180°. The muscles include flexor carpi radialis (F), extensor carpi radialis (E), biceps (B) and triceps (T). A "+" indicates elements whose activation was rewarded; a "-" indicates elements whose simultaneous suppression was required; 0 indicates elements whose activity was not included in the reinforcement contingency. (A-D) differential reinforcement of isolated bursts of EMG activity in each arm muscle with no contingency on the cortical unit activity; (E) operant unit bursts reinforced with no contingency on the muscle; (F) reinforcement of operant unit bursts and simultaneous muscle suppression; (G) response pattern when isolated biceps activity and simultaneous unit suppression were reinforced. Vertical bars calibrate firing rate of 50/sec. (Fetz & Finocchio, 1975.)

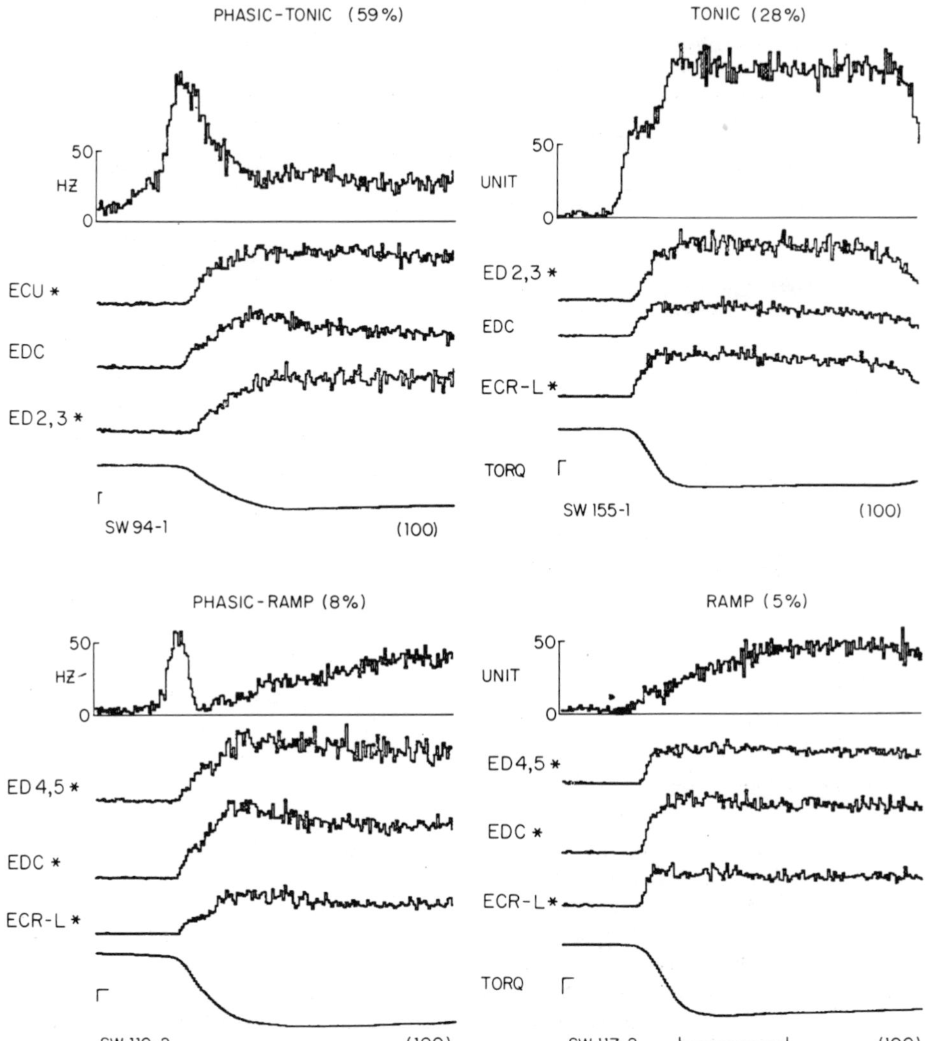

Fig. 3. Characteristic response patterns of CM cells during isometric ramp-and-hold torque trajectories. From top to bottom, each set illustrates averages of firing rate of CM cell, rectified EMG of identified agonist muscles and isometric torque response (from flexion to extension). The four types of response patterns are distinguished (a) by the presence (left set) or absence (right set) of a phasic burst of activity at movement onset and (b) by a constant (top set) or increasing (bottom set) discharge during the static hold period. Asterisks indicate target muscles that were facilitated in spike-triggered averages from each cell. Response averages include 100 events. (Cheney & Fetz, 1980.)

It is relevant to note that even if the monkey had suppressed this unit during activation of the biceps, there could be a simple explanation. The unit might have been associated with a synergist muscle, such as brachialis, that could be activated independently, or it might not have had any output to muscles whatsoever. To resolve such questions, we need an independent means of determining the output connections of cells under behavioral conditions. Such a test is provided by the technique of spike-triggered averaging of EMG activity (Woody & Black-Cleworth, 1973; Fetz & Cheney, 1979).

RELATIVE RECRUITMENT OF CM CELLS AND THEIR TARGET MUSCLE

In monkeys performing alternating flexion and extension of the wrist, it has been possible to identify those motor cortex cells that have output effects on agonist muscles by compiling spike-triggered averages of rectified EMG activity (Fetz & Cheney, 1979, 1980). Certain precentral cells generate a clear postspike facilitation (PSF) of motor unit activity consisting of a transient increase in the average EMG level, reaching a peak at about 10 msec after the spike. The latency and magnitude of such facilitation are consistent with the expected effects of corticomotoneuronal linkage, so we refer to the cells generating clear PSF as CM cells. To optimize chances of detecting CM cells, we recorded activity of several muscles simultaneously and found that over half of the CM cells facilitate more than one target muscle. The relative activation of CM cells and their target muscles is of particular interest, since the PSF indicates a direct correlational linkage.

The firing patterns of CM cells during ramp-and-hold wrist movements fall into four characteristic response patterns (Fig. 3). The most common type (59% of CM cells) is the phasic-tonic pattern, characterized by a phasic burst of activity at onset of movement, followed by a steady discharge during the static hold period. The next most common response pattern (28%) is tonic activity during the hold period, without any burst of activity at onset. The remaining CM cells have a gradually increasing firing rate during the hold period, which may or may not be preceded by a burst at onset.

With regard to the issue of their relative recruitment order, we have noted two conditions under which CM cells are active without their target muscles. As illustrated in Fig. 3, during ramp-and-hold movements many CM cells typically begin their firing pattern well before activation of their target muscles. Figure 4 plots the time of onset of activity in CM cells relative to onset of their target muscles. Many CM cells, particularly those whose firing begins with a burst, increased their firing rate several hundred milliseconds before their facilitated motor units became active. This would suggest that even motor cortex cells with direct linkages to motoneurons may be activated in the absence of any peripheral activity. The second condition in which CM cells can be activated without their target muscles is in response to adequate natural stimulation--usually

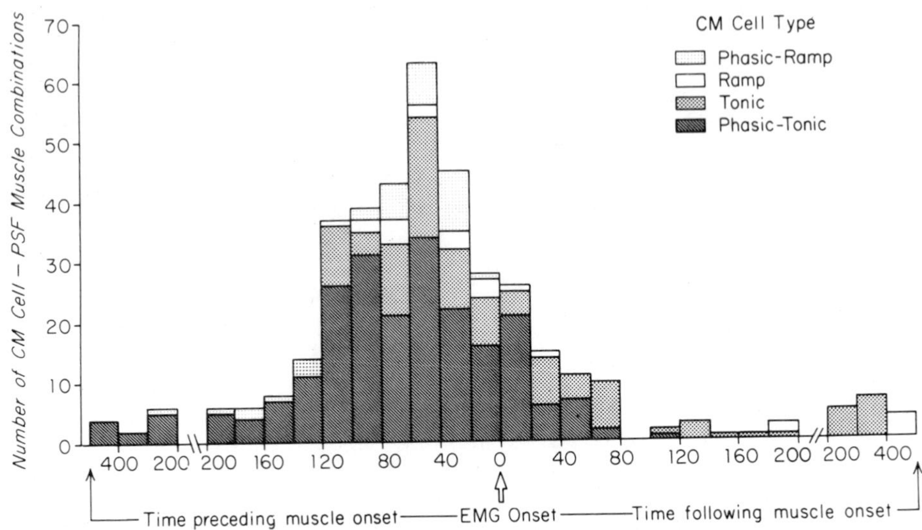

Fig. 4. Onset times of CM cell activity relative to onset of EMG activity in muscles facilitated by each cell. Origin of abscissa indicates time of onset of target muscle activity, and histogram plots relative onset time of CM cell preceding and following muscle onset (msec). Response pattern of CM cells during ramp-and-hold movements is indicated separately by shading. For CM cells that facilitated several muscles, the relative latencies are plotted for each muscle. (Cheney & Fetz, 1980.)

passive joint movements that stretch their target muscles. Since corticomotoneuronal EPSPs are not sufficiently large to activate the motoneurons by themselves, it is understandable that CM cells could be activated without necessarily recruiting their target muscles into activity.

There is also some evidence for the reverse dissociation, namely, activation of target muscles without activation of the CM cells that facilitate them. Under certain response conditions the target muscles were found to be activated in the relative absence of CM cell activity, viz., when the movement was ballistic rather than a controlled ramp-and-hold movement. Some CM cells observed under both types of movement conditions showed an appreciable discharge when the monkey carefully performed the ramp-and-hold movements; but when, in apparent frustration with the task, he alternately flexed and extended the wrist rapidly, the same CM cells remained paradoxically inactive, although their target muscle exhibited the most intense EMG activity (Cheney & Fetz, 1980). Presumably, the motor units activated during the ballistic responses included those that the CM cells facilitated; if so, this could indicate that the target motor units could be activated in the relative absence of CM cell activity during ballistic movements.

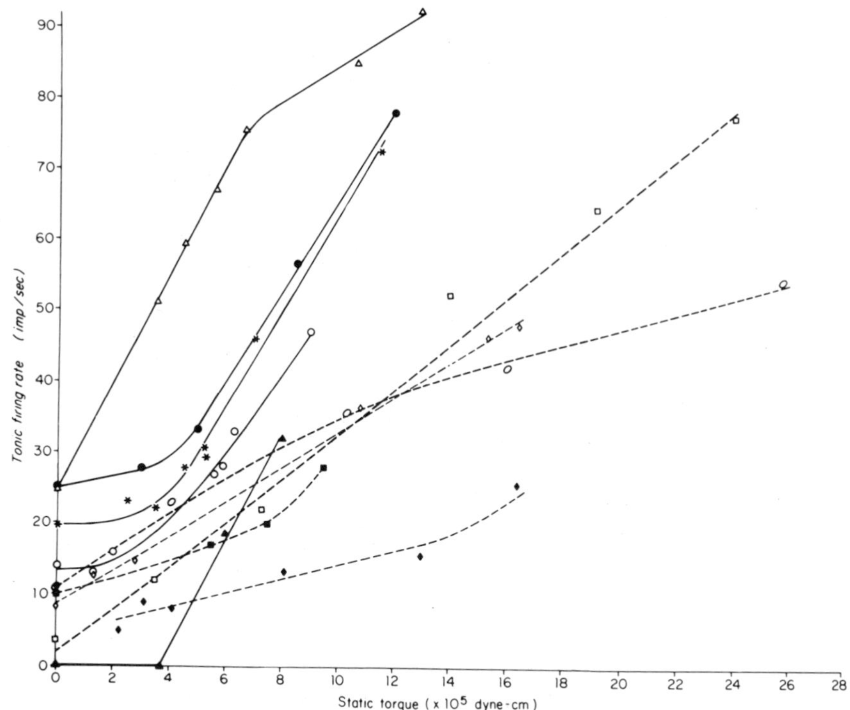

Fig. 5. Tonic firing rate of CM cells during static hold period plotted as a function of active torque. Representative examples of CM cells related to extension (———) and flexion (- - - -). Most CM cells were active even at lowest levels of active force; only one CM cell (▲) was recruited into activity at higher levels of static torque. (Fetz & Cheney, 1979.)

Even during controlled ramp-and-hold movements, there was some evidence of target muscle activity without CM cell firing. Some CM cells whose firing pattern had no burst at onset began to fire after their target muscles had become active (Fig. 4). When the activity of CM cells was documented during generation of increasing amounts of active force during the hold period, only one CM cell was recruited at a higher level of static force than its target muscle. While single motor units of agonist muscles are recruited sequentially as force is increased (Milner-Brown et al., 1973; Tanji & Kato, 1973), most CM cells appear to be recruited at the lowest levels of active force. They contribute to higher levels of force more by increasing their firing rate than increasing the number of active CM cells (Fig. 5). One observed exception was a CM cell that became active at higher force levels, well after its target muscles had been recruited into activity (▲ in Fig. 5). It may be possible to search out more such CM cells that are activated after their target muscles, but most of the CM cells observed to date were recruited at the lowest levels of muscular force.

Under normal conditions, then, the activation of CM cells without their target muscles occurs more commonly than the reverse dissociation. The final determination of the degree to which CM cells and their target muscles can be independently controlled awaits direct operant conditioning of their activity. This will confirm whether any CM cell can be bidirectionally dissociated from the motoneurons that it facilitates.

CONCLUSIONS

Taken together, these results suggest that precentral motor cortex cells undergo a much greater variety of activity than is reflected in the activity of motoneurons. The modulation of motor cortex cells without peripheral muscle activity has also been observed under other behavioral conditions. Following a cue for a delayed response, some precentral cells fire in anticipation of an intended movement (Tanji & Evarts, 1976; Thach, 1977). It seems likely that considerable subthreshold activity involved in integration and initiation of learned voluntary movements occurs in precentral motor cortex. The fact that many pyramidal tract neurons discharge more intensely with fine controlled movements than with ballistic responses (Fromm & Evarts, 1977; Cheney & Fetz, 1980) suggests that these cortical cells are particularly concerned with control of discrete learned movements. The interactions between motor cortex cells and muscles can be further analyzed by the application of operant conditioning techniques to control their activity directly.

Acknowledgments

These studies were supported in part by NIH grants RR00166 and NS12542.

The success of the experiments cited is due in large part to the skill and perseverance of my colleagues, Drs. Dom V. Finocchio and Paul D. Cheney. I thank Ms. Kate Schmitt for excellent editorial assistance.

REFERENCES

Basmajian, J. V., 1973, "Muscles Alive," Williams & Wilkins, Baltimore.

Cheney, P. D., and Fetz, E. E., 1980, Functional classes of primate corticomotoneuronal cells and their relation to active force, J. Neurophysiol., 44:773.

Desmedt, J. E., and Godaux, E., 1977, Ballistic contractions in man: characteristic recruitment pattern of single motor units of the tibialis anterior muscle, J. Physiol. (Lond.), 264:673.

Fetz, E. E., 1974, Operant control of single unit activity and correlated motor responses, in: "Operant Control of Brain Activity," M. Chase, ed., UCLA Press, Los Angeles.

Fetz, E. E., 1977, Biofeedback and differential conditioning of response patterns in the skeletal motor system, in: "Biofeedback and Behavior," J. Beatty and H. Legewie, eds., Plenum Press, New York.

Fetz, E. E., and Baker, M. A., 1973, Operantly conditioned patterns of precentral unit activity and correlated responses in adjacent cells and contralateral muscles, J. Neurophysiol., 36:179.

Fetz, E. E., and Cheney, P. D., 1979, Muscle fields and response properties of primate corticomotoneuronal cells, Progr. Brain Res., 50:137.

Fetz, E. E., and Cheney, P. D., 1980, Postspike facilitation of forelimb muscle activity by primate corticomotoneuronal cells, J. Physiol. (Lond.), 44:751.

Fetz, E. E., and Finocchio, D. V., 1975, Correlations between activity of motor cortex cells and arm muscles during operantly conditioned response patterns, Exp. Brain Res., 23:217.

Fromm, C., and Evarts, E. V., 1977, Relation of motor cortex neurons to precisely controlled and ballistic movements, Neurosci. Lett., 5:259.

Hannerz, J., 1974, Discharge properties of motor units in relation to recruitment order in voluntary contraction, Acta Physiol. Scand., 91:374.

Harrison, V. F., and Mortensen, O. A., 1962, Identification and voluntary control of single motor unit activity in the tibialis anterior muscle, Anat. Rec., 144:109.

Henneman, E., Shahani, B. T., and Young, R. R., 1976, The extent of voluntary control of human motor units, in: "The Motor System: Neurophysiology and Muscle Mechanisms," M. Shahani, ed., Elsevier, New York.

Milner-Brown, H. S., Stein, R. B., and Yemm, R., 1973, The orderly recruitment of human motor units during voluntary isometric contractions, J. Physiol. (London), 230:359.

Schmidt, E. M., Bak, M. J., McIntosh, J. S., and Thomas, J. S., 1977, Operant conditioning of firing patterns in monkey cortical neurons, Exp. Neurol., 54:467.

Tanji, J., and Evarts, E. V., 1976, Anticipatory activity of motor cortex neurons in relation to direction of intended movement, J. Neurophysiol., 39:1062.

Tanji, J., and Kato, M., 1973, Recruitment of motor units in voluntary contraction of a finger muscle in man, Exp. Neurol., 40:759.

Thach, W. T., 1978, Correlation of neuronal with pattern and force of muscular activity, joint position and direction of intended movement in motor cortex and cerebellum. J. Neurophysiol., 41:650.

Thomas, J. S., Schmidt, E. M., and Hambrecht, F. T., 1978, Facility of motor unit control during tasks defined directly in terms of unit behaviors, Exp. Neurol., 59:384.

Woody, C. D., and Black-Cleworth, P., 1973, Differences in excitability of cortical neurons as a function of motor projection in conditioned cats, J. Neurophysiol., 36:1104.

Wyler, A. R., and Burchiel, K. J., 1978, Factors influencing the accuracy of operant control of pyramidal tract neurons in monkey, Brain Res., 152:418.

Wyler, A. R., Lange, S. C., and Robbins, C. A., 1980, Operant control of precentral neurons: bilateral single-unit conditioning, Brain Res., 195:337.

CORTICAL NEURON ACTIVITY IN THE TEMPORAL ORGANIZATION OF BEHAVIOR

Joaquin M. Fuster

Department of Psychiatry and Brain Research Institute
School of Medicine, University of California
at Los Angeles, Los Angeles, CA 90024

SUMMARY. Neuropsychological studies in primates have implicated the prefrontal cortex and also (with regard to vision) the inferotemporal cortex in the integration of temporally separate items of sensory information. Single-unit studies support such evidence and point to the involvement of neurons in those neocortical regions in the mechanisms of temporal integration. Sustained elevations and diminutions of firing related to the retention of cues in delay tasks suggest participation of those neurons in the mnemonic process that makes that form of integration possible. Protracted and color-dependent changes of firing, after color cues to be provisionally retained by the animal in performance of a task, indicate that inferotemporal neurons are specifically involved in visual short-term memory.

INTRODUCTION

Most all prevalent models of learning share the concept of temporal contiguity as the basis for behavior formation. Whatever the mechanism of its formation, learned behavior presupposes the temporal coincidence or near-coincidence of certain events, such as conditioned and unconditioned stimuli, autonomic and skeletal responses, and reinforcement. The most irreducible unit of learned behavior, whether it is the conditioned reflex or some kind of cybernetic interaction with the environment, seems to rest by necessity on the principle of temporal contiguity. That principle may well apply also to more complex forms of behavior. Indeed, it is possible to conceptualize some patterns of behavior as the concatenation of temporally apposed behavioral units of smaller size.

However, in higher organisms, patterns of behavior emerge, or can be formed by conditioning, that are based on relationships of contingency between temporally separate events. In fact, at higher levels of the behavioral hierarchy one finds a wealth of behavioral structures that contain temporal discontiguities between their component elements. These structures may be considered as temporal gestalts that are defined mainly by goal or purpose and not by their individual components.

Although man is privileged with the ability to achieve the most elaborate forms of temporally integrated behavior (e.g., language), there is little doubt that the ability to integrate temporally discontiguous elements of sensorium or behavior is present in other species. Nonhuman primates have been shown to be fully capable of organizing behavior with temporal discontinuities between mutually dependent elements. At least two neural functions with an extended temporal dimension may be assumed to help the organism bridge those discontinuities: a prospective function of preparation (of receptors and motor apparatus), and a retrospective function of short-term memory. These two temporally "symmetrical" functions may possibly cooperate with one another to maintain the proper relationships of meaning and behavior between the temporally distant events of a behavioral gestalt. (For a more extensive discussion of these issues, see Fuster, 1980).

Delayed-response tests and variants thereof (e.g., delayed alternation, delayed matching-to-sample) are the best procedures thus far devised for testing an animal's capacity to temporally integrate behavior and for testing the two subordinate functions mentioned. Indeed, the narrow view of those tests as simply unnatural behaviors contrived by the experimenter, unjustly ignores the generality of the process and functions that they test.

All "delay tasks" share in common one important feature: a period of delay between a particular event (which can be a sensory stimulus, a motor act, or a combination of the two) and a behavioral response which in some critical respect depends on that event. The delay not only obliges the animal to retain information on that event but allows it to prepare for the eventualities to come. Even though the elements of the task may be thoroughly rehearsed and the events that constitute a trial repeat themselves innumerable times in the course of performance, each trial is essentially a unique temporal structure of behavior, inasmuch as it must be formed independently of all others (indeed, in spite of all others which may interfere "proactively" with it). That structure is not entirely reducible to its elements and critically depends on the potential to integrate temporally separate items of information.

Experimental evidence primarily from lesion studies indicates that associative areas of cortex constitute the substrate for temporal integration. The evidence is particularly strong and convincing in the case of the prefrontal cortex. Animals with lesions of this cortex are notoriously deficient at performance of delay tasks. For visual delay tasks, that is, tasks requiring the temporal integration of visual information, there is evidence that the inferotemporal cortex is also important (Delacour, 1977; Fuster et al., 1981; Kovner and Stamm, 1972).

In recent years a number of electrophysiological investigations have been conducted on animals and humans in behavioral paradigms that are predicated on temporal integration. The Contingent Negative Variation (CNV) or "expectancy" wave (Walter, 1967) was probably the first electrical correlate discovered of prefrontal function in temporal integration. Later, laboratories in Japan and ours in this country endeavored to explore the activity of single units of prefrontal cortex (Fuster, 1973; Fuster and Alexander, 1971; Kubota and Niki, 1971; Niki 1974b,c) and inferotemporal cortex (Fuster and Jervey, 1981; Mikami and Kubota, 1980) in monkeys performing delay tasks. What follows is a summary of some of our experiments on this subject. I will try to highlight, with the help of a few illustrations, the findings that most directly relate to temporal integration and, presumably, one of its auxiliary functions: short-term memory.

PREFRONTAL CORTEX

One of the most significant telltales of the involvement of prefrontal neurons in temporal integration is the observation, in prefrontal cortex, of cells that undergo sustained activation of discharge for the entire length of the delay period of delayed-response trials. What is peculiar about such activations, and makes them appear as something other than simply an "arousal" phenomenon, is the fact that oftentimes they are strictly circumscribed to the duration of that period. A unit may not show its firing altered either during presentation of the cue or during the period of choice at the end of the trial, yet be briskly active in the time between the two events (Fig. 1). As the delay is shortened or lengthened, so is the length of the activation. Furthermore, whatever is going on with the units during delay, it seems to depend on the recent exposure to a cue to be remembered (a cue "with a future", so to speak). The mere presentation of visual and auditory stimuli that ordinarily accompany the cue is not sufficient for subsequent activation (Fig. 2).

The sustained activation of prefrontal units during the delay may be at the foundation of the surface negativity, and thus the CNV, detected in delay paradigms in man and other primates (Borda, 1970; Donchin et al., 1971; Walter, 1967). However, activation of firing is not the only indicator, at the single-unit level, of prefrontal involvement in bridging temporal discontinuities. Some

Fig. 1. Firing of a prefrontal cell during five trials of a direct-method delayed-response task (delays: 32, 32, 32, 67, and 65 sec). At the time of the "cue", a food morsel is placed under one of two identical objects (right or left) in full view of the animal. At the end of the delay (arrow), the animal is given access to the two objects and has to choose the baited one for food reward. Bait position is randomly changed. Between trials and during the delay, a screen blocks the view of and the access to the objects.

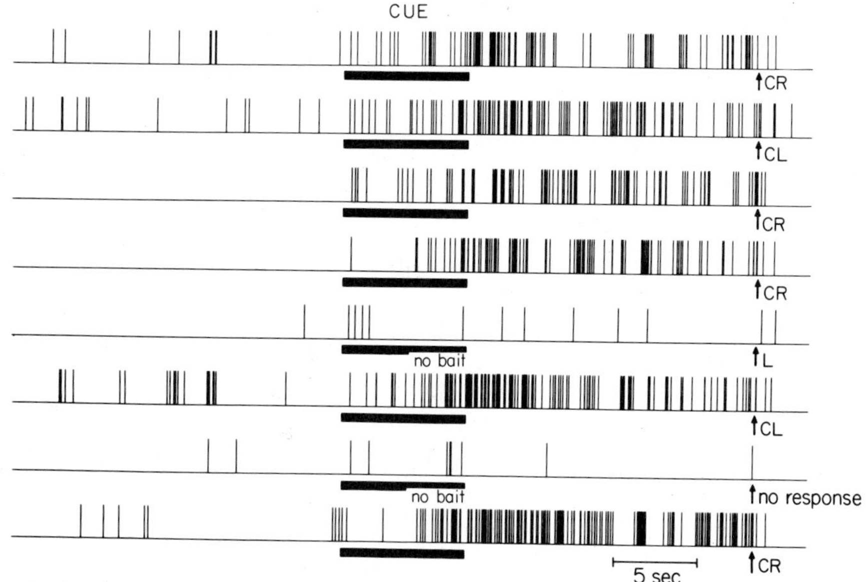

Fig. 2. Cell in prefrontal cortex during eight delayed-response trials. On trials fifth and seventh the screen was raised, as if for the regular cue, and the objects shown, but no bait was placed under either object. Notations at the end of the trials refer to the animal's response (C, correct; R, right; L, left). The unit is activated throughout each trial, except "no bait" trials.

units, a minority to be sure, show sustained delay inhibition (Fig. 3). Again, this inhibition of firing depends on the previous presence of a prospectively relevant cue.

The functional significance of delay activity, in terms of the task, is supported by the occasionally observed relationships between that activity and the level of performance (Fig. 4). Such relationships however, are in most units difficult to substantiate because of the usually excellent performance of the experimental animal.

In any case, the delay activity of prefrontal cells appears to have something to do with the bridging of two temporally separate events: the cue, on the one hand, and the stimulus combination demanding a choice at the end of the trial. On that basis, one may argue that the units showing sustained changes of activity during the delay are somehow involved in retention of the cue. But do they, themselves, retain the cue? In order to be able to answer

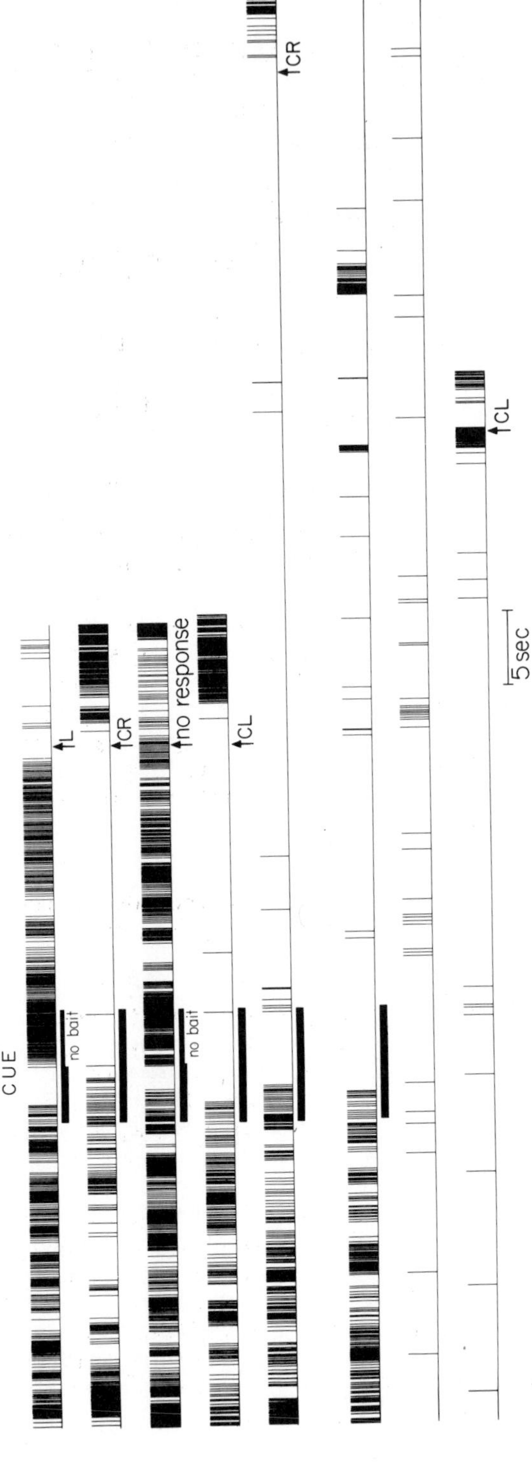

Fig. 3. Prefrontal unit during six delayed-response trials. The unit is inhibited during the entire delay, but not in "no bait" trials. The delay of the sixth trial is about 4 minutes long.

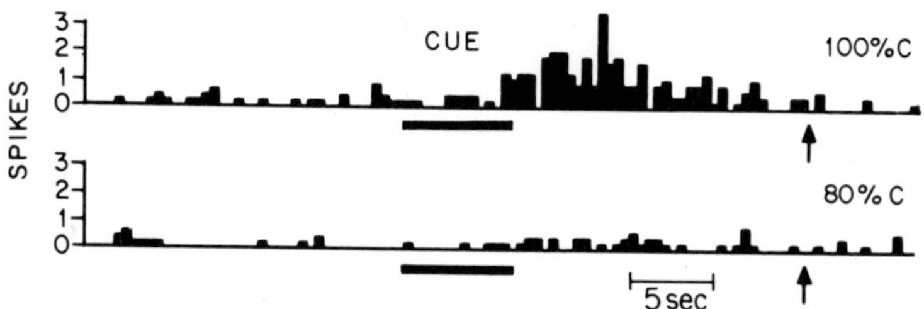

Fig. 4. Averaged activity of a prefrontal unit in two series of delayed-response trials at different levels of correct (C) performance.

this question in the affirmative it would seem necessary that the units show a clear difference of activity depending on the specific attribute of the cue that the animal must retain for optimal performance. We have found evidence of such units, particularly when using spatial delay tasks (Fig. 5), as Niki (1974a,b,c) has also.

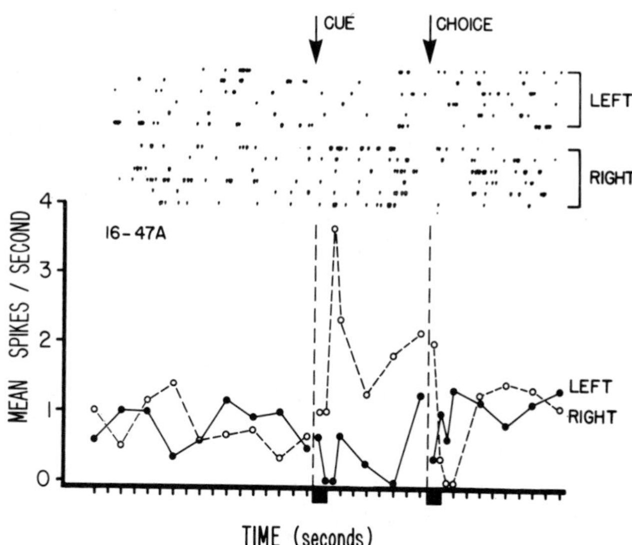

Fig. 5. Raster display and average curves of the activity of a prefrontal cell in an indirect-method spatial delayed-response task. (Left-cue trials separate from right-cue trials). Arrows mark the cue and choice periods. Note the higher probability of firing during the delay of right-cue trials.

However, the fact that the delay activation of a prefrontal unit is not cue-differential does not exclude it from participation in the memory process. For one thing, the unit may engage in retaining attributes of the cue that are common to the various cues (usually two) in the task. Retention of those attributes, we should not forget, is sufficient to ensure that the monkey emits responses on time and also ensures at least the bare minimum of correct responses (50% or whatever the chance level may be).

Furthermore, those nondifferential delay-activated cells (nearly one-half of all prefrontal units sampled by us) may well be exerting a facilitatory influence over cells in other brain structures that are even more deeply involved in retention of the cue in all its parameters. Among those structures we have to consider the parasensory areas of associative neocortex. In the case of visual tasks (most delay tasks in use have an important visual component), the area to consider is the inferior temporal cortex, which receives substantial input from prefrontal cortex (Jones and Powell, 1970; Pandya et al., 1971) and which lesion work suggests to be also involved in visual short-term memory.

INFEROTEMPORAL CORTEX

Following that rationale we have been exploring with microelectrodes the inferotemporal cortex (area TE of Bonin and Bailey, 1947) (Fig. 6) in animals performing delayed matching-to-sample, a visual short-term memory task without spatial cues (Fig. 7). As predicted from the research by Gross and others (Desimone and Gross, 1979; Gross et al., 1972; Sato et al., 1980), we have found units that are very reactive to the color-lighted disks serving the monkey as sample and matching stimuli in performance of his task. Here color seems to be, overall, a more powerful determinant of firing rate than in prefrontal cortex.

What is not so predictable from previous single-unit work is the finding, in inferotemporal cortex, of sustained and in some units color-dependent changes of firing during the retention periods of the task. Especially in the lower bank of the superior temporal sulcus, units may be found that not only react differently to the sample stimulus depending on its color, but show also color-dependent activity during the subsequent delay (Fig. 8).

It is possible that the delay discharge of some of the delay-activated cells represents a kind of sensory afterdischarge in response to the sample and, therefore, has nothing to do with the behavioral significance of that stimulus. However, visual afterdischarges of the length of our delays (16-20 sec) are most unusual anywhere in the brain of the normal drug-free animal. Anyway,

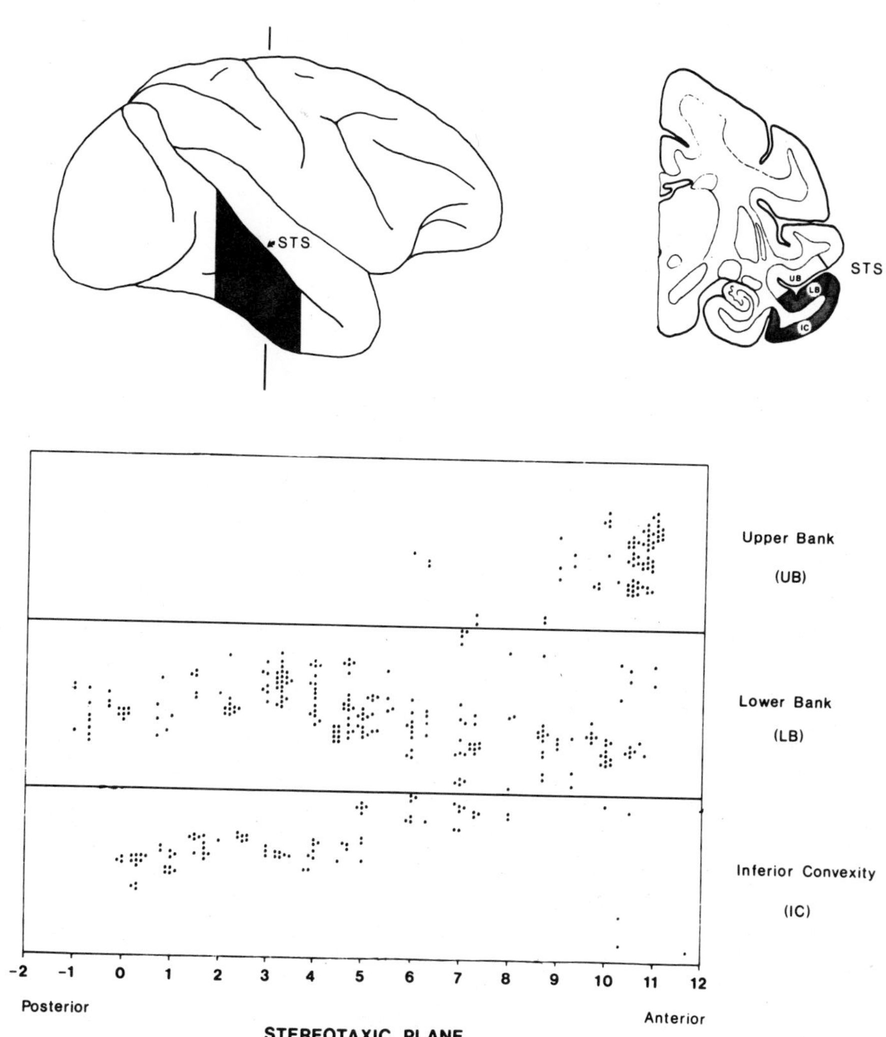

Fig. 6. Diagrams of monkey brain showing (by shading) the infero-temporal region from which single-unit activity has been recorded. The scatter plot below shows schematically the distribution of 452 units investigated. STS, superior temporal sulcus.

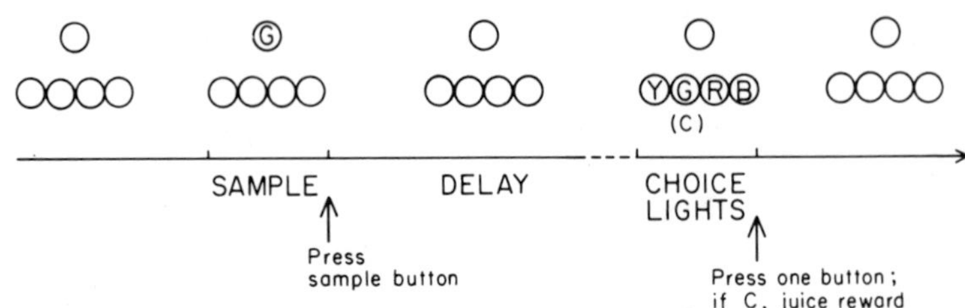

Fig. 7. Sequence of events in a delayed matching-to-sample trial (with green sample light). G, green; Y, yellow, R, red; B, blue; C, correct choice light.

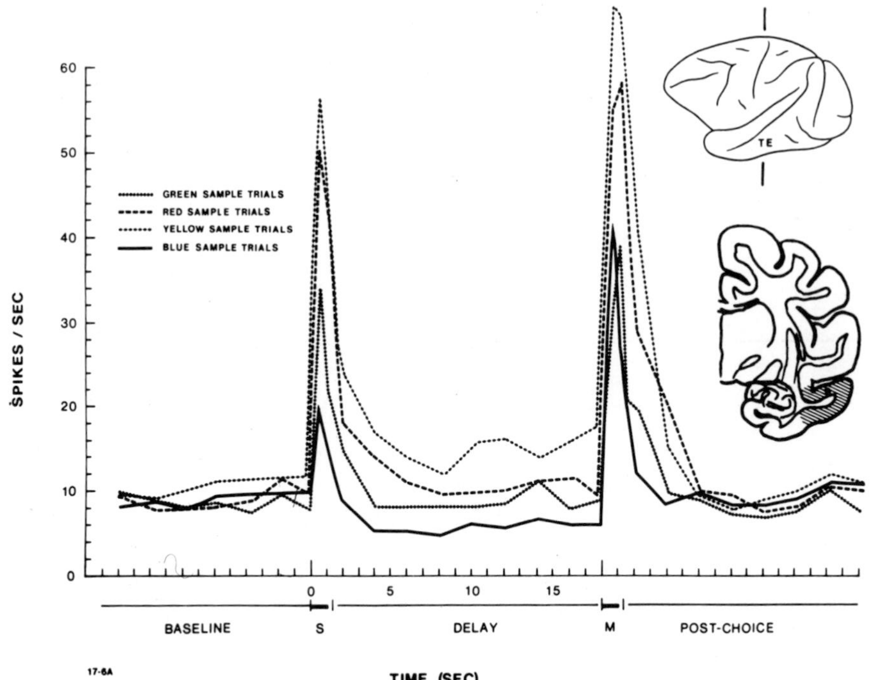

Fig. 8. Mean firing frequency of an inferotemporal unit in delayed matching-to-sample (four to seven trials with each color-sample). Sample (S) and match (M) periods marked by bars under the time base.

that interpretation does not easily apply to protracted excitation or inhibition that depends on the color of the stimulus. Furthermore, inferotemporal units need not react to the sample to undergo marked and differential changes of activity in the ensuing delay (Fig. 9).

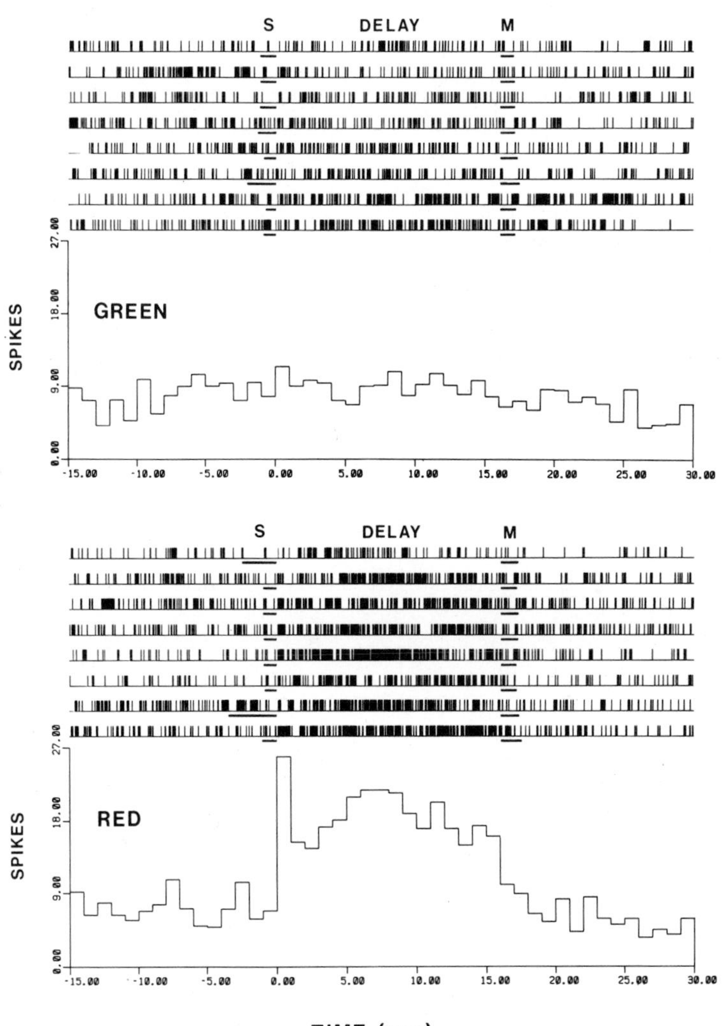

Fig. 9. Firing of an inferotemporal cell during green- and red-sample trials. Average frequency histograms are time-locked with the offset of the sample light.

We are inclined to think that the protracted and in many instances color-differential activation of inferotemporal units during the delay period of delayed matching-to-sample trials is probably related to their role in short-term memory. This interpretation is supported by evidence that the activation not only occurs during sample retention but rarely outlasts the trial. That is somewhat at variance with what has been observed in prefrontal cortex, where many units undergo increased discharge after the trial is over, apparently in relation to reinforcement (Rosenkilde et al., 1981). In inferotemporal cortex, elevated discharge usually terminates with the need to remember the sample, even though at trial's end the sample is again presented (together with other stimuli) and must be foveated by the animal for correct response (Figs. 8 and 9).

However, we need to be very cautious on attributing to inferotemporal units any form of color-specific memory. For one thing, our animals are only tested with a limited number of colors. At most, it seems, we can infer that the units in question take some part in representation and memory of the particular colored stimuli used by the animal in the task. Moreover, color is just one of the attributes of such stimuli, and the same units may also participate in representation and memory of other attributes.

In conclusion, it appears that neurons in inferotemporal cortex, like those in prefrontal cortex, are involved in the operations that allow the temporal integration of sensory data in the organization of purposeful, goal-directed behavior. This broad conclusion is in accord with the findings of lesion studies. However, it is not yet clear specifically which operations are subserved by the neural elements of either cortical region. By use of a behavioral task that requires retention of visual information with little possibility that this mnemonic function is aided by other than visual cues, we have obtained and shown some evidence of neuron participation in visual short-term memory, especially in inferotemporal cortex. Further research should clarify whether, as we suspect, this participation of cortical neurons in short-term memory reflects also their participation in the brain mechanisms that underly the formation of permanent, long-term memory.

ACKNOWLEDGEMENTS

This research was supported by grants BNS 76-16984 from the National Science Foundation and AA 3513 from the National Institute of Alcohol Abuse and Alcoholism. The author is the recipient of a Research Scientist Award (MH 25082) from the National Institute of Mental Health.

REFERENCES

Bonin, G. von, and Bailey, P., 1947, "The Neocortex of Macaca Mulatta," University of Illinois Press, Urbana.

Borda, R. P., 1970, The effect of altered drive states on the contingent negative variation (CNV) in rhesus monkeys. Electroencephalogr. Clin. Neurophysiol., 29:173-180.

Delacour, J., 1977, Cortex inférotemporal et memoire visuelle a court terme chez le singe. Nouvelles donnees, Exp. Brain Res., 28:301-310.

Desimone, R., and Gross, C. G., 1979, Visual areas in the temporal cortex of the macaque, Brain Res., 178:363-380.

Donchin, E., Otto, D., Gerbrandt, L. K., and Pribram, K. H., 1971, While a monkey waits: Electrocortical events recorded during the foreperiod of a reaction time study, Electroencephalogr. Clin. Neurophysiol., 31:115-127.

Fuster, J. M., 1980, "The Prefrontal Cortex," Raven, New York.

Fuster, J. M., 1973, Unit activity in prefrontal cortex during delayed-response performance: Neuronal correlates of transient memory, J. Neurophysiol. 36:61-78.

Fuster, J. M., and Alexander, G. E., 1971, Neuron activity related to short-term memory, Science, 173:652-654.

Fuster, J. M., Bauer, R. H., and Jervey, J. P., 1981, Effects of cooling inferotemporal cortex on performance of visual memory tasks, Exp. Neurol., 71:398-409.

Fuster, J. M., and Jervey, J. P., 1981, Inferotemporal neurons distinguish and retain behaviorally relevant features of visual stimuli, Science, 212:952-955.

Gross, C. G., Rocha-Miranda, C. E., and Bender, D. B., 1972, Visual properties of neurons in inferotemporal cortex of the macaque, J. Neurophysiol., 35:96-111.

Jones, E. G., and Powell, T. P. S., 1970, An anatomical study of converging sensory pathways within the cerebral cortex of the monkey, Brain, 93:793-820.

Kovner, R., and Stamm, J. S., 1972, Disruption of short-term visual memory by electrical stimulation of inferotemporal cortex in the monkey, J. Comp. Physiol. Psychol., 81:163-172.

Kubota, K., and Niki, H., 1971, Prefrontal cortical unit activity and delayed alternation performance in monkeys, J. Neurophysiol., 34:337-347.

Mikami, A., and Kubota, A., 1980, Inferotemporal neuron activities and color discrimination with delay, Brain Res., 182:65-78.

Niki, H., 1974a, Prefrontal unit activity during delayed alternation in the monkey. I. Relation to direction of response, Brain Res., 68:185-196.

Niki, H., 1974b, Prefrontal unit activity during delayed alternation in the monkey. II. Relation to absolute versus relative direction of response, Brain Res., 68:197-204.

Niki, H., 1974c, Differential activity of prefrontal units during right and left delayed response trials, Brain Res., 70:346-349.

Pandya, D. N., Dye, P., and Butters, N., 1971, Efferent cortico-cortical projections of the prefrontal cortex in the rhesus monkey, Brain Res., 31:35-46.

Rosenkilde, C. E., Bauer, R. H., and Fuster, J. M., 1981, Single cell activity in ventral prefrontal cortex of behaving monkeys, Brain Res., 209:375-394.

Sato, T., Kawamura, T., and Iwai, E., 1980, Responsiveness of inferotemporal single units to visual pattern stimuli in monkeys performing discrimination, Exp. Brain Res., 38:313-319.

Walter, W. G., 1967, Slow potential changes in the human brain associated with expectancy, decision, and intention, Electroencephalogr. Clin. Neurophysiol., Suppl., 26:123-130.

STUDIES OF AUDITORY CORTEX IN BEHAVIORALLY TRAINED MONKEYS

M. H. Goldstein, Jr., D. A. Benson and R. D. Hienz

Department of Biomedical Engineering
Johns Hopkins University School of Medicine
Baltimore, Maryland 21205

SUMMARY

Single-unit studies of neurons in the primary auditory cortex (AI) and surrounding belt areas of behaviorally trained rhesus monkeys are summarized. Responses of single cells to brief acoustic stimuli were recorded while the behavioral state of the animal was alternated between two different performing conditions or between a performing and a non-performing condition. In one study of 196 units the alternated performing tasks consisted of localizing one of 5 sound sources versus simply detecting the presentation of the same sounds. The second study concerned selective attention to one ear vs. the other. Stimuli were presented randomly to one ear or the other and monkeys were required to respond only to the stimuli in one ear, with the ear to be attended changed after a block of trials. For all comparisons more units showed no change than change. When responses in the Localize vs. Detect tasks were compared 8% of the units showed significant changes, and 29% of the units showed a change when these two tasks were compared to the non-performing condition. When monkeys selectively attended either left- or right-ear stimuli, only 18% of the population showed a statistically significant change between these two tasks, whereas 44% of the units showed a change when both attend conditions were compared with the non-performing conditions. Generally when there was a change in a unit's response to a given sound, the change was in strength of response, not in response pattern. Changes in evoked single-unit activity were not accompanied by changes in spontaneous activity.

INTRODUCTION

Single-unit studies of mammalian auditory cortex were initiated some years ago in our laboratory. We found that virtually all neurons in the primary auditory cortex (AI) are responsive to sound, and not at all responsive to visual stimulation (de Ribaupierre et al., 1973). A further salient feature was the individuality of certain response properties, and of evoked response patterns of the individual neurons. Tuning curves had quite varied shapes from cell to cell. Given stimuli (e.g., short bursts of tones or noise or clicks) evoked quite different response patterns for different units (Goldstein and Abeles, 1975).

More recently we have used behaviorally trained rhesus monkeys in our single-unit studies of cortical areas responsive to sound. Our principal interest has been in the cortical neurophysiological mechanisms involved in the localization of sound sources and in selective attention to sounds in one ear. Here we will briefly review studies employing: i) localization of sound sources (Benson et al., in press) and ii) selective attention to left or right ear stimuli (Benson and Hienz, 1978). The reader is advised to consult the cited references for detailed reports of these experiments.

In all of this work each unit served as its own control, in that comparisons were made between the evoked responses of a single unit to the same physical stimulus as an animal alternated between two behavioral conditions or between a performing and non-performing state. All animals were extensively trained to steady-state behavioral performances. Thus we were not studying the neurophysiology of learning.

After a monkey was behaviorally trained (and overtrained), surgery was performed to implant microelectrode chambers and a head restraint lug. Usually a few sessions were required for the monkey to adapt to the head restraint. Neural activity was recorded with metal microelectrodes, amplified and passed to a unit analyzer (Abeles and Goldstein, 1977). An on-line mini-computer was used to control the experiment and to display unit activity in dot display format. Off-line analysis included PSTH (peri-stimulus-time histograms) displays, histograms time-locked to response key presses, and statistical tests for significance of changes in evoked activity. Histological controls were used to determine the cortical areas (Sanides, 1972) in which the electrode tracks were made. In these studies all units were located in the primary auditory cortex or in the belt areas surrounding AI.

LOCALIZATION EXPERIMENT

In this experiment animals were situated in front of five sound sources (4-in. diameter speakers) located at ear level at azimuths of 0° (midline) and at 37.5° and 75° on either side of midline, as shown in Fig. 1. Animals were trained to press an observing key to produce a 100 msec sound burst randomly selected to come from one of the five speakers. Indicating the location of the sound burst by touching a key on the sound-producing speaker (Localize task) was rewarded with a 0.1 cc drop of water. A control task (called the Detect task) simply required an animal to touch the "detect" key following a sound presentation, as shown in Fig. 1. Thus, no active localization behavior was required in the Detect task. Animals were trained to perform the Localize task only when the speaker key lights were illuminated, and to perform the Detect task only when the Detect key was illuminated, allowing an animal's performance to be readily alternated between the Detect and Localize performances.

Comparisons were made of evoked activity recorded before the earliest motor activity, the observing key release, which never occurred before 200 msec after stimulus onset. Standard t-tests were used to compare evoked unit activity in the Localize and

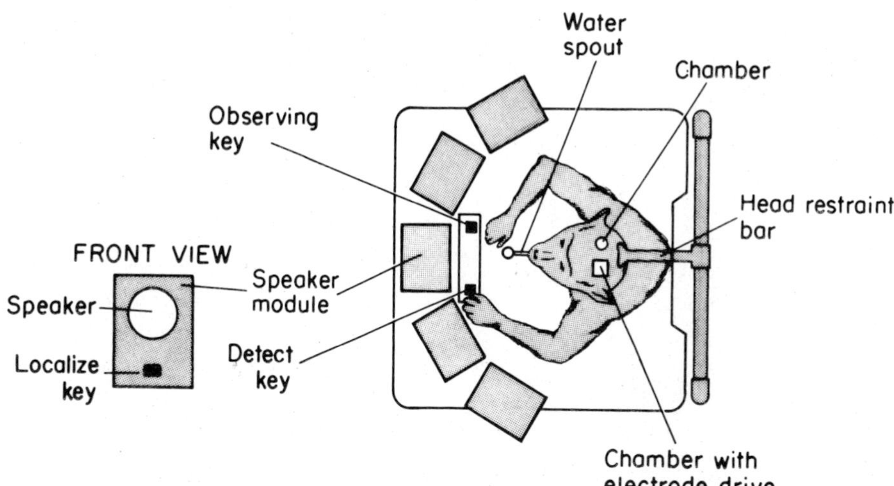

Fig. 1. Schematic view of sound localization apparatus. Both training and recording were conducted in sound-attenuating chambers. The electrode chambers and head restraint were implanted only after training was completed.

Detect conditions. For the great majority of comparisons there was little or no difference in the evoked responses obtained between these two conditions. Only sixteen of 196 units in the analysis population showed differences in activity which were statistically significant at the 0.01 significance level. Fifteen of the 16 units showing statistically significant changes had stronger responses in the Localize condition. Figure 2 gives two examples of such changes. It is worth emphasizing that the general finding, however, was of a population showing very little change in evoked activity that can be specifically related to localization behavior.

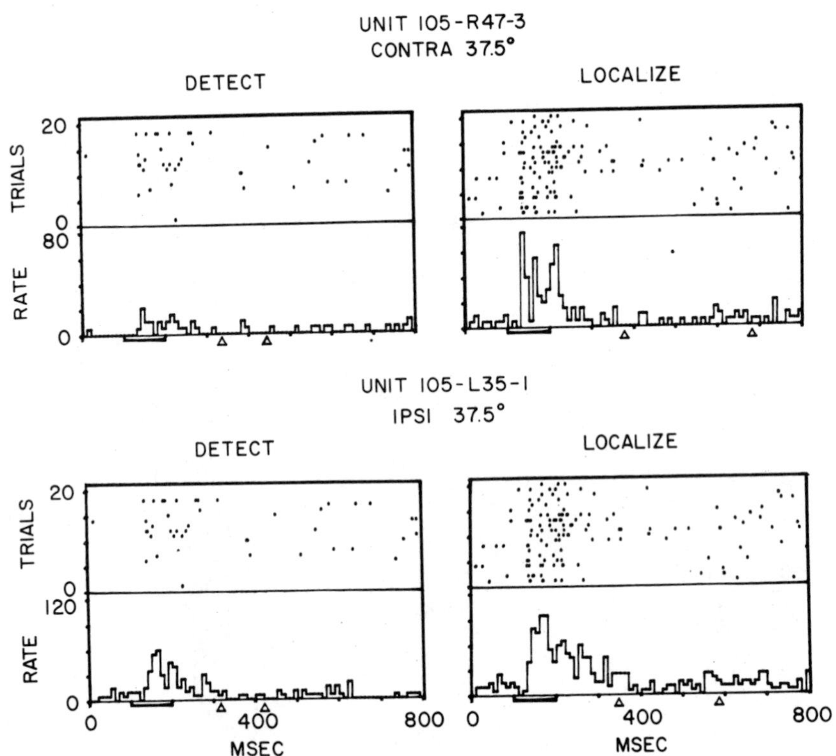

Fig. 2. Dot raster displays and corresponding PST histograms for two units which demonstrated significant increases in evoked activity during the Localize condition. The solid bars below the abscissae represent the acoustic stimulus; the triangles represent the median times of release of the observing key and press of the Detect/Localize keys, respectively. Stimuli were a 900 Hz square wave at 50 dB SPL (top panels) and a 730 Hz square wave at 55 dB SPL (bottom panels).

For those units exhibiting significant changes, the differences cannot likely be accounted for by such mechanisms as generalized arousal, middle-ear muscle contractions, or even hypothesized shifts in the "attentional state" of the animals. First, both the Localize and Detect conditions required an animal to be alert and active. Secondly, the observed changes were stimulus-dependent (i.e., a unit might show such a difference between the Localize and Detect conditions for a pure tone of a given frequency, but not for noise bursts). And finally, these Localize-Detect differences never occurred for all five speaker locations with a single unit, but were location-specific. These last two characteristics of the observed Localize-Detect differences, the location specificity and stimulus dependence of the effects, effectively rule out interpretations of the data based upon generalized arousal, middle-ear muscle contractions, and changes in attentional state. Since in a visual control task no alternation in unit activity appeared in the analysis period, the differences are specific to the auditory modality.

Another possibility that must be considered concerns the degree of correspondence between the behavioral procedures employed to obtain what have been thus far termed "Localize" and "Detect" behaviors, and what in actuality the animals were doing under these behavioral procedures. Thus one might well question whether the animals were simply detecting acoustic stimuli under the Detect condition, or whether they were in fact "localizing" the stimuli (i.e., they would have been able to report the locus of each stimulus, if required to do so) and then simply pressing the Detect key. Three pieces of evidence bear on this possibility. First, all animals performed with 100% accuracy on the Detect task, while performance of the Localize task varied from 92-96% correct, indicating that both tasks were fairly easy to perform, though not necessarily equivalent. Second, behavioral reaction times differed for the two conditions, with the release of the observing key consistently occurring earlier during the Detect condition than in the Localize condition. Third, on a few occasions EOG recordings were made while the animals performed the Localize/Detect task. These data indicated the occurrence of rapid saccades toward selected speakers at about 150-200 msec after stimulus onset during the Localize condition. During the Detect condition, however, there was a marked lack of correlation between speaker location and the direction of eye movement. While far from being definitive, these observations do indicate that the two tasks were performed differently.

Before and after a unit was studied in the alternated Detect and Localize behavioral conditions, evoked activity was recorded with the monkey awake but not performing. This Non-perform condition was indicated by turning off all key lights. Comparisons between performing and non-performing conditions were made only for those units in which no statistical differences in evoked firing rate occurred between the first and last non-performing condition. One hundred twenty-two of the 196 units in the sample met this test. Of these 122 units, 35 (29%) showed a significance difference ($p<0.01$) in evoked firing rate for one or more speaker locations, with 27 units having increased rates and 8 having decreased rates when the animal was performing.

An example of the differences in a unit's evoked firing rate between the performing and non-performing conditions for all five speaker locations is shown in Fig. 3. The evoked rate differences between the performing conditions and the non-performing conditions were significant ($p<0.01$) for all five speaker locations and ranged from a 100% increase in rate during the performing condition for the 75° ipsilateral location to a 25% increase for the 75° contralateral location. The increases in evoked rate were not accompanied by any change in the spontaneous rate. Figure 3 also illustrates what was commonly observed for most units, namely that the changes in firing rate between conditions did not selectively affect any single portion of the response pattern; instead the response pattern tended to remain fixed despite the change in overall rate of discharge. Nor were any abrupt changes in firing pattern observed, such as from an on-response to a through-response. When changes were observed in all of our studies of units in the superior temporal plane (AI and belt areas), they were in strength of response with no change in pattern of response.

SELECTIVE ATTENTION: LEFT EAR/RIGHT EAR

In the left ear/right ear selective attention task (Benson and Hienz, 1978) sounds were presented by earphones and were delivered randomly to either the left or right ear with equal probability, and with a variable interstimulus interval which averaged 1.4 sec. The ear to be attended was indicated by continuous illumination of one of a pair of response keys. The left key, for example, was illuminated for the "Attend-Left" condition, and vice versa. Monkeys were required to respond to stimuli presented to one ear and not to respond to stimuli presented to the opposite ear. These experimental conditions are referred to in terms of whether or not stimuli presented to a given ear were attended. Thus, for left-ear stimuli an Attend-Left condition was designated an "Attend" condition and an Attend-Right condition a "Non-Attend" condition (though in both the Attend and Non-Attend conditions the animal was attending acoustic stimuli). The ear to be attended was alternated in blocks of 100 trials until at least two Attend-Left and two Attend-Right conditions had been presented.

Fifty of the 77 units in the analysis populations had higher

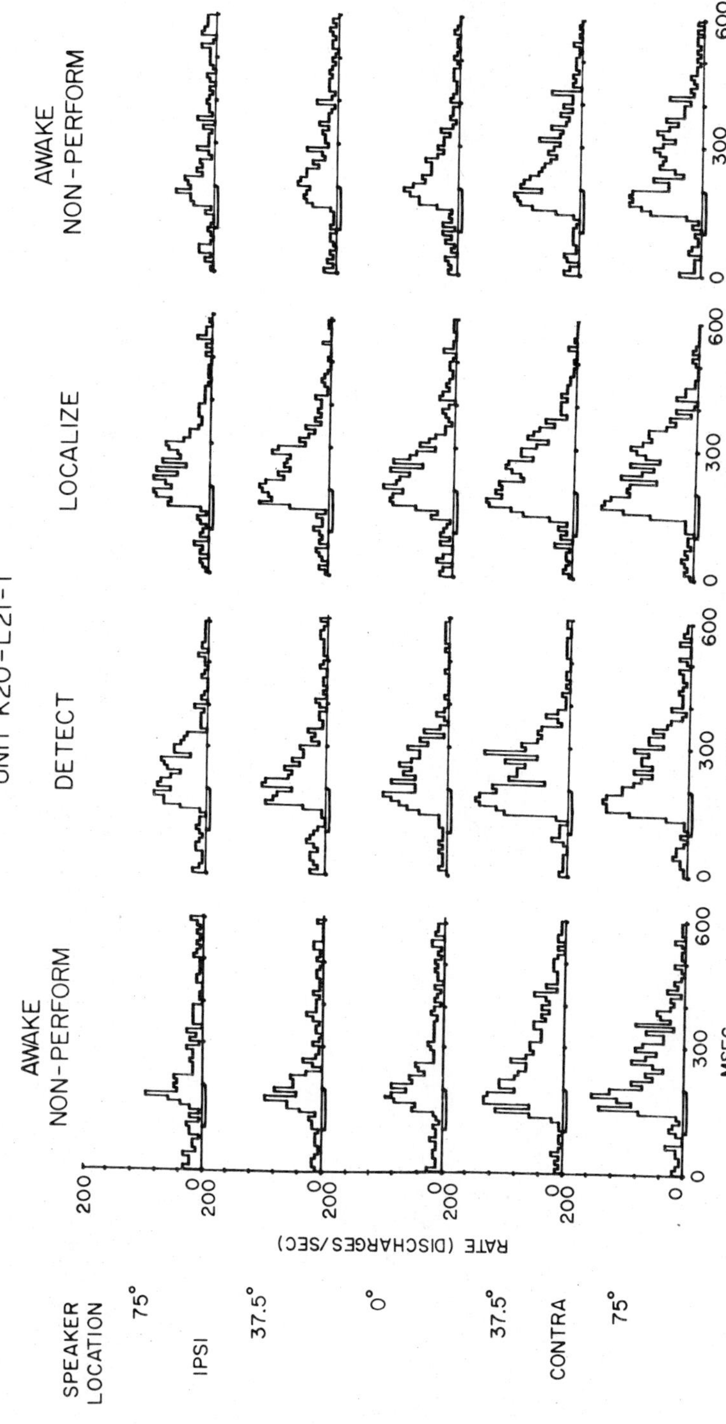

Fig. 3. PST histograms for 5 speaker locations as a function of the animal's behavioral state. The stimulus was identical for all conditions: a 70 Hz square wave of 28 dB SPL, presented at the time indicated by the bars below the abscissae. The sequence of recording conditions was: i) awake, non-perform (left column); ii) Localize/Detect interleaved; iii) awake, non-perform (right column).

rates of evoked activity during the Attend than during the Non-Attend conditions (Fig. 4). The differences in evoked rate were significant ($p<0.02$) for 14 units when t-tests were used to examine each unit separately. All 14 units had significantly higher evoked rates in the Attend condition; no units were found which had significantly less activity in the Attend condition.

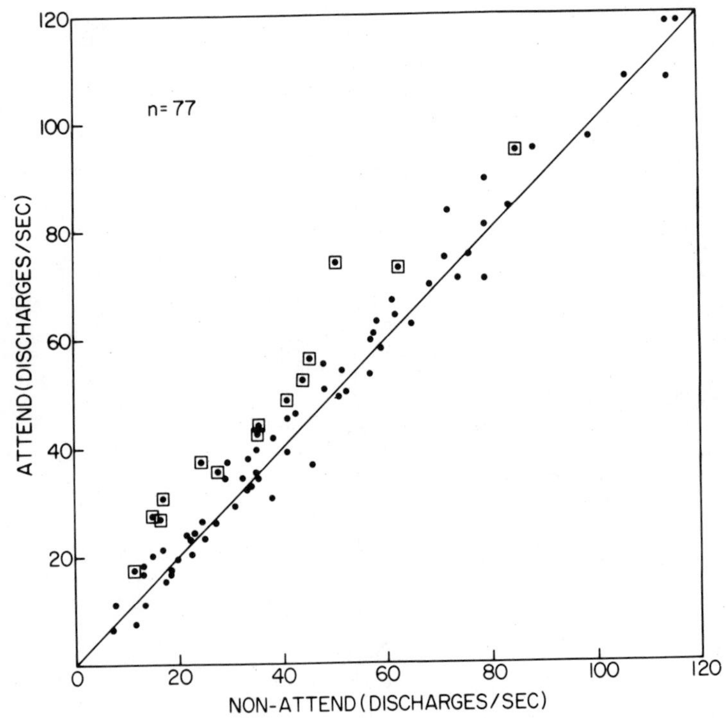

Fig. 4. Mean evoked discharge rate for each unit during the two behavioral conditions. Rates for the Attend condition are plotted along the ordinate; rates for the Non-Attend condition along the abscissa. Each point represents the mean of at least two Attend and two Non-Attend conditions. Points enclosed by boxes denote units with statistically significant ($p<0.02$) differences in discharge rate between the Attend and Non-Attend conditions.

Figure 5 shows an example of a unit with significantly greater evoked activity in the Attend condition. This unit responded with discharges shortly after the onset and again after the offset of the stimulus. Both the on and off components of the responses showed similar changes between the Attend and Non-Attend conditions.

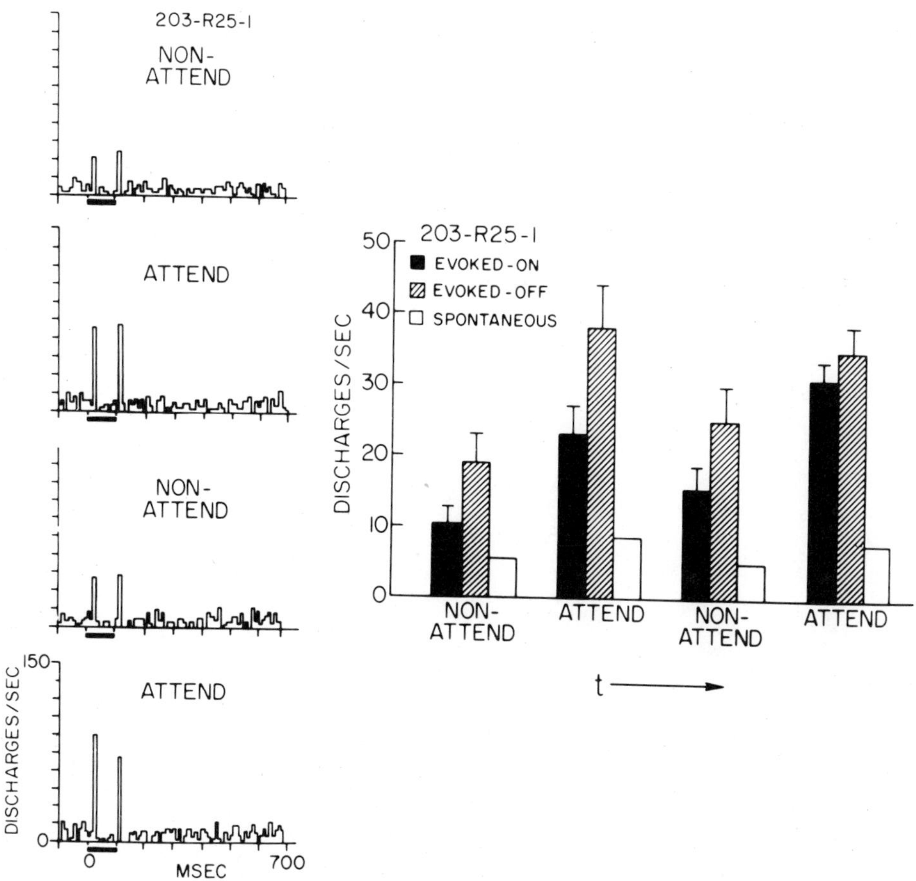

Fig. 5. Effects of Attend and Non-Attend conditions on responses of a single unit. Evoked activity for the on-response was sampled over a 20-50 msec period, for the off-response over a 100-120 msec period. Bar graphs represent the mean evoked activity and standard error of the mean. Spontaneous activity was sampled for the 100-msec period preceding stimulus onset. The behavioral conditions are arranged in chronological sequence beginning at the top for the histograms and at the left for the bar graphs. Stimulus: Click trains with 8 kHz repetition rate, 65 dB SPL peak equivalent, 100 msec duration.

The changes for both the _on_ and _off_ components of the response were statistically significant ($p<0.01$). Although the spontaneous activity showed systematic changes between conditions, these changes were considerably smaller than the changes in the evoked discharges. This particular unit also demonstrates that changes in evoked discharges could occur at very early latencies. In this case, significant differences occurred during the period of activity 10-40 msec after the onset of the stimulus. Four other units of the group of 14 units had changes which occurred earlier than 60 msec.

The evoked rate for the performing condition was derived from the mean of 2 Attend and 2 Non-Attend conditions and was compared to the mean rate during the non-performing condition using a standard t-test. The amount of evoked activity in the performing conditions was significantly greater ($p<0.02$) than in the non-performing conditions for 13 units (17% of the unit sample) but significantly less ($p<0.02$) for 21 units (27%).

Changes in latency to the initial discharge were observed between the performing and non-performing conditions, but these changes usually corresponded to changes in the amount of evoked activity. Latency changes were inversely correlated with changes in the evoked discharge rate ($r = 0.60$, $p<0.001$), so that shorter latencies occurred for conditions with the higher discharge rates. The mean and standard deviation of latencies for units with greater activity in the performing condition was 33.2 ± 10.6 msec in the performing condition and 37.2 ± 14.1 msec in the non-performing condition. The units with greater activity in the non-performing condition had latencies of 40.5 ± 11.5 msec and 35.1 ± 12.1 msec in the performing and non-performing conditions, respectively.

CONCLUSION

The results from our laboratory indicate that in the awake monkey, the evoked unit activity of the majority of neurons is not dependent upon the specific behavioral state of the animal. For those units showing such a behavioral dependency, however, differences in evoked activity between performing and non-performing conditions were larger and seen in more units than differences between specific behavioral conditions of both studies. These observations suggest that the general behavioral state accounts for the greater part of any change in the responsiveness of auditory cortical units, whereas the specific auditory task imposed on the animal is a secondary factor in modifying unit responsiveness.

ACKNOWLEDGEMENTS

The authors acknowledge the technical assistance of O. Asuncion and P. Taylor. Supported by NSF Grant Nos. BNS 81793 and 24519.

REFERENCES

Abeles, M. and Goldstein, M. H., Jr., 1977, Multispike train analysis, Proc. of the IEEE, 65: 762.

Benson, D. A. and Hienz, R. D., 1978, Single-unit activity in the auditory cortex of monkeys selectively attending left vs. right ear stimuli, Brain Res., 159: 307.

Benson, D. A., Hienz, R. D., and Goldstein, M. H., Jr., 1981, Single unit activity in the auditory cortex of monkeys actively localizing sound sources: spatial tuning and behavioral dependency, Brain Res. (in press).

Goldstein, M. H., Jr. and M. Abeles, 1975, Single unit studies of the auditory cortex, in: "Handbook of Sensory Physiology," W. D. Keidel and W. D. Neff, eds., Springer-Verlag, New York.

de Ribaupierre, F., Goldstein, M. H., Jr., and Yeni-Komshian, G., 1973, Lack of response in primary auditory neurons to visual stimulation, Brain Res. 52: 370.

Sanides, F., 1972, Representation in the cerebral cortex and its areal lamination pattern, in: "The Structure and Function of the Nervous Tissue," G. H. Bourne, ed., Academic Press, New York.

REFLECTIONS ON EARLY STUDIES OF CORTICAL UNIT ACTIVITY DURING CONDITIONING IN THE MONKEY

Herbert Jasper

Centre de recherche en sciences neurologiques Université de Montréal, and The Montreal Neurological Institute. 4501 Sherbrooke St. W., Montréal H3Z 1E7

SUMMARY

Retrospective review of early microelectrode studies (24 years ago) of firing patterns of cortical cells in occipital, parietal, sensory, motor, and frontal areas in the monkey during shock (UCS) avoidance conditioning to intermittent photic stimulation (full field, CS) has lead to the following conclusions.

1. Changes in cortical cell activity in all five areas studied was observed in response to both the UCS and the CS administered independently prior to associative conditioning.
2. The number, intensity, and pattern of these responses were reduced and altered by habituation to the CS alone without reenforcement, but some generalized responses remained.
3. Unit responses in the form of excitation, inhibition, or change in pattern occurred in a significant number of cells in all five cortical areas even after conditioned avoidance was well established.
4. Excitatory responses were most prominent in sensory and motor areas while inhibitory responses predominated in frontal and parietal areas, though both types of response occurred in all areas. The parietal area appeared to play a critical role in frequency selectivity of differential conditoning.
5. Attempts to differentiate processes of habituation, generalized arousal, mechanisms of motor response, and associative conditioning were not successful. It was concluded that they all participate in the conditioning process throughout.

Dr. Woody has asked me to review briefly some experiments carried out about twenty-four years ago with my colleagues Gianfranco Ricci and Ben Doane at the Montreal Neurological Institute (Ricci, Doane and Jasper, 1967; Jasper, Ricci and Doane, 1958, 1960). In these early studies, it may be recalled, we recorded from single cortical cells by means of tungsten microelectrodes * inserted with a microdrive into frontal, motor, sensory, parietal, and occipital areas in the unanaesthetized monkey sitting in a restraining chair during conditioning of a shock avoidance response (see Fig. 1). Surface cortical electrical activity was recorded simultaneously near the site of insertion of the microelectrodes and the EMG was recorded from flexors of the forearm. Intermittent photic stimulation at a frequency of 5/sec was the CS with a delay of 2-4 sec before the onset of a shock to the forepaw which could be avoided if the paw was withdrawn before this time. Higher frequencies of photic stimulation were used as a differential CS not followed by a shock. Response to the intermittent photic stimulus at 5/sec was used as a "tracer" in the attempt to follow the processing of information in the CS during the elaboration of the conditioned withdrawal response.

Since the results of these studies have been published in some detail, I shall present only a few illustrative examples to refresh your memory before presenting a few reflections upon their possible significance viewed from this considerable distance in time. The processing of our unit data was carried out by visual inspection of hundreds of meters of photographic film from a 4-beam oscilloscope, unfortunately without the aid of a computer.

In the design of the conditioning paradigm, we set for ourselves a rather ambitious objective in the attempt to investigate the following questions at the cellular level:

1) What changes in the firing pattern of cortical cells in various areas take place as the result of the generalized arousal effect of the conditioning or unconditioning stimulus as opposed to specific effects of the learning process itself.

2) What is the nature of the response relationship of sensory motor and other cortical areas to the conditioning stimulus before conditioning trials have been undertaken. In other words, are the connections already established before conditioning takes place between the visual cortex for example and the motor cortex.

3) What are the effects of habituation by prolonged repetition of the conditioning stimulus before administration of the

*I am pleased to acknowledge the assistance of David Hubel (1957) in the construction of the tungsten microelectrodes used in these studies.

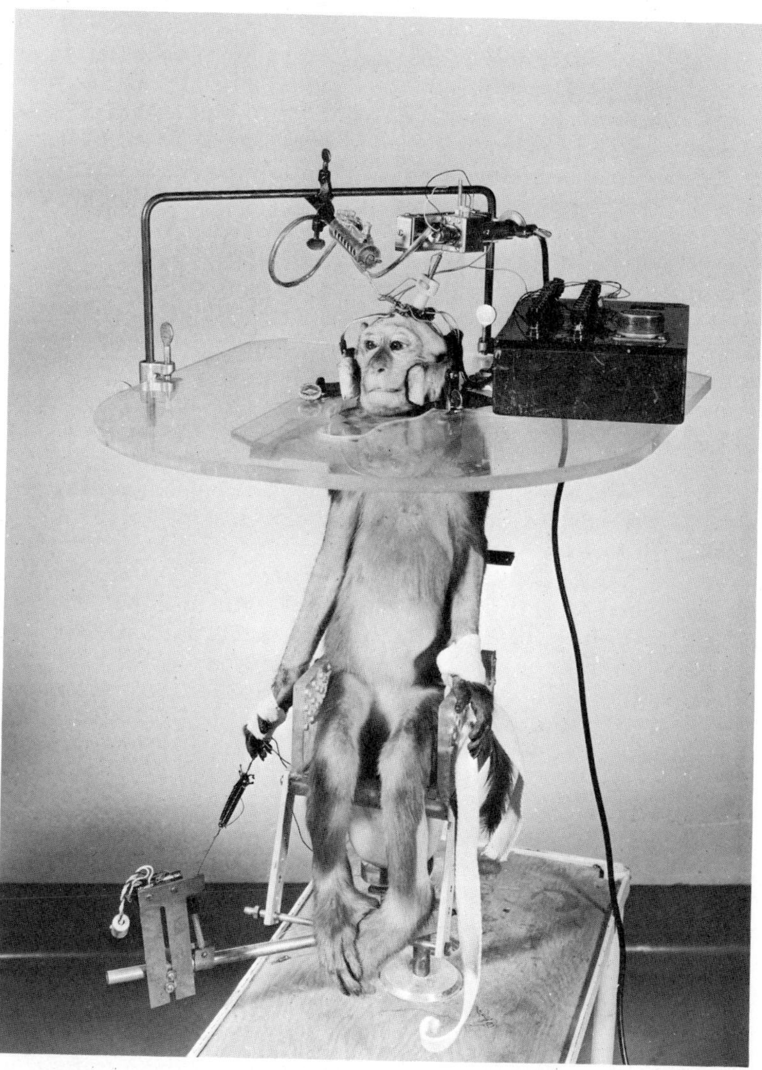

Fig.1. Monkey in restraining chair prepared for conditioning trials. Head is restrained with padded clamps. Arm is attached to a spring and a microswitch which disconnects shock to forepaw when it is withdrawn in response to the intermittent photic stimulus (CS). The diffusing screen for whole field illumination is not shown. Nylon plugs are screwed into skull over frontal, motor, sensory, parietal, and occipital areas to which may be attached the microdrive holding the tungsten microelectrodes. Silver surface electrodes were incorporated into the Nylon plugs to make possible surface recording adjacent to the site of insertion of the microelectrode. Surface electrodes were attached to the skin over the biceps muscle for the E.M.G.

unconditioned stimulus (shock). (We naively supposed that we would be able to differentiate habituation from conditioning as such).

4) By differential conditioning to two frequencies of a photic stimulus, we hoped to be able to trace the significant information in the conditioning stimulus to see to what cortical areas it was projected and whether it was included in the signal being delivered to the motor cortex.

5) What role is played by parietal and frontal areas in the conditioning process and in the motor response.

6) Is the somatosensory area involved in the establishment of conditioning connections or is it only passively involved in the feedback from the motor response itself.

7) In what way are the cells of the motor cortex themselves involved in the conditioning process as opposed to their function in eliciting the withdrawal motor response as such.

8) Is the sensory receiving area of the conditioning stimulus involved in any way in the elaboration of a conditioned reflex.

It became obvious early in the course of these studies that unitary records of firing of single cells during conditioning yielded far more significant and useful information than could be obtained by the gross surface electroencephalogram. The surface EEG was however useful in giving us an indication of the degree of arousal or alertness of the animal since the animals did tend to become drowsy with slow waves in their corticogram and low voltage fast activity when they were quite alert and aroused. The surface EEG from the occipital cortex was also most useful since it recorded the evoked potentials of the conditioning photic stimulus. To our surprise, occipital evoked potentials to the conditioning stimulus were very sensitive to the alertness of the animal and also gave the earliest and perhaps the most reliable indication of the establishment of a conditioned motor response (Jasper, 1963).

The occipital evoked potentials were always reduced in amplitude prior to the onset of a conditioned motor response marking an anticipatory state of responsiveness to the conditioned stimulus (see Fig. 2). This attenuation or decrement in the occipital evoked potentials was very marked preceding and during the conditioned motor response in all instances. It involved not only the later commponents of the evoked potentials but also the earlier components. It was not due to lid closure, direction of gaze or pupillary constriction.

Unitary analysis of the changes in cellular firing associated with this attenuation of the surface evoked response showed that unit responses could be completely inhibited prior to and during the conditioned motor response although this was not universally

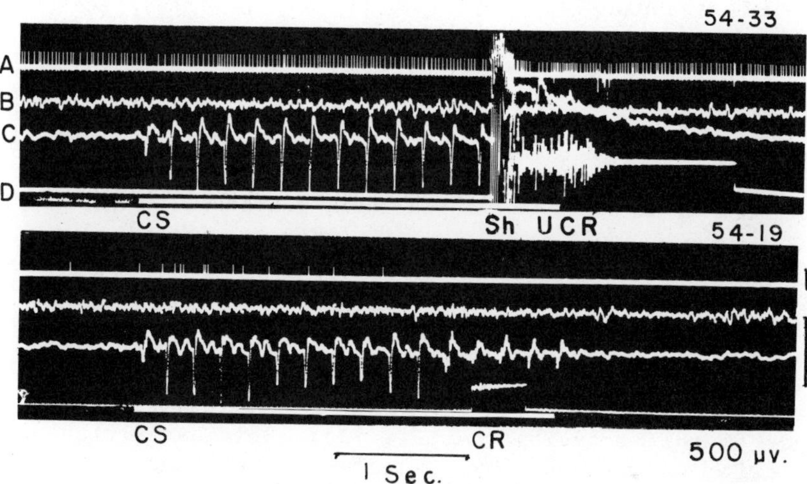

Fig. 2. Records of an unconditioned (shock) response after intermittent photic stimulation above, and a conditioned withdrawal response below. Unit activity in A and surface activity in B was from motor cortex. The third record was from visual cortex showing evoked potentials to light flashes. E.M.G. and microswitch were recorded in the fourth line (D). Note attenuation of evoked potentials in lower tracing just before and during a conditioned response.

the case. In other instances the cells would continue to fire, perhaps even more rapidly, but not grouped in bursts in response to the photic stimulus as though being activated by a generalized arousal rather than the flash stimulus itself. We were not able to completely resolve this question as to whether all of the attenuating action of the establishment of the conditioned response could be related to generalized arousal or perhaps to some extent a specific effect on the cortical receiving area of the conditioned response in some way related to conditioning itself or to the motor response as such.

Unit responses of one form or another were observed in response to the conditioning photic stimulus in parietal somatosensory motor and frontal areas before conditioning took place but tended to diminish with CS repetition during habituation. Frequency specific unit responses to the 5/sec photic stimulus were observed even occasionally in the motor cortex prior to conditioning but disappeared after prolonged habituation and the establishment of the conditioned motor response.

Unit responses which seemed peculiar to the conditioning process itself and persisted after conditioning had been established involved both excitation and inhibition as judged by increased or decreased unit firing. Excitation was more prominent in sensory and motor areas while inhibition was somewhat more marked in frontal and parietal areas as judged by change in frequency of unit activity (see Fig. 3). This was probably not a good criterion however since more important changes occurred in the pattern of responses as such rather than a simple change in frequency.

It seemed that all four cortical areas, the occipital, parietal, motor and frontal regions were actively involved in the conditioning response even after it had long been established. The somatosensory area appeared to respond only following motor response which would seem to indicate that it was not involved in the process of the conditioned response itself but only reacting to the motor response. In all other areas the unit changes anticipated the occurrence of the motor response itself and usually preceded the increase in unit discharge in the motor cortex. Examples of unit discharge during a CR in frontal, sensory, and parietal areas are shown in Fig.4.

The most critical changes related to conditioning appeared to be occurring in the parietal cortex where responses of cells would occur due to the conditioning stimulus after conditioning and cells would be inhibited to the differential unreenforced conditioning stimulus. These differential responses in the parietal lobe were reliably related to the occurrence or absence of a

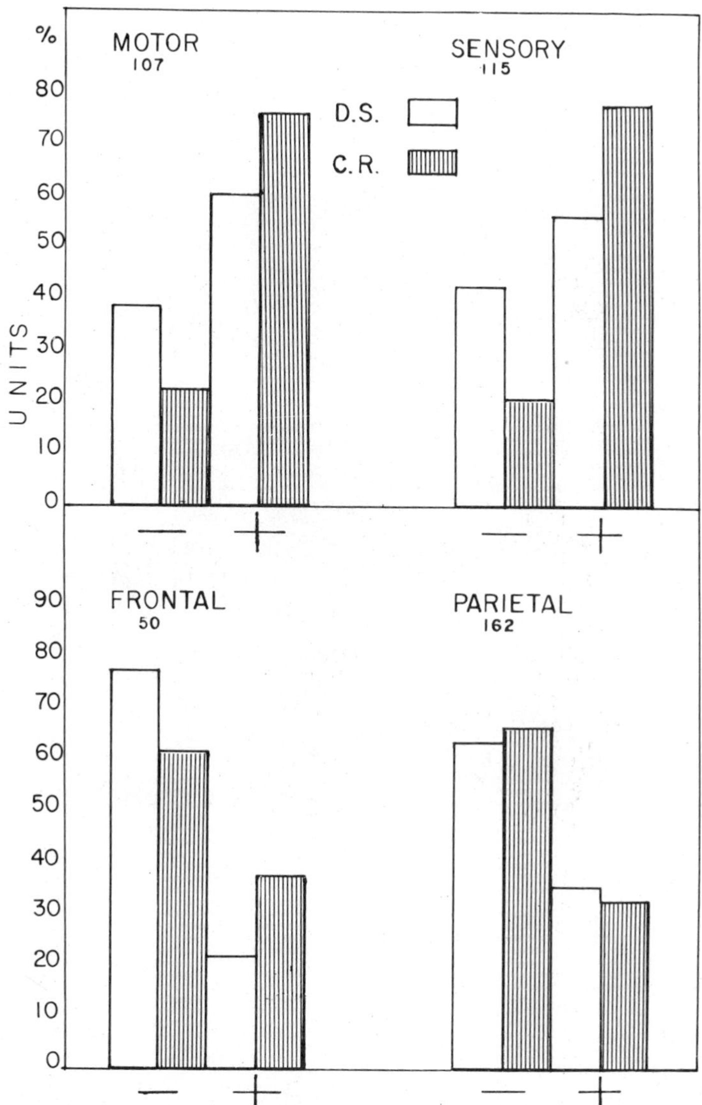

Fig. 3. Graph of percent of cells responding by a decrease (-) or an increase (+) in firing during a conditioned response (CR) and during a differential stimulus without a response (DS) in motor, sensory, frontal, and parietal cortical areas.

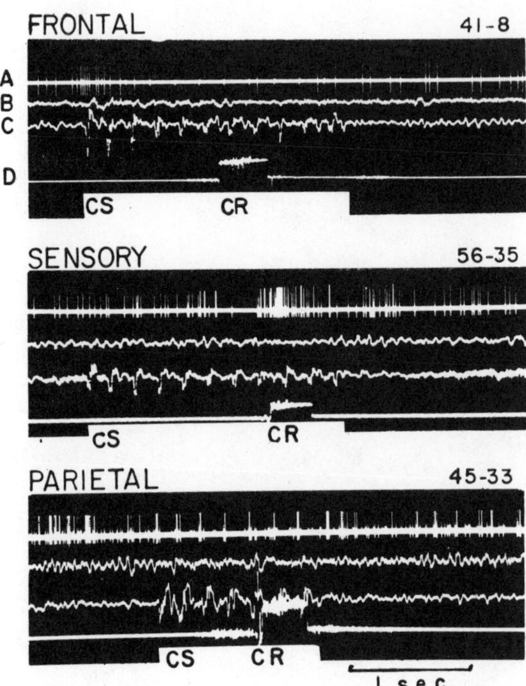

Fig. 4. Examples of conditioned unit responses in frontal sensory, and parietal areas when conditioned avoidance was well established.

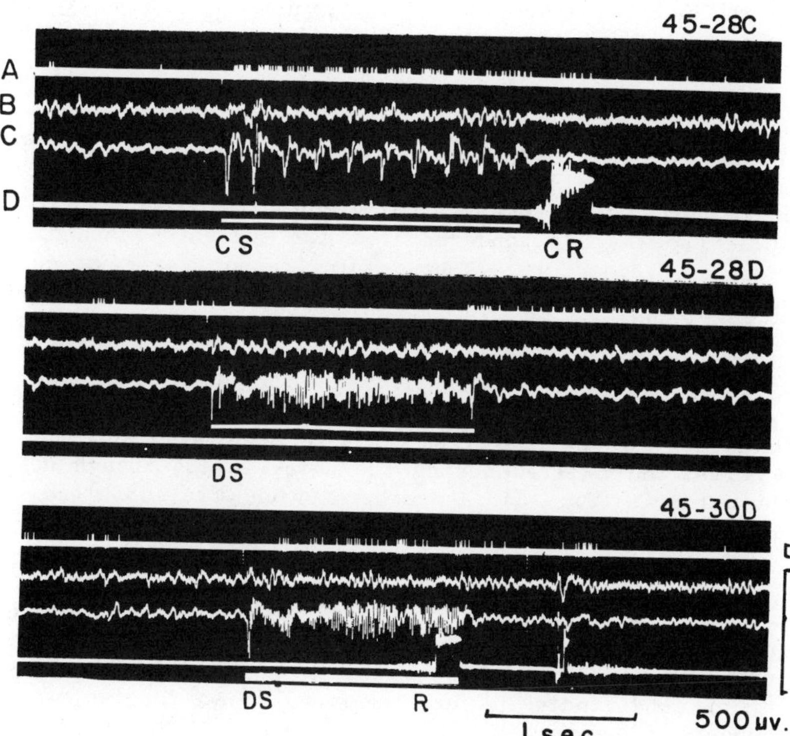

Fig. 5. Unit responses from the parietal lobe after establishment of CR to intermittent photic stimulus (CS) at 5H shown in upper 4 tracings. Note bursts of unit discharges with each photic stimulus marked by evoked potentials in tracing from visual cortex (C). Note also attenuation of visual evoked potentials during the delay period leading up to the CR. Below is shown a record from the same parietal cell inhibited during differential stimulus at 30H with no CR due to lack of reenforcement at this frequency. The lower tracings show firing of the same parietal cell when the animal responded in error to the DS frequency (30H).

conditioned motor response (see Fig.5).

The pattern of unit discharges in the motor cortex was variable with some cells, presumably the pyramidal tract cells, giving a faithful relationship to the electromyogram of the withdrawal response while other cells in the motor cortex could anticipate the motor response by inhibition during the delay period (see Fig. 6). There was no response, either excitatory or inhibitory, during a differential CS after it was established, thus giving no evidence for active inhibition in motor cortex in differential conditioning (Fig. 7).

There were no cells which seemed to be responding to the critical frequency of the conditioning stimulus after conditioning took place so that it appeared that the switching mechanism for the onset or decision regarding a motor response was not conveyed to the motor cortex but must have occurred at some prior station. There were however units which showed an initial short response to the onset of the conditioning stimulus and failed to respond during the motor activity itself (Fig. 8). These cells may have been signalling or commanding the motor response without actually participating in its execution. There were also some cells in motor cortex which fired during the delay period though not during the motor CR (Fig. 8), and others which were inhibited during the delay.

In general, it now seems in retrospect that it is not possible to study separately the processes of arousal and attention, habituation, the establishment of a conditioned response, and the mechanisms for the execution of the motor response itself independent of conditioning. These seem to be so interwoven in the development and execution of a conditioned motor response and they probably all play a role not only in its establishment but in its execution after it has been established. It seems apparent also that our attempt to differentiate habituation from positive conditioning of an avoidance response was naive in that the avoidance response itself seems to have been selected by habituation of irrelevant generalized motor responses, the habituation process being very important in this selection process so that it had to be included as a part of the learning as well as the establishment of the regular connection between the conditioned stimulus and the response.

Reflection on these early results leads to the impression, which may be confirmed by many results of the present workshop, that conditioning is a widely distributed function, involving the sensory receiving area of the CS, the parietal and frontal cortex, as well as subcortical structures (hippocampus, cerebellum, brain stem) each with its specialized contribution to the total

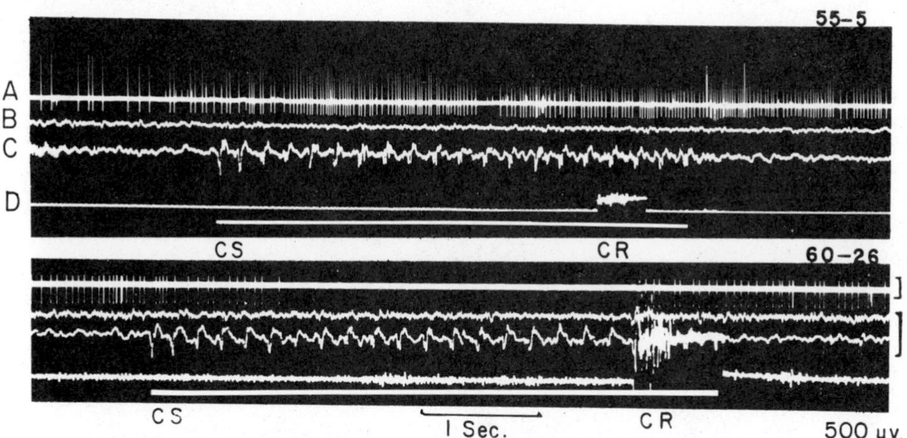

Fig. 6. Example of increased firing of motor cortical cell after conditioning was well established. Accelerated firing preceded the CR during the delay period, but did not follow the frequency of the CS as shown in the occipital evoked potentials in line C. Acceleration outlasted CR by several seconds. The tracings below show another motor cortical cell whose firing was arrested during the delay period prior to the CR, then resumed firing with the CR without acceleration.

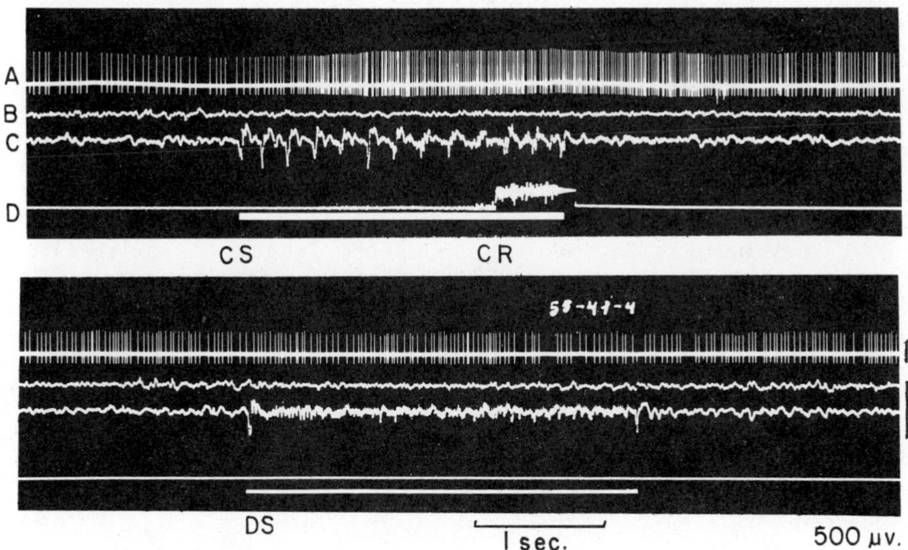

Fig. 7. Motor cortical cell responding actively to CS at 5H after differential delayed conditioned response was well established as shown in the upper tracing. The same cell in the lower tracing shows no response to the DS (30H) which has been repeated without reenforcement until it failed to evoke a motor response.

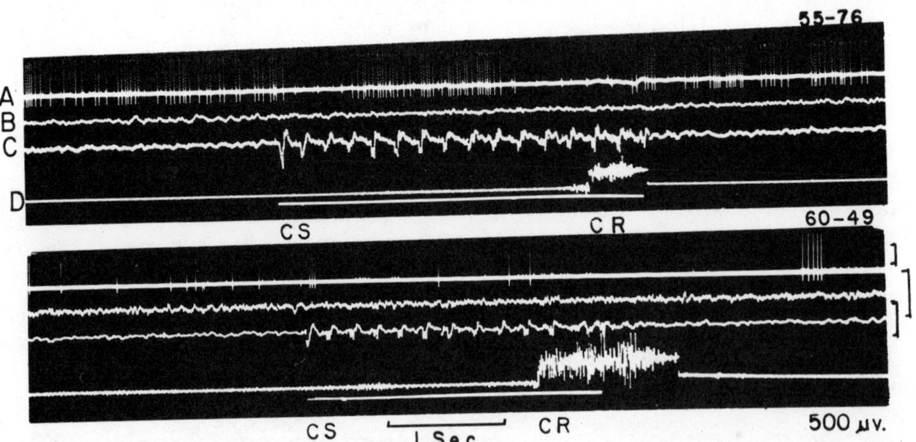

Fig. 8. Examples of motor cortical cells which, after thorough conditioning, fire during (above) or at the onset of the CS (below) but do not participate in the motor response itself (CR). They seem to be involved in events leading up to the CR, though not related to the frequency of the CS (5H).

process. The somato-sensory area did not seem to be involved except in response to the motor response itself. The motor cortex seemed involved only in the command and patterning of the motor response, not in the processing of the CS.

REFERENCES

Hubel, D.H., 1957, Tungsten microelectrode for recording from single units. Science, 125:549-550.

Jasper, H.H., 1963, Studies of non-specific effects upon responses in sensory systems, in: Progress in Brain Research, Vol.1, 272-286, Moruzzi, G., Fessard, A., and Jasper, H.H. eds., Elsevier, Amsterdam.

Jasper, H., Ricci, G.F., and Doane, B., 1958, Patterns of cortical neuronal discharge during conditioned responses in monkeys, in: Ciba Foundation Symposium on the Neurological Basis of Behaviour, 277-290.

Jasper, H. Ricci, G., and Doane, B., 1960, Microelectrode analysis of cortical cell discharge during avoidance conditioning in the monkey, in: Moscow Colloquium on Electroencephalography of Higher Nervous Activity. Jasper, H.H., and Smirnov, G.D, eds., J. Electroencephal. clin. Neurophysiol. Supp. 13, 137-155.

Ricci, G., Doane, B., and Jasper, H., 1957, Microelectrode studies of conditioning: technique and preliminary results, in: IV International EEG Congress, Brussels.

PREFRONTAL NEURON ACTIVITIES, REVERSAL AND ERROR PERFORMANCE

Kisou Kubota

Primate Research Institute
Kyoto University
Inuyama, Aichi, 484, Japan

SUMMARY

Single neuron activities were recorded from the dorsolateral and ventral convexities of the macaque prefrontal cortex, to analyze activities related to task reversal. A two-color discrimination reversal with Go-No Go performance was used. About 200 neurons of the two monkeys showed activity changes during events of the task. Fifty seven neurons of these showed activity changes related to reward reception and 36 neurons showed activity changes related to reversal. Three kinds of neurons were found when the monkey performed correctly with reward or incorrectly with no reward: reversal-related, reward-related and task-related.

Reversal-related neurons were activated when the task was reversed and the monkey made an erroneous response. One fourth of these neurons were activated transiently for 100-200 ms after incorrect responses and about half of them showed a steady activity until the onset of the cue stimuli of succeeding trials. Remaining one fourth showed an intermediate discharge pattern, that is, transient and steady. These reversal-related neurons behaved similarly when during a discrimination the monkey made erroneous responses, regardless of whether the error was commissional or omissional. Furthermore, if the reward was not given to a correct response, reversal-related neurons behaved as if the monkey had had made an error, that is, were activated.

Reward-related neurons (N=51) showed a rate increase when reward was presented after a correct response. Some task-related neurons (N=6) were activated whenever the task was performed regardless of whether the response was correct or incorrect, or regardless of whether the monkey was rewarded or not.

Because of timing relations, the activity of reward-related neurons is considered to induce activation of reversal-related neurons. It is suggested that the reversal-related neurons have the function of leading the monkey to correct the performance.

Activity changes of a prefrontal neuron designated as a visuokinetic neuron were compared between correct and incorrect trials during a visual delayed response (cue:left or right). Activities were less in cue and delay periods with increase of occurrences of erroneous performances. It was suggested that an attentive mechanism within the prefrontal cortex induced higher discharge rate of neurons involved in the correct performance.

INTRODUCTION

Damage given to the inferior or ventral convexity of the prefrontal cortex of the monkey induces a symptom called "perseverative interference" (5). The capacity of the prefrontal cortex to avoid this tendency may be tested by a reversal task.

The present study, the first of a series of similar studies, attempts to analyze neuronal mechanisms underlying the preseverative interference in the monkey. A two-color discrimination reversal task was employed (cf. 7). The monkey performed Go and No Go responses. Go-No Go performance was chose because a conventional conditioning, Go-Reward association, mostly employed in chronic unit studies (for example, 1,3,4,9) makes it difficult to abstract neuronal activities related to reward reception and unrelated to Go performance. Discrimination tasks were reversed after six consecutive correct performances so that the monkey recognized the task reversal through his erroneous unrewarded performance. Results show that neuronal discharges occurring during reversal are also activated after erroneous performances within-discrimination trials. Further, activity changes during correct and incorrect performances were compared in a prefrontal neuron and their implication was discussed. A preliminary report has been presented (2).

METHODS

Two young macaque monkeys were used. It took more than six months to perform a Go-No two-colored (red and green) discrimination (symmetrical) and its reversal at a criterion of 85% correct performance level (correction method). Fig. 1 illustrates the temporal sequence of a discrimination task (named here as schedule A) and a panel. In front of the monkey was there a panel with a central, two-colored LED and six yellow LEDs encircling the central LED. Manipulandum consisted of a lever placed between the panel and the monkey at waist level. After an intertrial interval period (ITI) of 2 s, yellow lamps (Start lamps) were on. If the monkey depressed the lever, the yellow lamps went off. If the monkey continued the lever press for 0.9 s, the Cue lamp (green or red) was on for 0.6-2.2 s (variable or fixed). The color was selected pseudo-randomly. Then yellow lamps were on again (Response lamps), indicating the monkey to respond. In schedule A, green cue stimulus was positive and red cue stimulus was negative. As soon as the yellow Response lamps were on after the green lamp was off, the monkey released the lever within 0.6 s. The monkey was rewarded by a drop of artificial orange juice (Go response). To the yellow lamps after the red lamp-off, the monkey continued to depress the key for one s (No Go response). Then the monkey was rewarded.

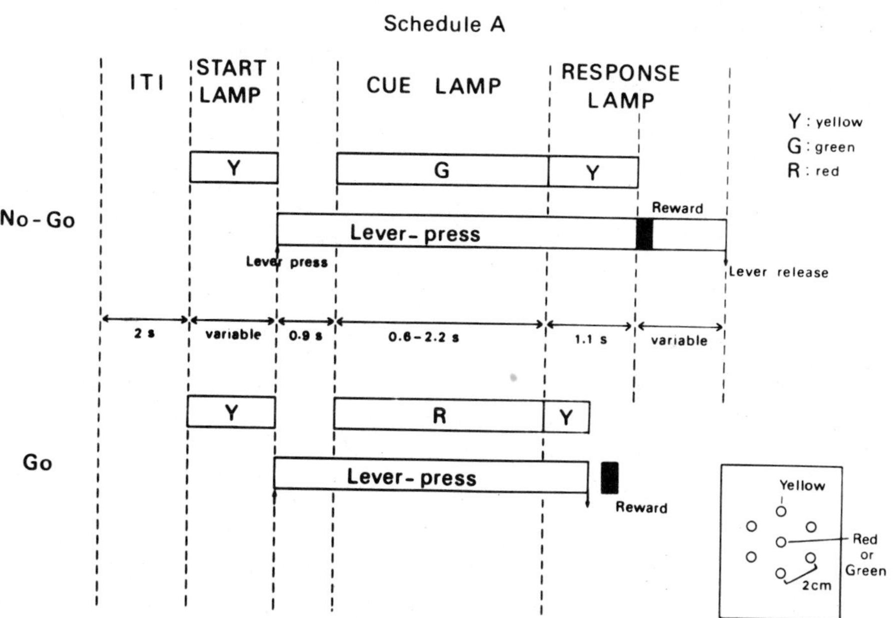

Fig. 1 Temporal sequence of a Go-No color discrimination task. The monkey faced a panel with one central LED and six surroundings LEDs (right bottom).
Manupulandum consisted of a lever placed between the monkey and a panel. To green Cue lamp the monkey continued to press the lever (No Go response) and red Cue lamp the monkey released the lever (Go response).
This combination was named as schedule A.
In schedule B, Cur lamp-Response relations were opposite to schedule A.
Schedules A and B were reversed after fixed number of correct performances, constituting a reversal task.

Furthermore neuron activities during a delayed response were presented from a prefrontal neuron. This sample was recorded during a previous study (3).

RESULTS

When the task was reversed from schedule A to B or schedule B to A, the reversal-related activity was found. During the reversal, the monkey made an erroneous performance, commissional or omissional, and neuronal dischargs appeared 100-500 msec after the onsets of these performances and often continued for several hundreds ms during the ITIs. In total, 36 neurons showed an activation after the reversal.

Figure 2 I and II illustrated from a prefrontal neuron, examples of the discharges activated at the reversal. In I, the task was reversed from schedule A to B at the fourth trial and in II it was reversed from schedule B to A also at the fourth trial.

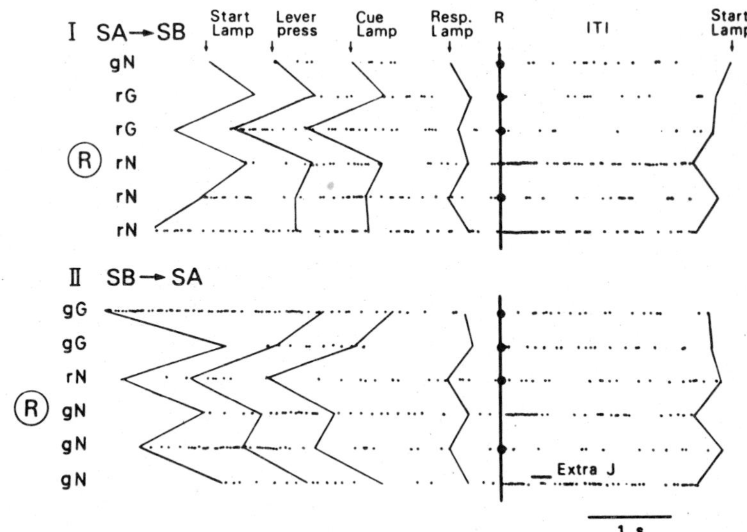

Fig. 2 Activities of a prefrontal neuron during a discrimination reversal.
I and II: in schedule A (B) the task was reversed to schedule B (A) in the fourth trial shown by (R). Traces are continuous and are aligned at moments of reward delivery R. Reward deliveries were indicated by filled circles along the vertical line. Bar with Extra J in II-sixth trial indicates extraneous juice delivery.

In both I and II, Nos. 1-3 were correct performances (I, No Go, Go and Go; II, Go, Go and No Go) and were reversed as indicated by encircled Rs.

In reversed trials of both I and II the burst discharges were followed by steady discharges through the succeeding ITI. Such bursts were not seen after the fifth correct trials.

A higher activity after the reversal (reversal burst), often reaching 30-50 sp/s, was observed. Its duration was variable in different neurons. Its onset timing adn time course were also variable in different neurons. These neurons were divided into three types, transient (N=13), intermediate (N=11) and sustained (N=12). The transient type showed the burst activity only for 200-500 ms with a latency of about 100 ms. The sustained type showed steady discharges at 10-20 sp/s, during ITIs and the activity started 300-400 ms after the reward time. Often it continued until Start lamp, through Leaver press, and Cur periods of succeeding trials.

Whether the neurons with reversal burst would show similar burst discharges in error performances in within-schedule trials was also investigated. The sixth trials in Fig. 2 I and II show responses in commissional error trials. The burst activity appeared, as seen in reversal trials. In the II-sixth trial the juice was given unexpectedly 1.5s later than presumed reward timing. The burst activity was not abolished.

All reversal activated neurons showed invariably identical responses in within-schedule error trials. As far as sampled neurons are concerned, neurons with activations after erroneous performances showed similar burst activations after the reversal. There were no differences in activations between commissional and omissional errors.

Recordings of an illustrated example in Fig. 2 were made in correction method, and in non-correction method no differences were seen. Furthermore, the burst appeared similarly if the reward was not delivered to correct performances. It was concluded that reversal activated discharges are identical to error activated discharges.

Reward-related neurons showed a rate increase transiently (N=43) or steadily (N=8) when reward was presented after a correct response. Most of these neurons were activated when reward juice was given. Prior to the reward, half of these neurons showed a gradually developing activity (reward expectancy activity). Its onset was usually 400-500 ms prior to the reward. If the monkey made an erroneous response, a clear transient suppression appeared for 100-300 ms in about one third of these neurons.

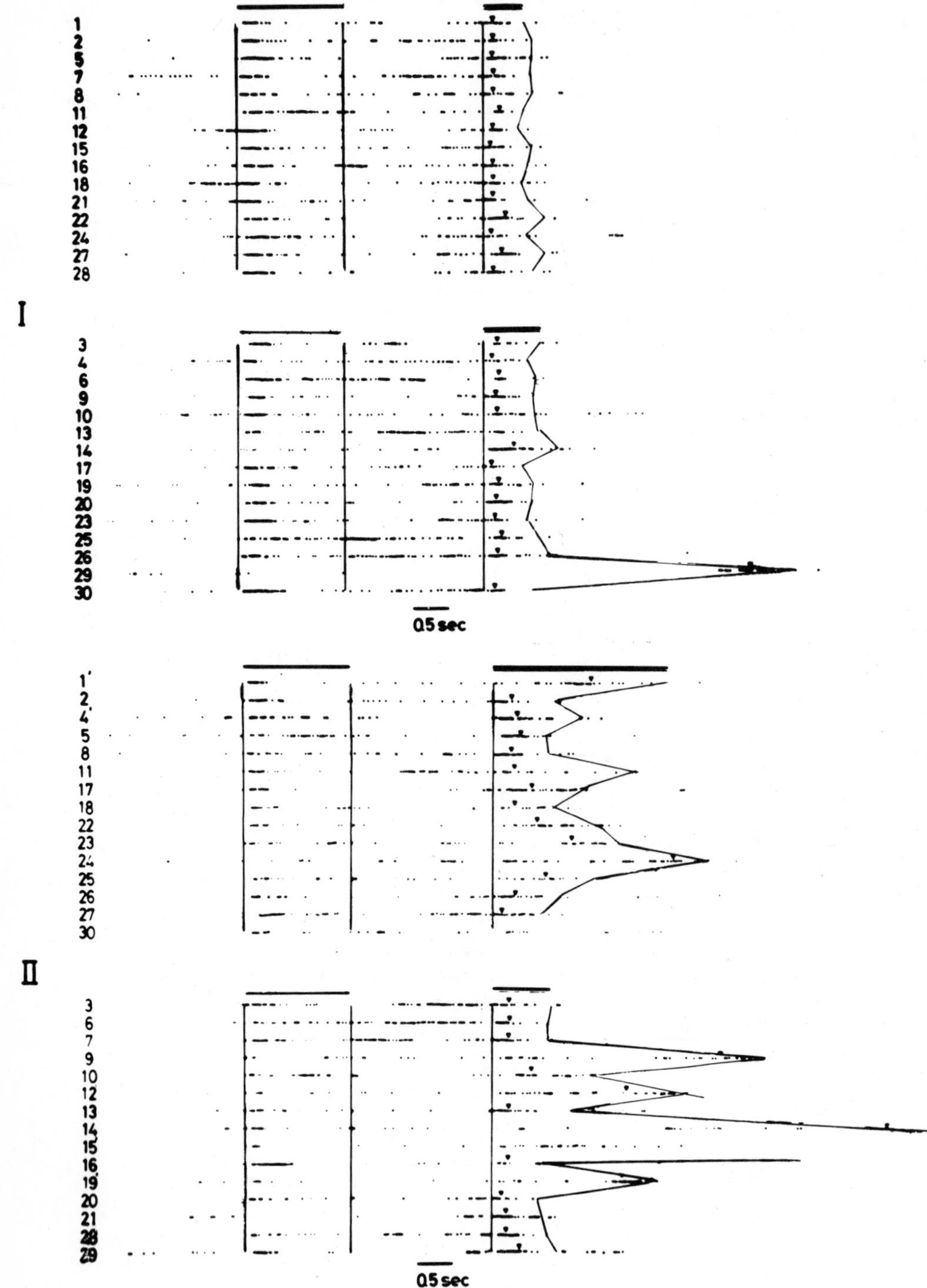
I
II
0.5 sec
0.5 sec

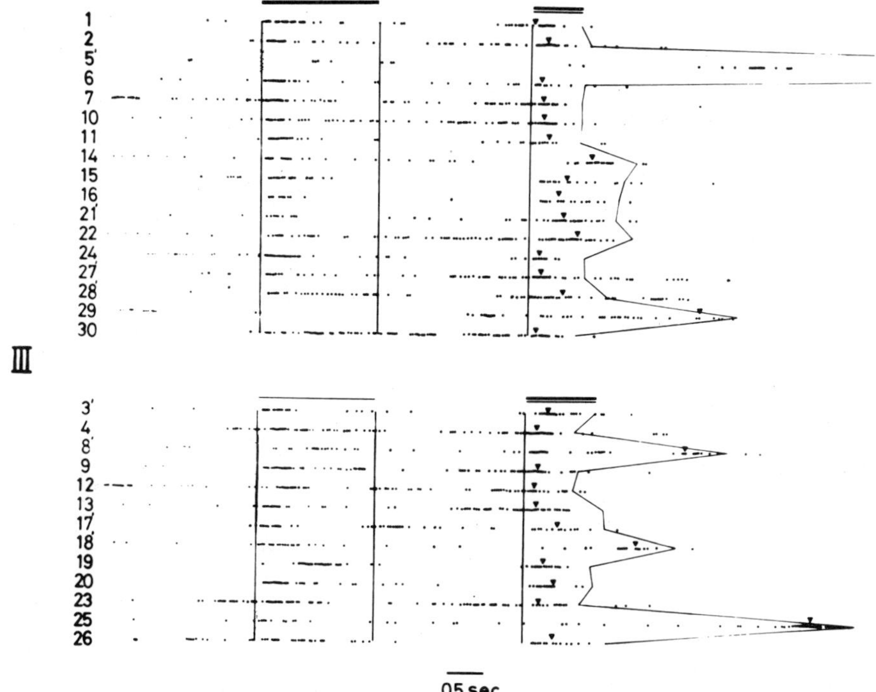

Fig. 3 Activities of a prefrontal neuron during a delayed response. Trials were performed from stage I, through II, to stage III in the sequence indicated by numerals to the left of each trial.
Each stage consisted of 30 trials and each trial consisted of 2 s of ITI, 0.5 s of cue time, 2 s of delay and response time lasting mostly for several hundred ms.,
were initiated with Hold key press by a monkey.
Two vertical lines with a line above indicate initial cue time.
Another vertical line at the right with two lines above indicats the onset of the response cue.
Broken line at the right in the response phase indicates the timing of the lever press.
Inverted triangles indicate onset of Hold key release.
In each stage of I-III, left cue trials are shown above and right cue trials are below.
Time bar: 0.5 s. Numerals with primes indicate erroneous trials.
Details of the task and manupulanda are described in (3).

A minor fraction of neurons (N=6) was activated whenever task was performed (task-related) regardless of whether the response was correct or incorrect, or regardless of whether the monkey was rewarded or not.

Activity Changes of PF Neuron Between Correct and Erroneous Performances

If a given neuronal activity is related to the execution of correct performance, it is expected that the activity before or during erroneous performance would be significantly different from the activity during correct performance. This would be particularly so if the activity was related to an attention mechanism. This aspect has to be studied in neurons involved in a G-No Go discrimination task.

Fig. 3 illustrates activities of a PF neuron recorded for relatively long periods during a visual two-choice delayed response (90 trials). Successive trials were divided into three stages with 30 trials each. While in stage I the monkey had a 100% correct performance level and in stage II, a 73% level; in stage III, the level dropped to 90%. Each trial was initiated with Hold key press by a monkey. As seen, this neuron was activated non-differentially by left and right visual cues and higher activities were sustained during delay periods. The activities were further increased after visual Go signals. Discharge peaks were around the Hold key release for the lever press. With increase of error trials, reaction times for the lever press became longer and discharge peaks appeared later.

This activity was the one designated as visuokinetic activity in a previous paper (3). Fig. 4 illustrates from the neuron shown in Fig. 3 graphically discharge rates of ITI (1.5 s), cue (1 s) and delay (2 s) periods of three stages. In stages II and III, rates of correct and incorrect trials were shown separately by continuous and broke columns respectively. Increases in cue and delay periods of correct trials of stages II and III were not different from those of respective periods of stage I, but increase in the same periods of incorrect trials of stages II and III was significantly lower than that of correct trials of respective stages. Discharge rates in ITIs for correct trials in stage III were slightly lower than those in stages I and II.

Thus, a visuokinetic neuron activated non-differentially during cue and delay periods showed a decreased activity during incorrect trials and this trend was amplified when the occurrences of erroneous performances were increased.

Although results of Fig. 3 and 4 are from a single neuron recorded for unusually long periods, they show the activity decrease related to erroneous performance.

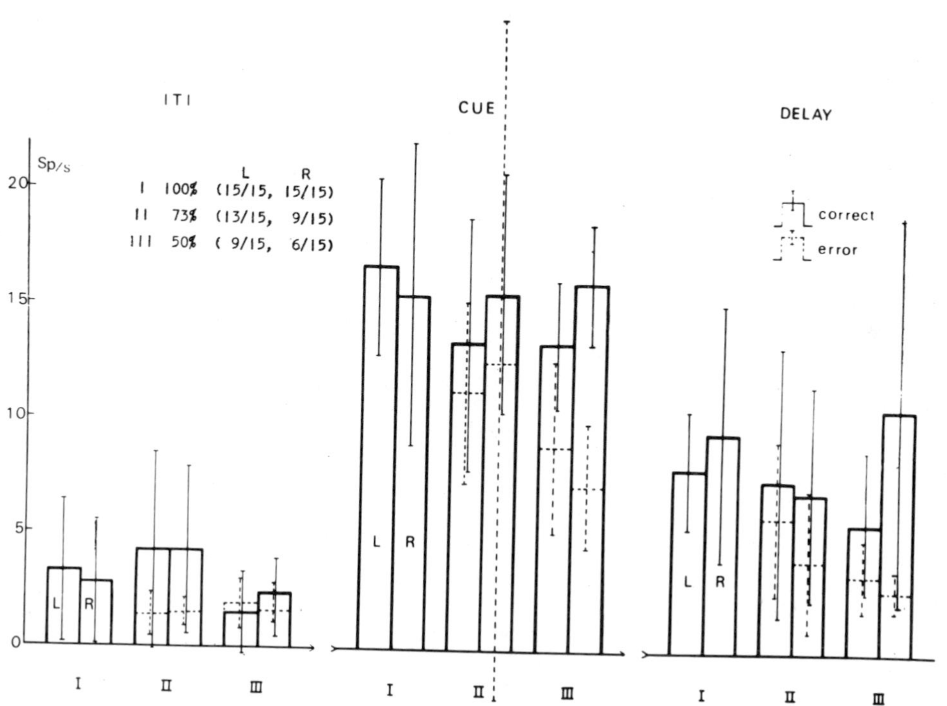

Fig. 4 Comparisons of averaged discharge rates of correct and incorrect trials in different stages (I, II and III) of the delayed response.
Calculations are from the data illustrated in Fig. 3.
Rates of correct and incorrect trials in ITI, Cue and Delay periods were compared.
SDs were also shown.
Rates for left (L) and right (R) trials are indicated separately.

DISCUSSION

In a two-color discrimination task, a burst-like activity was observed in the prefrontal cortex when the cue stimuli (green or red) choice relations (Go or No Go) were reversed. This burst was also observed when the monkey performed erroneous responses in intraschedule discrimination task trials. These two discharges were identical.

In previous studies on learned task situations of, prefrontal neuronal activities associated with error performance are reported (1, 6, 10, 11, 12) and it is noteworthy that observations are anecdotal and only suggestive of possible functions. There are two kinds of error related activities; one is related to cue and the other to performance. Niki(8) reported error related cingulate unit activity (N=12) in a differential reinforcement schedule of long latencies. This activity was not found in error trials of tone-response pairings in a classical conditioning paradigm. He suggested that error related units code "non-reinforcement after response" and may be involved in behavioral inhibition or unlearning (8). Niki and Watanabe (10) designated units with activations after erroneous performances as error-recognition units. These were also responsive to omission of reinforcement (Prefrontal=3; Cingulate=17,8). Rosenkindle, Bauer and Fuster (11) recorded single units in the ventral prefrontal cortex during short-term memory tasks (spatial delayed response and delayed matching to sample). Their type II units (N=13) were activated after un-reinforced correct trials. They said that these units appear to code deviations from expectancy of reward, rather than error-recognition, may be enabling the animal to withhold non-reinforced responses and to steer on-going behaviour to more reinforcing consequences. At present no evidence is presented to support these interpretations. How error related activities, as well as reversal-related activities, would revise the performance to a correct one is not known. It seems to me important to determine relationships between activities occurring at reward receptions and error or reversal related activities.

Activity changes of a PF neuron between correct and erroneous performance were only suggestive about functions in an execution of correct performance. It is expected that the activity before or during error performance would be significantly different from that before correct performance. This would be particularly so if the activity is related to an attention mechanism. Indeed, in an illustrated sample significantly lower activity was observed in cue and delay periods of error trials in stages II and III. Significant change was also observed in cue period of left correct trials in stage II. These indicate that an activity decrease occurs even in correct performance if the correct performance level approaches a chance level. Neuronal activities involved between correct and incorrect trials have to be studied in the future.

REFERENCES

K. Kubota, Prefrontal unit activity during delayed-response and delayed-alternation performances. Jap. J. Physiol., 25: 481-493 (1975).

K. Kubota and H. Komatsu, Prefrontal neuron activity related to task reversal. Neurosci. Abs., 7: 359 p (119.6) (1981).

K. Kubota, T. Iwamoto, and H. Suzuki, Visuokinetic activities of primate prefrontal neurons during delayed-response performance. J. Neurophysiol., 37: 1197-1212 (1974).

K. Kubota and H. Niki, Prefrontal cortical unit activity and delayed alternation performance in monkeys. J. Neurophysiol., 34: 337-347 (1971).

S. D. Iversen and M. Mishikin, Perseverative interference in monkeys following selective lesions of the inferior prefrontal convexity. Exp. Brain Res., 11: 376-386 (1970).

S. Kojima, M. Matsumura, and K. Kubota, Prefrontal neuron activity during delayed-response performance without imperative Go-signals in the monkey. Ex. Neurol., 74: 396-407 (1981).

H. J. Markowitsch and M. Pritzel, Single unit activity in cat prefrontal and posterior association cortex during performance of spatial reversal tasks. Brain Res., 149: 53-76 (1978).

H. Niki, Cingulate unit activity after reinforcement omission, in: "Integ. Contr. Func. of the Brain., Vol. I: 441-442," M. Ito, K, Kubota, N. Tsukahara, and K. Yagi, ed., Kodansha-Elsevier, Tokyo-Amsterdam (1979).

H. Niki, M. Sakai, and K. Kubota, Delayed alternation performance and unit activity of the caudate head and medical orbitofrontal gyrus in the monkey. Brain Res., 38: 343-353 (1972).

H. Niki and M. Watanabe, Prefrontal and cingulate unit activity during timing behavior in the monkey. Brain Res., 171: 213-224 (1979).

C. E. Rosenkilde, R. H. Bauer, and J. M. Fuster, Single cell activity in ventral prefrontal cortex of behaving monkeys. Brain Res., 209: 375-394 (1981).

M. Watanabe, prefrontal unit activity during delayed conditional discriminations in the monkey. Brain Res., 225: 51-65 (1981).

BEHAVIORAL MODIFICATION OF RESPONSE CHARACTERISTICS OF CELLS IN THE AUDITORY SYSTEM

Josef M. Miller, Bryan E. Pfingst and Allen F. Ryan

Department of Otolaryngology
and Regional Primate Research Center
University of Washington
Seattle, Wash.

SUMMARY

Response characteristics of cells in the auditory cortex and along the auditory pathway are significantly different in monkeys performing a behavioral task than in nonperforming monkeys. The differences, which include probability of response, evoked discharge rate, response latency, and response pattern, may be due to a number of behavioral as well as physiological factors. While some of the modifications may be related to conditioning and learning, most are more simply explained in terms of generalized or specific "arousal" or "attention." We will briefly review our work of the last ten years on questions related to response modification of cells of the auditory system with training and performance, and speculate on the possible mechanisms that underlie these changes.

METHODS

Our subjects were young, male rhesus macaques (Macaca mulatta). In aseptic surgery, a guide cylinder was anchored to the monkey's skull over the exposed dura with stainless steel screws and methyl methacrylate. The cylinder was sealed with silicone rubber to provide a closed system, and was stereotaxically oriented to guide tungsten microelectrodes to auditory cortex or to subcortical auditory centers down to the level of the cochlear nucleus (Evarts, 1968; Pfingst & O'Connor, 1980). We used standard methods and procedures for neurophysiological studies in unanesthetized mammals (see Hubel, 1959; Miller & Sutton, 1976). On-line data analysis employed dot raster displays and (in more recent studies) computer-generated poststimulus-time histograms. Digitized spike data were entered into a Prime 200 computer for quantitative analysis. For evaluation of discharge rate, spike activity during the first 200 msec following stimulus onset was analyzed.

During recording sessions, the monkey was seated in a primate restraint chair in a double-walled, sound-attenuated booth. Pure tone bursts were delivered via speakers that were modified so that the circum-aural ear cushions completely surrounded but did not distort the pinna. Calibration was performed with calibrated probe tubes attached to Brüel & Kjaer microphones introduced to a point approximately 2.3 cm lateral to the concha through the ear cushion (see Pfingst et al., 1975a,b).

Studies were performed in untrained monkeys and in monkeys trained to perform a variety of auditory reaction-time tasks. The animals were trained to depress a telegraph key to the onset of a visual stimulus, to hold the key down for a variable period of time, and then to release it rapidly at onset of an acoustic stimulus. Correct performance was rewarded with a small amount of apple or banana sauce. A well trained monkey's performance in such a task is similar to that of a human in a simple auditory reaction-time task: reaction time is long with weak-intensity stimulus, and decreases exponentially as stimulus intensity increases. Minimal reaction time varies according to the topography of motor response, and is somewhat longer than that seen in humans. The task yields precise measurements of psychoacoustic function in both human and nonhuman primates (Stebbins, 1966; Moody, 1970; Pfingst et al., 1975a,b; Marshall & Brandt, 1980).

Two modifications of the simple reaction-time task also were used in these studies. The first involved an auditory discrimination, the second a discrimination of auditory versus visual stimuli. In the auditory discrimination task (Beaton & Miller, 1975), the monkey was trained to perform under two conditions signaled by visual cues. In the "pan-reinforcement" condition, two stimuli varying in frequency were presented randomly and release of the telegraph key to either was reinforced. In the "frequency-discrimination" condition, the same two stimuli were presented, but release of the telegraph key to only one of the stimuli was reinforced. The intensities of the two stimuli were selected to yield equal-latency reaction times and thus were equally loud. With training, the monkeys recognized the visual cues and shifted readily between the two conditions: in the pan-reinforcement condition their reaction times were the same to both auditory stimuli, while under the frequency-discrimination condition, their reaction times to the reinforced stimulus were the same as under the pan-reinforcement condition but their reaction times to the unreinforced stimulus were significantly longer.

The second modification of the simple reaction-time task was termed the light-tone discrimination task (see Miller et al., 1980). This task was controlled by two additional cue lights as well as a neon light with a rapid onset and a 200-msec duration, which was used as a reaction-time stimulus. Four conditions were used in this task. In "condition 0001," 200-msec light and tone stimuli were presented randomly, but the monkey was reinforced only for responding to the tones; responses to the lights resulted in a brief time-out from reinforcement. In "condition 0002," the tones and lights were presented randomly, but the monkey was reinforced only for responding to the lights, with a brief time-out for responding to the tones. Thus, under these two conditions, auditory unit activity could be recorded in a constant auditory environment in which the monkey was "attending" to either the auditory or the visual stimulus. "Condition 0003" was a nonperformance condition in which the telegraph key was disabled, all cue lights were turned off, and auditory stimuli were presented randomly. "Condition 0004" was a simple reaction-time task using an auditory stimulus with no background visual stimuli. With extensive training, the monkeys readily changed their performance appropriately among the conditions of this light-tone discrimination task.

RESULTS

Figure 1 illustrates changes in discharge rate observed in a cell of the auditory cortex under three conditions: (1) while the monkey was performing a simple auditory reaction-time task, (2) while it was awake but not allowed to perform the task, and (3) while it was asleep. These observations followed directly from the gross potential findings in this preparation (Fig. 2) and findings reported by others. They contributed to our knowledge by combining adequate stimulus control, behavioral conditions that could be operationally defined, and a fairly unambiguous neurophysiological measure, single-unit activity (Miller et al., 1972; Pfingst et al., 1977). Interpretation of these results in terms of the underlying neurophysiological mechanisms or theoretical constructs regarding short-term behavioral changes (e.g., attention) versus long-term behavioral influences (e.g., learning) must be conditioned by (1) our observations in untrained animals, (2) further studies of the effects of performance, and (3) studies of selective attention.

Studies in Untrained Animals

In initial attempts to record single-cell activity in the auditory cortex in the unanesthetized primate using repetitive simple stimuli, we found significant variability in the response characteristics of these cells, as demonstrated in both short-term and long-term changes. One factor contributing to such variability was the effect of sleep versus wakefulness (Pfingst et al., 1977); Fig. 3 illustrates the clearly different responses of the same unit in the awake and asleep conditions. (In Fig. 3, the upper trace illustrates onset and duration of the CF tone-burst stimulus; unit sweep corresponds to the last trial of the stimulus illustrated in the dot raster pattern; superimposed traces are taken from the first spike discharge following stimulus onset on each trial.) As shown in Fig. 4, evoked discharges and probability of response usually decreased during sleep while initial latency and variability increased. Spontaneous activity did not vary with sleep state. Effects of sleep were seen in most of the units studied in primary auditory cortex and the surrounding belt areas, primarily area L.

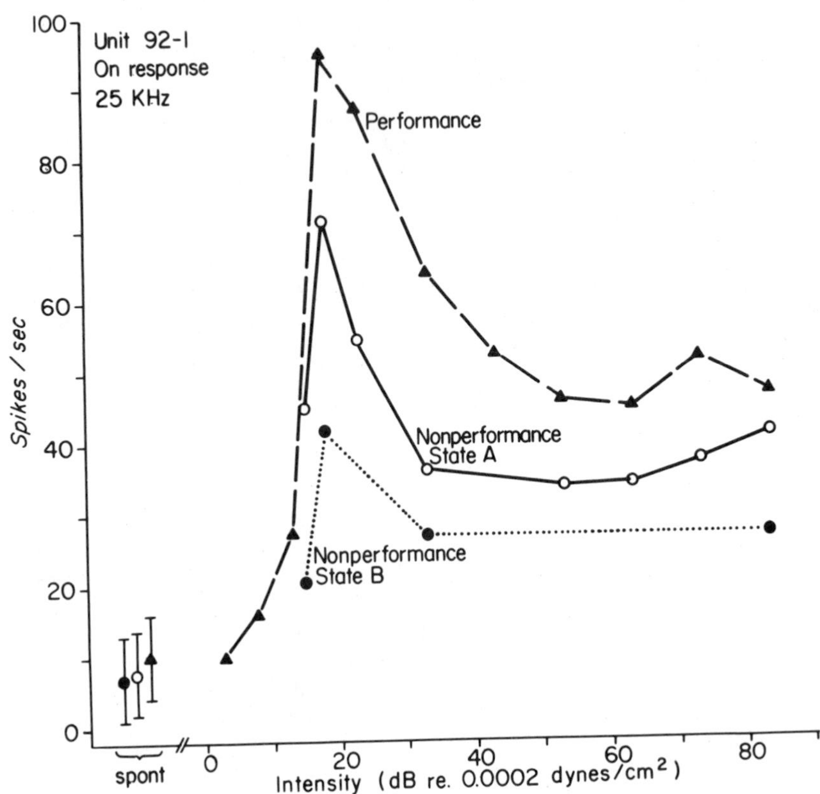

Fig. 1. Discharge rate vs. stimulus intensity functions for a cortical unit during task performance, and during nonperformance while awake (State A) and asleep (State B). (Pfingst et al., 1977.)

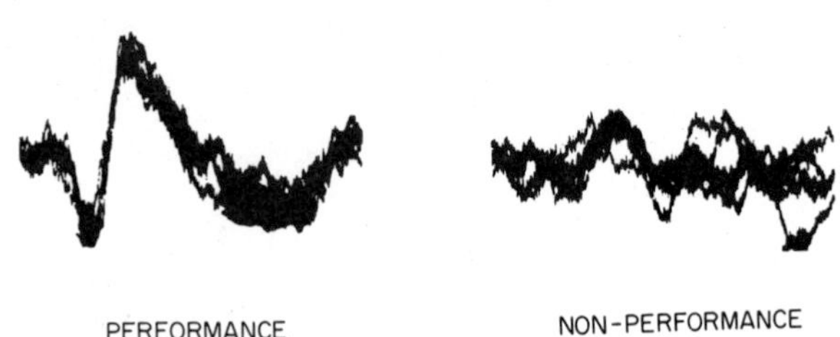

Fig. 2. Superimposed single traces of primary evoked auditory potentials recorded chronically during performance of a behavioral task and during a nonperformance, awake condition. (Miller, 1971.)

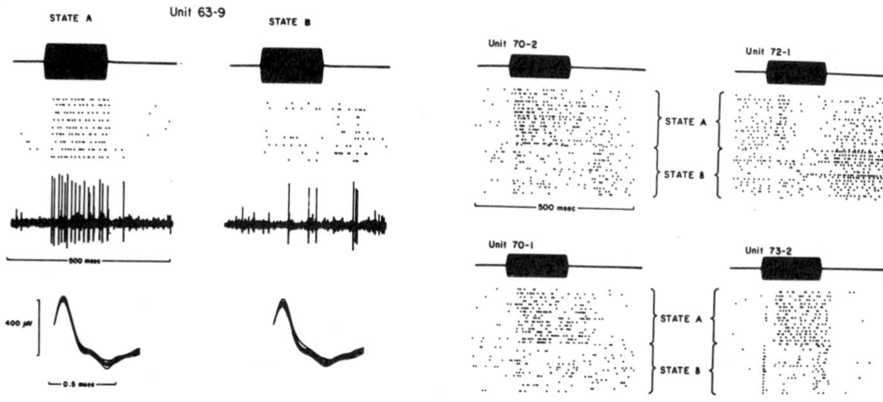

Fig. 3 Response of cortical unit during waking (State A) and sleeping (State B) conditions (see text). (Pfingst et al., 1977.)

Fig. 4. Pattern changes of cortical units during waking (State A) and sleeping (State B) conditions. (Pfingst et al., 1977.)

Changes in unit responsiveness may occur rapidly, or over more extended periods of time. Figure 5 illustrates the change in probability of response that occurred on successive trials over five sets of 15-trial blocks (Miller et al., 1972). The stimuli were simple, repetitive tonal pulses. The subject was awake and alert at the start of each block of trials. In many cases we saw fluctuations in response indicating that selective changes in attention, or changes in some other feature of cortical arousal under these nonbehaviorally controlled conditions, may also modify cortical cell activity. By contrast, long-term observations of cells in the inferior colliculus and cochlear nucleus of both untrained and trained monkeys under nonperformance conditions show minimal obvious fluctuations in evoked response over time.

In a few cells the effects of a short-acting nonbarbiturate anesthetic (ketamine hydrochloride) were examined (Pfingst et al., 1977). Figure 6 illustrates the effect of this drug on the nonmonotonic discharge rate versus intensity function of a cortical cell: evoked response was reduced uniformly across its dynamic range compared with that in the awake condition, and the "dominant intensity" remained the same. Moreover, spontaneous rate was not affected by the drug. The effect of the anesthetic on this cell was similar to that seen in the sleep condition, as described above.

Conclusion: Cells of the auditory cortex of the unanesthetized monkey exhibit significant lability of response characteristics. To some extent these changes can be accounted for in terms of the sleep/waking state of the animal. Additional factors related to selective changes in attention may play a role, particularly in the short-term changes. These

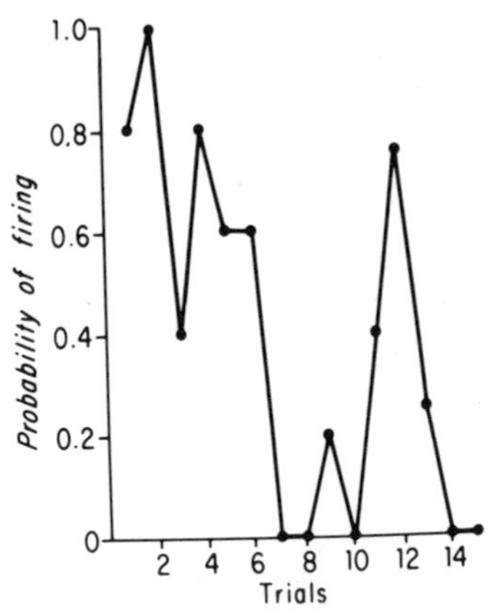

Fig. 5. Change in response probability over trials in a cortical unit of an awake subject with repetitive tonal stimuli. (Miller et al., 1972.)

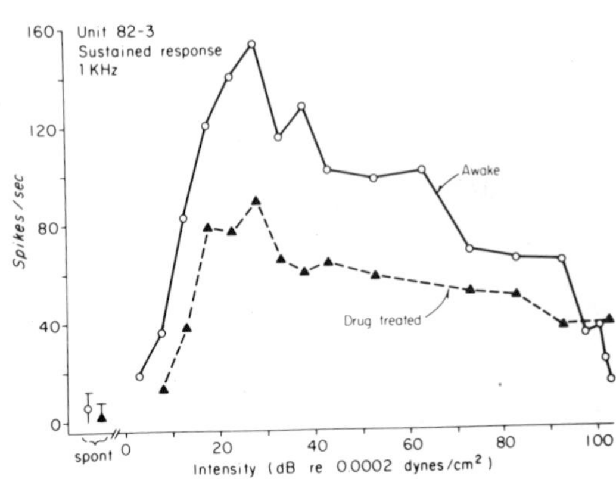

Fig. 6. Discharge rate vs. stimulus intensity for cortical unit before and after short-acting anesthetic.

changes in evoked responsiveness are not accompanied by change in spontaneous rate. Moreover, these changes either do not exist or are greatly reduced along the brain stem auditory pathway. Finally, nonbarbiturate anesthetic often produces changes in cortical unit activity similar to those induced by sleep.

Studies of Performance

The basic finding at the level of auditory cortex in regard to performance has been illustrated in Fig. 1. A similar, more elaborate set of observations is shown for another unit in Fig. 7, demonstrating responses when the monkey was required to perform in the simple auditory reaction-time task versus simply being presented with stimuli at the same rate as when performing in the task. The conditions were changed randomly every 1-3 min. Figure 8 summarizes the changes observed in evoked discharge rate, relative to spontaneous rate in a sample of cortical cells. Since the base rate of spontaneous activity is much lower than the evoked rate, plotting this change in terms of percent change rather than absolute spikes/sec gives a more conservative view of the evoked-to-spontaneous change. Figure 9 illustrates differences in initial latency of response to stimuli presented under performance and nonperformance conditions in a sample of cortical cells. The stimuli were presented at each cell's

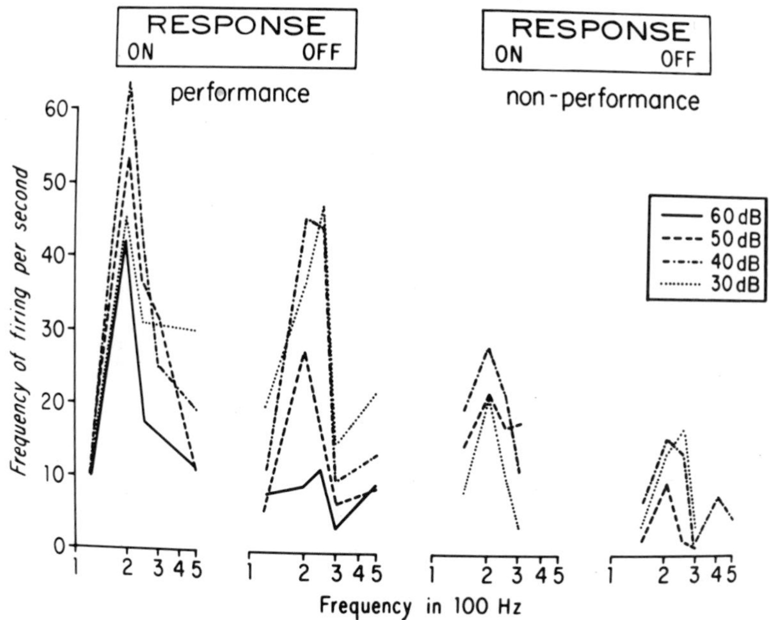

Fig. 7. Iso-intensity discharge rate contours for a sharply tuned low-frequency cortical unit under performance and nonperformance conditions. (Miller et al., 1972.)

characteristic frequency. While it is clear that most cells exhibited a shorter initial latency under the performance condition ($\bar{X}$ difference = 3.76 msec), this difference was not statistically significant.

Comparable studies have been performed at subcortical stations of the auditory pathway, including cochlear nucleus, superior olive, nuclei of the lateral lemniscus, inferior colliculus, and medial geniculate. Representative histograms from one inferior colliculus cell at different intensities are illustrated in Fig. 10. Figure 11 shows the mean percent change in discharge rate and latency that occurred at each station along the auditory pathway. The change in evoked discharge was statistically significant ($p < 0.05$) at the higher stations of the auditory system. These changes in evoked responsiveness with performance were not associated with a significant change in spontaneous activity. Over the entire sample, 50.5% of the cells exhibited an increase in spontaneous rate with performance, and 49.5% showed a decrease. At brain stem levels, initial latency of evoked discharge under conditions of performance (associated with an increase in discharge rate) consistently <u>increased</u>, while at the auditory cortex the performance condition was associated with an increase in evoked discharge and a <u>decrease</u> in initial latency. Thus, at inferior colliculus and medial geniculate levels, 76% and 86% of the cells showed increased latency, while at the cortical level, 71% showed decreased

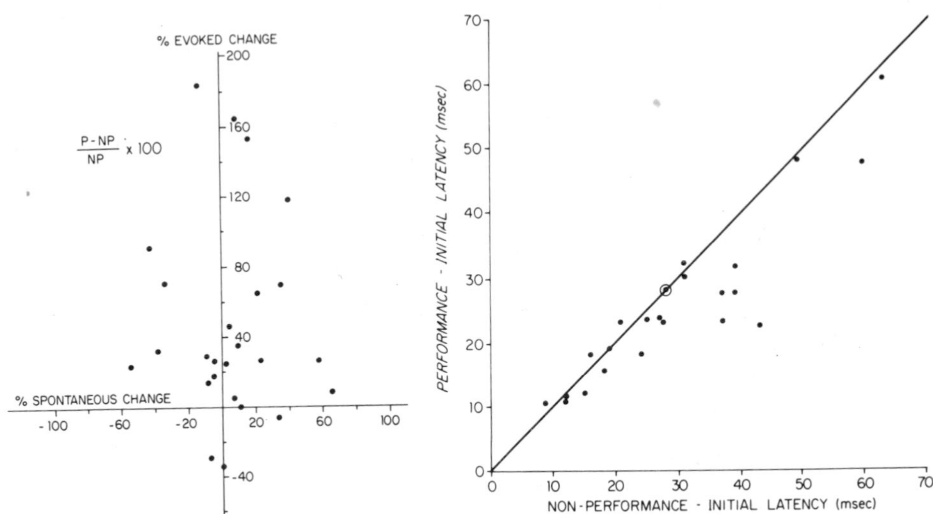

Fig. 8. Percent change in evoked discharge rate vs. spontaneous rate in cortical cells during performance vs. nonperformance.

Fig. 9. Initial latency of cortical cells under performance vs. nonperformance conditions.

latency. However, it must be noted that only the latency increase observed at the inferior colliculus was statistically significant.

Changes in responsiveness associated with performance are quite evenly distributed throughout the receptive field of the given unit. For example, Fig. 12 illustrates more or less parallel changes throughout the dynamic range of response at various intensity levels for an inferior colliculus cell. Similarly, Figs. 1 and 8 illustrate the change observed at various intensities and frequencies within the receptive field of the cortical units. Again, the effects are evenly distributed and parallel one another throughout the receptive field. This has also been observed for units with more complex receptive fields. These observations are similar in pattern to those resulting from sleep, as described above.

It should be noted that reductions in neural discharge rate associated with performance and nonperformance can have significant effects on sensory encoding. A change in evoked responsiveness can markedly affect the dynamic range of response (Fig. 1) and the size of the receptive field of a cell (Fig. 8).

Conclusion: Short-term reversible changes in evoked discharge rate occur throughout the auditory system with changes in performance in a simple auditory reaction-time task. The majority of cells at levels of the lateral lemniscus and above are affected by this change in performance. At brain stem levels, the discharge rate changes are associated with an

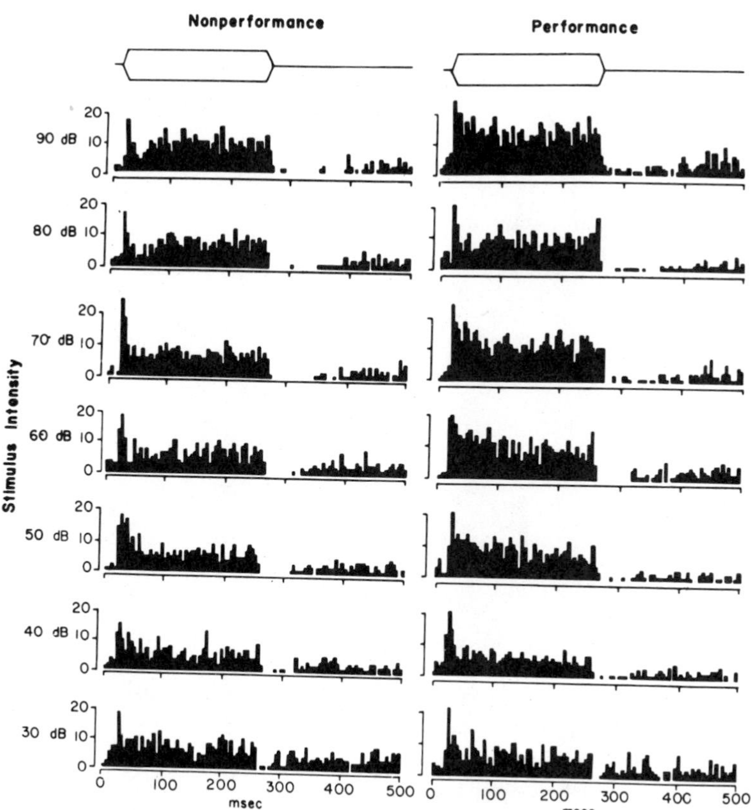

Fig. 10. Poststimulus-time histograms of inferior colliculus cell at various stimulus intensities under performance and nonperformance conditions. (Ryan & Miller, 1977.)

increase in latency of response and at cortical levels with a decrease in latency. At no site within the system are corresponding changes in spontaneous rate observed. The changes effected by such behavioral conditions usually are distributed uniformly within the cell's receptive field, and hence seldom introduce additional nonlinearities in the auditory system. However, the changes can be significant in their effect on cell sensitivity, dynamic range of response, and size of receptive field. Since the performance-versus-nonperformance conditions were varied randomly and frequently, these probably reflect short-term changes in CNS arousal associated with attention as opposed to changes in sleep-waking state of the preparation.

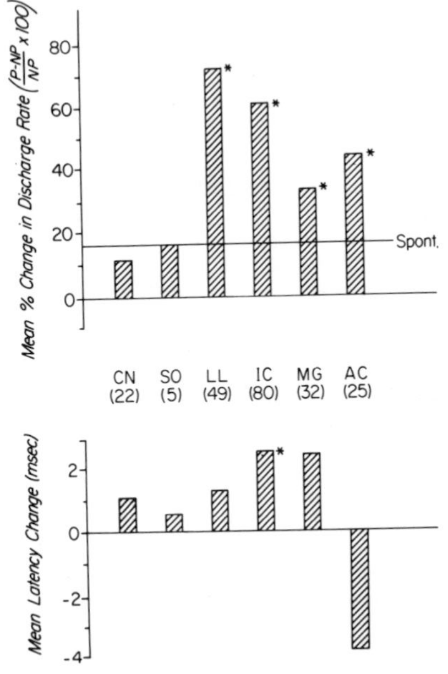

Fig. 11. Average percent change in discharge rate and latency for performance vs. nonperformance at each nucleus along the auditory pathway. (N=sample of cells studied.)

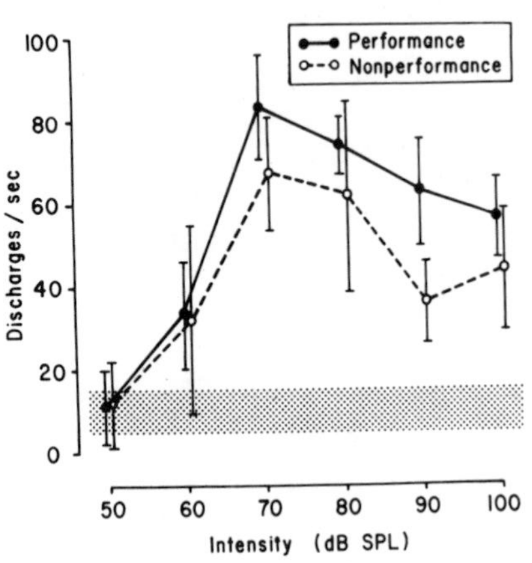

Fig. 12. Discharge rate vs. intensity functions for an inferior colliculus cell under performance and nonperformance conditions. (Ryan & Miller, 1977.)

Studies of Selective Attention

Figure 13 illustrates the response of a cortical cell to the same stimulus under the pan-reinforcement and frequency-discrimination conditions in the auditory discrimination task (Beaton & Miller, 1975). Unit activity and behavior were the same to the reinforced stimulus presented in each of these conditions. In the latter condition, there was a significant increase in evoked discharge rate for the unreinforced stimulus, and a significant decrease in initial latency. Figure 14 illustrates the effect of this behavioral modification on discharge rate for three frequencies of tonal stimulation. The number beside the mean discharge rate indicates the median reaction time associated with that stimulus. Thus, the discharge rate for the 1-kHz stimulus changed from a rate of about 15 spikes/sec under the pan-reinforcement condition to over 50 spikes/sec for the unreinforced stimulus under the frequency-discrimination condition. Of 60 auditory cortex cells so studied, 15 (25%) demonstrated a significant change under the frequency-discrimination condition, all in the direction illustrated. No change was observed in spontaneous rate.

A

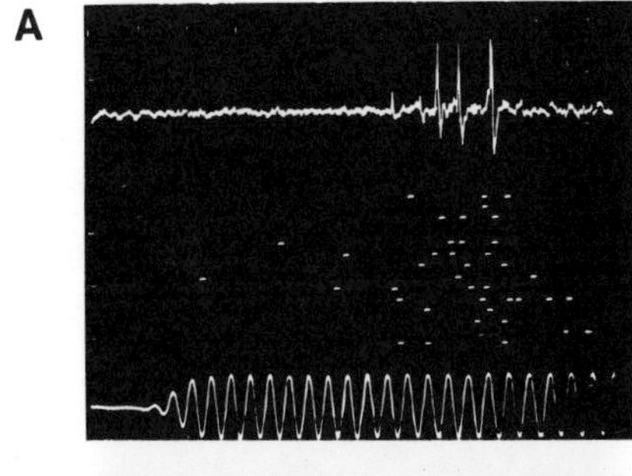

B

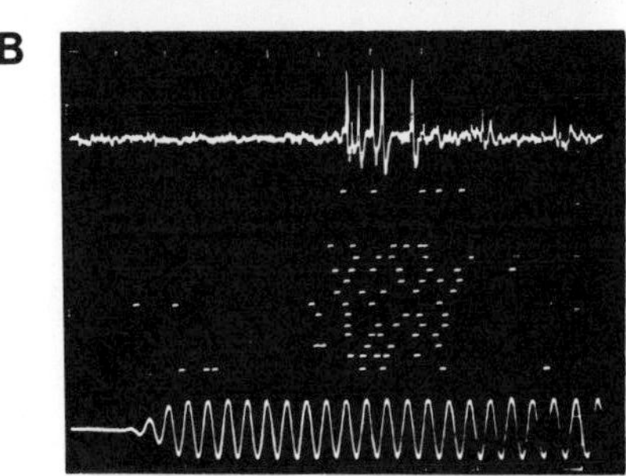

Fig. 13. Response of cortical cell during a simple auditory reaction-time task (A) and a frequency-discrimination task (B). Frequency of tonal sinusoid (lower traces) is 500 Hz. (Beaton & Miller, 1975.)

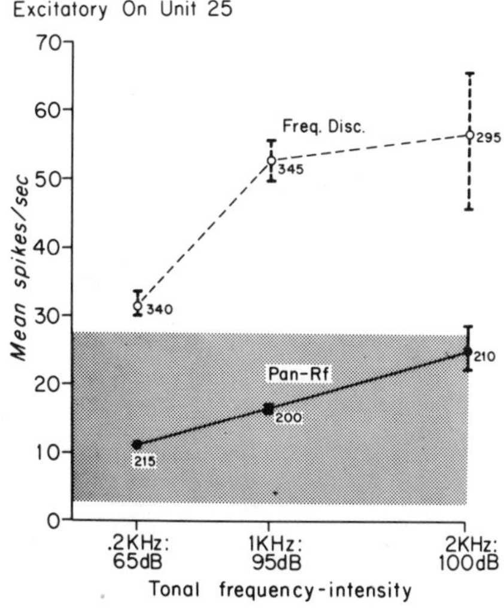

Fig. 14. Change in mean discharge rate evoked by three stimuli under pan-reinforcement and frequency-discrimination conditions. (Beaton & Miller, 1975.)

Figure 15 illustrates the evoked discharge rate and initial latency of cells under behavioral conditions requiring light-tone discrimination (conditions 0001 and 0002 described in Methods). Most cells exhibited an increase in evoked activity and a decrease in latency under the auditory reaction-time (0001) condition. Spontaneous rate did not vary under these two behavioral conditions. The overall change in the evoked discharge rate in the auditory reaction-time condition was approximately 20% over that seen in the visual reaction-time (0002) condition (significant at the 0.01 level). Of the cells studied, 53% demonstrated changes that were significant at the 0.05 level.

Figure 16 compares evoked discharge rate and initial latency under conditions in which the monkey was not performing (0003) versus a condition in which he was performing in the visual reaction-time task with background auditory stimuli (0002). Auditory stimuli were presented at the same random rate in both conditions. Evoked discharge rate did not seem to vary: three of 29 cells showed a significant increase under the

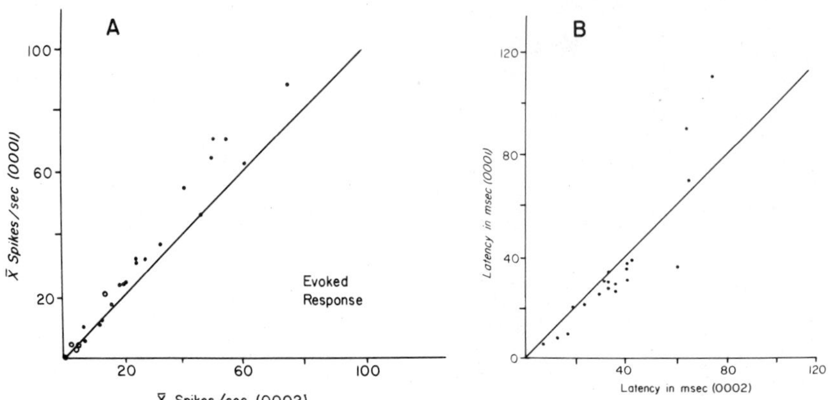

Fig. 15. Evoked discharge rate (A) and initial latency of response (B) of cortical cells to auditory stimulation when the animal was performing in an auditory reaction-time task (0001) with "background" visual stimuli vs. when it was performing in a visual reaction-time task (0002) with "background" auditory stimuli. (Miller et al., 1980.)

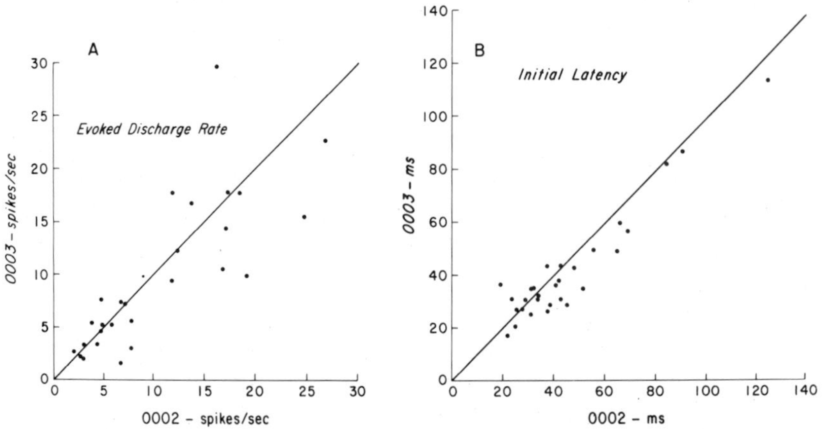

Fig. 16. Evoked discharge (A) and initial latency (B) of cortical units in a nonperformance, awake condition (0003) vs. a visual reaction-time task with "background" auditory stimulation (0002).

performance condition, while one cell showed a significant decrease ($p < 0.05$). On the other hand, 72% of the cells showed a decrease in latency under the performance condition. A statistically significant decrease occurred in six cells, and a significant increase occurred in one cell. The overall change ($\bar{X}$ difference 4.1 msec) was not statistically significant.

DISCUSSION

Results of the sleep-waking studies in untrained animals showed that general arousal of the organism results in increases in stimulus-evoked single-unit activity in most of the cells in the auditory cortex. In trained monkeys, performance in an auditory task also results in increased activity in a large proportion of cells compared with activity when the animal is not performing the task. To determine if the changs in stimulus-evoked activity were due to general arousal of the organism or to increased attention to the auditory stimulus, we designed two discrimination experiments. The results of these experiments indicated that selective attention in the presence of consistent behavioral arousal does result in increases in stimulus-evoked unit activity that are similar in nature to those accompanying general arousal of the organism. However, the number of neurons influenced by the selective attention condition is restricted compared with the number influenced by general arousal, and the magnitude of the effect within the affected sample population is also less. This indicates that in terms of cortical processing of sensory information, selective attention may be a restricted and refined case of arousal. Our working premise is that selective attention to various sensory stimuli results in increases responsiveness of selected cells in the sensory cortex.

This premise raises two questions: How does this model of sensory cortex plasticity relate to learning processes? and What are the neurophysiological mechanisms that underlie these changes in responsiveness? We may first ask whether observed changes in neural activity associated with a learning process reflect learning per se or are actually the result of changes in the subject's attention. In fact, as far as the sensory cortex is concerned, this question may pose an artificial distinction. If sensory cortex is what we imagine it to be, namely, a processor of <u>sensory</u> information, then selective attention and learning may be very closely intertwined. The enhancement of sensory-evoked neural activity associated with selective attention may be part and parcel of the learning process itself, and thus will inevitably reflect this process.

The site and mechanisms by which selective attention influences sensory-evoked responses have been the subject of several experiments and many discussions in our laboratory. If we assume an increase in complexity of neuroanatomical circuits as we ascend the auditory pathways, we may hypothesize an increase in elaboration of plasticity and behavioral influence on cells at higher stations of the auditory system. While long-term nonperformance observations indicate that general lability of response may differ at brain stem versus cortical levels, the systematic performance versus nonperformance observations are not consistent with this hypothesis. Behavioral effects are equally great for levels of the auditory system from lateral lemniscus through auditory cortex. Our sample size is too small at superior olive to evaluate this question at that level. The cochlear nucleus, however, does show a smaller influence of performance in an auditory task. Given the extensive descending influences that may affect all levels of the auditory system (Harrison & Howe, 1974), it is perhaps surprising that greater performance effects are not observed at the cochlear nucleus. This may reflect the fact that the majority of our recordings at this level were made from cells of the anterior ventral cochlear nucleus. These cells demonstrate fewer descending and interneuron contacts than other nuclei of the auditory pathway (Lorente de No, 1981). Certainly, they show the simplest electrophysiological response patterns, similar to those of 8th nerve fibers (Pfeiffer, 1966; Kiang et al., 1973). In the somatosensory system, behavioral modulation of unit responses has been observed as far peripheral as the dorsal horn in the medulla (Hayes et al., 1981).

It is clear that the observed changes in neural activity associated with behavioral state are due to neural mechanisms, not to peripheral mechanisms such as middle ear contractions or pinna movements. The clearest evidence against these motor mechanisms, which would reduce the sound intensity reaching the cochlea, is that rate and/or latency of neural activity can be altered in the absence of changes in the intensity encoding in the neuron. For example, the lack of a shift of the dominant intensity of the neurons shown in Figs. 1 and 6 indicates that the reductions in activity observed in these cells were not due to a reduction in the sound pressure level reaching the cochlea.

Neural circuits underlying observed plasticity may be considered in two classes, (1) intrinsic and (2) extrinsic to the auditory system. The descending influences considered above would fall in the former category. Influences from the reticular formation and other generalized projection systems classically associated with arousal would form the extrinsic circuits. Additional study of cells at the level of auditory cortex may lead to some better understanding of the influence of these two systems. Such study would be based on careful anatomical specifications of the cortical layer within which each isolated cell was located. Thus, the primary auditory projections from the thalamus are known to terminate in cells of layer III of the auditory cortex. Within the koniocortex, they also terminate in layer IV (Jones & Burton, 1976). The medial division of the medial geniculate nucleus, which is strongly influenced by descending projections from the cortex as well as other thalamic nuclei, projects sparsely to layer I in all areas. Primary contralateral projections of the auditory cortex terminate on layers II, III and IV of the auditory cortex (Pandya & Sanides, 1973), while generalized thalamic projection systems, associated with the ascending reticular formation, primarily terminate on layers I and II. Variation in behavior-induced cell activity, restricted to particular cortical areas and layers, may shed light on the systems mediating these changes.

Specification of synaptic mechanisms underlying these behaviorally induced changes must take into account the lack of change in spontaneous rate, the increase in latency associated with rate increases at the level of brain stem versus the decrease in latency at the level of auditory cortex under the same conditions, the uniformity of effect throughout the receptive field of response of these cells, and the observation that behavior may influence initial components of a cell's temporal response pattern.

The consistently observed lack of influence of behavioral state on spontaneous activity at all levels of the auditory pathway must be contrasted with observations in other systems. In visual cortex, Evarts (1960) found both increases and decreases in spontaneous activity during sleep but the majority of neurons (10 of 15) showed decreases in spontaneous activity. Motor units show changes in pattern of spontaneous activity when the subject goes to sleep (Evarts, 1964).

In general, it seems that performance versus nonperformance affects primarily sustained components of each cell's evoked discharge pattern. This is true for cells of both the brain stem and the auditory cortex. It is not true, however, for all cells. Our figure in the appendix illustrates the poststimulus instantaneous spike rate for two cells under varying behavioral conditions. For cell Z63-1D, 0003 illustrates the discharge rate pattern in the nonperformance condition. With behavioral performance to a visual stimulus, a responsiveness to an auditory "background" stimulus increases the overall rate of response more or less uniformly over the response pattern. With attention to the auditory stimulus in the presence of background visual stimuli, the late component of the response is principally affected. For unit H45-5B, attention to an auditory (0001) versus visual (0002) stimulus primarily resulted in an effect on initial discharge rate.

Certainly, these changes in cell activity, which are associated with short-term, rapidly reversible modification in performance, must be considered within a separate category from the long-term changes associated with learning and conditioning. However, the overlap in neurophysiological mechanisms that may underlie these changes in evoked unit activity may be significant.

Acknowledgments

This research was supported by NIH grants NS08181 and RR00166, and by Office of Naval Research grant N00014-75-C-0463. We express appreciation to Mia O'Neill for typing, Pat Roberts for preparation of figures, and Kate Schmitt for editing and formatting the paper.

REFERENCES

Beaton, R., and Miller, J. M., 1975, Single cell activity in the auditory cortex of the unanesthetized, behaving monkey: correlation with stimulus controlled behavior, Brain Res., 100:543.

Evarts, E. V., 1960, Effects of sleep and waking on spontaneous and evoked discharge of single units in visual cortex, Federation Proc., 19:828.

Evarts, E. V., 1964, Temporal patterns of discharge of pyramidal tract neurons during sleep and waking in the monkey, J. Neurophysiol., 27:152.

Evarts, E. V., 1968, A technique for recording activity of subcortical neurons in moving animals, Electroenceph. Clin. Neurophysiol., 24:83.

Harrison, J. M., and Howe, M. E., 1974, Anatomy of the descending auditory system (mammalian), in: "Handbook of Sensory Physiology," Vol. V, Auditory System, W. D. Keidel and W. D. Neff, eds., Springer-Verlag, New York.

Hayes, R. L., Dubner, R., and Hoffman, D. S., 1981, Neuronal activity in medullary dorsal horn of awake monkeys trained in a thermal discrimination task. II. Behavioral modulation of responses to thermal and mechanical stimuli, J. Neurophysiol., 46:428.

Hubel, D. H., 1959, Single unit activity in striate cortex of unrestrained cats, J. Physiol. (Lond.), 147:226.

Jones, E. G., and Burton, H., 1976, Areal differences in the laminar distribution of thalamic afferents in cortical fields of the insular, parietal and temporal regions of primates, J. Comp. Neurol., 168:249.

Kiang, N. Y. S., Morest, D. K., Godfrey, D. A., Guinan, J. J. Jr., and Kane, E. C., 1973, Stimulus coding at caudal levels of the cat's auditory nervous system: I. Response characteristics of single units, in: "Basic Mechanisms in Hearing," A. R. Møller, ed., Academic Press, New York.

Lorente de No, R., 1981, "The Primary Acoustic Nuclei," Raven Press, New York.

Marshall, L., and Brandt, J. F., 1980, The relationship between loudness and reaction time in normal hearing listeners, Acta Oto-laryng. (Stockh.), 90:244.

Miller, J. M., 1971, Single unit discharges in behaving monkeys, in: "The Physiology of the Auditory System," M. B. Sachs, ed., National Educational Consultants, Baltimore.

Miller, J. M., Dobie, R. A., Pfingst, B. E., and Hienz, R. D., 1980, Electrophysiologic studies of the auditory cortex in the awake monkey, Amer. J. Otolaryng., 1:119.

Miller, J. M., and Sutton, D., 1976, Techniques for recording single cell activity in the unanesthetized monkey, in: "Handbook of Auditory and Vestibular Research Methods," C. A. Smith and J. A. Vernon, eds., Thomas, Springfield.

Miller, J. M., Sutton, D., Pfingst, B., Ryan, A., Beaton, R., and Gourevitch, G., 1972, Single cell activity in the auditory cortex of rhesus monkeys: behavioral dependency, Science, 177:449.

Moody, D. B., 1970, Reaction time as an index of sensory function, in: "Animal Psychophysics: The Design and Conduct of Sensory Experiments," W. C. Stebbins, ed., Appleton-Century-Crofts, New York.

Pandya, D. N., and Sanides, F., 1973, Architectonic parcellation of the temporal operculum in rhesus monkey and its projection pattern, Z. Anat. Entwickl.-Gesch., 139:127.

Pfeiffer, R. R., 1966, Classification of response patterns of spike discharges for units in the cochlear nucleus: tone-burst stimulation, Exp. Brain Res., 1, 220.

Pfingst, B. E., Hienz, R., Kimm, J., and Miller, J. M., 1975a, Reaction time procedure for measurement of hearing: I. Suprathreshold functions, J. Acoust. Soc. Amer., 57:421.

Pfingst, B. E., Hienz, R., and Miller, J. M., 1975b, Reaction time procedure for measurement of hearing: II. Threshold functions, J. Acoust. Soc. Amer., 57:431.

Pfingst, B. E., and O'Connor, T. A., 1980, A vertical stereotaxic approach to auditory cortex in the unanesthetized monkey, J. Neurosci. Meth., 2:33.

Pfingst, B. E., O'Connor, T. A., and Miller, J. M., 1977, Response plasticity of neurons in auditory cortex of the rhesus monkey, Exp. Brain Res., 29:393.

Ryan, A., and Miller, J., 1977, Effects of behavioral performance on single unit firing patterns in inferior colliculus of the rhesus monkey, J. Neurophysiol., 40:943.

Stebbins, W. C., 1966, Auditory reaction time and the derivation of equal loudness contours for the monkey, J. Exp. Anal. Behav., 9:135.

NEURONAL MECHANISMS UNDERLYING THE FORMATION AND DISCONNECTION OF ASSOCIATIONS BETWEEN VISUAL STIMULI AND REINFORCEMENT IN PRIMATES

Edmund T. Rolls

Oxford University
Department of Experimental Psychology
South Parks Road
Oxford, U.K.

SUMMARY

Damage to the temporal lobe neocortex or to the amygdala impairs the ability of primates to perform tasks which require the formation of learned associations between complex visual stimuli and reward or punishment. Analysis of the responses of single neurons in the anatomically connected sequence inferior temporal visual cortex / amygdala / hypothalamus in the monkey showed that neuronal responses to visual stimuli were not related in the inferior temporal cortex to whether the stimuli were associated with reinforcement, were partly related to this in some amygdaloid neurons, and were related to reinforcement in a population of hypothalamic neurons. Damage to the primate orbitofrontal cortex impairs the performance of tasks which require the disconnection of associations between stimuli and reinforcement. Neuronal responses recorded in this region were related for example to whether particular visual stimuli had been reinforced previously, or for different subsets of neurons to whether reward or punishment had been obtained, or reward had been omitted. These findings thus provide evidence on how associations are formed and broken between stimuli normally of importance to primates and reinforcement, and indicate that the formation and disconnection are separable processes.

INTRODUCTION

The capacity to form learned associations between visual stimuli and reinforcement is highly developed in primates including monkeys and man. It is used for example during learning that something seen is food, and monkeys moving through their natural habitat may select from the rich visual scene up to 200 different foods to eat in a day. Similarly, humans learn reinforcement associations for a very wide range of foods, and in general this type of association will be formed whenever learning occurs that one stimulus is pleasant or should be approached, or that a stimulus is unpleasant or should be avoided. It is also very important to be able to break these associations, so that for example if one type of object becomes inedible, or poisoning arises from its ingestion, that type of object is no longer associated with reward, and it is no longer approached and selected. This ability to form and disconnect associations between stimuli and reinforcement is also basic to learned emotional responses, which can be considered as responses which occur to stimuli previously associated with reinforcement. This capacity is also required for classically conditioned responses such as salivation which might occur to the sight of stimuli associated with food but not to other visual stimuli.

Evidence on which parts of the primate brain are involved in these types of learning, and on neuronal activity in these regions during this learning, is discussed in this paper. It is shown that there are different neural mechanisms for the formation and disconnection of stimulus-reinforcement associations, so that these must be separable processes, and that these two types of learning are separable from other types of learning.

Because the visual stimuli which primates must normally treat as foods or as emotional are complex, cortical mechanisms are essential for their analysis, in that, as shown below, cortical lesions impair this processing. It will also be shown that the cortical outputs are directed towards limbic structures which are important in this processing. In fact, these pathways normally used for this processing can probably be bypassed if simple stimuli such as flashes of light or tones are used in conditioning studies, in that conditioning to such simple stimuli can occur even with a total ablation of the neocortex (Oakley, 1981). It seems possible that if such simple stimuli are used experimentally, the neuronal mechanisms involved may not be the same as those used with more normal, complex, stimuli, in which the well-developed neocortical inputs to limbic structures in primates participate.

THE FORMATION OF STIMULUS-REINFORCEMENT ASSOCIATIONS.

Lesions

Bilateral damage to the temporal lobes of primates leads to the Kluver-Bucy syndrome, in which lesioned monkeys for example select and place in their mouths non-food as well as food items shown to them, and repeatedly fail to avoid noxious stimuli (Kluver and Bucy, 1939; Jones and Mishkin, 1972). The lesioned monkeys have a visual discrimination deficit, in that they are impaired in learning to select one of two objects under which food is found, and thus fail to form correctly an association between the rewarded stimulus and reinforcement (Jones and Mishkin, 1972). This syndrome is produced by lesions which damage the cortical areas in the anterior part of the temporal lobe and the underlying amygdala (Jones and Mishkin, 1972), or by lesions of the amygdala (Weiskrantz, 1956), or of the temporal lobe neocortex (Akert et al, 1961). Lesions to part of the temporal lobe neocortex, damaging the inferior temporal visual cortex and extending into the cortex in the ventral bank of the superior temporal sulcus, produce visual aspects of the syndrome, seen for example as a tendency to select non-food as well as food items (L. Weiskrantz, personal communication). Anatomically, there are connections from the inferior temporal visual cortex to the amygdala (Jones and Powell, 1970; Herzog and Van Hoesen, 1976), which in turn projects to the hypothalamus (Nauta, 1961), and lesions of the hypothalamus produce a severe disruption of feeding (see Rolls, 1981b).

This evidence thus indicates that there is a system which includes visual cortex in the temporal lobe, projections to the amygdala, and further connections to structures such as the lateral hypothalamus, which is involved in behavioral responses made on the basis of learned associations between visual stimuli and reinforcement. Given this evidence from lesion studies, it is next possible to consider whether there is any evidence from studies in which the activity of single neurons has been recorded in these regions which is consistent, and how each of these regions might be involved in the formation of learned associations between visual stimuli and reinforcement.

Inferior temporal visual cortex

Recordings were made from single neurons in the inferior temporal visual cortex while rhesus monkeys performed visual discriminations, and while they were shown visual stimuli associated with positive reinforcement such as food, with negative reinforcement such as aversive hypertonic saline, and neutral visual stimuli (Rolls, Judge and Sanghera, 1977). It was found that during visual discriminations inferior temporal neurons often had sustained visual responses with latencies of 100-140 ms to the discriminanda, but that these responses did not depend on whether the visual stimuli were associated with reward or punishment (in that the neuronal responses did not alter during reversals, when the previously rewarded stimulus was made to signify aversive saline, and the previously punished stimulus was made to signify reward) (Rolls, Judge and Sanghera, 1977). The conclusion, that the responses of inferior temporal neurons during visual discriminations do not code for whether a visual stimulus is associated with reward or punishment, is also consistent with the findings of Ridley, Hester and Ettlinger (1977), Jarvis and Mishkin (1977), Gross, Bender and Gerstein (1979), and Sato et al (1980). Further it was found that inferior temporal neurons did not respond only to food-related visual stimuli, or only to aversive stimuli, and were not dependent on hunger, but rather that in many cases their responses depended on physical aspects of the stimuli such as shape, size, orientation, color, or texture (Rolls, Judge and Sanghera, 1977).

These findings thus indicate that the responses of neurons in the inferior temporal visual cortex do not reflect the association of visual stimuli with reinforcement. Given these findings and the lesion evidence described above, it is thus likely that the inferior temporal cortex is an input stage for this process. The next structure on the basis of anatomical connections (see above) is the amygdala, and this is considered next. In the context of the functions of the inferior temporal cortex, which has outputs to the amygdala, orbitofrontal cortex, tail of the caudate nucleus, entorhinal cortex and thus the hippocampo-septal system, each one of which is specialized for a different type of learning (see Rolls, 1981a), it may be important that the responses of inferior temporal neurons are not specialized for each of these types of learning.

Amygdala

In recordings made from 1754 amygdaloid neurons, it was found that 113 (6.4%), of which many were in a dorsolateral region of the amygdala known to receive directly from the inferior temporal visual cortex (Herzog and Van Hoesen, 1976), had visual responses which in most cases were sustained while the monkey looked at effective visual stimuli (Sanghera, Rolls, and Roper-Hall, 1979). The latency of the responses was 100-140 ms or more. The majority (85%) of these visual neurons responded more strongly to some stimuli than to others, but physical factors which accounted for the responses such as orientation, color and texture could not usually be identified. It was found that 22 (19.5%) of these visual neurons responded primarily to foods and to objects associated with food, but for none of these neurons did the responses occur uniquely to food-related stimuli, in that they all responded to one or more aversive or neutral stimuli. Further, although some neurons responded in a visual discrimination to the visual stimulus which indicated food reward, but not to the visual stimulus associated with aversive saline, only minor modifications of the neuronal responses were obtained when the association of the stimuli with reinforcement was reversed in the reversal of the visual discrimination. A comparable population of neurons with responses apparently partly but not uniquely related to aversive visual stimuli was also found (Sanghera, Rolls and Roper-Hall, 1979).

These findings thus suggest that the amygdala could be involved at an early stage of the processing by which visual stimuli are associated with reinforcement, but that neuronal responses here do not code uniquely for whether a visual stimulus is associated with reinforcement. Neurons with responses more closely related to reinforcement are found in an area to which the amygdala projects, the lateral hypothalamus and substantia innominata, as described next.

Lateral Hypothalamus and Substantia Innominata

In recordings made in the lateral hypothalamus and substantia innominata of the monkey, a population of neurons was found which responded to the sight of foods, and to stimuli associated with foods such as a syringe from which the monkey was fed orally, but did not respond to neutral or to aversive stimuli, or in relation to arousal or movements (Rolls, Burton and Mora, 1976). These neurons comprised 9.3% of those in one sample of 764 neurons, and a further 2.5% had responses which occurred to the sight or to the taste of food (Rolls, Burton and Mora, 1976, 1980). The responses of these hypothalamic neurons became associated with food-related visual stimuli as a result of learning, in that during visual discrimination learning their responses became associated with the sight of the stimulus which indicated that food was available, in that their responses reversed during visual discrimination reversal so that they occurred to whichever visual stimulus was associated with food reinforcement, and in that their responses declined in extinction when a visual stimulus previously associated with food was presented without reinforcement (Mora, Rolls and Burton, 1976). The latency of the responses of these neurons was 140-200 ms, and thus in a visual discrimination task, the responses of these neurons preceded and predicted the behavioral responses of the monkey to the food-associated stimulus, which had latencies of 350-450 ms (Rolls, Sanghera and Roper-Hall, 1979). Because the only behavioral response relevant to the visual discrimination task was a lick response made by tongue protrusion, it was also possible to obtain EMG recordings which showed that these neuronal responses preceded the earliest EMG signs of the initiation of the behavioral response to the food-associated stimulus.

These findings thus showed that the responses of these hypothalamic neurons which occurred to visual stimuli associated with reinforcement could be involved in the behavioral responses made to these reinforced stimuli. Further evidence for this is that it has been possible to show in recent experiments by E.T.Rolls, E.Murzi and C.Griffiths that these neurons project this reinforcement-associated information directly to the cerebral cortex, in that at least some of these neurons can be antidromically activated by stimulation of such regions of the cortex as the dorso-lateral prefrontal cortex, the supplementary motor cortex, and the parietal cortex. At least some of these neurons are therefore those in the Basal Magnocellular Forebrain Nuclei of Meynert, which have direct projections to the cerebral cortex (Kievit and Kuypers, 1975; Divac, 1975). Further evidence that the responses of these neurons are related to reinforcement processes is that their responses only occur to food-associated stimuli if the monkey is hungry (Burton, Rolls and Mora, 1976), that these neurons are activated by positively reinforcing stimulation of some brain sites, and that brain-stimulation reward occurs in the region of these neurons (Rolls, Burton and Mora, 1980). It is also likely that some of the neurons in this region with visual responses related to reinforcement mediate autonomic and endocrine responses to patterned visual stimuli associated with reinforcement, and consistent with this there are projections from the hypothalamus to the brainstem autonomic centers (Saper et al, 1976, 1979). It may well be that part of the function of these hypothalamic neurons may be to bring complex stimuli analysed by the cerebral cortex and processed through limbic, e.g. amygdaloid, reinforcement-association learning mechanisms into contact with brainstem autonomic motor centers. Consistent with this evidence that these hypothalamic neurons are one stage in a system involved in behavioral and autonomic responses to food is that hypothalamic lesions disrupt feeding and autonomic responses (see Rolls, 1981a,b).

These findings thus indicate that there is a population of hypothalamic neurons with responses which are determined by whether visual stimuli are associated with reinforcement, and suggest that these neurons mediate some of the responses of primates to such conditioned complex visual stimuli. The effective stimuli and the response latencies of neurons recorded in the anatomical sequence inferior temporal cortex / amygdala / hypothalamus, suggest that visual processing along this pathway becomes related to reinforcement, with little relation to reinforcement in the inferior temporal visual cortex, with some effect of reinforcement becoming evident in the amygdala, and with full elaboration of neuronal responses in relation to reinforcement becoming evident only in the hypothalamus, from which outputs reflecting whether a stimulus is associated with reinforcement proceed. The gap in response characteristics and latencies between amygdaloid and hypothalamic neurons suggests that intermediate processing is taking place between these structures in relation to the formation of associations between visual stimuli and reinforcement, which it will be of interest to investigate further given the responses found in these two regions.

THE DISCONNECTION OF ASSOCIATIONS BETWEEN VISUAL STIMULI AND REINFORCEMENT

Lesions

The disconnection of associations between visual stimuli and reinforcement may involve separate mechanisms from those involved in their formation. The orbitofrontal cortex is implicated by lesion evidence in these disconnection processes. Lesions of the orbitofrontal cortex impair (a) reversals of visual discriminations, in that the monkeys make responses to the previously reinforced stimulus or object, (b) extinction, in that responses continue to be made to the previously reinforced stimulus, (c) Go/Nogo tasks, in that responses are made to the stimulus which is not associated with reward, and passive avoidance, in that responses are made when they are punished (Butter, 1969; Iversen and Mishkin, 1970; Jones and Mishkin, 1972; Tanaka,1973; see also Rosenkilde, 1979; Fuster, 1980). In contrast, the formation of associations between visual stimuli and reinforcement is much less affected by these lesions than by temporal lobe lesions, as tested during visual discrimination learning; and the reversal of a spatial response task, in which responses must be prevented to a position rather than to an object previously associated with reinforcement, is much less impaired by orbitofrontal than by hippocampal lesions (Jones and Mishkin, 1972).

Neuronal activity in the orbitofrontal cortex

To investigate the possible functions of the orbitofrontal cortex in the disconnection of stimulus-reinforcement associations, recordings were made of the activity of 494 orbitofrontal neurons during the performance of a Go/Nogo task, reversals of a visual discrimination task, extinction, and passive avoidance (Thorpe, Maddison and Rolls, 1979; Thorpe, Rolls and Maddison, in preparation; see Rolls, 1981a). First, neurons were found which responded in relation to the preparatory auditory or visual signal used before each trial (15.1%), or non-discriminatively during the period in which the discriminative visual stimuli were shown (37.8%). These neurons are not considered further here. Second, 8.6% of neurons had responses which occurred discriminatively during the period in which the visual stimuli were shown. The majority of these neurons responded to whichever visual stimulus was associated with reward, in that the stimulus to which they responded changed during reversal. However, 6 of these neurons required a combination of a particular visual stimulus in the discrimination <u>and</u> reward in order to respond. Further, none of this second group of neurons responded to all the reward-related stimuli including different foods which were shown, so that in general this group of neurons coded for a combination of one or some visual stimuli <u>and</u> reward. Thus information that particular visual stimuli which had previously been associated with reinforcement was represented in the responses of orbitofrontal neurons. Third, 9.7% of neurons had responses which occurred after the lick response was made in the task to obtain reward. Some of these responded independently of whether fruit juice reward was obtained, or aversive hypertonic saline was obtained on trials on which the monkey licked in error or was given saline in the first trials of a reversal. Through these neurons information that a lick had been made was represented in the orbitofrontal cortex. Other neurons in this third group responded only when fruit juice was obtained, and thus through these neurons information that reward had been given on that trial was represented in the orbitofrontal cortex. Other neurons in this group responded when saline was obtained when a response was made in error, or when saline was obtained on the first few trials of a reversal (but not in either case when saline was simply placed in the mouth), or when reward was not given in extinction, or when food was taken away instead of being given to the monkey, but did not respond in all these situations in which reinforcement was omitted or punishment was given. Thus through these neurons task-selective information that reward had been omitted or punishment given was represented in the responses of these neurons.

These three groups of neurons found in the orbitofrontal cortex could together provide for computation of whether the reinforcement previously associated with a particular stimulus was still being obtained, and generation of a signal if a match was not obtained. This signal could be partly reflected in the responses of the last subset of neurons with task-selective responses to non-reward or to unexpected punishment. This signal could be used to alter the monkey's behavior, leading for example to reversal to one particular stimulus but not to other stimuli, to extinction to one stimulus but not to others, etc. It could also lead to the altered responses of the orbitofrontal differential neurons found as a result of learning in reversal, so that their responses indicate appropriately whether a particular stimulus is now associated with reinforcement.

Thus the orbitofrontal cortex contains neurons which appear to be involved in altering behavioral responses when these are no longer associated with reward or become associated with punishment. In the context of the disconnection of stimulus-reinforcement associations, it appears that without these neurons the primate is unable to correct his behavior when disconnection becomes appropriate, and the orbitofrontal neurons could be involved in the actual breaking of the association, or in the alteration of behavior when other neurons signal that the connection is no longer appropriate. The observation that humans with damage to the frontal lobe may know that a particular strategy is inappropriate, and be able to verbalize the correct solution, and yet be unable to correct their inappropriate responses (Teuber, 1964), suggests that the ability to unlearn the association is intact, but that with damage to the frontal lobe this particular type of unlearning cannot influence behavioral response mechanisms. On the other hand, as shown here, the orbitofrontal cortex contains neurons with responses which could provide the information necessary for, and the basis for, the unlearning. In relation to how associations between stimuli and reinforcement are broken and the way in which this influences behavioral responses, it will clearly of importance to investigate further with the lesion and recording techniques the orbitofrontal neurons described here, which are implicated in at least one of these processes by the evidence presented.

REFERENCES

Akert,K., Gruesen,R.A., Woolsey,C.N., and Meyer,D.R., 1961, Kluver-Bucy syndrome in monkeys with neocortical ablations of temporal lobe, Brain, 84:480-98.

Burton,M.J., Rolls,E.T. and Mora,F., 1976, Effects of hunger on the responses of neurons in the lateral hypothalamus to the sight and taste of food. Exptl. Neurol., 51:668-77.

Butter,C.M., 1969, Perseveration in extinction and in discrimination reversal tasks following selective prefrontal ablations in Macaca mulatta, Physiol. Behav., 4:163-71.

Divac,I., 1975, Magnocellular nuclei of the basal forebrain project to neocortex, brain stem, and olfactory bulb. Review of some functional correlates. Brain Res., 93:385-98.

Fuster,J.M., 1980, "The Prefrontal Cortex", Raven Press, New York.

Gross,C.G., Bender,D.B. and Gerstein,G.L., 1979, Activity of inferior temporal neurons in behaving monkeys, Neuropsychologia, 17:215-29.

Herzog,A.G. and Van Hoesen,G.W., 1976, Temporal neocortical afferent connections to the amygdala in the rhesus monkey, Brain Res., 115:57-69.

Iversen,S.D. and Mishkin,M., 1970, Perseverative interference in monkey following selective lesions of the inferior prefrontal convexity. Exp. Brain Res., 11:376-86.

Jarvis,C.D. and Mishkin,M., 1977, Responses of cells in the inferior temporal cortex of monkeys during visual discrimination reversals. Soc. Neurosci. Abstr., 3:1794.

Jones,B. and Mishkin,M., 1972, Limbic lesions and the problem of stimulus-reinforcement associations. Exptl. Neurol., 36:362-77.

Kievit,J. and Kuypers,H.G.J.M., 1975, Subcortical afferents to the frontal lobe in the rhesus monkey studied by means of retrograde horseradish peroxidase transport, Brain Res., 85:261-6.

Kluver,H. and Bucy,P.C., 1939, Preliminary analysis of functions of the temporal lobes in monkeys. Arch. Neurol. Psychiatr., 42:979-1000.

Mora,F., Rolls,E.T. and Burton,M.J., 1976, Modulation during learning of the responses of neurons in the hypothalamus to the sight of food, Exptl. Neurol., 53:508-19.

Nauta,W.J.H., 1961, Fiber degeneration following lesions of the amygdaloid complex in the monkey. J.Anat., 95:515-31.

Oakley,D.A., 1981, Brain mechanisms of mammalian memory, Brit. Med. Bull., 37:175-180.

Ridley,R.M., Hester,N.S. and Ettlinger,G., 1977, Stimulus- and response-dependent units from the occipital and temporal lobes of the unanaesthetized monkey performing learnt visual tasks. Exp. Brain Res., 27:539-52.

Rolls,E.T., 1981a, Processing beyond the inferior temporal visual cortex related to feeding, memory, and striatal function. Ch. 16, pp. 241-69 in "Brain Mechanisms of Sensation", Y.Katsuki, R.Norgren and M.Sato, eds., Wiley, New York.

Rolls,E.T., 1981b, Central nervous mechanisms related to feeding and appetite, Brit. Med. Bull., 37:131-4.

Rolls,E.T., Burton,M.J. and Mora,F., 1976, Hypothalamic neuronal responses associated with the sight of food, Brain Res., 111:53-66.

Rolls,E.T., Judge,S.J. and Sanghera,M.K., 1977, Activity of neurons in the inferotemporal cortex of the alert monkey. Brain Res., 130:229-38.

Rolls,E.T., Sanghera,M.K. and Roper-Hall,A., 1979, The latency of activation of neurons in the lateral hypothalamus and substantia innominata during feeding in the monkey. Brain Res., 164:121-35.

Rolls,E.T., Burton,M.J. and Mora,F., 1980, Neurophysiological analysis of brain-stimulation reward in the monkey, Brain Res., 194:339-57.

Rosenkilde,C.E., 1979, Functional heterogeneity of the prefrontal cortex in the monkey: a review. Behav. Neural Biol., 25:301-45.

Sanghera,M.K., Rolls,E.T. and Roper-Hall,A., 1979, Visual responses of neurons in the dorsolateral amygdala of the alert monkey. Exptl. Neurol., 63:610-26.

Saper,C.B., Loewy,A.D., Swanson,L.W. and Cowan,W.M., 1976, Direct hypothalamo-autonomic connections. Brain Res., 117:305-12.

Saper,C.B., Swanson,L.W. and Cowan,W.M., 1979, An autoradiographic study of the efferent connections of the lateral hypothalamic area in the rat. J. Comp. Neurol., 183:689-706.

Sato,T., Kawamura,T., and E.Iwai, 1980, Responsiveness of inferotemporal single units to visual pattern stimuli in monkeys performing discrimination. Exp. Brain Res., 38:313-9.

Tanaka,D., 1973, Effects of selective prefrontal decortication on escape behavior in the monkey. Brain Res., 53:161-73.

Teuber,H.-L., 1964, The riddle of frontal lobe function in man. Pp. 410-77 in "The Frontal Granular Cortex and Behavior", eds. J.M.Warren and K.Akert, McGraw-Hill, New York.

Thorpe,S.J., Maddison,S. and Rolls,E.T., 1979, Single unit activity in the orbitofrontal cortex of the behaving monkey. Neurosci. Lett., S3:S77.

Weiskrantz,L., 1956, Behavioral changes associated with ablation of the amygdaloid complex in monkeys, J. Comp. Physiol. Psychol., 49:381-91.

FUNCTIONAL SIGNIFICANCE OF VISUALLY TRIGGERED DISCHARGES IN EYE MOVEMENT RELATED NEURONS

John Schlag and Madeleine Schlag-Rey

Department of Anatomy and Brain Research Institute
UCLA Medical School, Los Angeles, CA

SUMMARY

Gaze orientation is a quick, natural, almost automatic reaction. Yet, in the couple of hundred milliseconds that separate the appearance of a photic target and the orientation of the gaze to it, the CNS has to make a number of delicate computations and decisions. The where, how, and when of the movement have to be determined. Analysis of single-unit events occurring during this period suggests that the spatial coordinates of the goal are calculated immediately upon stimulus presentation. The information predictive of the trajectory of the orienting movement to be performed appears already available in what, on the basis of fixed latency, would be considered stimulus-locked visual response. The actual launching of the saccade is a separate, subsequent decision.

INTRODUCTION

Most of the data that we shall use in this presentation derive from microelectrode recordings from a central thalamic region in alert cats (Schlag et al., 1974; Schlag-Rey and Schlag, 1977) and monkeys (Schlag-Rey and Schlag, in press). Anatomically, this region corresponds approximately to the domain of the internal medullary lamina (IML). The lamina separates the external sector of n. medialis dorsalis which, classically, is known as the source of thalamic afferents to the frontal eye field (FEF) of the cortex, and the most medial sector of n. ventralis lateralis which projects to the face and neck area of the motor cortex. There is now ample evidence to regard the cell populations in this region as the most likely center concerned with gaze control at the thalamic level, in much the same way as the frontal eye field is the most likely area concerned with eye movements at the cortical level. FEF, IML, and superior colliculus are reciprocally linked. Interestingly, in the monkey, a major contingent of FEF projections to the tectum has been shown to pass through the IML to which they distribute terminal collaterals (Leichnetz et al., 1981). This is a quite unusual arrangement for corticofugal efferents to transit through the thalamus in their way to a further station. It means that, at least, some IML neurons receive the same cortical input as collicular neurons. But this is not the sole supply of afferents to the IML. It also receives afferents from several pre-oculomotor centers of the brain stem (e.g. Kotchabhakdi et al., 1980) and it entertains reciprocal connections with other cortical areas such as the parietal lobe (e.g. Kasdon and Jacobson, 1978). It may be premature at this stage to propose any scheme specifying the location of IML units in a functional diagram of gaze control involving the forebrain. It is clear, however, that in close proximity to each other in the IML, are cell types also found in other structures with which the IML has relations. For instance, in the monkey, there are in and around the IML: presaccadic units as in the brain stem (Luschei and Fuchs, 1972), eye-position units as in the frontal eye field (Bizzi, 1968) and visually responsive units similar to those of the frontal eye field (Mohler et al., 1973) and inferior parietal lobule (Hyvarinen and Poranen, 1974; Lynch et al., 1977). Whether or not the patterns of activity characterizing these cell types arise in the IML or are transmitted from elsewhere, one can safely assert, at least, that the IML is a node of the forebrain-midbrain circuit involved in gaze mechanisms. This view is further substantiated by lesions of the IML which produce transient signs of contralateral visual neglect in cats (Orem et al., 1973) and monkeys (Watson et al., 1978), and by electrical stimulation which evokes contraversive saccades in cats (Schlag and Schlag-Rey, 1971). Working with cats whose head was free to move in a horizontal plane, we now know that such saccades are accompanied by contraversive head turning (Maldonado et al., 1981). Thus, it is suggested that it is the gaze - rather than simply the eyes - which is controlled from this region. The idea that a structure at the level of the thalamus would be involved in the initiation of gaze movements is consistent with current views on movement initiation since, for other kinds of movement too, it has been shown that thalamic neurons are among the earliest in the forebrain to show movement-related discharges (e.g. Horne and Porter, 1980).

IML UNITS VISUALLY RESPONSIVE AND ACTIVE WITH SACCADES

What seems to be a particular opportunity to study the neuronal events occurring during visuo-oculomotor orientation is that many IML units discharge both at the time of presentation of a visual target and starting just before an orienting saccade. The two events occur successively in the same cells: one time-locked to the stimulus, the other to the movement. They can be distinguished when the delay of orienting is long enough.

In our experiments, the animals had their head fixed and they faced a tangent screen in an ambient, homogeneous, red lighting. Two miniature green light-emitting diodes (LEDs) were placed behind the translucent screen, one at 15° left, the other at 15° right from the center. The animals were trained to look alternately at these sites. When the gaze, monitored with electrooculographic (EOG) electrodes, was correctly adjusted at the site of the anticipated target, the LED at that site was turned on and a few drops of milk delivered as reinforcement. This procedure kept the cats attentive to their environment and it encouraged their visual exploration (for further procedural details, see Schlag-Rey and Schlag, 1977).

Sometimes, one LED was turned on unexpectedly, eliciting a quick orienting response in a thirsty animal. The reaction time was typically as shown in Fig. 1.

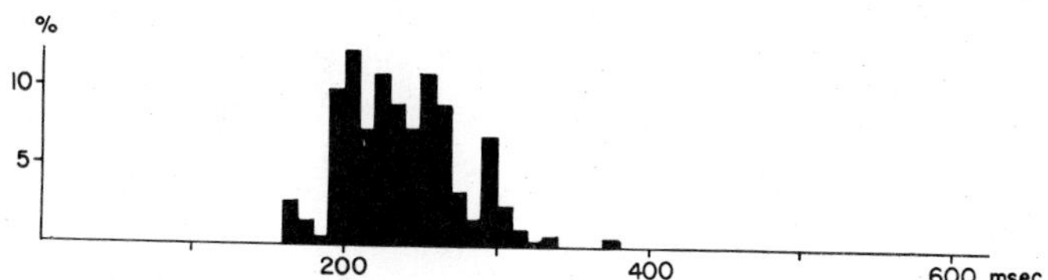

Fig. 1. Reaction time of targeting to a rewarded stimulus.

During the periods of unit recording in the same sessions, a 1.5° annulus of dim blue light was back-projected on the screen from a cathode-ray scope to test the cell visual responsiveness. This test stimulus was quite different from the LED, it could appear anywhere on the screen, and it was so dim that only its presence, but not its features, could be perceived by peripheral vision. Orientation to this stimulus was never rewarded by milk. Nevertheless, probably out of curiosity, cats tried to acquire it most of the time. Reaction times of orientation toward an unreinforced stimulus were somewhat more scattered. The distribution shown in Fig. 2 concerns reaction times obtained under this conditon in the same session as Fig. 1.

If the annulus was turned off as soon as the animals oriented to it, they were hardly given a chance to observe it at their leisure. Soon they developed a strategy of feigning to ignore the stimulus as they so frequently do when playing with a prey, presumably in order to catch it later by surprise. Then, orientation times could become even longer: delays as long as 10 sec were not unusual.

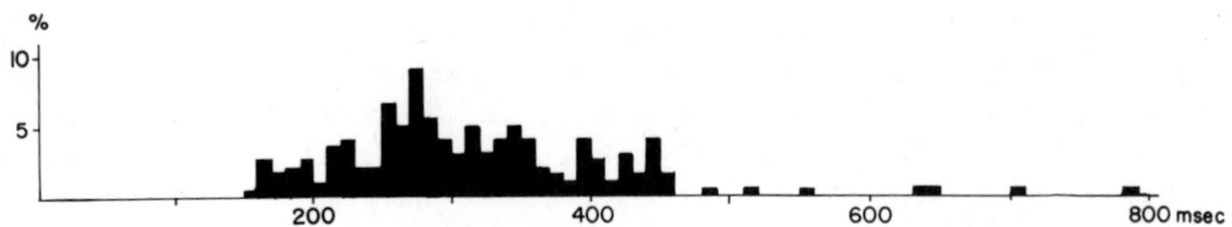

Fig. 2. Reaction time of targeting to an unrewarded stimulus in the same animal and the same session.

Let us note that long orientation times did not correspond to artificial conditions. In fact, the situation was probably more natural than when the reinforcement pressed the subject to react quickly. The cats had free control of their behavior. In the neurophysiological analysis of the sequence of neuronal events occurring in a sensory-motor paradigm like this one, it is important to consider - not only minimal - but also normal, sometimes very long time intervals. In cats, the situation described here made it possible to show a clear distinction between 3 IML unit types according to the timing of the activity patterns. The first type (about 25%) were cells responding at target presentation (T) not with the eye movement (EM in Fig. 3).

The second type (about 10%) were cells active with targeting saccades (EM) but not at target onset (Fig. 4). Clearly their firing started before saccades (i.e. presaccadic burst).

The third type which was the most common (about 65%) responded, first, to target onset and then again, later, when an orienting saccade became imminent (Fig. 5). In order to demonstrate the time

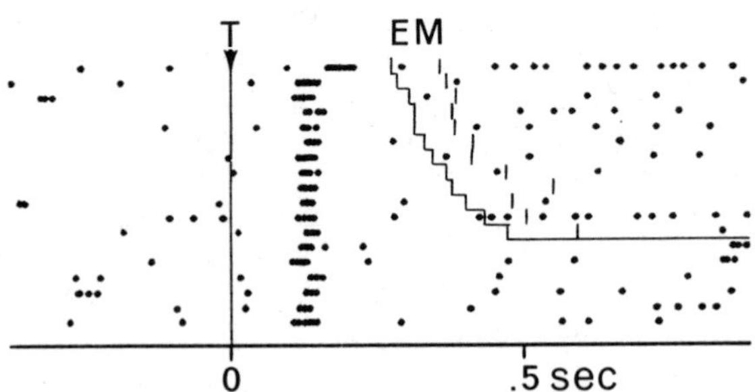

Fig. 3. Visual responses of an IML unit. Raster synchronized on target onset. Onset and offset of subsequent eye movements indicated by bars. Ranking by increased reaction times.

relations with each of these events, the same traces in Fig. 5 have been displayed twice: once, in a raster synchronized on target onset (T) and, second, in a raster synchronized on eye movement onset (EM).

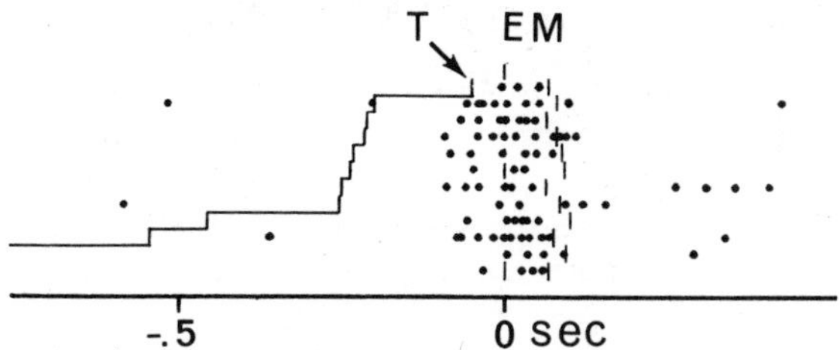

Fig. 4. Eye-movement IML unit. Raster synchronized on targeting eye movements.

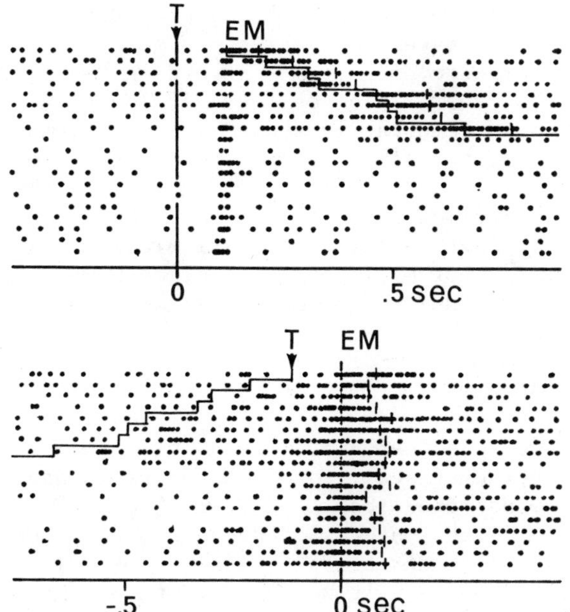

Fig. 5. Visual-and-presaccadic IML unit. Rasters synchronized as in Fig. 3 and Fig. 4.

Fig. 6 presents 8 sec of an original record showing another visual-and-presaccadic IML unit with the vertical (V) and horizontal (H) EOG and stimulus coordinates displayed under the unit trace. This particular cell had a sustained firing in the presence of a stimulus. It was most excitable from the center of the retina which explains the high frequency of firing during fixation, that is after the targeting movement. Note, however, that the frequency increase precedes the movement.

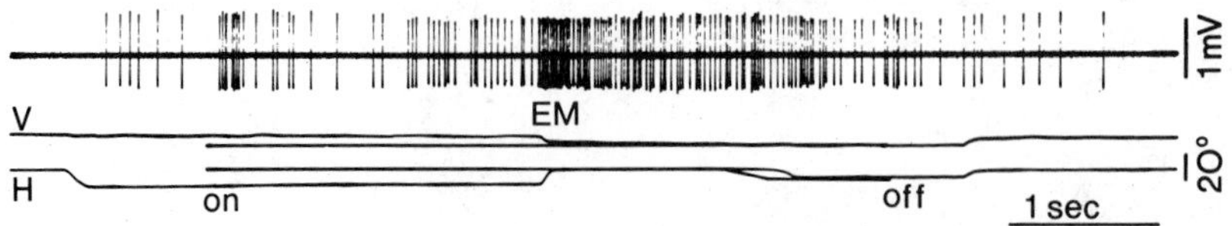

Fig. 6. Another visual-and-presaccadic unit shown with vertical and horizontal coordinates of EOG and target.

In the IML of cats and monkeys - and elsewhere - there are indeed cells which fire tonically or are continuously silenced by the presence of a photic stimulus, however faint, in their receptive field. Such changes of activity can perdure very long (e.g. 20 sec). Therefore, it is not gratuitous to assume that a stimulus trace may be stored. It would be available to specify target location when the "go" decision to make the movement is generated later. Although there may be divergence of opinions regarding the mode of spatial coding in the CNS, there is no serious difficulty in conceiving that this information is temporarily stored in cell firing. What seems interesting is that, at stimulus onset - and time-locked to it - one finds patterns of unit activity indicative of the targeting movement to be performed even if this movement is not immediately released. In the next Section, we shall present some data suggesting that the programming of movement takes place immediately upon stimulus presentation whether the movement is made or not.

ON THE SIGNIFICANCE OF THE "VISUAL" ON-RESPONSE

The correspondence between stimulus time-locked and eye-movement time-locked patterns of activity in IML units is striking. As we have already demonstrated (Schlag-Rey and Schlag, 1977), IML units have a preferred direction of saccades and their receptive field extends in a preferred direction. We always found these directions to be the same. Thus, a unit which would fire maximally for rightward saccades would have its receptive field on the right side. Reciprocally, a unit which would pause for rightward saccades would be inhibited by presenting a stimulus on the right side. Units which had a clear zone of higher responsiveness within their receptive field displayed the most profuse bursts with saccades directed to that zone (Schlag and Schlag-Rey, 1977). In other words, the patterns of activity were similar when the target was offered and when the movement to acquire it was produced.

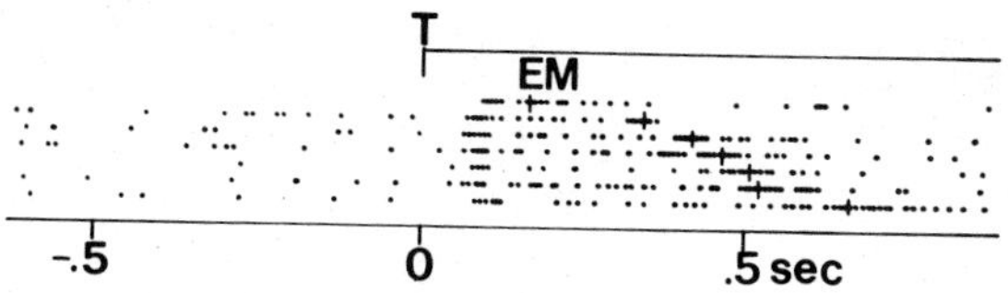

Fig. 7. Visual-and-presaccadic IML unit shown during targeting. Figs. 8 to 11 will exhibit other properties of the same cell.

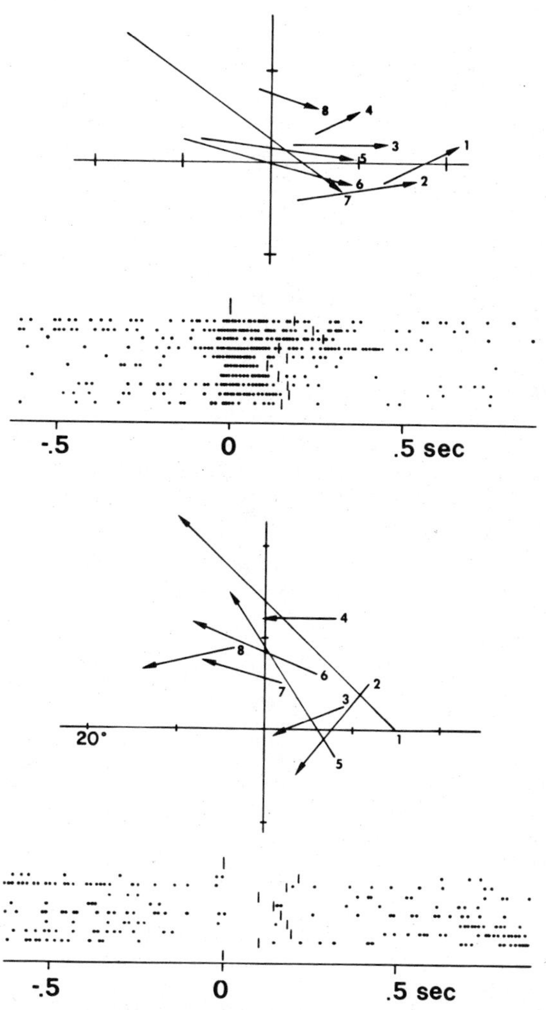

Fig. 8. Activity during spontaneous saccades in darkness. Saccade vectors shown above rasters and numbered in the order of traces in rasters.

The unit shown in Fig. 7 responded at target onset (T) when the annulus was presented to the right of the point of fixation. It also discharged with eye movements (EM) directed to the stimulus, i.e. with rightward targeting saccades. To study the spatial relations in the properties of the cell, the background light and stimuli were turned off. Fig. 8 presents samples of burst discharges occurring with spontaneous eye movements in complete darkness. Saccade vectors are numbered in the order of lines in the raster. Clearly, this cell was presaccadic and its firing was restricted to saccades directed rightwards, whether they were visually evoked or self-generated.

Fig. 9 shows the on-responses of the same cell to annuli successively placed at different points on the screen. Their retinocentric location is specified by numbers corresponding to the order of lines in the raster. To map the receptive field, trials such as those shown here were selected because no targeting occurred and thus no contamination of on-responses by saccade-related activity could be suspected. The receptive field included points 1 to 10. It encompassed the center of the retina but extended asymmetrically to the right side. In can be seen in the raster that the latency of response was longer for stimulus locations at the border of the field (i.e. trials 1, 2, 9 and 10). This fact was verified in repeated testing.

The stimulus was then left on continuously and moved linearly at constant speed (48°/sec) across the screen. Again, for analysis of the response induced by stimulus movement, trials were selected in which no eye movements occurred. The cell was found to be preferentially responsive to rightward stimulus movements, as seen by comparing the 2 rasters of Fig. 10.

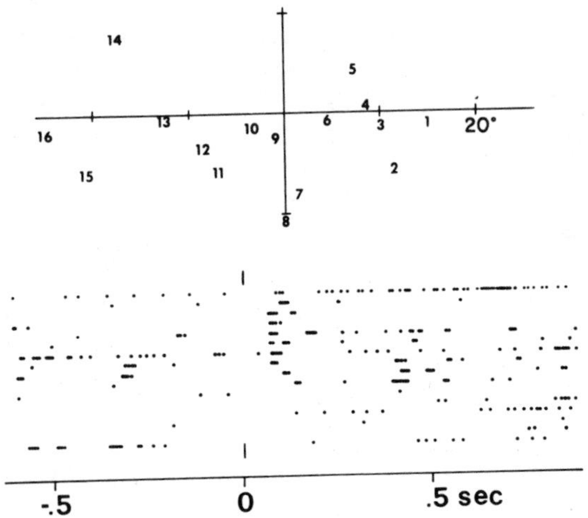

Fig. 9. Same as Fig. 7 but no eye movements in these trials. Positions of stimulus with respect to point of eye fixation, numbered in the order of traces in raster.

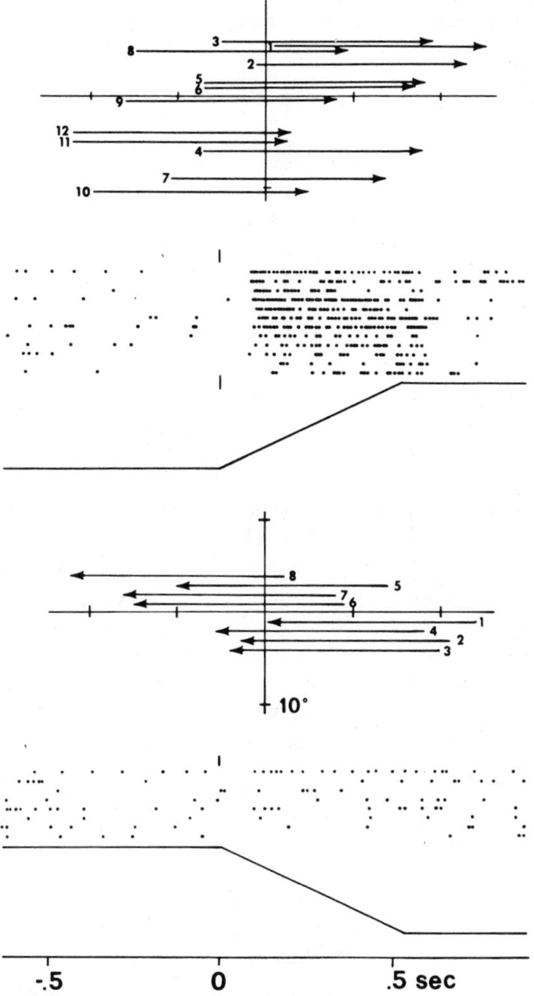

Fig. 10. Activity produced by stimuli moving as indicated on retinocentric maps above rasters. Time course of stimulus movement below rasters. No eye movements in these trials.

Directional specificity is not the only significant feature demonstrated in Fig. 10. A careful inspection will reveal that cell activation started well before the stimulus entered the receptive field during rightward stimulus movement and, reciprocally, that the cell did not fire even though the stimulus was still in the receptive field, about to leave it in a leftward direction. This can be seen by comparing the latencies of activity even in the last lines of the upper raster, Fig. 10 with those of Fig. 9. At the beginning of these experiments, it was a puzzling finding that IML units particularly sensitive to stimulus displacement seemed to have non-coextensive receptive fields for stationary and moving stimuli. The results from many units were consistent, particularly with respect to the relative spatial relation of these receptive fields.

Such a systematic discrepancy in field location may be difficult to account for in terms of stimulus characteristics because it depended on several parameters: position, direction, and velocity in a way which escapes any simple formulation. But we noticed that, whenever the animals tried to acquire the flying target crossing its field of vision, it always did it by eye movements directed to catch up with it as it moved away, rather than to encounter it as it approached. This strategy was clearly adapted to target velocity: when the velocity was high enough as in this case, the animal had no time to make a saccade toward the target starting position. Eventual eye movements were all aimed in the direction in which the target travelled. A sample of this kind of movements is shown in Fig. 11. These movements had variable delays. Here again, as in Fig. 10, one can recognize in the upper raster the activity triggered by the moving target but, in contrast with Fig. 10, there were secondary increases of firing accompanying the eye movements.

It can be said that the type of unit activity elicited by a moving stimulus is consistent with the preferred direction of its saccadic activity. If this observation is valid, it means that the photic events are immediately analyzed in terms of the motor demands of the situation.

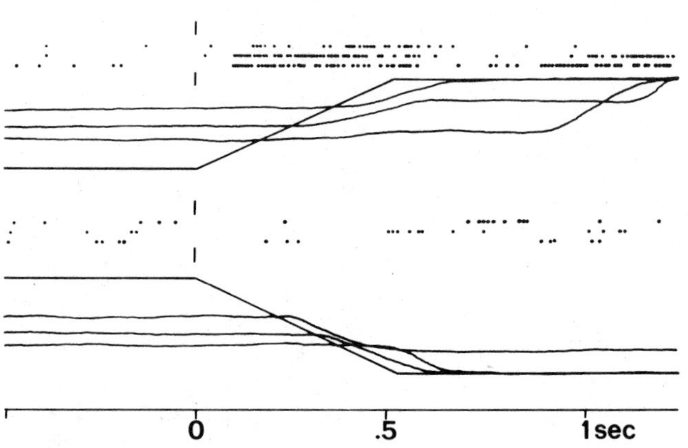

Fig. 11. Same as Fig. 10 to show the direction of eye movements, when they occurred. Three trials in each direction with the horizontal EOG and stimulus coordinates.

Time-wise, the unit activity seen in Fig. 10 has all the characteristics of a visual response because it is linked to stimulus presentation. Any other interpretation would be anyway difficult since there were no movements in these trials. But the response of the cell was contingent upon the orient-to-the right versus orient-to-the left motor alternative. We are familiar with the usual categories that visual physiologists use to describe stimulus properties such as color, size, contrast, line orientation, spatial frequencies, etc... Such categories are meaningful to explain perception. Alternatively, categories that make more sense for the motor apparatus would seem more pertinent to explain motor guidance (see Thompson, 1980). Such a category would be, for instance: "A moving object such that, if I want to see it, I would have to direct my gaze 20° up-right". This may be the message that the IML units studies were conveying. Is such a message sensory or motor? On one hand, it is stimulus time-locked; on the other hand, its content relates to action. The cell is better specified by the "adequate response" than by the "adequate stimulus".

Another characteristic that all such cells have is insensitivity to eye-movement induced stimulation. For instance, if responding to a rightward stimulus displacement and active with a rightward saccade, what would a unit do when a leftward saccade sweeps across a stationary stimulus? The apparent (or virtual) stimulus displacement is rightward, that is: in the on-direction. We have tested this situation, using stimulus velocities in the range of saccadic velocities, and we found that eye-movement generated visual stimulation never gave responses. This makes sense because one would not expect a cell active with saccades in one direction to react to saccades in the opposite direction.

Finally, let us again stress that the neuronal events discussed here occurred irrespective of whether a movement was actually performed or not. If the movement occurred after the unit activity predictive of the characteristics of that movement had been emitted, the same cells were again firing with the movement. This suggests that the decision to move is made secondarily and, when it is made, the program is probably already existing.

ACKNOWLEDGEMENTS

This work was supported by U.S.P.H.S. Grants NS 04955 and EY 02305. We are grateful to Mr. V. Pagano, MS. D. Blanco and B. Truex for their assistance, and to Drs. H. Maldonado and B. Merker for useful comments on the manuscript.

REFERENCES

Bizzi, E., 1968, Discharge of frontal eye field neurons during saccadic and following eye movements in unanesthetized monkeys, Exp. Brain Res., 6:69.

Horne, M. K., and Porter, R., 1980, The discharges during movement of cells in the ventrolateral thalamus of the conscious monkey, J. Physiol. (London), 304:349.

Hyvarinen, J., and Poranen, A., 1974, Function of the parietal association area 7 as revealed from cellular discharges in alert monkeys, Brain, 97:673.

Kasdon, D. L., and Jacobson, S., 1978, The thalamic afferents to the inferior parietal lobule of the rhesus monkey, J. comp. Neurol., 177:685.

Kotchabhakdi, N., Rinvik, E., Yingchareon, K., and Walberg, F., 1980, Afferent projections to the thalamus from the perihypoglossal nuclei, Brain Res., 187:457.

Leichnetz, G. R., Spencer, R. F., Hardy, S. G. P., and Astruc, J., 1981, The prefrontal corticotectal projection in the monkey: an anterograde and retrograde horseradish peroxidase study, Neurosci., 6:1023.

Luschei, E. S., and Fuchs, A.F., 1972, Activity of brainstem neurons during eye movements of alert monkeys, J. Neurophysiol., 35:445.

Lynch, J. C., Mountcastle, V. B., Talbot, W. H., and Yin, T. C., 1977, Parietal lobe mechanisms for direct attention, J. Neurophysiol., 40:362

Maldonado, H., and Schlag, J., 1981, Head and eye movements evoked by electrical stimulation of thalamic gaze center, Neurosci. Abstr., (in press).

Mohler, C. W., Goldberg, M. E., and Wurtz, R. H., 1973, Visual receptive fields of frontal eye field neurons, Brain Res., 61:385.

Orem, J., Schlag-Rey, M., and Schlag, J., 1973, Unilateral visual neglect and thalamic intralaminar lesions in the cat, Exp. Neurol., 40:784.

Schlag, J., Lehtinen, I., and Schlag-Rey, M., 1974, Neuronal activity before and during eye movements in the thalamic internal medullary lamina of the cat, J. Neurophysiol., 37:982.

Schlag, J., and Schlag-Rey, M., 1971, Induction of oculomotor responses from thalamic internal medullary lamina in the cat, Exp. Neurol., 33:498.

Schlag, J., and Schlag-Rey, M., 1977, Visuomotor properties of cells in the cat thalamic internal medullary lamina, in: "Control of gaze by brain stem neurons," R. Baker and A. Berthoz, eds., Elsevier, Amsterdam, pp. 453-462.

Schlag-Rey, M., and Schlag, J., 1977, Visual and presaccadic neuronal activity in the thalamic internal medullary lamina of cat: A study of targeting, J. Neurophysiol., 40:156.

Schlag-Rey, M., and Schlag, J., Eye-movement related neuronal activity in the central thalamus of monkeys, in: "Progress in oculomotor research," A. Fuchs and W. Becker, eds., Elsevier, Amsterdam, (in press).

Thompson, J. A., 1980, How do we use visual information to control locomotion?, TINS, 3:247.

Watson, R. T., Mohler, B. D., and Heilman, K. M., 1978, Nonsensory neglect, Ann. Neurol., 3:505.

NEURONAL ACTIVITY IN CENTRAL THALAMUS OF PRIMATES AND THE VOLUNTARY CONTROL OF THE GAZE

Madeleine Schlag-Rey and John Schlag

Department of Anatomy and Brain Research Institute

UCLA School of Medicine, Los Angeles, CA 90024

SUMMARY

Most electrophysiological studies on central mechanisms of gaze control (in looking) have been concerned with experimental situations where the movement of the eyes is entirely controlled, temporally and spatially, by a visual stimulus. We have recorded single units in a thalamic region of alert monkeys, where cells active with self-initiated eye movements are found. Neuronal activation could anticipate contraversive saccades by 200-300 ms. In this region, we have studied cells while the animal made intermittent attempts to track a target or even shifted its gaze voluntarily between two targets. The pattern of activity of some of these cells appeared indicative of the decision by the animal to make a target the goal of its oculomotor apparatus.

INTRODUCTION

Little is known about central mechanisms that enable us to order the priorities of competing visual stimuli and to explore our visual world with eye movements (EM) initiated on our own. Most electrophysiological studies of the gaze have been concerned with orienting or tracking movements of the eyes rather than with their voluntary control; this may be due to the fact that no known cortical area plays, for the gaze, a role analogous to that of motor area 4, for limb movements. While both the inferior parietal lobule and the frontal eye fields, area 8, have been implicated in the control of visually evoked EMs, neither one was found activated before spontaneous saccades (Bizzi and Schiller, 1970; Mountcastle et al., 1975; Goldberg and Bushnell, 1981).

"Spontaneous saccades" is a confusing term, it evokes wanderings of the gaze that have little or no behavioral significance as well as eye movements purposefully aimed at remembered or anticipated target locations. The latter, in fact, represent one of the highest forms of voluntary control of movement.

Our research, in the past decade, has been geared toward discovering neurons that might be responsible for the initiation of such movements.

A prerequisite to this work was the finding of forebrain neurons involved in the decision to make a saccade not contingent on present visual cues. As improbable as it may be, the central thalamus is still - as far as we know - the only part of the forebrain where neurons were found discharging before spontaneous EMs in complete darkness.

Our initial discovery of EM-related neurons in the region of the thalamic internal medullary lamina (IML) was made in cats (Schlag et al., 1973). We have recently duplicated this finding in monkeys (Schlag-Rey and Schlag, 1981); however, it is already clear that the primate oculomotor thalamus extends beyond the limits of the IML proper.

This report focuses on some properties of thalamic EM-related neurons that appear relevant to voluntary control.

The methods of eye movement and unit recording have been described previously (Schlag-Rey and Schlag, 1977; Schlag et al., 1980). The reconstruction of microelectrode tracks was greatly facilitated by using a new silver staining technique (Merker, 1979).

Prior to recording sessions the monkeys were trained to fixate a dim 1.5° annulus, presented at various locations on a tangent screen and to keep the gaze fixated on this target, stationary or moving, for a duration randomly varied (1-10 s). The amount of reward (juice) was proportional to the duration of the fixation required on a given trial. Note that in this situation the monkeys did not know where nor when the fixation target would appear.

In a variant of this simple task the monkey turned on the fixation target (annulus) by depressing a panel and holding it down until the annulus was replaced by a square. The appearance of the square was always followed by a juice reward. Note that in this situation the monkeys knew when but not where the fixation target would appear.

The present results are based on a sample of 156 units found related to EMs, to the onset of the fixation target, or to both. All of these units had directional preferences, some very broad, some more finely tuned.

IML LONG LEAD BURST NEURONS

It is customary to classify units discharging before saccades in short and long lead burst neurons. An example of long presaccadic activation, before spontaneous contraversive saccades, is provided in Fig. 1. The existence of such long presaccadic activations suggest that self-initiated EMs may be prepared quite a long time before they are actually executed. The discharge pattern of long lead burst units was found depending on saccade parameters, not on the task, not on ambient illumination (light vs. dark), not on trigger mode (spontaneous vs. evoked) except for the fact that in visually evoked saccades the reaction time of the monkey drastically shortened otherwise long presaccadic activations.

LATENCY OF DISCHARGE OF PRESACCADIC UNITS IN TARGETING EMS

Whether expecting or not expecting the onset of the stimulus, well trained monkeys usually initiated a targeting saccade with a latency of 130-150 ms.

Since thalamic long lead burst units could start discharging as early as 300 ms before a spontaneous saccade, it is relevant to ask how fast the activity of such a unit can be triggered by a visual stimulus attracting the eyes in the unit's preferred direction. This information provides an estimate of the shortest time required for the visual signal to reach a neuron whose firing is consistently related to the motor output but still must be remote from the final common pathway. Fig. 2 shows responses visually evoked in the unit of Fig. 1. The raster has been ordered according to the latencies of targeting saccades (indicated by the tick marks) in the preferred direction. The shortest unit latencies were found to be less than 100 ms.

This unit was tested in the simple fixation task, in which the monkey did not know when the fixation stimulus would appear, and therefore, was sometimes making a spontaneous saccade away from the stimulus at the time of its onset. When this happened, as was the case in the first trial of Fig. 2, the monkey quickly reversed the direction of the ongoing spontaneous EM and made an appropriate targeting saccade. As can be seen in this particular instance, the presaccadic burst started less than 80 ms after stimulus onset.

SEPARATE SYSTEMS FOR VISUALLY EVOKED AND SPONTANEOUS SACCADES?

In cats we found that most IML EM-related neurons discharged before saccades in specific directions, regardless of whether the saccade was visually triggered, visually guided, anticipatory or spontaneous (Schlag and Schlag-Rey, 1981). In monkeys, this type of unit is well represented by very long lead burst neurons just described.

However, we also found units that had opposite firing patterns depending on whether saccades were visually evoked or self-initiated.

Fig. 3 provides a typical example of a unit bursting in response to contralateral visual stimuli. In order to see whether the

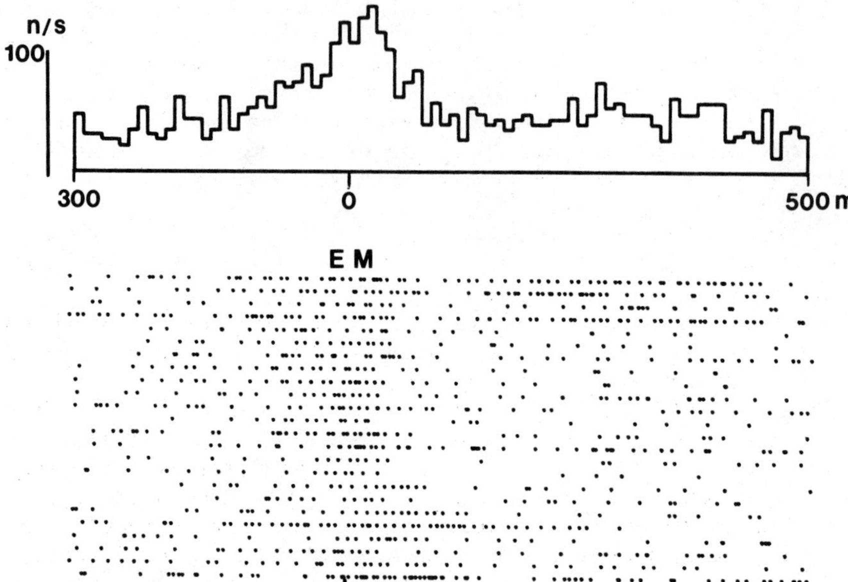

Fig. 1. Activity of a long lead burst neuron during contraversive spontaneous EMs. Raster synchronized on the start of EMs (time = 0 ms).

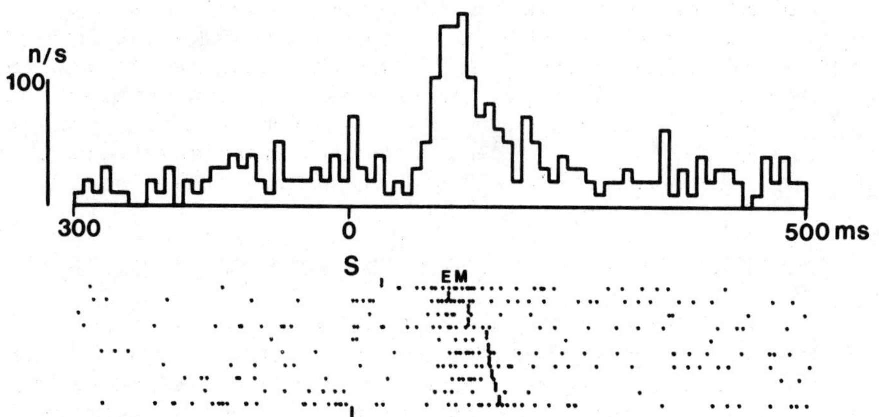

Fig. 2. Visually evoked activity of same cell as in Fig. 1 prior to a targeting EM in the preferred direction. Raster synchronized on stimulus onset. Tick marks indicate onset of EM.

occurrence of the burst was temporally linked to the fixation stimulus onset or to the targeting EM, we ranked the raster according to the latencies of targeting EMs in individual trials. This procedure revealed in this case as in many others, that the bursts were more closely related to the timing of the targeting saccade than to the onset of the stimulus. This unit, apparently saccade-related, was never seen discharging before any spontaneous saccade. Such "visually triggered EM units" exist in the superior colliculus (Mohler and Wurzt, 1976), the parietal cortex (Mountcastle et al., 1975) and the frontal eye fields (Goldberg and Bushnell, 1981).

One can then wonder whether the central thalamus also contains neurons activated before spontaneous saccades but not before visually evoked saccades with similar vectors. Such units should exist but they have never been reported. The patterns of firing of such a unit, for saccades in the preferred direction, are illustrated in Fig. 4.

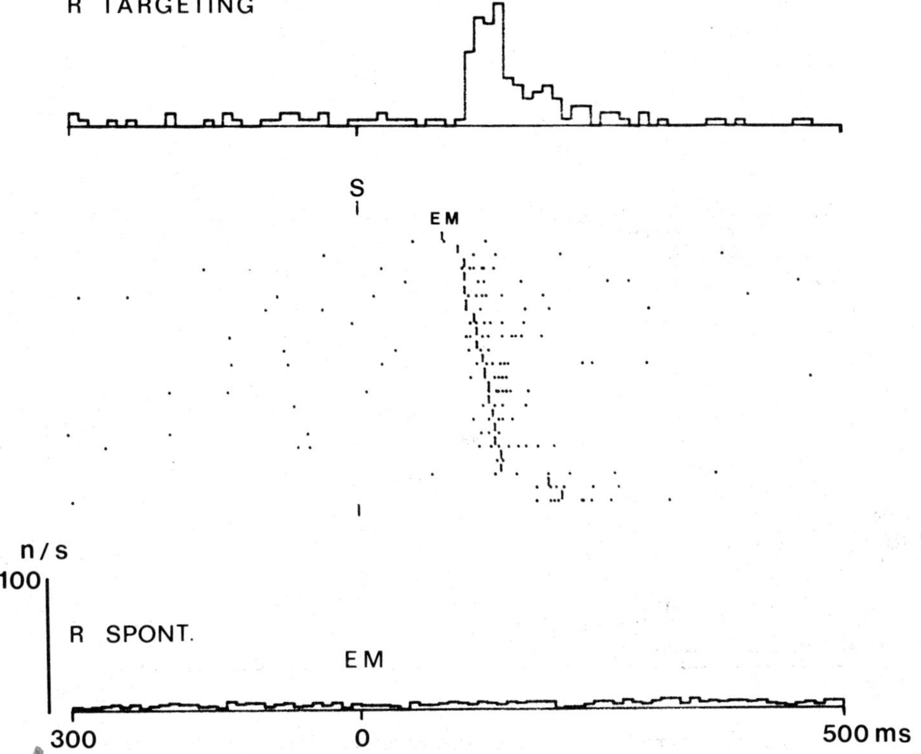

Fig. 3. Unit discharging before visually evoked EMs (raster and upper histogram), not before spontaneous EMs (lower histogram). Tick marks in raster indicate onset of EM.

This should still be viewed as a preliminary finding, but if confirmed it would provide a grip on the problem of competition between various command signals for the gaze.

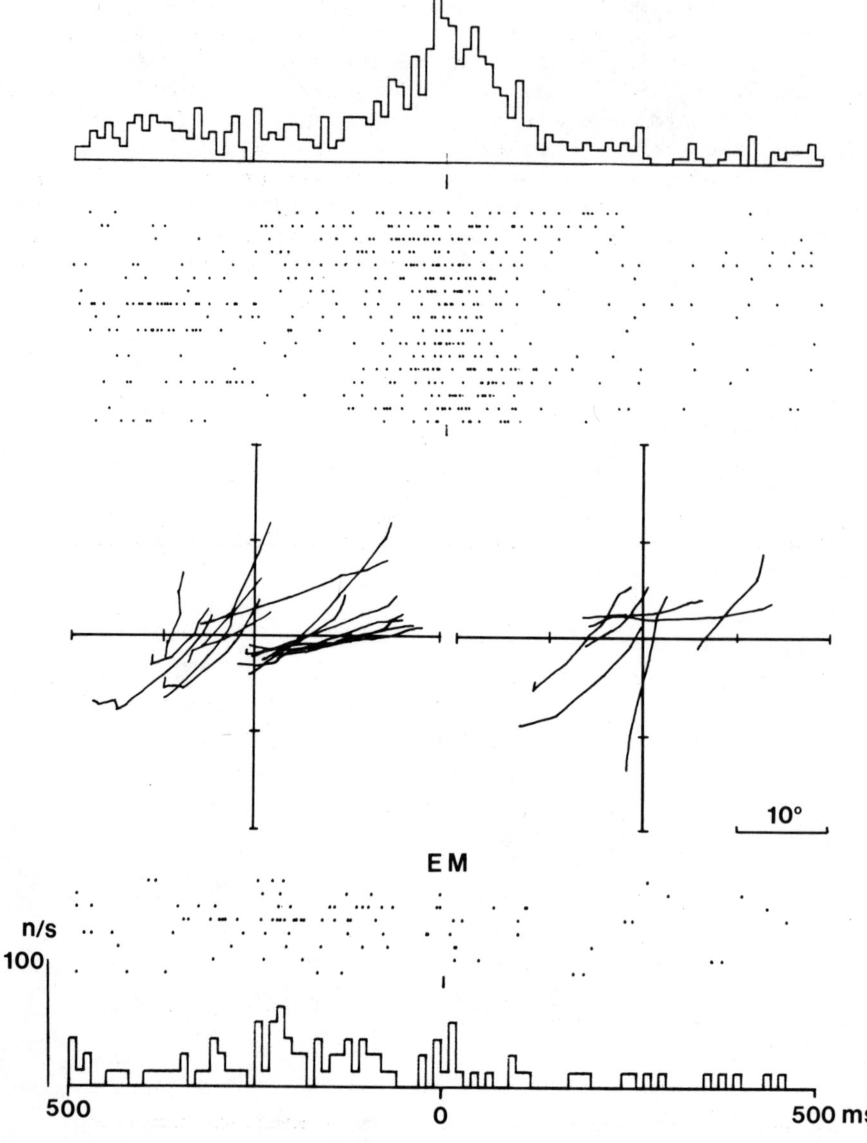

Fig. 4. Unit discharging before spontaneous EMs (upper raster), not before visually evoked EMs (lower raster). Between rasters: computer plots of the spontaneous EMs (left diagram) and visually evoked EMs (right diagram), all directed left and downward.

TONIC ACTIVITIES RELATED TO ACTIVE FIXATION

The same region of the thalamus where transient signals have been observed also contain units whose pattern of discharge was sustained.

Among tonic units an interesting class consisted of units either activated or inactivated when the animals fixated or pursued visual targets. Fig. 5 illustrates changes in the firing rate of two units during active fixation of the target. The rasters were synchronized on target onset and ranked in order of increasing stimulus duration, to demonstrate the relation existing between the

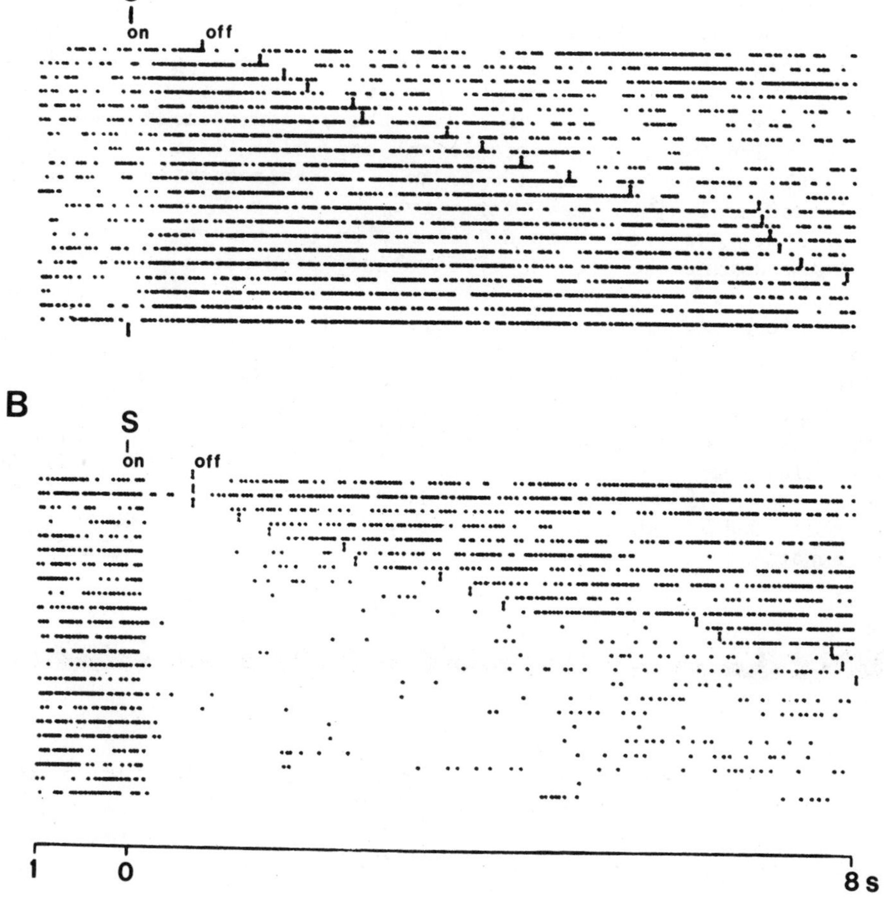

Fig. 5. Two types of sustained changes of activity during stimulus fixation. Rasters synchronized on stimulus onset (on) and ranked in order of stimulus duration (off stimulus tick marks). Unit A activated and unit B inactivated for whole period of fixation.

duration of activation (or inactivation) and the presence of the stimulus on the screen. The animal looked at the target as was indicated by EOG records (not shown). There were occasional perturbations of the pattern of firing which could be linked to relaxations of fixation (see below). But overall it is clear that the units were affected by the presence of a stimulus.

We analyzed in detail 11 activated units (as in the upper raster) and 23 inactivated units (as in the lower raster). Fig. 6 presents actual records during an experiment in which one of the stimulus-inactivated cells was submitted to different tests. In this figure, we have information on the vertical (V) and horizontal (H) coordinates of stimulus and eye positions. Periods of fixation are recognizable by the fact that the EOG and stimulus lines coincide. To clarify the presentation, the areas where these lines separate have been stippled; thus the stippling marks the discrepancy of gaze adjustment in no-fixation. The monkey was still in an early stage of training. Its attempts to follow the target(s) moving linearly back and forth across the screen as indicated in the bottom drawings, were intermittent and, altogether, not plainly successful. Advantage will now be taken of this erratic ocular behavior to analyze the cell activity.

Clearly, the cell stopped firing when the target appeared; it was silent during the periods of fixation; resumption of activity only occurred when the animal looked away from the target. Roughly, this is consistent with the hypothesis of a visual cell having a foveal receptive field. The hypthesis, however, is not tenable when latencies of responses are taken into consideration.

First, the latency of the inactivation was measured with precision taking into account both the stimulus onset and the timing of the initial targeting saccade. Were the inactivation due to irruption of the stimulus within the hypothetical foveal receptive field, its start would be expected some time, i.e., at the least, 50 ms (by comparison with other visual responses in the same thalamic

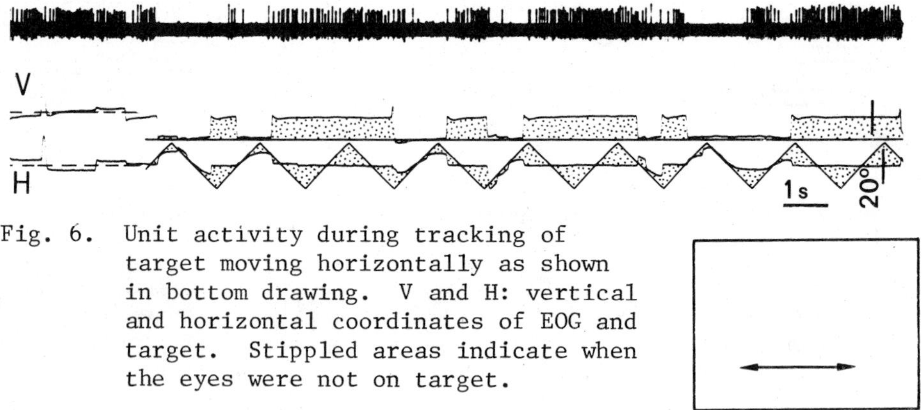

Fig. 6. Unit activity during tracking of target moving horizontally as shown in bottom drawing. V and H: vertical and horizontal coordinates of EOG and target. Stippled areas indicate when the eyes were not on target.

region) after the saccade. The histogram of Fig. 7 shows the inactivation being already quite pronounced when that saccade terminated.

Second, the firing should have resumed in temporal relation, i.e. within a delay of 50-150 ms, with the stimulus offset. In fact, the animal continued to fixate for 200-500 ms the site where the target had been projected and the resumption of activity was temporally linked - not to stimulus offset - but to the post-stimulus saccade that broke this fixation (not illustrated).

The behavior of this unit was not dependent on the location of the stimulus on the screen or on the direction of its movement. Thus, for example, in the trial of Fig. 8, the target was moved vertically on the right side of the screen and, as in Fig. 6, it can be seen that the inactivation started with the onset of fixation.

Two targets were then offered, moving horizontally, parallel to each other (Fig. 9). The monkey attempted to track them, shifting its gaze alternately between them. The vertical excursion of the gaze was the same as in Fig. 6. However, here in contrast to Fig. 6

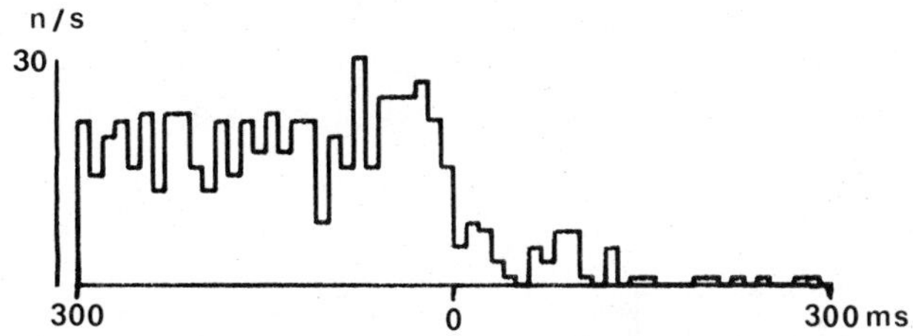

Fig. 7. Latency of unit of Fig. 6. Time zero in the histogram corresponds to the end of the initial targeting saccade, i.e., to the time when the eyes arrive on target.

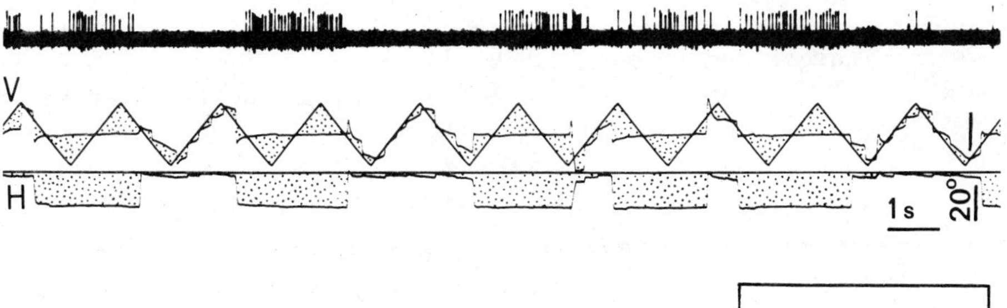

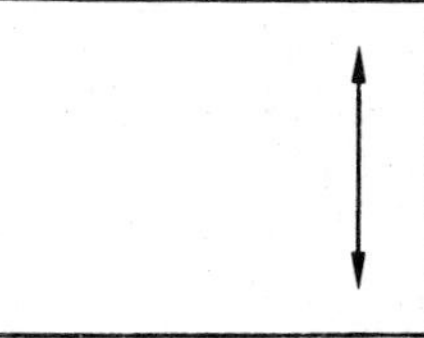

Fig. 8. Same unit as in Fig. 6 during tracking of a vertically moving target.

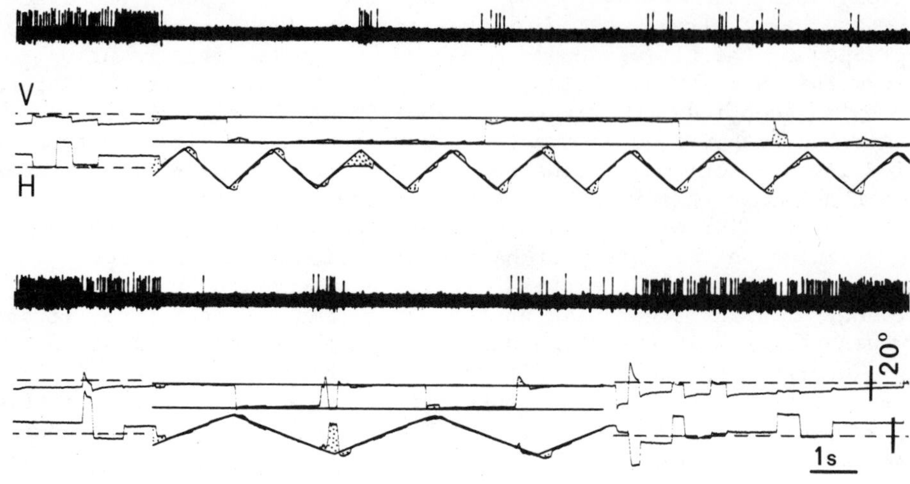

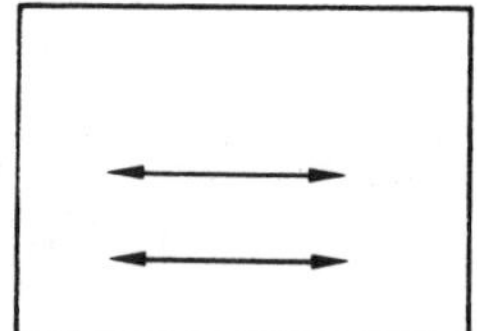

Fig. 9. Same unit as in Figs. 6 and 8 during tracking of 2 targets moving horizontally in parallel. Velocity was lower in bottom record. Note that the gaze shifted vertically between the 2 targets.

the gaze was on target (one of the two targets) practically all the time and the cell remained almost continuously silent.

In some units, such as the one illustrated in Fig. 10, we found a close relation of the firing with minute errors of tracking. This record was obtained in an animal whose tracking performance was quite good.

It seems obvious that the significance of the types of units described here cannot be understood in terms of either stimulus or gaze parameters alone. The unit activity depended on the relation between stimulus and gaze. A particular pattern appeared when the gaze was on target and wore off when a discrepancy occurred. Could it be a signal indicating an error of targeting? The fact is that for many cells the latencies did not fit with this hypothesis:

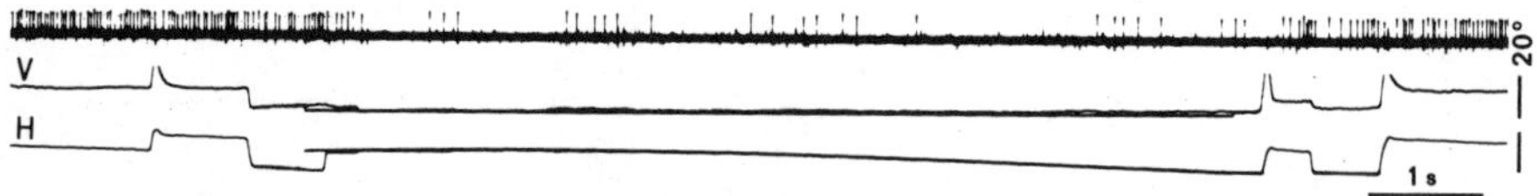

Fig. 10. Unit inactivation during fixation of a slowly moving target. Note resumptions of activity concomitant with slight errors of tracking.

namely, the pattern (e.g. the inactivation in Fig. 7) started before the error of gaze adjustment became zero. In other words, the cell activity was not likely to be a consequence of the animal's behavior, it must have been related to the preparation of this behavior. The notion of goal-directed behavior, obviously, implies a goal with respect to which motor aiming is adjusted. Error measurements cannot be made without a goal. In many experimental situations, the goal is imposed by the experimenter. If the goal is not imposed or, even more, if there are several goals (as in the case of Fig. 9), we must postulate that the goal signal is internally generated in the subject's brain. It is suggested that the units described participate in the decision to make a visual target the immediate goal of the oculomotor apparatus and, thereby, to take purposeful control of this apparatus.

ACKNOWLEDGEMENTS

This work was supported by U.S.P.H.S. Grants EY 02305 and NS 04955. We are grateful to Mr. V. Pagano, Ms. D. Blanco and B. Truex for their assistance.

REFERENCES

Bizzi, E., 1968, Discharge of frontal eye field neurons during saccadic and following eye movements in unanesthetized monkeys, Exp. Brain Res., 6:69.

Goldberg, M.E., and Bushnell, M.C., 1981, Role of the frontal eye fields in visually guided saccades, in: "Progress in oculomotor research", A. Fuchs and W. Becker, eds., Elsevier, Amsterdam.

Merker, B.H., 1979, Physical development: new applications to silver staining of neural tissue, Neurosci. Abstr. 1455.

Mohler, C.W., and Wurtz, R.H., 1976, Organization of monkey superior colliculus: intermediate layer cells discharging before eye movements, J. Neurophysiol., 40:74-94.

Mountcastle, V.B., Lynch, J.C., Georgopoulos, A., Sakata, H., and Acuna, C., 1975, Posterior parietal association cortex of the monkey: command functions for operations within extrapersonal space, J. Neurophysiol., 38:871-908.

Schlag, J., Lehtinen, I., and Schlag-Rey, M., 1974, Neuronal activity before and during eye movements in the thalamic internal medullary lamina of the cat, J. Neurophysiol., 37:982.

Schlag, J., Schlag-Rey, M., Peck, C., and Joseph, J.P., 1980, Visual responses of thalamic neurons depending on the direction of gaze and the position of targets in space, Exp. Brain Res., 40:170-184.

Schlag, J., and Schlag-Rey, M., 1977, Visuomotor properties of cells in the cat thalamic internal medullary lamina, in: "Control of gaze by brain stem neurons", R. Baker and A. Berthoz, eds., Elsevier, Amsterdam, pp. 453-462.

Schlag-Rey, M., and Schlag, J., 1977, Visual and presaccadic neuronal activity in the thalamic internal medullary lamina of cat: A study of targeting, J. Neurophysiol., 40:156.

Schlag-Rey, M., and Schlag, J., 1981, Eye-movement related neuronal activity in the central thalamus of monkeys, in: "Progress in oculomotor research", A. Fuchs and W. Becker, eds., Elsevier, Amsterdam.

CEREBELLAR LEARNING IN LIMB MOVEMENTS?

W.T. Thach, M.H. Schieber, P.F.C. Gilbert,
and R.J. Elble, R.J.

Departments of Neurobiology and Neurology
Washington University School of Medicine
Saint Louis, MO

SUMMARY

Evidence is given for the dissociation of activity of alpha and gamma motor neuron activity during slow precise pursuit tracking, in which the cerebellum may play a role. Questions are raised as to whether this is a learned phenomenon, how the cerebellum might participate in the learning, and what is needed to find out.

Five features of cerebellar circuitry figure prominently in physiological theory: 1) cerebellar neurons fire at high frequency and modulate up (500/s) and down (o/sec) from a maintained "center" frequency (25-100/s); 2) all nuclear cell output is excitatory; 3) the cortical circuitry is much the same in all parts of the cortex, and all cortical output (Purkinje cells) is inhibitory; 4) the two inputs to the cerebellum (mossy fibers and climbing fibers) both go to the deep nuclei and to the cerebellar cortex and both are excitatory; 5) the two inputs contrast: the climbing fiber-Purkinje cell connection is 1:1 and causes "complex spikes" in the Purkinje cell at around 1/s, while the granule cell-Purkinje cell connection is >200,000:1 and causes simple spike discharge in the Purkinje cell at high frequencies.

Ito (8) has proposed that a fundamental function of the vestibulocerebellum is to adapt and maintain the gain of the vestibulo-ocular reflex (VOR) such that any given head movement results in an eye movement of equal amplitude in the opposite direction. This reflex can maintain the stability of gaze fixation on a distant target during head movement. The reflex is adaptable so that it can be changed to compensate for early life growth, late life

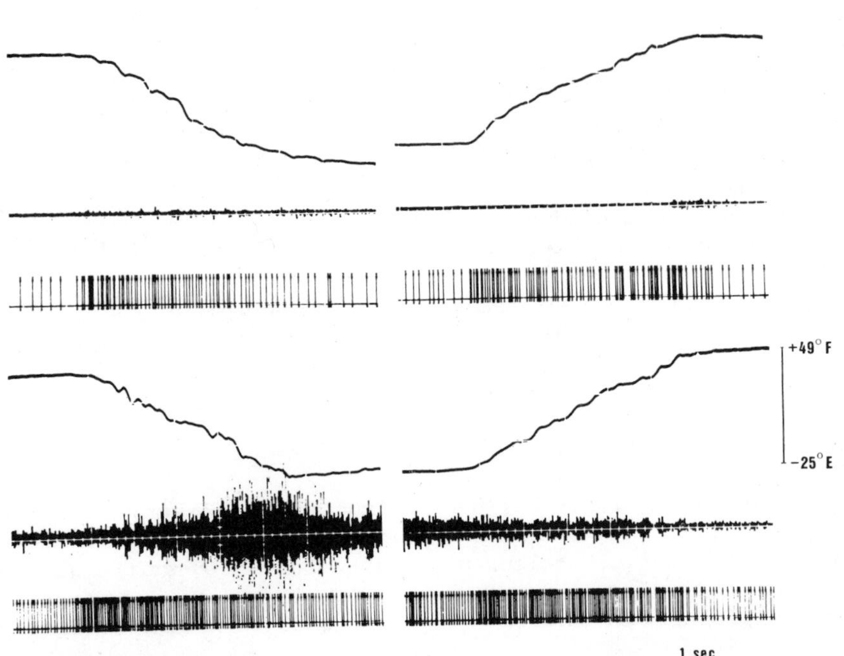

Fig. 1. Spindle afferent activity and EMG recorded from the parent muscle, extensor carpi radialis (ECR), during hold-ramp-hold tracking movements. To the left are extension ramps and to the right flexions; the upper frames were performed under flexor load, the bottom under extensor load. Each frame shows an individual trial: the top trace represents angular wrist position, the middle trace is EMG recorded via wire electrodes inserted percutaneously on either side of the unit's receptive field in ECR, and the bottom trace is the discriminated activity of a DRG unit identified as a spindle afferent. Average velocity of each ramp is 28°/sec. From Schieber and Thach (18).

damage, and any intervening novel demands placed on the system (16). The cellular mechanism that has been proposed is that a basic VOR is produced by a labyrinth-vestibular nuclei-oculomotor neuron excitatory "main line" that has tonic activity which modulates up and down during the reflex. Superimposed on this is the inhibitory "side loop" through the cerebellar cortex; it also is driven by tonic mossy fiber labyrinthine input, and it returns to exert an inhibitory signal onto the tonically firing vestibular nuclei. The sensitivity (gain) of the inhibitory side loop determines the amount of the excitatory output in response to a given input. The low frequency inferior olive climbing fiber system functions (1,12) to change (adjust and maintain) the side loop sensitivity to a given head movement input, and thus to control the overall gain (eye movement/head movement) of the reflex. The theory has been supported by the observation that in rabbits (9) and cats (10) in whom the reflex has been experimentally altered by the animals' adaptation to spectacles or other visual novelty, cerebellar ablation returns the reflex to near its initial gain and makes it unalterable.

Does this input/output adaptability exist for other parts of the cerebellum, as a general fundamental function? By what other experimental strategies might the theory be tested? The experiments briefly mentioned below were conducted on rhesus monkeys as they performed highly trained movements of the wrist. Single unit activity was recorded in cerebellar cortex (Purkinje cells) and in the interposed (spinocerebellum) and dentate (neocerebellum) nuclei during movement. The patterns of neural discharge suggest to us additional kinds of adaptive control by the cerebellum.

Monkeys were trained to observe a slowly moving (8°-28°/sec) target on an oscilloscope and to track it accurately with ramp movement of the wrist (17,18,21). This was difficult for both humans and monkeys to do, as evidenced by frequent errors, and by a remarkable physiological tremor (10-13 Hz) during the ramp; monkeys were trained for as long as 2 years. Recordings were then made of unit discharge in cerebellum, motor cortex, dorsal root ganglia (c_7 and C_8; primary spindle afferents from the arm) as well as arm muscle EMGs during the monkeys' movement performance. Fig. 1 shows the discharge of a spindle afferent (bottom line), EMG of extensor carpi radialis (in which the spindle lay - middle line), and the position trace (top line). The left graphs are during wrist extension (position moves down) and the right graphs during wrist flexion (position moves up); the upper graphs are under flexor torque load, and the lower graphs under extensor torque load. One can see that the extensor muscle is active only under extensor load (bottom graphs), and that the EMG increases for extensor directed movements (left graph) and decreases for flexor directed movement (right graph). Under extensor load the flexor muscles were silent, as the extensors did all the work; the reverse was true under flexor load. In sum, this is the expected EMG pattern of a well behaved wrist extensor muscle. In sharp contrast was the pattern of firing of the spindle afferent: despite the marked variation in EMG activity under the different conditions, the spindle afferent discharge is of one remarkably constant pattern - a sharp increase <u>before</u> the onset of movement and of EMG change, a downward sloping plateau as the movement was performed, and a further lowering on completion of the movement. We can think of no other way to explain this except by assuming that an elevated discharge in gamma motor neurons, sharply dissociated from activity in alpha motor neurons, in large part caused the change. This is most striking for the extreme situation in the upper left graphs: during extension, the extensor spindle is shortening; under flexor load, the extensor muscle is silent. One would therefore expect no excitation of the spindle by stretch and no excitation via gamma motor neurons if they are obligatorily coupled to alpha motor neurons in a pattern of coactivation (13,22). Yet the spindle discharge is much the same as in the other conditions, and under no conditions does it resemble the pattern of EMG activity in the muscle. This was true of all 5 units identified as spindle afferents in the dorsal root ganglia; no exceptions were found. Can one generalize from the observation of 5 units? The certainty of the DRG unit receptor identity and location, together with the uniformity of their striking response pattern, lead us cautiously to assume that this was the general pattern for all primary spindle afferents from the principle active muscles moving the wrist.

Whether or not "alpha-gamma dissociation" exists has been a controversial subject. Merton (with Granit and Holmgren) advanced the idea of an extreme sort of dissociation, in which the CNS might initiate and control limb movement by commands sent directly to the gamma motor neurons (7,14). The gamma motor neuron-spindle-spindle afferent-alpha motor neuron loop would operate as a servomechanism that would automatically compensate for length disturbances during the course of movement. The idea was discredited by the observations of Vallbo (22) and others (13) in peripheral nerve recordings in man, in which there always appeared to be simultaneous coactivation of gamma and alpha motor neurons - apparently ruling out the role of the gamma motor neuron as an initiator, but permitting that of a "servo-assister" (13). The observation reported here again raises the question of the functional purpose and the effect of this increased spindle (and presumed gamma motor neuron) activity; this will be addressed shortly.

What of the activity patterns of neurons in the CNS during these movements? Fig. 2 shows graphs for a flexor muscle (Fig. 2A), one type of motor cortex neuron (Fig 2B) another type of motor cortex neuron (Fig. 2C), a cerebellar nuclear neuron (Fig. 2D), and the extensor muscle and extensor spindle afferent (previously shown - Fig. 2E). The limb traces are averages of 8 or more trials, the left during extensor and the right during flexor slow ramp tracking movements. The middle two traces are under no load; the upper two are under flexor and the lower two under extensor loads. Fig. 2B shows a "flexor" neuron in motor cortex with a pattern that is markedly changed by the direction and the loading of movements in a pattern similar to the flexor muscle shown in Fig. 2A and just opposite that of the extensor muscle shown in Fig. 2E. This pattern was characteristic of about half the wrist-related neurons recorded in motor cortex. In sharp contrast is the discharge pattern of another type of motor cortex neuron shown in Fig. 2C: as for the spindle afferent, there is an abrupt increase in frequency before the start of the movement, a downward sloping plateau during and a drop at the end of the ramp movement. The discharge pattern is bidirectional and relatively constant despite marked variation in movement direction and loading. This was seen for the remaining half of motor cortex neurons. Discharge of a cerebellar dentate neuron is shown in Fig. 2D: quite surprisingly, nearly all of the units (which were identified as being well related to arm movement by several criteria 13,18,22) in both dentate and interpositus showed this same bidirectional discharge pattern that was seen for half the "wrist" neurons in motor cortex and all of the DRG neurons identified as forearm spindle afferents. Since all the cerebellar nuclear "wrist" neurons and half the motor cortex "wrist" neurons discharged in a pattern similar to that of all the forearm spindle afferent neurons, we assume that these neurons may be influenced by spindle feedback, or may influence gamma (and inter) neurons, or both. They seem much less directly concerned with the discharge of alpha motor neurons. What is the meaning of these patterns of discharge?

Interpositus and motor cortex neurons both are influenced by a fast path from somatosensory afferents - including spindles (10,11, 15) - at minimum latencies of about 15 msec (20). Both sets of neurons discharged (Fig. 4) as did spindle afferents (Fig. 3) in relation to the tremor and had a phase lag consistent with the possibility that they were driven by sensory feedback from the tremor. By contrast, the dentate nucleus has no such rapid somatosensory input, and its activity was not modulated in relation to the tremor, yet it did have the same pattern of bidirectional discharge. Was it playing a role in generating a similar pattern in gamma motor neurons? Since both ablation (6) and stimulation (7) studies have shown a path from cerebellar nuclei to gamma motor neurons, this is quite possible.

What would be the purpose of elevated gamma motor neurons and spindle afferent discharge? There has been a recent tendency to regard spindle afferents, and especially the primaries, as preferentially sensitive to length perturbations that are small in amplitude, as opposed to large (13). One of the striking observations in the 4 monkeys that have so far been trained to this task is that

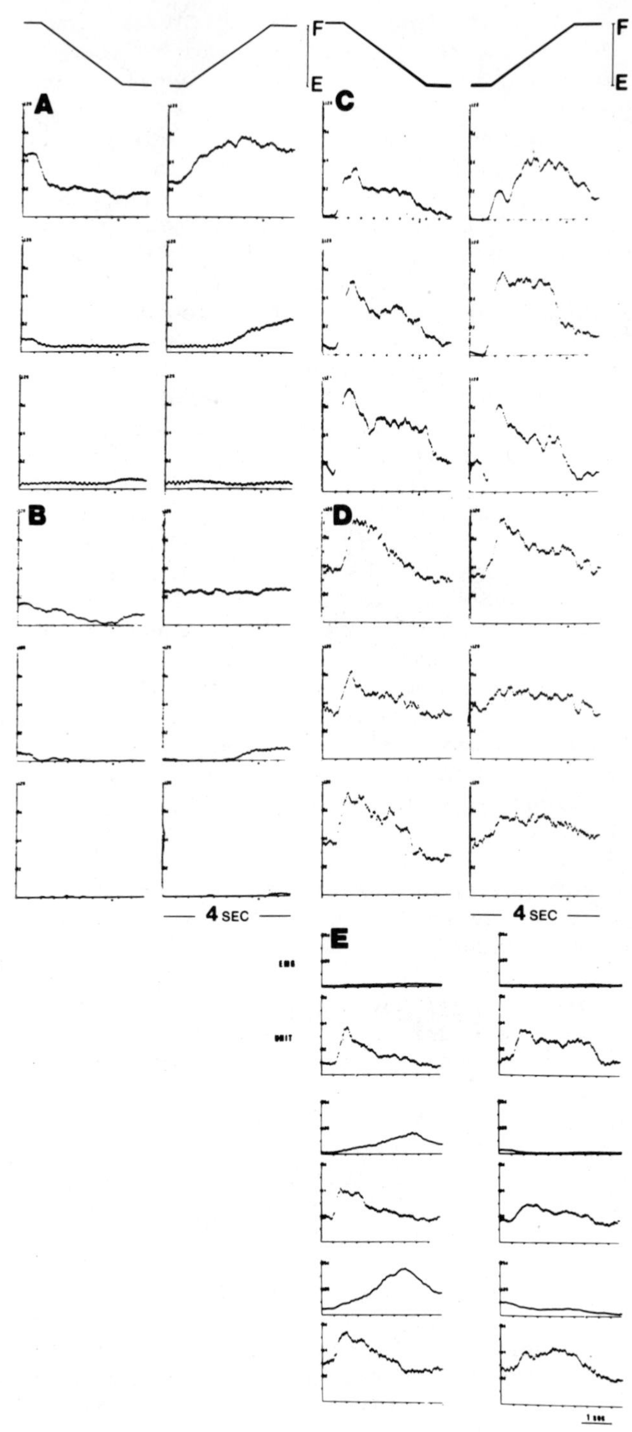
F
E
F
E
A
C
B
D
4 SEC
4 SEC
E
EMG
UNIT
1 sec

Fig. 2 α-γ-Motoneuron dissociation and the α-γ-motoneuron relation
← of motor cortex and cerebellar nuclear neurons. A: EMG of wrist flexor in forearm during slow wrist tracking. Top: schematic hold-ramp-hold tracking for extension (left) and flexion (right). Graphs are of EMG intensity (ordinate) versus time (abscissa) during extension (left) and flexion (right). Top graphs show discharge under flexor load; middle graphs, under no load; and bottom graphs, under extensor load. EMG was related to direction of load and to position. B: discharge of one type of precentral cerebral cortex neuron during slow wrist tracking. This neuron shows patterns of discharge under different conditions that are similar to activity of a wrist flexor muscle. C: discharge of second type of precentral cerebral neuron. This neuron shows pattern of bidirectional discharge that is remarkably constant under all conditions. D: discharge of a cerebellar nuclear neuron. This nuclear neuron and all others showed bidirectional discharge like second category of neurons in motor cortex. E: discharge of extensor muscle EMG (upper trace) and unit discharge (lower trace) of neuron in C8 dorsal root ganglion. Unit was identified as primary afferent from spindle within extensor muscle. EMG discharge resembles directional discharge of type I precentral cerebral cortex neurons. By contrast, activity of this spindle afferent and of all others resembled bidirectional discharge of type II precentral cerebral cortex neurons and of all cerebellar nuclear neurons. From Thach et al. (21).

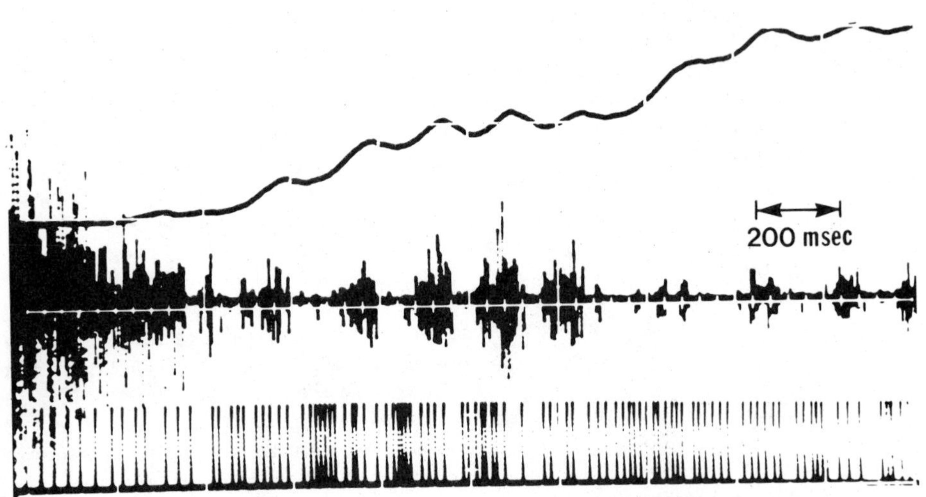

Fig. 3. Spindle afferent and EMG recordings during tremor. Simultaneous position, extensor digitorum EMG (middle tracing), and extensor-related muscle spindle (lower tracing) recordings obtained during a flexor ramp maneuver under an extensor torque load. Two definite (and 3 probable) muscle spindles were studied, one flexor and one extensor. Each was modulated by the tremor, and their modulations were 180 degrees out of phase. Phase analysis was performed, and the bursts in the spindle afferents led peak muscle stretch by an average of 150 degrees (range 133-167). The EMG bursts therefore followed the spindle bursts by approximately 39 msec (84 degrees). From Elble et al. (4).

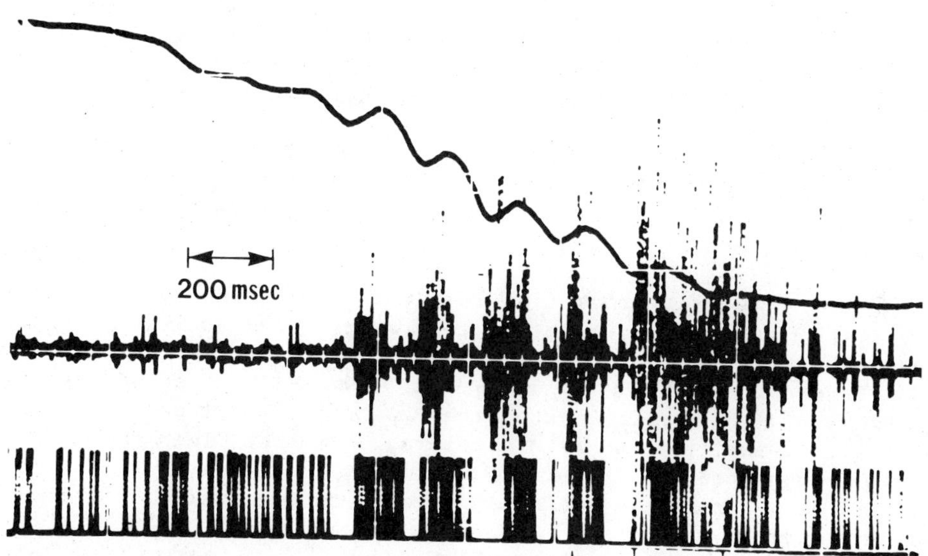

Fig. 4. Cerebellar interpositus neuron and EMG recordings during tremor. Simultaneous position, extensor digitorum EMG (middle trace), and extensor related interpositus neuron (lower trace) recordings obtained during a extensor ramp maneuver. By applying extensor and flexor torque pulses to the wrist, 6 of 14 tremor-related interpositus neurons could be classified as excited by stretch of either the extensor or the flexor muscles. The tremor bursts of these interpositus neurons led the peaks in muscle stretch by an average of 51 degrees (range 19-86). The interpositus tremor bursts therefore lagged the EMG bursts by an average of 12 sec (range 4-22 msec). From Elble et al. (4).

they all developed a small (<5°) fast (10-13 Hz) tremor, with reciprocal alternating agonist-antagonist EMG discharge, during the course of the ramp movements. The tremor does not occur in the holds prior to or following the ramp movement. There is evidence that the normal or "physiological" tremor consists of a natural tendency of the limb to oscillate because of its inertial and the elastic properties of the limb, and that it may be amplified by the action of the segmental stretch reflex (3,19,24). Consistent with this view is the fact that the spindle afferents discharged in full-range modulation in relation to the tremor, and were time locked to and we presume the cause of subsequent EMG bursts. The EMG bursts in turn were so timed as to augment (rather than restrain) the tremor. Further, the tremor was slowed (as low as 2.5 Hz) with inertial loads, and was eliminated with large viscous loads, suggesting that the tremor was at least in part caused by a peripheral mechanism, and was not generated by a central oscillator (19,24).

Interpositus neurons (and some motor cortex neurons) were exquisitely modulated in relation to tremor: peak activity followed peak EMG activity by 12 ms and peak spindle activity by 50 msec. Was interpositus discharge triggered (like EMG) by spindle activity? Did it then act to stop the EMG burst, and thus to restrict the tremor amplitude to within tolerable limits? That this may be so is suggested by the experiments of Vilis and Hore (23) who cooled deep cerebellar nuclei of monkeys and observed during tremor a prolonged discharge of motor cortex neurons, which was in turn thought to cause the prolonged EMG bursts that resulted in large amplitude, low frequency tremor. In our own monkey, after a number of interpositus penetrations without other damage to the animal, the tremor frequency dropped suddenly to 5-7 Hz and increased by fivefold in amplitude. From these observations, we tentatively conclude that interpositus acts to limit tremor amplitude, and that it uses afferent input to do so. How it does so is unclear: does it act to turn off the alpha motor neuron and the EMG soon after its onset? Does it quicken the response of the motor cortex neurons to stretch and/or inhibit their prolonged discharge? Does it increase the gain of the segmental stretch reflex, and the sensitivity of the spindle, by increasing gamma neuron discharge frequency? We do not yet know the answers to these questions, yet they would seem to be at the heart of an important aspect of normal cerebellar function.

We suspect that several crucial aspects of the performance of slow precise ramp tracking are that it is both difficult and takes a long time to learn. This may be why alpha-gamma dissociation has not been observed in those non-trained, casual movements made by men and walking cats (22,13). Another possibly crucial aspect is the tremor, which if uncontrolled, could hamper performance. We theorize that if the alpha-gamma dissociation is used to prevent errors and improve performance, it may develop only through learning and through the experience of whatever error (e.g. tremor) it is that occurs during the performance of that task. Different tasks may predispose to different types of error. One might further speculate that a fundamental feature that distinguishes "skilled" from "unskilled" movements is the degree to which the subject has optimized the dissociated alpha, gamma, and interneuronal firing pattern to offset anticipated errors. These are testable speculations. In such a role, the cerebellum would operate in a fashion analogous to its putative role of adjusting, through learning from the experience of errors in performance, the gain of the VOR.

A single-neuron recording experiment has given some results consistent with the notion of adaptive motor control (5). Monkeys were trained to hold a lever in the hand fixedly in a central position in return for fruit juice. Loads were imposed by a torque motor on the hand alternately against flexors and extensors. A shift in load at some unpredictable time knocked the lever and the hand out of the position and the monkey had to return to the position quickly to get a reward. During initial behavioral training both the flexor and the extensor loads were fixed at the same magnitude. When the monkey was prepared for Purkinje cell recording, the task was changed. The monkey performed for 25 or so trials against flexor and extensor loads that were "familiar". Then, without warning, one of the loads was changed to a "novel" value and the monkey's performance suddenly deteriorated: if the load were greater than that given previously, the hand would undershoot the central positions; if the load were lighter, the hand would overshoot. With practice, over 12-100 trials, the return to the central position became as quick and as smooth as it had been previously (Fig. A). For the Purkinje cells that changed at all in relation to the task performance, the clearest and greatest pattern of change was as shown in Figure B. Following the change to a novel load there was an increase in the complex-spike occurrence just after the load switch that persisted for many trials before returning to base line, and there was also a concurrent decrease in the simple-spike occurrence. Simple-spike frequency gradually decreased over successive trials and remained decreased after the complex-spike firing frequency had returned to its baseline level. Finally, these changes occurred over a time course similar to that of the improvement in motor performance. A diagram of the time course of the change in complex- and simple-spike discharge frequencies and the behavior is given in Figure 5. The pattern is that which would be predicted by the Albus model (1) of cerebellar participation in adaptive motor control.

Before concluding that learning takes a place in the cerebellar control of limb movements, we should like answers to the following questions:

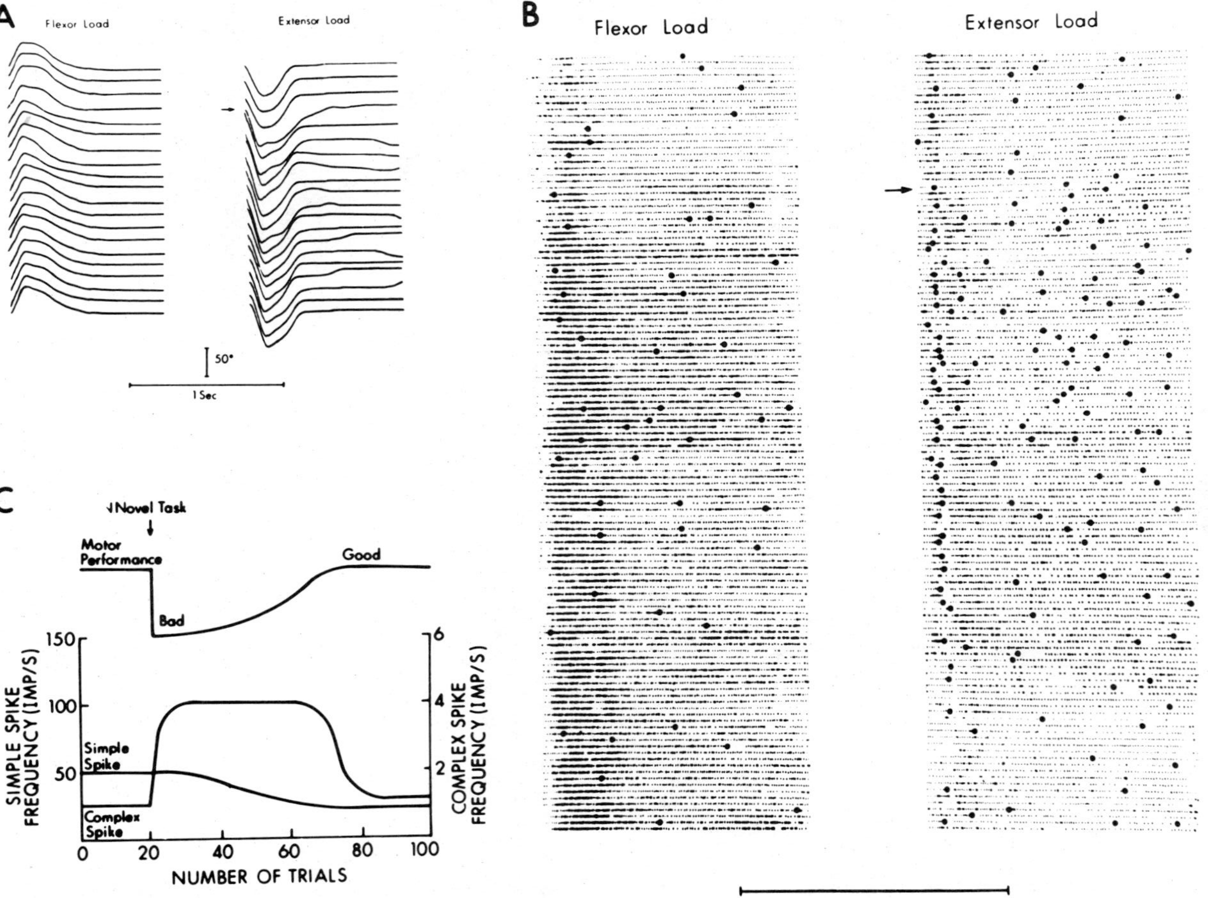
A
Flexor Load
Extensor Load
50°
1 Sec
B
Flexor Load
Extensor Load
1 Sec
C
Novel Task
Motor Performance
Good
Bad
SIMPLE SPIKE FREQUENCY (IMP/S)
150
100
50
Simple Spike
Complex Spike
COMPLEX SPIKE FREQUENCY (IMP/S)
6
4
2
0
20
40
60
80
100
NUMBER OF TRIALS

Fig. 5. Cerebellum in adaptive motor control. A: changes in task performance with introduction of a novel load. Task was to move a handle in horizontal arc by flexing or extending wrist to central position and to try to hold it there despite flexor and extensor loads applied to handle. Each trace starts as load switched to one in opposite direction, displacing handle from the central position for a transient period of about 300 ms. Position traces of handle are shown for successive trials (top to bottom) alternately against flexor and extensor loads. Each flexor trace on left is followed by extensor trace on right. With known loads, position traces were smooth and reproducible from trial to trial (above arrow). When extensor load was increased from known 300 g to novel 450 g (arrow), there were immediate irregularities in position traces during transient and maintained periods, which gradually diminished with further trials (below arrow). For flexor trials there were a few irregularities in transient period only as load switched from novel to known. B: complex (CS) and simple (SS) spike frequency changes for Purkinje cell after change in load. Each dot represents spike potential (SSs, small dots; CSs, large dots); each row of dots represents the discharge during a trial, beginning at change in direction of load. Successive trials represented top to bottom, each flexor trace on left followed by an extensor trace on right. This cell was load-related with higher SS frequency in maintained period for flexor than for extensor trials. At arrow, known extensor load of 300 g was changed to a novel 450 g while known flexor load of 310 g was kept constant. Before load change (above arrow), there was a low frequency of related CS activity at about 100 ms after start of extensor trials. AFter load change (below arrow) CS frequency at that time increased greatly and persisted for about 70 trials. There was also an increased CS frequency in the extensor maintained period for about 40 trials. Associated with these transient increases in CS frequency there were decreases in SS frequency that persisted. C: relationship of motor performance and complex- and simple-spike frequencies over multiple trials. From Brooks and Thach (2).

1) What is the cause of the increased spindle afferent discharge? Is it driven from gamma motor neurons as we deduce, and can this be proven directly by recording from gamma motor neurons under these conditions?

2) What is the effect of increased spindle afferent discharge? Increased spindle sensitivity to perturbation or tremor? Increased alpha motor neuron excitability? Increased motor cortex excitability? Increased gain of segmental and/or "long loop" reflexes? Increased stiffness of the limb?

3) Is the dissociated spindle (and presumably alpha and gamma motor neuron) activity only the result of learning? Can one demonstrate a gradual change through the process of learning?

4) Does the dissociation depend on the function of the cerebellum? Does cerebellar ablation prevent it from occurring and abolish it if it has occurred?

5) What is the mechanism of the putative cerebellar control over dissociation of activity of alpha and gamma motor neurons?

6) What is the mechanism of the change in cerebellar control? Does the climbing fiber reduce Purkinje cell sensitivity to mossy fiber input?

And most important, 7) Can experiments be designed to answer these questions?

REFERENCES

1. Albus, J.S.A. (1971) A theory of cerebellar cortex. Math. Biosci. 10:25-66.
2. Brooks, V.B. and Thach, W.T. (1981) Cerebellar control of posture and movement. In: Handbook of Physiology. Section I. The Nervous System. Vol. II. Motor control. Ed. by Brookhart, J.M., Mountcastle, V.B., Brooks, V.B., Geiger, S.R. American Physiological Society, Bethesda, MD. pp. 877-946.
3. Elble, R.J. and Randall, J.E. (1976) Motor unit activity responsible for the 8- to 12-Hz component of human physiological finger tremor. J. Neurophysiol. 39:370-383.
4. Elble, R.J., Schieber, M.A., and Thach, W.T. (1981) Involvement of nucleus interpositus in action tremor. Soc. Neurosci. Abstr. 7:691.
5. Gilbert, P.F.C. and Thach, W.T. (1977) Purkinje cell activity during motor learning. Brain Res. 128:309-328.
6. Gilman, S., Marco, L.A., and Ebel, H.C. (1971) Effects of medullary pyramidotomy in the monkey. II. Abnormalities of spindle afferent responses.

7. Granit, R., Holmgren, B., and Merton, P.A. (1955) The two routes for the excitation of muscle and their subservience to the cerebellum. J. Physiol. (Lond.) 130:213-224.
8. Ito, M. (1972) Neural design of the cerebellar motor control system. Brain Res. 40:81-84.
9. Ito, M., Shiida, N., Yagi, N. and Yamamoto, M. (1974) The cerebellar modification of rabbits horizontal vestibulo-ocular reflex induced by sustained head rotation combined with visual stimulation. Proc. Jap. Acad. 50:85-89.
10. Lucier, G.E., Ruegg, D.C., and Wiesendanger, M. (1975) Responses of neurones in motor cortex and in area 3a to controlled stretches of forelimb muscles in Cebus monkeys. J. Physiol. (Lond.) 251:833-853.
11. Mackay, W.A. and Murphy, J.T. (1974) Response of interpositus neurons to passive muscle stretch. J. Neurophysiol. 37:1410-1423.
12. Marr, D. (1969) A theory of cerebellar cortex. J. Physiol. (Lond.) 202:437-470.
13. Matthews, P.B.C. (1981) Muscle spindles: their messages and their fusimotor supply. In: Handbook of Physiology. Sect. I. The Nervous System. Vol. II. Motor control. Ed. by Brookhart, J.M., Mountcastle, V.B., Brooks, V.B. and Geiger, S.R. American Physiological Society, Bethesda, Maryland. pp. 189-228.
14. Merton, P.A. (1953) Speculations on the servocontrol of movement. In: The Spinal Cord, ed. by J.L. Malcolm, J.A.B. Gray, and G.E.W.Wolstenholme. Boston, Little, Brown & Co., pp. 183-198 (Ciba Foundation Symp.)
15. Phillips, C.G., Powell, T.P.S., and Wiesendanger, M. (1971) Projection from low-threshold muscle afferents of hand and forearm to area 3a of baboons cortex. J. Physiol. (Lond.) 217:419-446.
16. Robinson, D.A. (1976) Adaptive gain control of vestibulo-ocular reflex by the cerebellum. J. Neurophysiol. 39:954-969.
17. Schieber, M.H. (1981) Muscle, motor cortex, cerebellar nucleus and spindle afferent activity during slow hold ramp hold position tracking movements of the monkeys wrist. Doctoral dissertation, Washington University, Program in Neural Science, St. Louis.
18. Schieber, M.H., and Thach, W.T. (1980) Alpha-gamma dissociation during slow tracking movements of the monkeys wrist: preliminary evidence from spinal ganglion recording. Brain Res. 202:213-216.
19. Stein, R.B., and Lee, R.G. (1981) Tremor and clonus. In: Handbook of Physiology. Section I. The Nervous System. Vol. II. Motor Control. Ed. by Brookhart, J.M., Mountcastle, V.B., Brooks, V.B. and Geiger, S.R. American Physciological Society, Bethesda, Maryland. pp. 189-228.
20. Thach, W.T. (1978) Correlation of neural discharge with pattern and force of muscular activity, joint position, and

direction of intended next movement in motor cortex and cerebellum. J. Neurophysiol. 41:654-676.

21. Thach, W.T., Perry, J.G., and Schieber, M.H. Cerebellar output: body maps and muscle spindles. In: The Cerebellum: New Vistas, ed. by S. Palay and V. Chan-Palay. New York: Springer-Verlag. In press.

22. Vallbo, A.B. (1971) Muscle spindle response at the onset of isometric voluntary contraction in man. Time difference between fusimotor and skeletomotor effects. J. Physiol. 318:405-431.

23. Vilis, T. and Hore, J. (1980) Central neural mechanisms contributing to cerebellar tremor produced by limb perturbations. J. Neurophysiol. 43:279-291.

24. Hagbarth, K.E. and Young, R.R. (1979) Participation of the stretch reflex in human physiological tremors. Brain 102: 509-526.

SEPTO-HIPPOCAMPAL ACTIVITY AND LEARNING RATE

Stephen D. Berry

Department of Psychology
Miami University
Oxford, Ohio

SUMMARY

This paper presents the results of experiments investigating the relationships between hippocampal unit and slow wave activity and classical conditioning of the nictitating membrane (NM) response in rabbits. In Experiment 1, a strong, predictive correlation was found between frequency components of slow wave activity and the rate of acquisition of a conditioned response. Animals displaying higher proportions of 2-8 Hz hippocampal EEG learned more quickly, while those with more 8-22 Hz activity required more trials to reach asymptotic criterion. These groups also showed opposite across-training changes in EEG: the faster group shifted towards higher frequencies, and the slower group towards lower frequencies. Significant differences in the responsiveness of hippocampal multiple unit activity to the conditioning stimuli were also observed between the two groups. It was concluded that the state of the hippocampal EEG prior to training predicts both cellular responsiveness and the rate of behavioral learning.

In experiment 2, small lesions were made in the medial septal nucleus to disrupt the frequency "pacemaker" of the hippocampal EEG. Relative to controls, the lesion group displayed higher EEG frequencies, reduced neuronal responsiveness to conditioning stimuli, and slower acquisition of the conditioned response. Taken together, these data support the idea of hippocampal involvement in classical NM conditioning and suggest that one determinant of learning rate is the state of the hippocampus as modulated by the septal pacemaker.

INTRODUCTION

One aspect of learning that has important implications for both behavioral and psychobiological studies of conditioning is the occurrence of individual differences in learning rate. Even in well-controlled animal classical conditioning experiments, such as the rabbit nictitating membrane (NM) preparation, it is not uncommon to observe substantial variations between subjects in the number of trials required to display consistent conditioned responding. Such variations are especially important in seeking the neural bases of learning since differences in behavior should correlate highly with variations in relevant neural processes. This paper presents the results of two experiments demonstrating that differences in the activity of the hippocampus are related to the rate of acquisition in rabbit NM conditioning, and that manipulation of the septo-hippocampal system alters the rate of learning.

A number of studies have implicated the rodent hippocampus, especially as measured by multiple unit activity, in learning or closely related processes (Olds et al., 1972; Berger and Thompson, 1978; Phillips et al., 1980). A particularly striking form of hippocampal activity is the high amplitude, rhythmic slow activity (RSA) or "theta" rhythm that has been correlated with movement (Vanderwolf, 1975), attention or orienting (Bennett, 1975; Coleman and Lindsley, 1977; Grastyan et al., 1959), and learning (Adey, 1966). The first experiment reported here attempted to assess any learning-related changes in hippocampal EEG that accompany the changes in unit activity during rabbit NM conditioning reported by others (Berger and Thompson, 1978). The second experiment investigated lesion-produced disruption of septo-hippocampal activity and its relation to conditioning. In both experiments, recordings were taken of hippocampal multiple unit activity and slow waves (EEG), as well as of the behavioral responses during training. Some of these data have been published elsewhere (Berry and Thompson, 1977, 1978, 1979, 1982).

EXPERIMENT 1

Methods

The standard NM conditioning procedure developed by Gormezano (1966) was used. Animals were given 13 blocks of trials, with each block consisting of 8 paired (tone-air puff) trials and one test trial (tone alone). The conditioned stimulus (CS) was a 1 KHz, 85 dB, 350 msec tone. The unconditioned stimulus (UCS), a 210 g/cm^2 corneal air puff, was given 250 msec after tone onset. The mean intertrial interval was 60 sec, varying randomly between 50 and 70 sec. Control animals received a random sequence of tone and air puff presentations explicitly unpaired with a 30 sec mean intertrial interval.

Under halothane anesthesia, 16 subjects were implanted with chronic, stainless steel multiple unit electrodes in area CA1 of the dorsal hippocampus. After a 1 week recovery period, the rabbits were given 1 session of adaptation to the conditioning apparatus, followed by up to 4 days of paired training. Unit spike discharges (from small clusters of neurons) and slow waves were recorded on magnetic tape for off-line analysis on a PDP-12 computer. Two-min samples of spontaneous EEG and unit activity were recorded from the awake, restrained rabbits before and after each training session. The analysis of unit activity changes during trials consisted of converting spikes exceeding a preset discriminator level into standard pulses. The data collection program counted the number of unit discharges in each 3 msec time bin throughout the trial. Data collection began 250 msec prior to CS onset (PreCS period or baseline), continued through 250 msec of the CS period (tone on), and ended with a 250 msec sample after UCS onset (UCS period). Thus, each trial yielded 750 msec of data, which were accumulated across 8 trials to produce peristimulus time histograms of multiple unit activity. These data were converted into standard scores for the CS and UCS periods for each block of trials. Each score consisted of the mean change in unit counts (CS or UCS minus PreCS baseline) divided by the standard deviation of the PreCS activity.

Analysis of slow wave frequencies used a zero crossing program that measured the period between successive positive-going baseline crossings in the EEG, converted this to frequency, and accumulated the number of waves in each frequency during a 2-min sample. The records were band-pass filtered from 0.1-22 Hz for this analysis. The NM extension response was measured with a transducer connected to a nylon loop in the nictitating membrane. The output was recorded on magnetic tape with the neuronal records of each trial. In analysis, the NM activity was digitized at 3 msec intervals and stored as an average response along with the 8 trial averages of unit activity. Subjects were trained to a criterion of 8 conditioned responses (CRs) in 9 consecutive trials, or for a maximum of 4 training sessions. A CR was defined as ½ mm of NM extension prior to UCS onset or, on test trials, within 500 msec of CS onset.

Results and Discussion

The analysis of hippocampal EEG frequencies led to a completely unexpected finding: a 2 min baseline sample of spontaneous EEG, recorded prior to training, predicted the subsequent rate of NM conditioning. Noticing a systematic difference in the shape of frequency histograms between fast- and slow-learning subjects, we correlated the number of trials to reach asymptotic criterion (TTC) with the amount of activity in successive frequencies from 2 to 22 Hz. Table 1 shows the coefficients obtained in this analysis. Since

Table 1. Correlations Between EEG Frequencies and Trials to Criterion

Hz	from	2	4	6	8	10	12	14	18
	to	4	6	8	10	12	14	18	22
r		-.33	-.50[a]	-.39	+.61	+.45	+.59	+.68[b]	+.60

Sum of 2-8 Hz: r = -.66

Sum of 8-22 Hz: r = +.64

High/Low Ratio: r = +.72

[a] $r_{.05}$ = .497.

[b] $r_{.01}$ = .623.

trials to criterion is the inverse of learning rate, the negative correlations relate 2-8 Hz activity with faster learning (r = -.66), while the total of higher frequencies (8-22 Hz) predicted slower learning (r = +.64). An index of the overall distribution of EEG frequencies, the proportion of high to low, was significantly correlated with TTC (r = +.72), as shown in the scatterplot in Figure 1.

There is a striking correspondence between the change in the type (sign) of correlation at or near 8 Hz that we found and the discovery of pharmacologically distinct systems controlling hippocampal EEG in rats and rabbits. Briefly, Vanderwolf and his colleagues (1978) have shown that hippocampal activity below 7 Hz can be blocked by atropine but not urethane, while activity from 7 to about 12 Hz is unaffected by atropine but blocked by urethane. Our data provide support for this dichotomy on behavioral grounds. Operation of the atropine-sensitive system correlates with rapid CR acquisition, while the presence of frequencies not blocked by atropine (8-22 Hz) predicts slower learning. Figure 2 (top row) illustrates the average frequency histograms for fast (column 1; less than 120 TTC; N = 3), medium (col. 2; 120-240 TTC; N = 9), and slow learners (col. 3; more than 240 TTC; N = 4). Note the clear reduction in 2-8 Hz activity across groups and the corresponding increase in higher frequencies.

The bottom row in Figure 2 shows the mean histograms for fast, medium, and slow groups derived from a 2-min sample taken at the end of the training session in which each subject reached criterion.

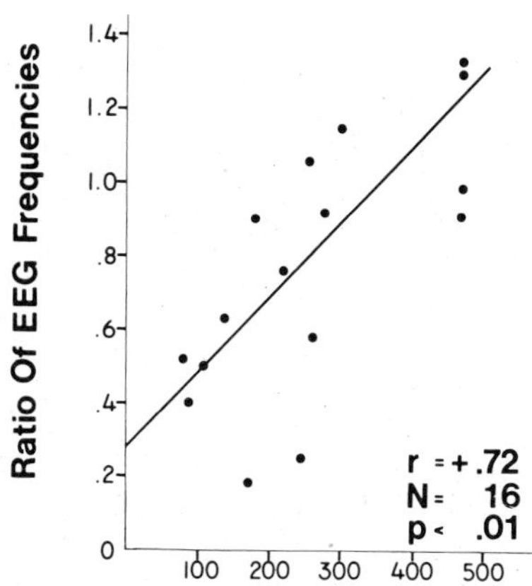

Figure 1. Scatterplot showing the relationship between trials to criterion and a ratio index of EEG frequencies.

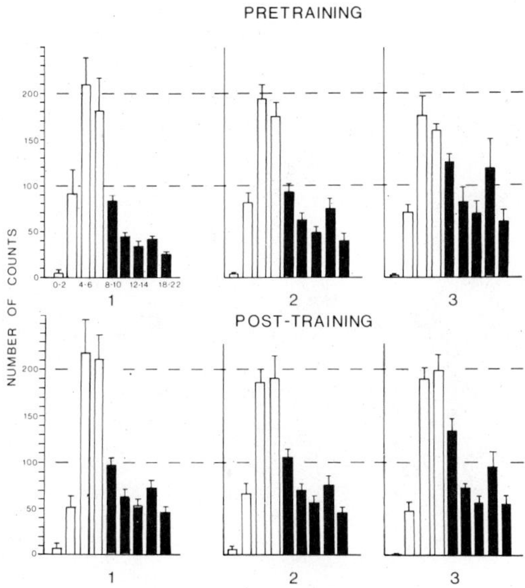

Figure 2. Averaged frequency histograms for animals grouped according to learning rate. (White bars: 0-2, 2-4, 4-6, 6-8 Hz; Black bars: 8-10, 10-12, 12-14, 14-18, 18-22 Hz.)

The differences between groups are not as strong as above, a fact borne out in the lack of correlation (r = .01) between the post-criterion frequency index (defined above) and TTC. Evaluation of slow wave changes across training showed that there were between-groups differences in the type of change observed, with the fast- and slow-learning subjects actually shifting in opposite directions. Figure 3 shows "difference histograms" derived by subtracting the pretraining EEG sample from the post-criterion frequency histogram. On the left are the differences in total 2-8 Hz and 8-22 Hz activity for the 3 learning-rate groups. Note the opposite changes in groups 1 _vs_ 3. On the right, the pre-post changes are shown for each frequency category, again illustrating the qualitative difference in the type of shift seen. In order to correlate the type of EEG shift with each subject's behavior, we computed the EEG frequency index (high/low ratio) for the post-criterion sample, and subtracted the pretraining index from it. We then correlated this new value, the "EEG ratio difference," with TTC. Figure 4 is a scatterplot showing the strength of the EEG shift-TTC relationship (r = -.86). It is interesting to note that several subjects showed no shift in EEG index across training. (Four unpaired control animals also showed no consistent shift during 2 sessions of CS and UCS presentations.) The occurrence of such different EEG changes in one species during one task, and their correlation with learning _rate_, may help explain some of the differing reports concerning hippocampal EEG changes across training (Adey, 1966; Coleman and Lindsley, 1977; Grastyan et al., 1959).

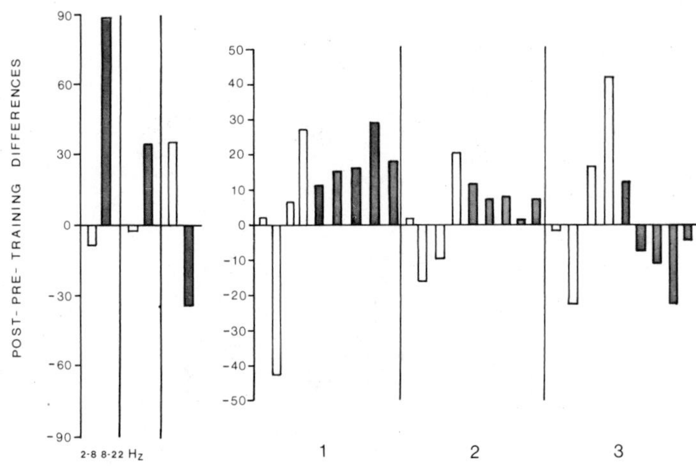

Figure 3. Pretraining vs post-criterion differences in EEG frequencies for (1) fast, (2) medium, and (3) slow learning subjects. Left, differences in the 2-8 Hz and 8-22 Hz totals for each group; right, differences in individual frequency categories.

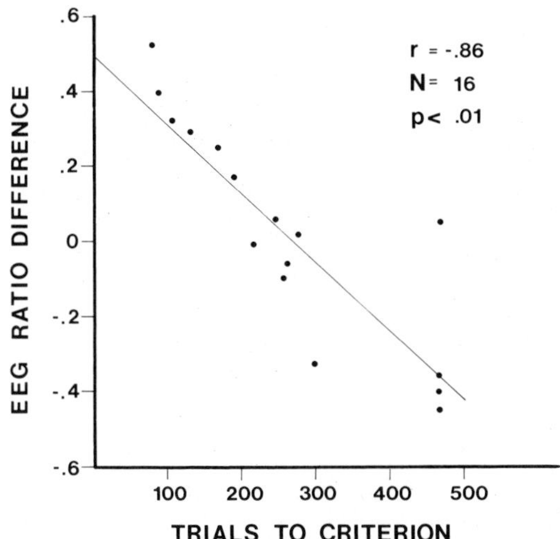

Figure 4. Scatterplot of the relationship (r = -.86) between TTC and the frequency shift in hippocampal EEG across training.

The examination of multiple unit activity with respect to the learning rate of individual subjects indicated that the EEG predictors of behavioral learning also predicted the growth of unit activity in the hippocampus. Figure 5 illustrates the differences in multiple unit standard scores for the 3 groups on the last day of training. The scores are for the last 125 msec of the CS period (left) and the first 125 msec of the UCS period, times during which conditioned responses were most likely. It is interesting to note that some animals not displaying a great increase in standard scores across training still performed at post-criterion levels behaviorally. That is, the Day 2 and 3 criterion groups were performing learned behaviors even though their standard scores were significantly lower than those of faster learning animals. These data reflect the differences seen throughout training in the responsiveness of hippocampal cells to the conditioning stimuli, differences that were predicted, along with learning rate, by the state of hippocampal EEG prior to the start of training. Since standard scores reflect mean activity change divided by baseline variability, these lowered standard scores during training could be due to either a lack of responsiveness or an increase in variability of hippocampal cells (both have been observed). The fast learning group had the greatest mean percent increase in multiple unit firing, accompanied by the lowest mean standard deviation in the baseline period. This was reversed in the slowest group, with the median group falling between. Thus, the differences in unit activity reflected a combination of responsiveness and variability.

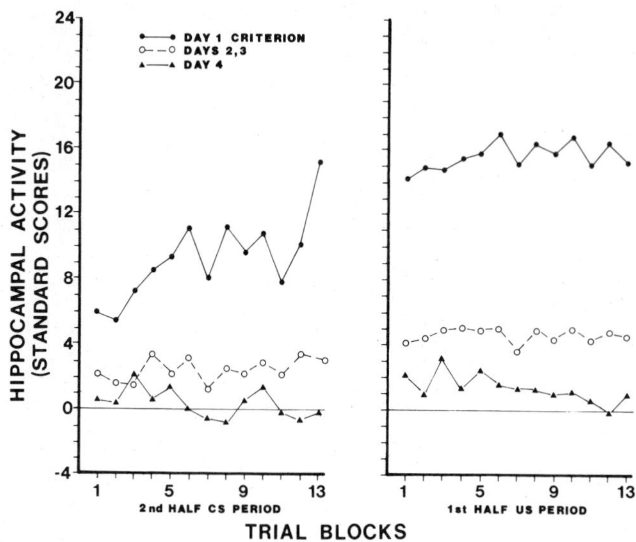

Figure 5. Standard scores of multiple unit activity for 13 blocks of trials on the last day of training for the fast (Day 1 criterion), medium (Days 2, 3), and slow (Day 4) groups. Each point represents an 8-trial average score for the change in activity during the last ½ (125 msec) of the CS period or the first ½ (125 msec) of the UCS period.

Figure 6 illustrates the type of histogram variability that can be seen in slow-learning subjects. Shown are consecutive 8-trial averages of multiple unit activity accompanying NM responses. In each trace, the cursors indicate (left) tone onset and (right) air puff onset. Note the variability across blocks in the amount of PreCS activity (baseline) and the presence of a clear post-UCS response in most, but not all, averages. This pattern illustrates both variability and below-normal responsivity of hippocampal activity in this animal, who failed to reach criterion in 468 trials.

In examining the way in which EEG frequencies relate to unit activity, we found a relationship between the EEG frequency index and the PreCS standard deviation. Although not significant ($r = +.274$, $N = 15$), this statistic suggests a positive relationship between EEG frequencies and variability of baseline unit activity. This variability (as reflected in baseline S.D.) also correlated with the percent increase in unit activity during both the tone ($r = -.379$) and air puff periods ($r = -.394$). Finally, the magnitude of unit response to the tone CS was a highly significant negative correlate of trials to criterion ($r = -.668$, $N = 15$, $p < .01$).

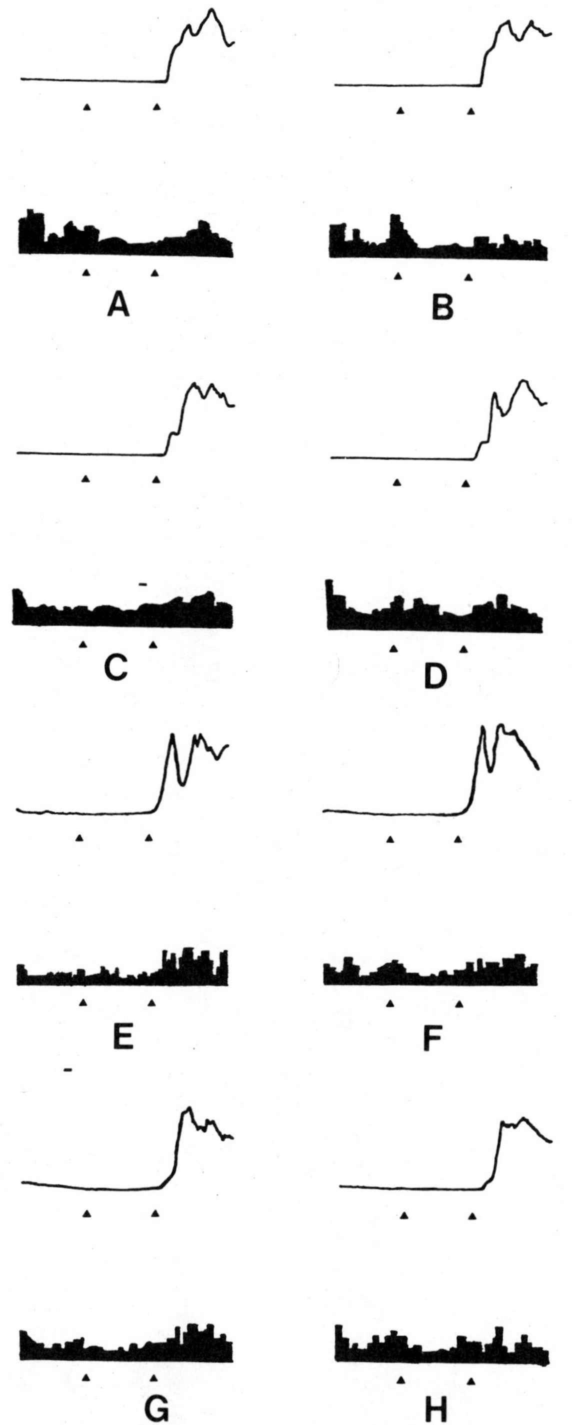

Figure 6. Unit histogram variability (see text for details).

Thus, the mechanism by which hippocampal EEG predicts learning rate may be that it corresponds to (a) greater variability in the background rate of unit activity which, in turn, predicts (b) reduced responsiveness to the conditioning stimuli, leading to (c) slower acquisition.

EXPERIMENT 2

Methods

The subjects were 7 New Zealand White rabbits given the same surgical and training treatments as in experiment 1, with the exception that they received small, electrolytic lesions of the medial septal nucleus during the surgical implantation of the hippocampal recording electrodes. Lesion current was 0.8-1.0 ma for 8-10 sec, through a stainless steel electrode insulated except for 0.2 mm at the tip. Controls were 7 of the subjects from experiment 1 that were being trained at the same time as the lesion group.

Results and Discussion

Medial septal lesions were very small (see Berry and Thompson, 1979) in order to insure that the lateral septal region was fully spared (i.e., leaving subcortical hippocampal output intact). As a result, the disruption of hippocampal EEG was significant, but lower frequencies were still present as shown by averaged pretraining histograms (see Figure 7). The frequency index used to predict learning in experiment 1 differed significantly between groups [$t_{(11)} = 2.42$, $p < .05$]. The behavioral effect of these lesions was a delay in the appearance of conditioned responses (see Berry and Thompson, 1979), a type of behavioral deficit seen in NM conditioning following electrical disruption of the hippocampus (Salafia and Allan, 1980), cholinergic blockade of the septum (Solomon and Gottfried, 1981), or systemic drug treatments that probably disrupt hippocampal EEG (Moore et al., 1976). Briefly, these disruptions do not prevent conditioning completely, but they significantly prolong the phase of training prior to emergence of conditioned responses. Other experiments on the effects of septal lesions on rabbit conditioning provide mixed results. Lockhart and Moore (1975) found no behavioral effect on acquisition (but poorer discrimination performance), while Powell et al. (1976) found both impaired acquisition and poor discrimination performance. In both studies, the lesions were larger than those reported here, and the Powell et al. study used a slightly different behavior, the corneoretinal potential.

Medial septal lesions also attenuated the responses of hippocampal cells, as reflected by lower standard scores of multiple unit activity (see Figure 8). During the CS period, several subjects in

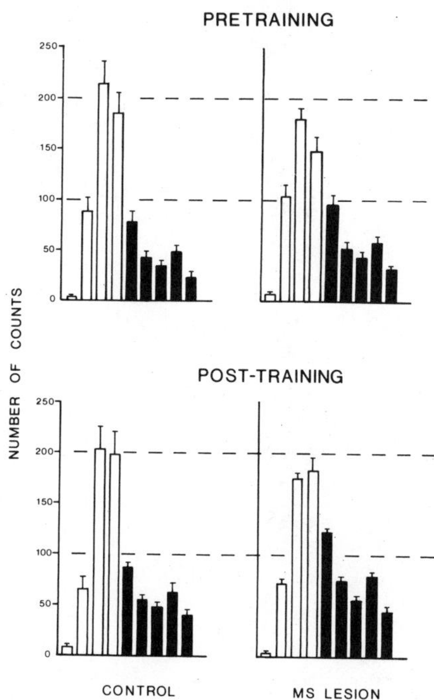

Figure 7. Average hippocampal EEG frequency histograms from two-min samples recorded just prior to training and at the end of the session in which criterion was reached. Histograms on the left are from controls, those on the right from the septal lesion group.

the septal group showed slightly suppressed activity in response to the tone, and none showed normal levels of response to either stimulus. One interesting effect of medial septal lesions was an increase in the variability of the baseline rate of unit activity. The standard deviation of the prestimulus period was almost twice (185%) that of the control group. Since hippocampal activity is normally related to the rate of learning, it is possible that this variability was a factor in the slowing of the learning process.

GENERAL DISCUSSION

The major findings in these two experiments underscore the involvement of the hippocampus in rabbit NM conditioning. First, the distribution of frequencies in the hippocampal EEG in a pre-training sample predicts not only the responsiveness of cells, but also predicts the behavioral rate of learning. Changes in EEG frequencies across training are also highly related to the rate of

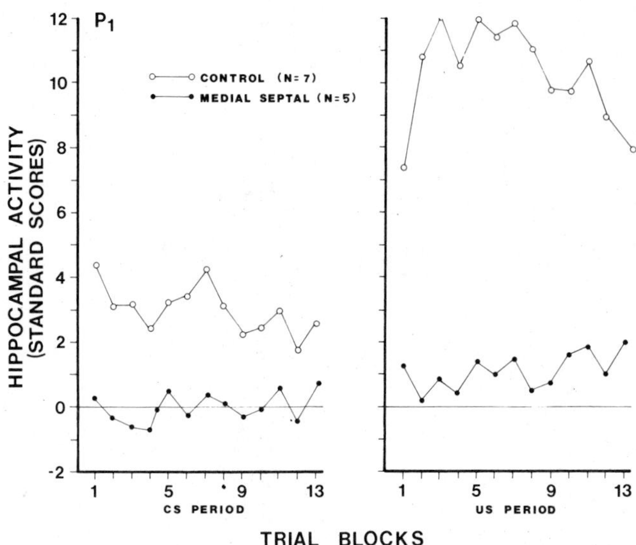

Figure 8. Standard scores of hippocampal unit activity during CS and UCS periods on the first day of training for animals in the control and medial septal lesion groups.

conditioning, with fast and slow learners showing opposite shifts. Second, manipulations of hippocampal activity (as exemplified by the medial septal lesions used here) tend to retard, but not always prevent, acquisition of a classically conditioned response in the rabbit. Interestingly, the form of the impairment is usually a delay in the appearance of conditioned responses, followed by a relatively normal increase to asymptotic levels. This form of disruption suggests a role for the hippocampus in the early stages of conditioning, termed phase 1 in Prokasy's (1972) two-phase model of conditioning. The finding of increased variability in baseline unit activity presents a possible mechanism for the disruptive effects of these small lesions.

Our conclusion from this pattern of results is that our measures reflect some type of arousal or attentional processes, rather than learning or memory itself. The major reasons for this conclusion are (1) the predictive measure is recorded prior to training, i.e., there are no stimuli to remember; (2) posttraining correlations show a relationship between EEG shift and rate of learning, not its occurrence or absence; and (3) the lesions retard acquisition rate, but do not prevent learning from taking place. Our data on unit responsiveness are compatible with a "tuning out irrelevant stimuli" function for the hippocampal formation (Solomon, 1979), although they fit equally well with a schema using the hippocampus to enhance the salience of biologically important stimuli.

Although the hypothesized role of hippocampal EEG in movement systems (Vanderwolf, 1975) does not easily fit our data, it raises an interesting issue. His finding of a relationship between hippocampal EEG frequencies and modes of behavior suggests that our findings might have been due to the fact that the EEG reflected the occurrence of incompatible, or competing, behaviors that interfere with the rate of NM conditioning. On the other hand, if EEG in the 8-22 Hz range reflects an attentional or arousal process that normally accompanies movements (whereas 2-8 Hz EEG reflects a non-movement attention process), our prediction of rabbit conditioning based on EEG frequencies could have been due to slower-learning animals being in an improper (movement-related) attentive state for learning a response under conditions of restraint. The concept of movement-specific arousal states was suggested by Schwartzbaum (1975), who found that the responses of reticular formation units, presumably involved in arousal, were constrained by qualitative aspects of ongoing behavior (i.e., immobility). Kandel (1980) has also suggested a refinement of the arousal concept to include response modes, citing data indicating that not all behaviors are affected equally by "arousing" stimulation. In *Aplysia*, noxious stimuli that enhance siphon withdrawal depress biting, whereas food stimuli that depress siphon withdrawal enhance biting. Thus, at least two types of arousal may occur in *Aplysia*, each occurring in conjunction with a different response mode. A similar relationship between arousal and movement may exist in mammals. If rabbit hippocampal EEG frequencies differ with respect to various movement-related arousal (or attentional) states, correlations with both movements *and* learning rate would be expected.

The issue of why hippocampal EEG activity predicts NM acquisition rate is still an open question. Experiments with the possible contributions of competing responses and multiple arousal systems in mind should be done. We are currently studying further manipulations of septo-hippocampal activity during NM conditioning and have begun to examine hippocampal activity during appetitive learning.

ACKNOWLEDGMENTS

I would like to thank Richard F. Thompson for his support and guidance throughout these experiments and for critique of some of the ideas in this paper. I also thank Cathy Berry for illustrations, and Celia Oliver and Betty Marak for assistance with the manuscript. The research projects and preparation of this manuscript were supported in part by grants to Richard F. Thompson from NSF (BMS 7500453), NIH (NS12268 and MH26530), and the McKnight Foundation. Additional support (to S.D.B.) came in the form of postdoctoral fellowship 5 F32 MH05052, and grants from the Miami University Faculty Research Committee.

REFERENCES

Adey, W. R., 1966, Neurophysiological correlates of information transaction and storage in brain tissue, in: "Progress in Physiological Psychology" (Vol. I), E. Stellar and J. M. Sprague, eds., Academic Press, New York.

Bennett, T. L., 1975, The electrical activity of the hippocampus and processes of attention, in: "The Hippocampus" (Vol. 2), R. L. Isaacson and K. H. Pribram, eds., Plenum Press, New York.

Berger, T. W., and Thompson, R. F., 1978, Neuronal plasticity in the limbic system during classical conditioning of the rabbit nictitating membrane response. I. The hippocampus, Brain Res., 145:323-346.

Berry, S. D., and Thompson, R. F., 1977, Hippocampal EEG predictors of learning rate in rabbits, Soc. Neurosci. Abstr., 3:230.

Berry, S. D., and Thompson, R. F., 1979, Medial septal lesions retard classical conditioning of the nictitating membrane response in rabbits, Science, 205:209-2111

Berry, S. D., and Thompson, R. F., 1978, Prediction of learning rate from the hippocampal electroencephalogram, Science, 200: 1298-1300.

Berry, S. D., and Thompson, R. F., 1982, Interrelations among hippocampal EEG activity, hippocampal unit activity, and medial septal nuclei in classical conditioning of the rabbit nictitating membrane response (in preparation).

Coleman, J. R., and Lindsley, D. B., 1977, Behavioral and hippocampal electrical changes during operant learning in cats and effects of stimulating two hypothalamic-hippocampal systems, EEG Clin. Neurophysiol., 42:309-331.

Gormezano, I., 1966, Classical conditioning, in: "Experimental Methods and Instrumentation in Psychology," J. B. Sidowski, ed., McGraw-Hill, New York.

Grastyan, E., Lissak, K., Madarasz, L., and Donhoffer, H., 1959, Hippocampal electrical activity during the development of conditioned reflexes, EEG Clin. Neurophysiol., 11:409-430.

Kandel, E. R., 1980, Cellular insights into the multivariant nature of arousal, in: "Neural Mechanisms in Behavior," D. McFadden, ed., Springer-Verlag, New York.

Lockhart, M., and Moore, J. W., 1975, Classical differential and operant conditioning in rabbits (Oryctolagus cuniculus) with septal lesions, J. Comp. Physiol. Psychol., 88:147-154.

Moore, J. W., Goodell, N. A., and Solomon, P. R., 1976, Central cholinergic blockade by scopolamine and habituation, classical conditioning, and latent inhibition of the rabbit's nictitating membrane response, Physiol. Psychol., 4:395-399.

Olds, J., Disterhoft, J. F., Segal, M., Kornblith, C. L., and Hirsh, R., 1972, Learning centers of rat brain mapped by measuring latencies of conditioned unit responses, J. Neurophysiol., 35:202-219.

Phillips, J., Eichenbaum, H., and Kuperstein, M., 1980, Hippocampal unit activity related to sensory, motor, and EEG events during odor discrimination learning, Soc. Neurosci. Abstr., 6:425.

Powell, D. A., Milligan, W. L., and Buchanan, S. L., 1976, Orienting and classical conditioning in the rabbit (Oryctolagus cuniculus): Effects of septal lesions, Physiol. Behav., 17:955-962.

Prokasy, W. F., 1972, Developments with the two-phase model applied to human eyelid conditioning, in: "Classical Conditioning (Vol. II) Current Research and Theory," A. H. Black and W. F. Prokasy, eds., Appleton-Century-Crofts, New York.

Salafia, W. R., and Allan, A. M., 1980, Conditioning and latent inhibition with electrical stimulation of hippocampus, Physiol. Psychol., 8:247-253.

Schwartzbaum, J. S., 1975, Interrelationships among multiunit activity of the midbrain reticular formation and lateral geniculate nucleus, thalamocortical arousal, and behavior in rats, J. Comp. Physiol. Psychol., 89:131-157.

Solomon, P. R., 1979, Temporal versus spatial information processing views of hippocampal function, Psych. Bull., 86:1272-1279.

Solomon, P. R., and Gottfried, K. E., 1981, The septo-hippocampal cholinergic system and classical conditioning of the rabbit's nictitating membrane response, J. Comp. Physiol. Psychol., in press.

Vanderwolf, C. H., Kramis, R., Gillespie, L. A., and Bland, B. H., 1975, Hippocampal rhythmic slow activity and neocortical low-voltage fast activity: Relations to behavior, in: "The Hippocampus" (Vol. 2), R. L. Isaacson and K. H. Pribram, eds., Plenum Press, New York.

Vanderwolf, C. H., Kramis, R., and Robinson, T. E., 1978, Hippocampal electrical activity during waking behavior and sleep: Analyses using centrally acting drugs, in: "Functions of the Septo-Hippocampal System," CIBA Foundation Symposium 58, Elsevier, New York.

ANALYZING THE RABBIT NM CONDITIONED REFLEX ARC

John F. Disterhoft, Michael T. Shipley and Nina Kraus[1]

Department of Cell Biology and Anatomy
Northwestern University Medical School
Chicago, Illinois 60611

SUMMARY

The nictitating membrane (NM) conditioned reflex arc in rabbit is being analyzed with neurophysiological recording and anatomical tracing techniques. Current studies focus on the tone conditioned stimulus (CS) afferent pathway and the NM extension conditioned response (CR) output motoneurons. Studies are underway to locate and characterize CS-CR linkage regions at the brainstem level.

Single neurons in rabbit auditory association cortex have been monitored during the course of nictitating membrane conditioning. Tone CS evoked unit activity was compared before and after behavioral acquisition. Units from pseudoconditioned rabbits and from rabbits which did not acquire the conditioned response served as controls. The conditioned rabbits had more than twice as many significantly altered responses (51% vs. 19%) during the 250 msec CS-US interval. The whole CS evoked response, or components of it, either increased or decreased. Most changes occurred with a latency of 21-40 msec. Some were as early as 11-20 msec, the latency at which tone information reaches auditory cortex in the naive, conscious rabbit. Auditory cortex unit changes were not evident in the trial sequence until after behavioral acquisition.

The output motoneurons for NM extension have been localized in accessory abducens nucleus with HRP retrograde tracing from the retractor bulbi muscles (whose contraction causes NM extension). Coagulation of the abducens nerve branch traveling to the lateral rectus muscle, with the branch to retractor bulbi left intact, indicated that there may be a few abducens motoneurons which send axons to retractor bulbi. But the primary locus of the motoneurons is clearly accessory abducens. Accessory abducens motoneurons were also shown to be strongly acetylcholinesterase positive, as are other brainstem and spinal motoneurons.

INTRODUCTION

Our physiological and anatomical analyses of rabbit nictitating membrane (NM) conditioning are aimed at delineating the processes and circuitry underlying the acquisition of this simple association at the cellular level. Previous multiple unit recording studies have cast considerable light on neural correlates of the learning process in various brain regions (Buchwald, Halas and Schramm, 1966; Olds, et al., 1972; Disterhoft and Olds, 1972; Oleson, Ashe and Weinberger, 1976; Segal, 1975; Gabriel, 1975; Berger, Alger and Thompson, 1976; Disterhoft and Stuart, 1976; Birt, Nienhuis and Olds, 1979). This work has given us "boundary conditions" which can guide better focused, single cell recording studies. For example, we might expect "lemniscal adjunct" sensory regions to be very much involved in early stages of associative learning. Specifically, posterior nucleus of thalamus (Olds, et al., 1972; Disterhoft and Stuart, 1976) and magnocellular portions of medial geniculate (Ryugo and Weinberger, 1978; Weinberger, 1979) are thalamic auditory lemniscal adjunct regions where multiple unit studies have demonstrated considerable plasticity in sensory input processing during conditioning. We have examined single units in auditory association cortex, to which these thalamic regions project (Winer, Diamond, and Raczkowski, 1977), during NM conditioning.

In order to map out the circuit by which the NM conditioned reflex arc is formed, we must link up the tone CS input pathway with the output motoneurons causing NM extension. Our first step has been to anatomically locate and characterize the neurons in accessory abducens nucleus which are the principle source of axons to the retractor bulbi muscles. Retractor bulbi contraction pulls the eyeball back into the orbit and causes NM extension as a passive result (Cegavske, Harrison, and Torigoe, 1981). We have some working hypotheses about how the auditory CS and corneal air puff US are linked up with the NM conditioned response output motoneurons at the brainstem level which guide our ongoing studies.

AUDITORY ASSOCIATION CORTEX

Previous work showed that multiple units in auditory cortex demonstrate "response plasticity" to an invariant acoustic stimulus as that CS gains behavioral significance during learning (Buchwald, Halas and Schramm, 1966; Halas, Beardsley and Sandlie, 1970; Olds, et al., 1972; Disterhoft and Stuart, 1976; Oleson, Ashe, and

Weinberger, 1976). The alterations observed were generally increases in the number of CS-evoked spikes as learning progressed. Auditory cortex single unit studies done in previously conditioned cats (Woody, et al., 1976; Kitzes, Farley and Starr, 1978) and primates (Miller, et al., 1972; Beaton and Miller, 1975; Hocherman, et al., 1976; Benson and Heinz, 1978; Benson, Heinz and Goldstein, 1979; Pfingst and O'Connor, 1981) have shown much greater variation in the patterns of neuronal response plasticity to a behaviorally significant auditory stimulus (i.e., responses increased or decreased in whole or in part) than did the multiple unit work. The variability observed in the single unit studies seemed more consistent with the "lability" of responsivity which has been reported for single units in auditory cats cortex of conscious primates (Merzenich and Brugge, 1973), cats (Goldstein, 1975) and rabbits (Kraus and Disterhoft, 1981a).

Our study of single neurons in rabbit auditory association cortex during the course of NM conditioning (Kraus and Disterhoft, 1981b) was an attempt to bridge the gap between the previous multiple unit and single unit studies done on auditory cortex in learning contexts. We wished to determine if the CS evoked response changes in single neurons during learning were relatively heterogeneous or homogeneous; to assess how many neurons exhibited plasticity; and to get an idea when auditory cortex began showing changes in the trial sequence.

Methods

Albino rabbits were prepared by surgically implanting restraining headbolts and placing a recording chamber over auditory association cortex. After recovery from surgery, each rabbit was given 2 hour habituation sessions on two successive days. The rabbit was placed in a cloth bag, his head was bolted to a bar attached to a stereotaxic, and his body strapped down for restraint. Corneal air puffs to elicit the NM unconditioned response were presented at intervals which varied from 20 to 100 sec and averaged 60 sec.

On the conditioning day, the rabbit was again restrained. A tungsten microelectrode was driven into auditory cortex with a hydraulic microdrive system controlled from outside the acoustically isolated recording chamber. A standard amplication system and amplitude-time window discriminator were used. Pure tone and white noise search stimuli were delivered to the ear contralateral to the recording chamber, through a closed concentric sound system which used a dynamic earphone for stimulus transduction and incorporated a probe tube for measuring sound intensity (Kraus and Disterhoft, 1981a). The sound delivery tube passed through a silastic insert molded to fit the rabbit's external auditory meatus and terminated close to the tympanic membrane. The ipsilateral ear was plugged with a silastic earmold.

A unit was isolated and its best frequency was determined. The pure tone CS frequency was set at the neuron's best frequency at 80 db re 20 $\mu N/m^2$. NM conditioning was done with procedures described previously (Disterhoft, Kwan and Lo, 1977). The CS was 400 msec long and the air puff was 150 msec long. During conditioning, the CS-US interval was 250 msec and the stimuli terminated simultaneously. The intertrial intervals varied randomly and averaged 60 sec. 100 conditioning trials were given. During the pseudoconditioning control procedures, 100 tones and 100 puffs were presented in a random, unpaired fashion at intertrial intervals averaging 30 sec. NM extension was measured with an infrared light reflection transducer.

Complete behavioral and neural data were obtained from 35 neurons in 35 rabbits during conditioning. One neuron was studied per rabbit because the animals were naive only once. Twenty-six neurons were recorded from 4 rabbits during pseudoconditioning. A second serendipitous control group consisted of 15 neurons recorded from 9 rabbits which did not acquire the conditioned response.

PST histograms were constructed for each neuron in the conditioning group in relation to the trial-by-trial course of acquisition. "Initial trials" were the last 20 trials when a CR occurred less than 20% of the time. "Trained" trials began with the 11th CR. The CR usually occurred more than 80% of the time in this 20 trial group. Previous behavioral work had shown that the trial of the 10th CR is a useful index of asymptotic NM acquisition during the first training day (Frey and Butler, 1973; Disterhoft, Kwan and Lo, 1977). Our present studies confirmed this. T-tests were used to compare the significance of changes in the neuronal responses (PST histograms) between initial and final trials. There were no behaviorally defined break points in the pseudoconditioning and nonlearning control groups, so these neurons were randomly matched to a conditioning neuron for determining trial intervals.

Results

Conditioning units showed more than twice as many significant changes as the pseudoconditioning units in the CS-US interval as a whole(51% vs. 19%)and in its early (0-60 msec, 46 vs. 15%) and late (60-250 msec, 43% vs. 23%) components when the "initial" and "trained" trial groups were compared. The latency to onset of CS evoked changes in the conditioning group were concentrated in the 21-40 msec time period. The earliest changes occurred at 11-20 msec, the shortest latency of cortical neuron response to tone onset in the naive, alert rabbit (Kraus and Disterhoft, 1981a). The animals that did not learn showed percentages similar to the pseudoconditioning group. Spontaneous rates during the background period varied little in both conditioning and pseudoconditioning groups (14% and 8%, respectively).

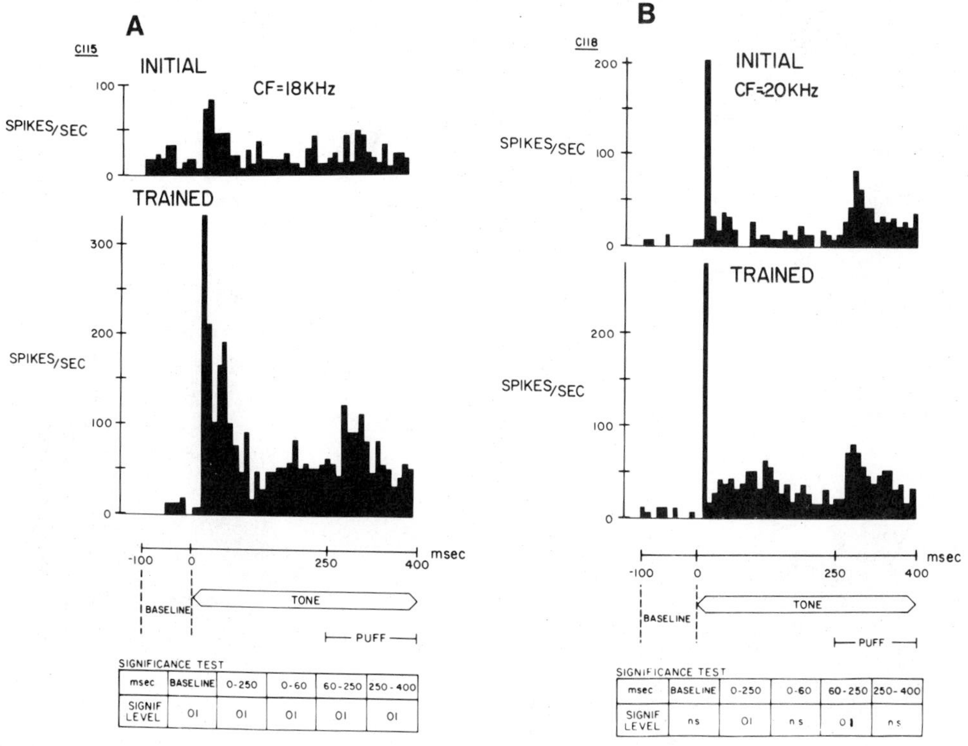

Fig. 1. Neural activity occurring during "initial" trials (rabbit behaviorally naive) is shown for comparison with that occurring during "trained" trials (CR has been learned). Each histogram consists of firing rate summed over 20 trials. The stimulus configuration and statistical changes in neural activity occurring during various components are illustrated. The CF of each unit is indicated. A. Generalized increase in CS-evoked firing rate with training. Note the accompanying decrease in spontaneous firing rate. B. Increase in CS-evoked activity selective to the late (60-250 msec) portion of the CS-US interval.

In most neurons that changed, the rate during the whole CS period either increased or decreased (Fig. 1A). In some neurons, only one component of the response changed (Fig. 1B). About the same number of neurons increased (47%) as decreased (53%) during the CS-US interval. We made a composite map of the conditioning neurons but could detect no tendency for changed neurons to group on the "Standard" cortical surface (Fig. 2).

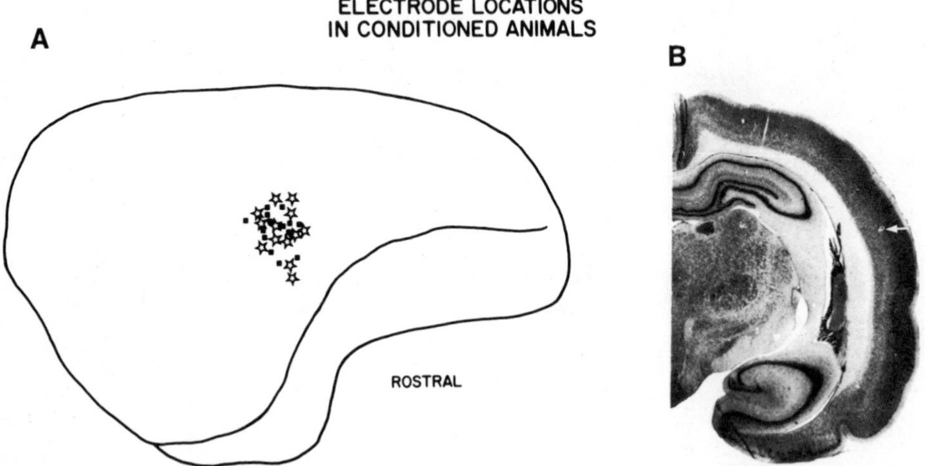

Fig. 2. A. Electrode locations in conditioned animals are shown on the lateral surface of the right cerebral hemisphere. Stars indicate neurons that showed significant changes in firing rate with learning. Dots mark the location of neurons that did not change. B. Coronal section of a rabbit's right hemisphere. An electrode lesion, located deep in the granular layer (IV), is indicated with an arrow.

Histograms were also constructed for the "transition" trials, the 20 trials between the "initial" and "trained" trial groups. No significant differences between conditioned and pseudoconditioned units were seen in this period. That is, auditory cortex neurons showed response plasticity only after the NM conditioned response had become well established. They tended to lag, rather than lead, behavioral acquisition.

Comments

Single neurons in auditory association cortex show a more heterogeneous pattern of change during tone signalled conditioning than the multiple unit data had suggested. Neurons either increased and decreased. The whole response, as well as individual components of it changed. These data agree with previous reports of single neurons recorded in auditory cortex of previously conditioned animals (Woody, et al., 1976; Kitzes, Farley and Starr, 1978). Importantly, not all neurons changed during conditioning. About 50% of the neurons we recorded changed, which was more than twice as many as in the pseudoconditioning group.

Neurons in auditory cortex showed response plasticity only after behavioral learning had been established. Decorticate rabbits can acquire the NM conditioned response (Oakley and Russell, 1972; Moore, et al., 1980), so we know _a priori_ that the cortex is not necessary for acquisition. But our data clearly indicate that auditory cortex neuron responses were related to the behavioral state of the rabbit. Response plasticity did not occur in the pseudoconditioned rabbits or in the animals which failed to acquire the response. In this sense, our data confirm the single unit data in previously trained primates, i.e., behavioral state or signal value affects neuronal processing of an auditory signal (Beaton and Miller, 1975; Hocherman, et al., 1976; Benson and Heinz, 1978; Pfingst, O'Connor and Miller, 1977; Pfingst and O'Connor, 1981). Our data also confirm the multiple unit studies which have shown that auditory cortex neurons tend to change after, not before, behavioral acquisition (Oleson, Ashe and Weinberger, 1975; Disterhoft and Stuart, 1976). We can also conclude that auditory cortex neurons change later than hippocampal neurons in the trial sequence, since neurons in hippocampus usually change before CR acquisition during NM conditioning (Thompson, 1980).

We predict that single neurons in posterior thalamus and magnocellular medial geniculate regions which project to auditory association cortex, will also be shown to precede cortex in the trial sequence of conditioning. Previous multiple unit studies in rat (Disterhoft and Olds, 1972; Disterhoft and Stuart, 1976; Birt, Nienhuis and Olds, 1978) and cat (Ryugo and Weinberger, 1978) support this assumption. We have also recently recorded neurons in external nucleus of inferior colliculus of rabbit. Some cells in this midbrain auditory structure change prior to NM acquisition in the trial sequence. External nucleus is a component of the lemniscal adjunct system which projects to posterior nucleus and magnocellular medial geniculate.

Hopkins and Weinberg (1980) have recently done a study of single neurons in auditory cortex of paralyzed cat during pupillary conditioning. Their conclusions, in regard to response change patterns, both increased and decreased changes, and overall percentage of neurons which change, are very similar to ours.

Finally, it is interesting to compare our findings with the sensory-sensory conditioning studies that Morrell and his colleagues have done in parastriate cortex in paralyzed cats and rabbits

(Morrell, 1967; Morrell, Hoepner, and de Toledo-Morrell, 1981). Although their paradigm has not related unit changes to behavioral learning, there are some intriguing parallels between our results. Morrell found neuronal alterations which were quite specific and varied among neurons. Components of, as well as whole responses, changed after sensory pairing. Response increments and decrements were seen. About the same percentage of neurons changed in the visual cortex (45% in their last study) as we found in the auditory cortex. Plastic neurons were observed to group together within columns in the visual cortex - we have no data on a possible columnar organization of plastic neurons in the auditory system since we only studied one neuron per rabbit. But it is appealing to think that the principles of sensory plasticity may be similar for both auditory and visual cortices.

NM FINAL OUTPUT MOTONEURONS

A complete analysis of the NM conditioned reflex arc requires a knowledge of its underlying neuroanatomical circuitry. We have started an experimental series using HRP to trace the arc in a retrograde fashion. Nictitating membrane (NM) extension is a passive result of eyeball retraction to corneal irritation (Cegavske, Harrison, and Torigoe, 1981). The retraction is caused by simultaneous contraction of four parallel muscles, the retractor bulbi. They arise in the rear of the orbit and insert into the sclera around the optic nerve, posterior to the insertions of the recti. Cegavske, et al. (1976) reported that multiple units in abducens nucleus fire in close correlation with NM extension and that section of the abducent nerve eliminated NM extension. They concluded, quite reasonably, that the final output motoneurons for NM extension lie in the abducens nucleus. We hypothesized that there well might be a specific subregion of abducens nucleus given over to retractor bulbi control. We injected horseradish peroxidase (HRP) into the retractor bulbi muscles in an attempt to delineate such a regional specialization (Disterhoft and Shipley, 1980).

→

Fig. 3. A. Coronal section through rabbit brainstem. Abducens nucleus (Abd), Accessory Abducens nucleus (Acc Abd), and Lateral Superior Olive (LSO) are indicated. Fascicles of nerve VI may be seen exiting toward the base of the brainstem. Bar = 0.5 mm. B. Polarized light (PL) photomicrograph at same level as 3A. HRP was injected into the Retractor Bulbi muscles (RB). Cells in Acc Abd nuclei are heavily labeled. Bar = 0.5 mm. C. Higher power, PL view of Abd shown in 3B. Bar = 0.1 mm. D. Higher power, PL view of Acc Abd shown in 3B. Bar = 0.1 mm.

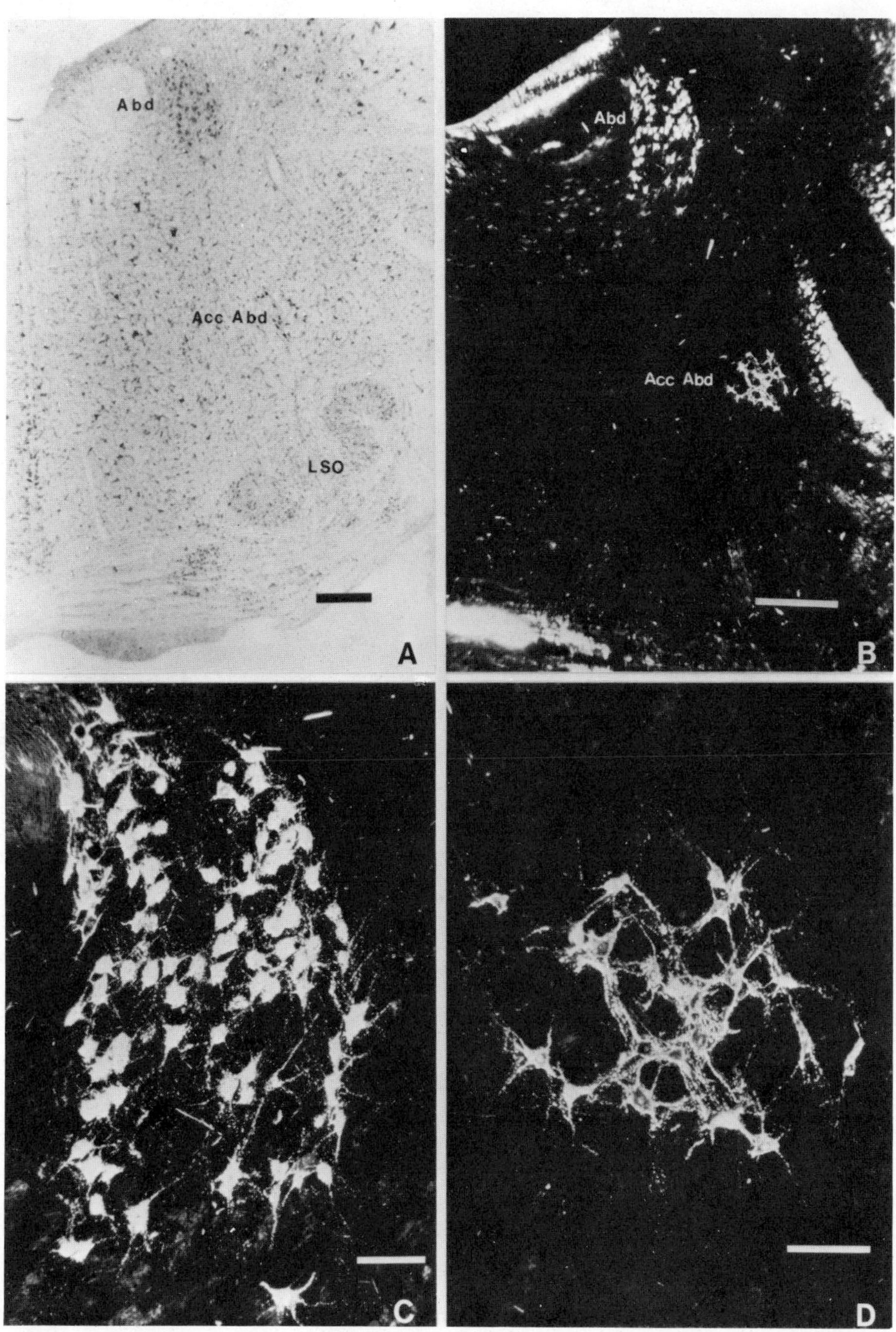
Abd
Acc Abd
LSO
A
Abd
Acc Abd
B
C
D

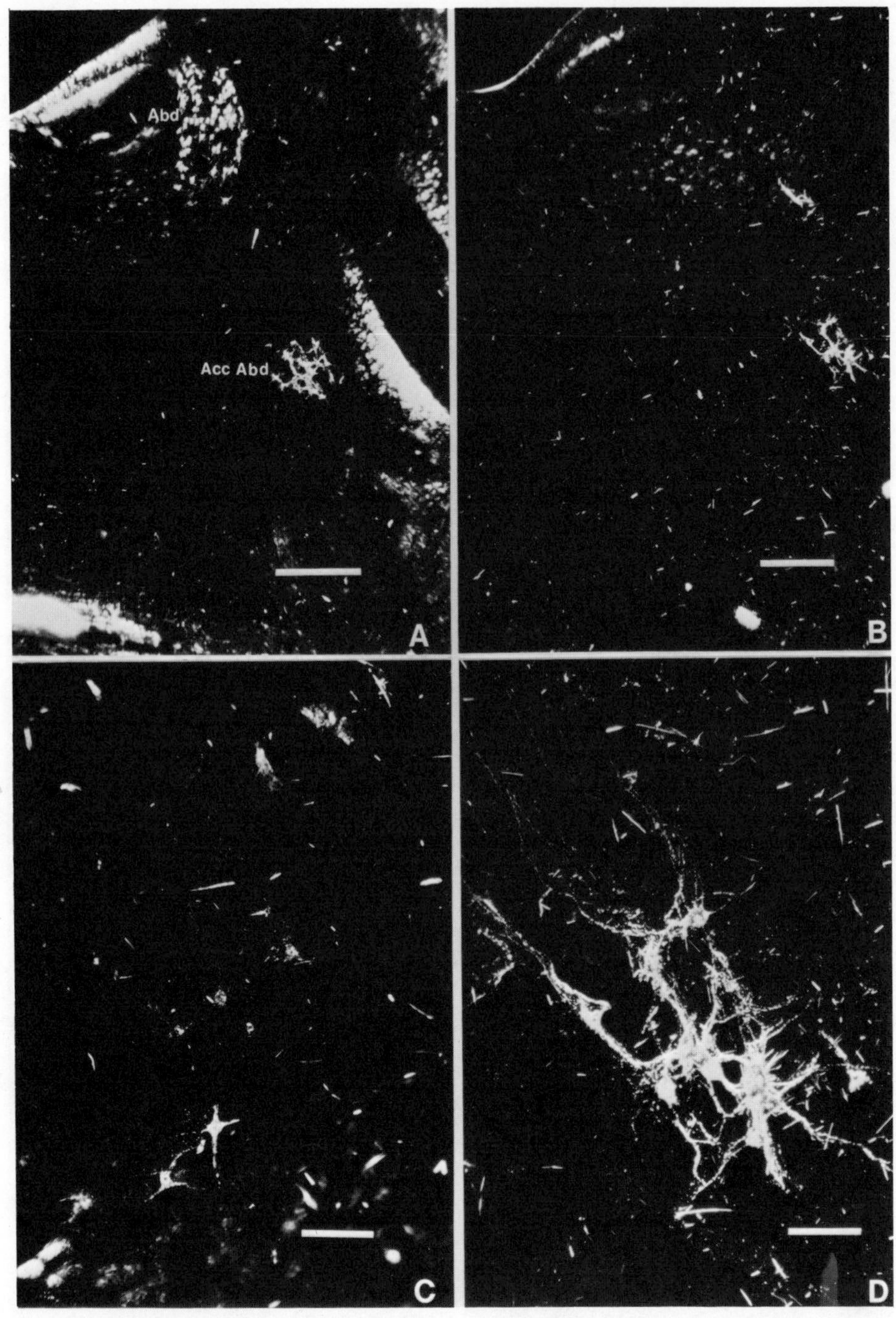
Abd
Acc Abd
A
B
C
D

Fig. 4. ← A. Normal: Polarized light (PL) view of coronal section similar to 3A showing HRP labeling after retractor bulbi (RB) injection in a non-cauterized rabbit. Both abducens (Abd) and Accessory Abducens (Acc Abd) are heavily labeled. Bar = 0.5 mm. B. Experimental: PL view showing retrograde HRP transport from RB after the abducens fibers going to lateral rectus had been cauterized. Labeling in Abd is very weak, only one or two cells show the profile-filling commonly seen in these preparations. (See 3A.) The labeling in Acc Abd nucleus is of normal intensity. Bar = 0.5 mm. C. PL view of labeling in Abd in 3B. This section contained the greatest number of labeled cells of any section through Abd. Bar = 0.1 mm. D. PL view of Acc Abd after cauterization. Labeling is normal for Acc Abd. (Compare with Fig. 3D.) Bar = 0.1 mm.

Methods

Fifteen male Dutch and 6 male albino rabbits were used. The retractor bulbi were exposed by incising the sclera, collapsing the eyeball and cutting the insertions of the other extraocular muscles. A 50% solution of HRP in 2% DMSO was injected into the retractor bulbi under visual control. The animals were sacrificed after 48 hours. Procedures for perfusion and tetramethylbenzidine (TMB) reactions were those described by Mesulam (1978).

Results

Accessory abducens nucleus motoneurons were, in fact, the most heavily and reliably labeled group after retractor bulbi injections. This nucleus is a concentrated group of large cells ventral and slightly caudal to the abducens nucleus and just dorsal to lateral superior olive. Axons from it course dorsal and rostrally through the manin abducens nucleus to exit the brainstem with the sixth nerve (Fig. 3).

Abducens motoneurons were also labeled after our retractor bulbi injections, but these abducens neurons may have been labeled by leakage of HRP from retractor bulbi into the region of lateral rectus. To test this possibility, we cauterized the lateral rectus before retractor bulbi injections in three experiments. After this procedure, abducens uptake was slight while accessory abducens labeling was complete (Fig 4).

Further supporting the idea that accessory abducens cells are the motoneurons for the retractor bulbi, we showed that they are as strongly acetylcholinesterase positive as other known motoneurons in the brainstem (Fig. 5).

Both nictitating membrane extension and eyelid closure occur as a defensive reflex response to irritating corneal stimuli. Thus another important group involved includes those motonerons innervating as a defensive reflex response to irritating coreal stimuli. Thus another important group involved includes those motoneurons innervating the orbicularis oculi muscle. A discrete group of motoneurons in the facial motor nucleus were filled following HRP injections into orbicularis oculi. They cluster as a dorsomedial cap in the facial nucleus. This region was shown previously to contain motoneurons of facial muscle aroun d the eye (Van Gehuchten, 1906).

Comments

These experiment show that motoneurons controlling NM extension are located primarily, if not exclusively, in accessory abducens nucleus. The fact that accessory abducens is involved in retractor bulbi control has been reported recently in both cat (Grant, et al., 1979; Huston, Glendenning and Masterton, 1979; Spencer, Baker and McCrea, 1980) and rabbit (Gray, et al., 1980;

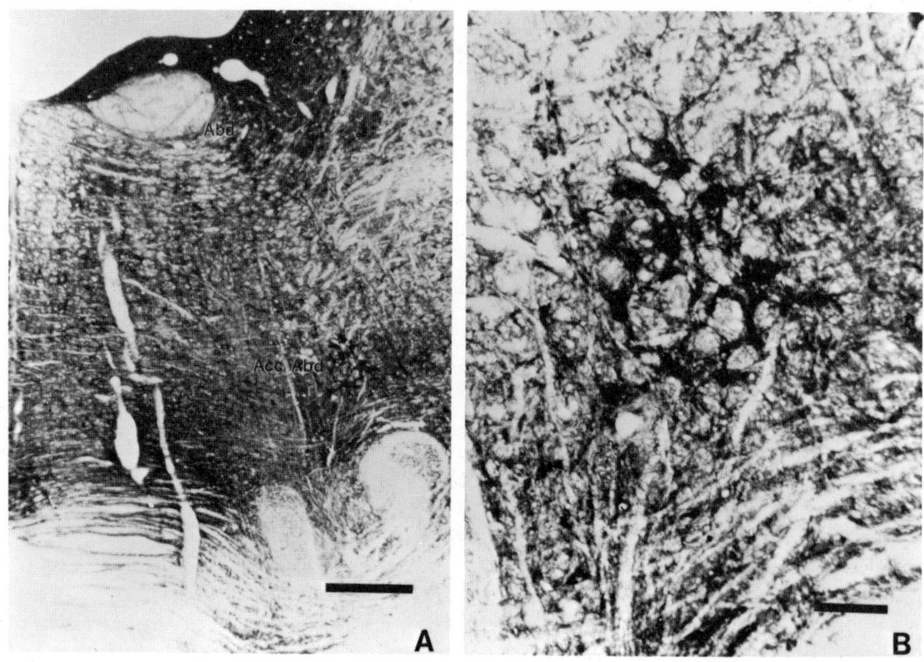

Fig. 5. Neurons in both Abd and Acc Abd are Acetylcholinesterase positive. A. Coronal section through the brainstem at the level of Abd and Acc Abd. LSO is clearly visible. (See Figure 3A for comparable cresyl section.) Bar = 0.5 mm. B. Higher power view of 5A showing the neurons in Acc Abd intensely stained for acetylcholinesterase. Bar = 0.1 mm.

Cegavske, Harrison, and Torigoe, 1981; Berthier, 1981). Experiments are underway to assess accessory abducens functional involvement in NM extension with physiological recording and with lesions of the nucleus. Our next step in this retrograde analysis of rabbit NM conditioning will be to inject HRP into the accessory abducens nucleus to determine its source of afferent input.

Conclusions

The data we have obtained thusfar in auditory cortex and brainstem indicate that rabbit nictitating membrane conditioning is an extremely useful system in which to explore the substrates of learning in mammalian brain. The data which Thompson and his colleagues have been gathering in hippocampus and limbic system give us further encouragement (Thompson, 1980).

We intend to concentrate our own work on circuit analysis of the substrates of simple, non-discriminative NM conditioning at the brainstem level. Chronically maintained decorticate and thalamic rabbits can acquire NM conditioned responses (Oakley and Russell, 1972; Enser, 1976; Moore, et al., 1980). Decorticate and precollicular decerebrate cats can form conditioned eyeblinks, a similarly simple conditioned response (Norman, et al., 1974, 1977). Therefore, the brainstem contains integrative circuitry sufficient for NM conditioning.

Our working hypothesis is that brainstem premotor, integrative regions exist which are necessary and perhaps sufficient to mediate NM conditioned reflex formation. These integrative regions must have access to tone CS and/or corneal air puff US information and project to the final output motoneurons in accessory abducens nucleus. We hypothesize further that these sites are located in brainstem reticular formation. We are attempting to use straightforward single unit recording and light microscopic pathway tracing techniques in an attempt to characterize the integrative regions which subserve this simple association.

ACKNOWLEDGEMENTS

This research was supported by NIH Grants 5 R01 NS 12317, 1 T32 MH 16097 and 2 S07 RR05370.

[1] Dr. Kraus is currently at Siegel Hearing Institute, Michael Reese Hospital, Chicago, IL 60616.

REFERENCES

Beaton, R., and Miller, J.M., 1975, Single cell activity in the auditory cortex of unanesthetized, behaving monkey: correlation with stimulus controlled behavior, Brain Res., 100:543-562.

Benson, D.A., and Heinz, R.D., 1978, Single unit activity in the auditory cortex of monkeys selectively attending left vs. right ear stimuli, Brain Res., 159:307-320.

Berger, T.W., Alger, B., and Thompson, R.F., 1976, Neuronal substrates of classical conditioning in the hippocampus, Science, 192:482-485.

Berthier, N.E., 1981, The unconditioned nictitating membrane response: The role of the abducens nerve and nucleus and the accessory abducens nucleus in rabbit, Doctoral Dissertation, University of Massachusetts, Amherst.

Birt, D., Nienhuis, R., and Olds, M., 1979, Separation of associative from non-associative short latency changes in medial geniculate and inferior colliculus during differential conditioning and reversal in rats, Brain Res., 167:129-139.

Buchwald, J.S., Halas, E.S., and Schramm, S., 1966, Changes in cortical and subcortical unit activity during behavioral conditioning, Physiol. and Behav., 1:11-22.

Cegavske, C.F., Harrison, T.A., and Torigoe, Y., 1981, Identification of the substrates of the unconditioned response in the classically conditioned, rabbit, nictitating membrane preparation, Submitted for publication.

Cegavske, C.F., Thompson, R.F., Patterson, M.M., and Gormezano, I., 1976, Mechanisms of efferent neuronal control of the reflex nictitating membrane response in rabbit (Oryctolagus cuniculus), J. Comp. Physiol. Psychol., 90:411-423.

Disterhoft, J.F., Kwan, H.H., and Lo, W.D., 1977, Nictitating membrane conditioning to tone in the immobilized albino rabbit, Brain Res., 137:127-143.

Disterhoft, J.F. and Olds, J., 1972, Differential development of conditioned unit changes in thalamus and cortex of rat. J. Neurophysiol., 35:665-679.

Disterhoft, J.F. and Shipley, M.T., 1980, Accessory abducens nucleus innervation of rabbit retractor bulbi motoneurons localized with HRP retrograde transport, Neuroscience Abstracts, 6:478.

Disterhoft, J.F. and Stuart, D.K., 1976, The trial sequence of changed unit activity in auditory system of alert rat during conditioned response acquisition and extinction, J. Neurophysiol., 39:266-281.

Enser, L.D., 1976, A study of classical nictitating membrane conditioning in neodecorticate, hemidecorticate and thalamic rabbits, unpublished doctoral dissertation, U. of Iowa, Iowa City.

Frey, P.W. and Butler, C.S., 1973, Rabbit eyelid conditioning as a function of unconditioned stimulus duration, J. Comp. Physiol.

Psychol., 83:289-294.

Gabriel, M., Saltwick, S.E. and Miller, J.D., 1975, Conditioning and reversal of short latency multiple unit responses in the rabbit medial geniculate nucleus, Science, 189:1108-1109.

Goldstein, M.H. and Abeles, M., 1975, Single unit activity of the auditory cortex, in: "Handbook of Sensory Physiology, Volume V/2, Auditory System", W.D. Keidel and W.D. Neff, eds., Springer-Verlag, Berlin, 199-218.

Grant, L, Gueritaud, J.P., Horcholle-Bossavit, G., and Tyc-Dumont, S., 1979, Anatomical and electrophysiological identification of motoneurons supplying the cat retractor bulbi muscle, Exp. Brain Res., 34:541-550.

Gray, T.S., McMaster, S.E., Harvey, J.A. and Gormezano, I., 1980, Localization of the motoneurons which innervate the retractor bulbi muscle in the rabbit, Neurosci. Abs., 6:16.

Graybiel, A.M., 1973, The thalamo-cortical projection of the so-called posterior nuclear group: A study with anterograde degeneration methods in the cat, Brain Res., 49:229-244.

Graybiel, A.M., 1974, Studies on the anatomical organization of posterior association cortex, in: "The Neuroscience Third Study Program", F.O. Schmitt and T.G. Worden, eds., MIT Press, Cambridge, 205-214.

Halas, E.S., Beardsley, J.V. and Sandlie, M.E., 1970, Conditioned neuronal responses at various levels in conditioning paradigms, Electroenceph. clin. Neurophysiol., 28:468-477.

Hocherman, S., Benson, D.A., Goldstein, M.H., Jr., Heffner, H.E., and Heinz, R.D., 1976, Evoked unit activity in auditory cortex of monkeys performing a selective attention task, Brain Res., 177:51-68.

Hutson, K.A., Glendenning, K.K., and Masterton, R.B., 1979, Accessory abducens nucleus and its relationship to the accessory facial and posterior trigeminal nuclei in cat, J. Comp. Neurol., 188: 1-16.

Kitzes, L.M., Farley, G.R., and Starr, A., 1978, Modulation of auditory cortex unit activity during the performance of a conditioned response, Exp. Neurol., 62:678-697.

Kraus, N., and Disterhoft, J.F., 1981a, Location of rabbit auditory cortex and description of single unit activity, Brain Res., 214:275-286.

Kraus, N. and Disterhoft, J.F., 1981b, Response plasticity of single neurons in rabbit auditory cortex during tone-signalled learning, submitted for publication.

Merzenich, M.M. and Brugge, J.F., 1973, Variation of excitability of neurons in primary auditory cortex in the unanesthetized macaque monkey: effects of sleep and body movement, J. Acoust. Soc. Amer., 53:1.

Mesulam, M.M., 1978, A tetramethyl benzidine method for the light microscope tracing of neural connections with horseradish peroxidase (HRP) neurohistochemistry, in: "Neuroanatomical Techniques", Soc. for Neuroscience Short Course.

Miller, J.M. Beaton, R.D., O'Connor, T. and Pfingst, B.E., 1974, Response pattern complexity of auditory cells in the cortex of unanesthetized monkeys, Brain Res., 69:101-113.

Moore, J.W., Yeo, C.H., Oakley, D.A. and Russell, I.S., 1980, Conditioned inhibition of the nictitating membrane response in neodecorticate rabbits, Behav. Brain Res., 1:397-410.

Morrell, F., 1967, Electrical signs of sensory coding, in: "The Neurosciences: A Study Program," G.C. Quarton, T. Melnechuk, and F.O. Schmitt, eds., Rochefeller University Press, Ney York, 452-469

Morrell, F., Hoeppner, T.J., and deToledo-Morrell, L., 1981, Conditioning of single units in visual association cortex: Cell specific behavior within a small population, submitted for publication.

Norman, R.J., Buchwald, J.S. and Villablanca, J.R., 1977, Classical conditioning with auditory discrimination of the eye blink in decerebrate cat, Science, 196:551-553.

Norman, R.J., Villablanca, J.R., Brown, K.A., Schwafel, J.A. and Buchwald, J.S., 1974, Classical eyeblink conditioning in the bilaterally hemispherectomized cat, Exp. Neurol., 44:363-380.

Oakley, D.A. and Russell, I.S., 1972, Neocortical lesions and Pavlovian conditioning, Physiol. Behav., 8:915-926.

Olds, J., Disterhoft, J.F., Segal, M., Kornblith, C.L. and Hirsh, R., 1972, Learning centers of rat brain mapped by measuring latencies of conditioned unit responses, J. Neurophysiol., 35:202-219.

Oleson, T.D., Ashe, J.H., and Weinberger, N.M., 1975, Modification of auditory and somatosensory system activity during pupillary conditioning in the paralyzed cat, J. Neurophysiol., 38:1114-1139.

Pfingst, B.E., O'Connor, T.A., 1981, Characteristics of neurons in auditory cortex of monkeys performing a single auditory task, J. Neurophysiol., 45:16-34.

Pfingst, B.E., O'Connor, T.A. and Miller, J.M., 1977, Response plasticity of neurons in auditory cortex of the rhesus monkey, Exp. Brain Res., 29:393-404.

Ryugo, D.K. and Weinberger, N.M., 1978, Differential plasticity of morphologically distinct neuron populations in the medial geniculate body of the cat during classical conditioning, Behav. Biol., 22:275-301.

Segal, M., 1973, Flow of conditioned responses in the limbic telencephalic system of the rat, J. Neurophysiol., 36:840-854.

Spencer, R., Baker, R., and McCrea, R.A., 1980, Localization and morphology of cat retractor bulbi motoneurons, J. Neurophysiol., 43:754-770.

Thompson, R.F., 1980, The search for the engrám, II., in: "Neural Mechanisms of Behavior", D. McFadden, ed., Springer-Verlag, New York, 172-222.

Van Gehuchten, A., 1906, "Anatomie du Systeme Nerveux de l'Homme", (4th ed.), Uystpruyst-Dieudonne, Louvain.

Weinberger, N.M., 1979, Effects of arousal and attention on the auditory system, presented at DuPont Symposium on the Neural Basis of Behavior.

Winer, J.A., Diamond, I.T., and Raczkowski, D., 1977, Subdivisions of the auditory cortex of the cat: The retrograde transport of horseradish peroxidase to the medial geniculate body and posterior thalamic nuclei, J. Comp. Neurol., 176:387-418.

Woody, C.D., Knispel, J.D., Crow, T.J., and Black-Cleworth, P.A., 1976, Activity and excitability to electrical current of cortical auditory receptive neurons of awake cats as affected by stimulus association, J. Neurophysiol., 39:1045-1061.

EXCITABILITY CHANGES OF FACIAL MOTONEURONS OF CATS RELATED TO CONDITIONED AND UNCONDITIONED FACIAL MOTOR RESPONSES

Michikazu Matsumura and Charles D. Woody

Depts of Anatomy and Psychiatry
UCLA Medical Center
Los Angeles, CA 90024

SUMMARY

The electrical excitability of facial motoneurons changes after Pavlovian conditioning ("Conditioned" group) and after repetitive presentation of USs such as glabella tap ("US-only" group). Measurements were made in awake, unparalyzed cats using intracellular recording and stimulation techniques. Threshold currents required to elicit action potentials were significantly lower in "Conditioned" and "US-only" groups than in a "Naive" control group. A decrease in the threshold of depolarizing current required to produce spike discharges was correlated with an increase in input resistance. The increase in excitability to intracellularly injected current persisted for more than four weeks in cells of the "Conditioned" group, but decayed in cells recorded from the "US-only" group. The transient increase in excitability after presentation of USs coincided with behavioral facilitation of subsequently acquired Pavlovian eyeblink conditioning. This facilitation of learned motor performance produced by prior, repeated presentations of USs may be analogous to the phenomena of reflex dominance and latent facilitation.

INTRODUCTION

Cortical neuronal excitability, measured by levels of intracellularly applied depolarizing current required to generate action potentials, increases after acquisition of a Pavlovian conditioned eyeblink response (Woody and Black-Cleworth, 1973). Brons and Woody (1980) showed that the development of the increases in excitability of neurons of the motor cortex was contingent on presentations of USs alone. The changes persisted for more than four weeks if the USs were associated with CSs.

In the present study, changes in neuronal excitability were investigated using two different approaches. The first was physiologic, involving direct experimental determination of whether or not the excitability of facial motoneurons was altered. Intracellular recording and stimulation were used to compare the levels of neuronal excitability among different behavioral groups.

The second approach was behavioral, examining how repetitive presentations of USs would affect rates of subsequent eyeblink conditioning.

METHODS

Intracellular recordings from facial motoneurons were obtained from unanesthetized, awake cats of three different behavioral groups: I. "Conditioned" group - cats were trained by repeatedly presenting a click as a CS, followed by a glabella tap US (ISI: 400 msec). One hundred and fifty pairings of CS and US were presented per day at 10 second intertrial intervals. Training was continued for 10 to 12 days, allowing each cat to reach a criterion of greater than 80% conditioned response performance level. II. "US- only" group - cats received glabella tap only, presented repetitively every 10 seconds over a period of 10 days; 150 USs were given daily. III. "Naive" group - cats were not given presentations of either CS or US.

After training, intracellular recording was attempted from the facial nucleus of each cat with the head fixed and body loosely restrained using techniques described by Woody and Black-Cleworth (1973). Facial motoneurons were identified by (1) antidromic spikes on stimulating the zygomatic branch of the facial nerve and (2) collision between orthodromic and antidromic spikes. During intracellular recording, 10 msec depolarizing current pulses were injected every 100 msec to determine the threshold level of current required to elicit action potentials and to measure input resistance.

Another group of cats was given repetitive presentations of USs according to the same training paradigm used for cats of the "US-only" group. The rate of spontaneous eyeblink was counted repeatedly over three different days before and after the training. The cats were then divided into two sub-groups. The first was given a CS-US conditioning paradigm similar to that given to the "Conditioned" group <u>7 days</u> after the US presentations; the second sub-group was given the same CS-US conditioning paradigm <u>4 weeks</u> after the US presentations. Levels of CR acquisition were compared between these groups and with control groups which did not receive any presentations of the US before conditioning.

RESULTS

One hundred and forty neurons were recorded intracellularly from the facial nuclei of 19 cats. Fifty-nine of these neurons were identified as motoneurons by antidromic activation (latencies ranged from 0.6 to 2.6 msec) and by collision between orthodromic and antidromic spikes. The others responded orthodromically (trans-synaptically) to stimulation of the facial nerve. The mean membrane potentials and sizes of action potentials (±SD) were -57±11 mV and 33±12 mV, respectively.

Less Current Required for Spike Initiation After CS-US or US Presentations

Neurons of the "Conditioned" and "US-only" groups were divided into sub-groups according to the day recorded after training: 1) neurons recorded 3 to 9 days after CS-US presentations (Conditioned, 1 week), 2) neurons recorded 26 to 29 days after CS-US

Table 1. Neural Changes after Behavioral Training. Means ± SDs are Shown.

Experimental Group	No. of Neurons Moto-neurons/ total*	Threshold Current (nA)	Input Resistance (MΩ)	Threshold De-polarization (mV)
Conditioned				
1 week	18/35	1.3±1.2	4.8±2.5	5.6±3.8
4 weeks	7/23	1.3±0.8	4.6±2.1	5.0±1.9
US-only				
1 week	17/39	0.9±0.5	4.5±2.4	4.1±2.8
4 weeks	4/13	3.0±2.0	3.2±1.7	7.0±2.2
Naive	13/24	3.0±2.0	3.8±2.4	7.4±3.9

*(The total number is less than 140 because six neurons were recorded at periods between one week and four weeks after training.)

presentations (Conditioned, 4 weeks), 3) neurons recorded 1 to 12 days after US presentations (US-only, 1 week), and 4) neurons recorded 28 to 30 days after US presentations (US-only, 4 weeks). As shown in Table 1, mean threshold currents required for spike generation in the "Conditioned, 1 week" and "US-only, 1 week" groups were significantly lower than those in the "Naive" group ($p<0.01$, analysis of variance). No differences were found between the neurons of the "Conditioned, 1 week" and "US-only, 1 week" groups. Mean threshold currents were also lower in the "Conditioned, 4 weeks" group, but currents in the "US-only, 4 weeks" group were not. The latter were not significantly different from means of the "Naive" group. There were no significant differences in threshold currents between motoneurons and orthodromically activated neurons.

Increases in Input Resistance

As shown in Table 1, input resistances of the neurons of the

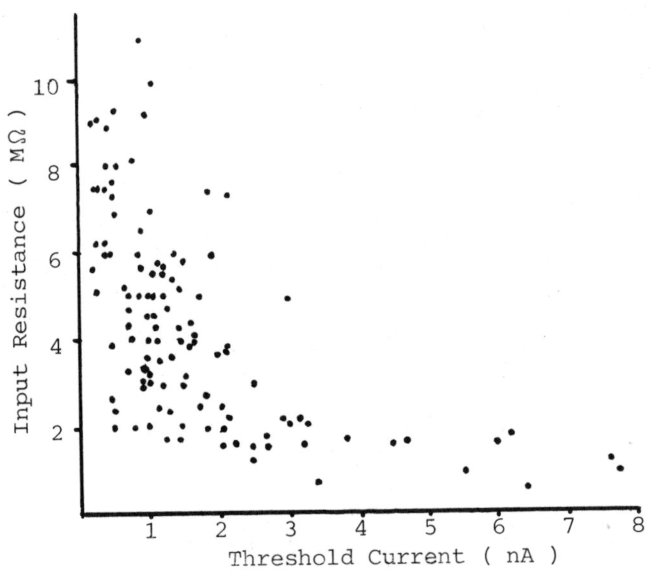

Figure 1. Relationship between threshold current (abscissa) and input resistance (ordinate) recorded from neurons in and near the facial nucleus.

"Conditioned" and "US-only, 1 week" groups tended to be higher than those of the "Naive" group ($0.05< p <0.10$). This trend reflected an inverse correlation between threshold current and input resistance (Figure 1). Neurons which had higher levels of threshold current had lower values of input resistance, and vice versa. Neurons of the "US-only, 4 weeks" group showed levels of input resistance slightly lower than those of the "Naive" group.

Decreases Threshold Depolarization

The threshold depolarization (the potential difference between the potential at threshold and the resting potential) was calculated as follows:

$$\text{Threshold depolarization } (\Delta V) = V_{th} - V_m = I_{th} \times R_m ,$$

where V_{th} was the potential at threshold current, V_m was the resting potential, I_{th} was the threshold current, and R_m was the input resistance. As shown in Table 1, the threshold aepolarization showed a significant decrease after CS-US presentations and one week after US presentations. However, four weeks later, the mean value of the threshold depolarization in the "US-only" group returned to the naive level.

Behavioral Effects of US Presentation

Rates of spontaneous eye blinking were measured in six cats before and after 10 daily sessions of US presentation. Each cat showed some increase of spontaneous blink rate after US presentation. The increases were significantly greater than initial values in four of the cats. The rate of acquisition of CRs during Pavlovian conditioning was accelerated above that in naive control cats when repetitive presentations of USs were given 7 days prior to the conditioning paradigm. Animals which were given USs 7 days beforehand reached 90% CR performance levels on the 5th day of conditioning, while naive control animals reached but 85% CR performance levels on the 9th day. Animals which were given USs 4 weeks before conditioning did not show any facilitation of the rate of CR acquisition, and did not reach 80% CR performance levels even on the 10th day of training. The latter may reflect a separate latent inhibition arising from US instead of CS presentations [Kimble, 1961; Leonard et al 1972; Brons and Woody, 1978].

DISCUSSION

In the present study, changes in electrical excitability were found in facial motoneurons and other, unidentified neurons in or near the facial nucleus after cats learned a conditioned behavior. Threshold currents required to elicit action potentials in these cells decreased after repetitive presentations of paired CS-USs or USs alone. The increase in neural excitability lasted for more than four weeks when USs were paired with CSs. A similar result was found in neurons of the motor cortex (Brons and Woody, 1980). The change in threshold current of the motoneurons was correlated with an increase in their input resistance. The threshold depolarization required for spike initiation also decreased after presentations of CS-US or US. Although steadily increased presynaptic activity could have led to a sustained postsynaptic depolarization in the cells that were studied herein, this is not the only possible explanation for the decreases in threshold depolarization that were found. Neurons having higher input resistances might have had more depolarized membrane potentials even with the same levels of presynaptic input. Conductance decreases in potassium channels, with resulting changes in the space constant of the cells, could have produced this effect.

The rate of spontaneous blinking increased after repetitive presentation of USs. The rate also increases after Pavlovian conditioning with presentations of paired CS-USs (Woody et al., 1974). These results are well correlated with the finding of increased neural excitability along corticomotoneuronal pathways. Both the increase in spontaneous blink responses and in the ability to learn conditioned blink responses after US presentations are consistent with a latent facilitation of motor behavior analogous to that described by other investigators (see discussion in Woody, 1982). Facilitation of the acquisition of CR performance was lost four weeks after presentation of USs. This was in good accordance with the time course of the excitability increase found along corticomotoneuronal pathways after US presentations. In summary, transient changes in the electrical excitability of neurons along corticomotoneuronal pathways are produced by repeated presentations of USs. The changes have facilitatory effects on motor performance. Temporal association of CS and US appears to be important for the retention of increased excitability in motoneurons as well as in neurons of the motor cortex and for the long-term maintenance of conditioned behavior.

ACKNOWLEDGEMENTS

We gratefully acknowledge the pilot study of chronic intra-cellular recording from facial motoneurons done by Dr. S. Jordan and colleagues (1976). We also thank Dr. N. Allon for his contribution to the behavioral studies. This research was supported by US Public Health Service Grant HD-05958.

REFERENCES

Brons, J. and Woody, C.D., 1978, Decreases in excitability of cortical neurons to extracellularly delivered current after eyeblink conditioning, extinction, and presentation of US alone, Soc. Neurosci. Abs. 4:255

Brons, J.F. and Woody, C.D., 1980, Long-term changes in excitability of cortical neurons after Pavlovian conditioning and extinction, J. Neurophysiol. 44:605

Jordan, S.E., Jordan, J., Brozek, G., and Woody, C.D., 1976, Intracellular recordings of antidromically identified facial motoneurons and unidentified brain stem interneurons of awake, blink conditioned cats, Physiologist 19:245

Kimble, G.A., 1961, Hilgard and Marquis' Conditioning and Learning, Appleton-Century-Crofts: New York (Second Edition)

Leonard, D.W., Fischbein, L.C., and Monteau, J.E., 1972, The effects of interpolated US alone (USa) presentations on classical nictitating membrane conditioning in rabbit (Oryctolagus cuniculus), Conditional Reflex 7:107

Woody, C.D. and Black-Cleworth, P.A., 1973, Differences in the excitability of cortical neurons as a function of motor projection in conditioned cats, J. Neurophysiol., 36:1104

Woody, C.D., Yarowsky, P., Owens, J., Black-Cleworth, P.A., and Crow, T.J., 1974, Effect of lesions of cortical motor areas on acquisition of conditioned eye blink in the cat, J. Neurophysiol. 37:385

Woody, C.D., 1982, Neurophysiologic correlates of latent facilitation. In: "Conditioning: Representation of Involved Neural Function", C.D. Woody, ed., Plenum, New York

THE METENCEPHALIC BASIS OF THE CONDITIONED NICTITATING MEMBRANE RESPONSE

John W. Moore, John E. Desmond, and Neil E. Berthier

Department of Psychology
University of Massachusetts
Amherst, Massachusetts 01003

SUMMARY

The classically conditioned nictitating membrane response of the rabbit has evolved into a useful model system for neurobiological studies of associative learning. Converging methodologies from behavioral, physiological, and anatomical approaches indicate key roles in conditioning for the limbic system, especially the hippocampus, and the brain stem. This article presents evidence that the metencephalon contains neural elements essential for generation and performance of conditioned responses in this preparation.

Recordings of multiple-unit activity from chronically implanted microelectrodes during conditioning in alert animals suggest that the dorsolateral pons at the level of the trigeminal nerve contains populations of neurons which are a substrate of the conditioned response. Lesions in this region virtually abolish conditioned responding while leaving the unconditioned response to eye shock intact. This observation suggests that components of the reflex arc of the unconditioned response, including rostral elements of the sensory trigeminal system and of the accessory abducens nucleus, are not crucial for learning. Instead, associative convergence between conditioned and unconditioned stimuli appears to occur in an adjacent interneuron system of the supratrigeminal reticular formation.

INTRODUCTION

The classically conditioned nictitating membrane response (NMR) in rabbit has proven to be an attractive system for neurobiological studies of associative learning in a mammalian species (Thompson, 1976). The behavioral parameters of this preparation have been thoroughly investigated, and its applicability to both physiological investigations and the advance of learning theory has been amply demonstrated (Moore, 1979a).

Neurobiologists concerned with mammalian learning and memory are often hard pressed to demonstrate that particular regions of the brain subserve the acquisition and performance of a particular behavior (Lashley, 1950). With but few exceptions (e.g., Woody et al., 1974), this has been particularly the case with simple associative learning as exemplified by classical Pavlovian conditioning, and the conditioned NMR in rabbit has been no exception. Until now no region of the brain has proven essential for conditioning of the rabbit NMR. Electrophysiological activity correlated with this conditioned response (CR) has been demonstrated by recording from neocortex (Kraus Perkins and Disterhoft, 1979), hippocampus (Thompson et al., 1980), septal nuclei (Berger et al., 1980), and the abducens nucleus or the pons (Cegavske et al., 1979). However, when a conditioned stimulus (CS) and unconditioned stimulus (US) are programmed in a manner conducive to robust conditioning, lesions and ablations of these and other brain structures (e.g., mesencephalon) do not typically eliminate CRs or prevent their acquisition. What has been lacking is evidence that relatively discrete brain damage can selectively disrupt CRs without also interrupting sensory or motor pathways necessary for the unconditioned response (UR).

Some relevant literature (see Moore, 1979a; Norman, et al., 1977) suggests that neural elements essential for conditioning are located in the pons of the brain stem. This chapter reviews evidence that this is indeed the case. This evidence derives from experiments employing a variety of techniques in connection with behavioral conditioning of the NMR: 1) stimulation 2) lesions 3) electrophysiological. These studies of conditioning can best be understood from the perspective of the anatomy and physiology of the UR.

ANATOMY AND PHYSIOLOGY OF THE UNCONDITIONED NMR

The NMR in rabbit is a passive consequence of eyeball retraction. Eyeball retraction occurs reflexively to tactile and nociceptive stimulation to the cornea or facial tissue marginal to the eye. The principal muscles producing eyeball retraction are the retractor bulbi muscles--four slips of muscle encapsulating the optic nerve. The principal innervation of these muscles is by way of the abducens (sixth cranial) nerve. There is some uncertainty as to whether fibers for the oculomotor (third cranial) nerve also provides some innervation (e.g., see Disterhoft and Shipley, 1980; Gray, et al., 1980). What does seem clear, however, is that extraocular muscles in addition to those innervated by the sixth nerve participate in eyeball retraction, although their role is thought to be secondary to that of the retractor bulbi muscles (see Berthier and Moore, 1980a).

The location of motoneurons that contribute to eyeball retraction has recently become clarified. Studies involving HRP techniques (e.g., Berthier and Moore, 1980; Disterhoft and Shipley, 1980; Gray et al., 1980) have shown that the rabbit resembles the cat in possessing two distinct populations of motoneurons that contribute to the sixth nerve. One population lies in the abducens nucleus in the dorsal pons--just ventral to the genu of the facial (seventh cranial) nerve. This nucleus is thought to contain motoneurons for both the ipsilateral lateral rectus and retractor bulbi muscles. The other population of motoneurons lie in a recently rediscovered accessory abducens nucleus (Baker, et al., 1980). These cells are thought to contribute only to retractor bulbi muscles.

Physiological evidence suggests that these motoneurons are principally involved in defensive retraction of the globe; with those in the abducens nucleus proper having the primary role in coordinating the retractor bulbi muscles with those of the other extraocular muscles in visual motor pursuit and gaze (see Delgado-Garcia et al., 1980).

Defensive eyeball retraction to electro-stimulation of the marginal region of the eye is very rapid: Accessory abducens motoneurons fire with a latency of roughly 5 ms to a single suprathreshold pulse of dc shock to the eye, and corresponding action potentials can be recorded from the sixth nerve as it exits the ventral pons with a latency of 5 ms following stimulation (Berthier, 1981).

Berthier (1981) investigated the electrophysiology of the abducens nerve and its motoneurons in anesthetized and paralyzed rabbits. While moderate single-pulse shocks (2.5 mA, 1 ms duration) to the eye readily elicited unit discharges from the accessory abducens nucleus, shocks of twice this intensity did not elicit unit discharges from cells of the abducens nucleus. This observation is consistent with reports from cat that the threshold of contraction of retractor bulbi muscles trigeminal stimulation is much lower than that of lateral rectus muscles (Baldissera and Broggi, 1968). It therefore reinforces the conclusion that motoneurons of the accessory abducens nucleus are the primary source of retractor bulbi innervation for defensive reflexes.

Thus, the principal output component of the defensive NMR to electrostimulation appears to be the accessory abducens motoneurons. The sensory side of the reflex arc was further investigated by

Berthier (1981) by simultaneously recording from trigeminal (fifth cranial) and the abducens nerve. These experiments indicated that the threshold of activation of the abducens nerve was the same as that for elicitation of Aα fiber potentials observed in the trigeminal nerve. The difference in latency between Aα potential and sixth-nerve activation (central delay) was approximately 1.8 ms., suggesting a disynaptic pathway from the primary afferent units to the motoneurons. Moreover, this pathway involves secondary afferent neurons that are activated by Aα fibers. The location of these secondary afferents appears to lie rostral to the motoneurons, as transection of the brain stem at the border between trigeminal subnuclei oralis and interpolaris did not affect the reflex. Subsequent experiments have indicated that large ipsilateral lesions of the principal sensory trigeminal nucleus eliminates the reflex.

The picture that emerges is of a reflex arc involving a fast-conducting primary afferent component synapsing on secondary afferent neurons located in the principal trigeminal nucleus rostral to the motoneurons of the accessory abducens nucleus.

THE METENCEPHALIC BASIS OF THE CONDITIONED NMR

Lesion and ablation experiments have excluded much of the brain from consideration as the site of crucial events involved in acquisition and performance of the CR. These considerations led Moore (1979a) to suggest that these events may occur rather near to the reflex arc of the NMR, i.e., in close proximity to the neural circuits that mediate the response, i.e., in the vicinity of the sensory trigeminal complex and/or the motoneurons of the abducens nerve.

ESB as the US

Three groups of investigators have reported that electrical brain stimulation (ESB) via electrodes chronically implanted with tips near the abducens nuclei can reinforce the acquisition and performance of normal appearing CRs to auditory CSs (Martin et al., 1980; Mis et al., 1979; Powell and Moore, 1980).

Powell and Moore (1980) also demonstrated the CRs can be established to CSs of other sensory modalities (visual and tactile) using ESB as the US and that these procedures yield normal differential conditioning performance and stimulus generalization gradients. The rate of conditioning with ESB was very retarded when compared to that obtained using electro-stimulation of the orbit of the eye or corneal air puff: Where eye shock typically yields CRs within 100 pairings with the CS, ESB at current levels sufficient to produce a full response might not yield CRs after 2000 pairings. Although ESB was as likely to be ineffective in reinforcing CRs as not, there was clear evidence of positive transfer or savings when normal eye shock was substituted for ESB. In addition, ESB could substitute for eye shock in maintaining a previously established CR, thereby preventing extinction. It is difficult and inappropriate to over interpret such findings (see O'Brien et al., 1977) beyond the support they provide for the idea of a metencephalic basis for the conditioned NMR.

Brain Stem Correlates of Conditioning

To date we have obtained recordings of multiple-unit activity (MUA) from the midbrain and pons of 15 rabbits undergoing various conditioning procedures. Of these, 6 have shown unit activity that closely parallels the behavioral CR in latency and other topographical features and 7 have not. Two additional animals yielded "noisy" artifactual recordings.

The electrodes were tungsten low-impedance (approximately 80-100 KΩ) monopolar microelectrodes obtained from Frederick Haer & Co. A few days after implantation of one or two electrodes plus a cranial ground, animals began a series of training sessions in an electrically shielded chamber. The animal was restrained in Gormezano-type Plexiglas boxes that permit little movement. Sutures sewn into the right and left nictitating membranes provided attachment to low-torque rotary potentiometer transducers for simultaneous polygraphic recording of NMRs from both eyes.

In addition, eye-shock electrodes (9 mm wound clips) were crimped into the dorsal and ventral aspect of the right eye, approximately 3 mm from the margin. These electrodes provided the US, which consisted of a 50 ms train of square-wave pulses (60 pps, pulse duration = 8.3 ms, 1-2.5 mA) generated by a Grass S88 stimulator and associated isolation and constant-current unit.

Leads from recording electrodes and a ground lead from a safety-pin chronically implanted in the skin on the animal's back provided inputs to a grass P15 preamplier filtered from 300 to 10 KHz. The output of these preamplifiers could be displayed on an oscilloscope (Tektroniks 502A). A parallel circuit provided input to a Grass 5P3 integrator preamplifiers for polygraphic display. Thus, integrated unit activity from one or two microelectrodes could be displayed together with NMRs from one or both eyes.

Procedures varied but slightly from animal to animal: Each session lasted 50 minutes, intertrial (CS-US) intervals were constant at 500 msec, CS and the US were always presented in a forward-delay arrangement with the two stimuli terminating together, and intertrial intervals were constant at 30 sec. The first phase of training consisted of 2-4 sessions of 100 reinforced trials, 50 to a light CS and 50 to a pure-tone CS. The light was a dim spot with slow rise time in an otherwise dark chamber, and the tone was an 85 dB (SPL) sinewave of 1200 Hz presented over white masking noise of 65 dB (SPL). With these stimulus parameters, the tone is far more salient than the light, leading to relatively rapid acquisition of CRs in comparison with the light. This mismatch in the effectiveness of the light and tone for conditioning provided for relatively rapid acquisition of conditioned inhibition to the tone in a later stage of training (for CI methodology, see, e.g., Moore et al., 1980).

Following acquisition training, all animals received a sufficient number of nonreinforced trials, often extending beyond one session, to produce extinction of CRs to both CSs. This training was followed by conditioned inhibition (CI) training in which reinforcement to the light CS was reinstated while the tone, now paired with the light, was not reinforced. With the institution of CI training, CRs gradually returned to the light. This is followed by a gradual and progressive decline of CRs on nonreinforced light-tone trials while CRs are maintained on the reinforced light trials. Conditioned inhibition training, in addition to serving as a within-animal control for pseudo-conditioning, provides potential evidence of the role of various brain regions in learned inhibition.

With concurrent recording of NMRs and integrated unit activity from the brain providing trial-by-trial "hard copy", it is possible to determine the degree of coupling between unit activity and the behavioral CR. From these observations, illustrated in Fig. 1, it was possible to categorize electrode placements as hits or misses as far as correlated activity is concerned. Typical misses are illustrated in Fig. 2 c, d. The location of electrode tips was determined for 12 cases, 5 hits and 7 misses. Though providing only the sketchiest of outlines of a map that separates regions of highly correlated activity from those of low correlation, the clear impression is that of a band of tissue extending ipsilaterally from the rostral pons to the level of the abducens nerve and in the dorsolateral gradient (see Fig. 3).

Electrodes of animals 34 and 41 are typical hits. The tip of electrode of animal 34 was approximately 1.5 mm rostal to the level of the abducens nerve and within a band of tissue that Mizuno (1970) defines as the supratrigeminal reticular formation, and interneuron system intercalcated between the principal sensory nucleus of the trigeminal nerve and various cranial motor systems. Unit activity of late acquisition trials (Fig. 1, column 1, rows a, b), early extinction (Fig. 1, column 1, row c), and late extinction (Fig. 1, column 1, row d) closely parallel the corresponding behavioral CRs (Fig. 1, column 3). The integrated unit activity corresponding to these trials is illistrated in Fig. 1, column 2. Columns 4-5 of Fig. 1 show similar recordings of integrated unit

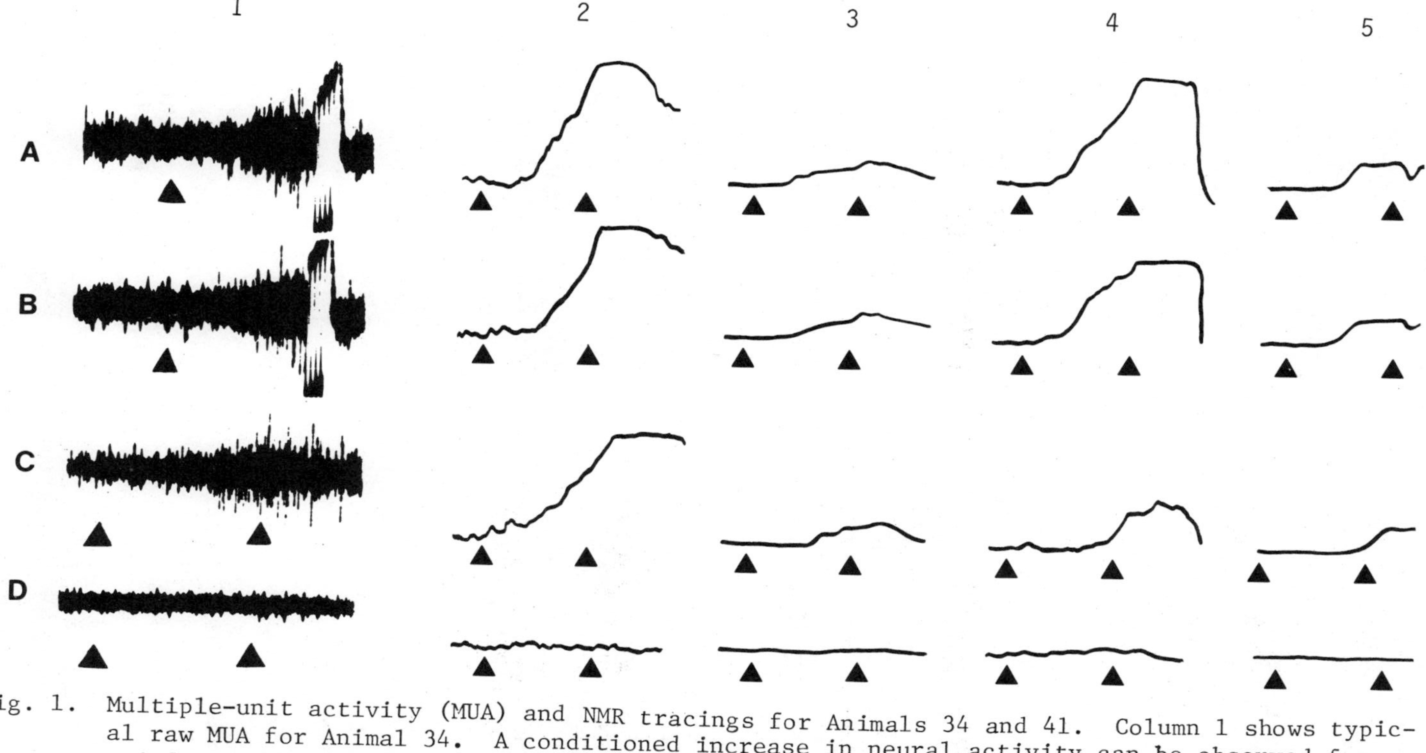

Fig. 1. Multiple-unit activity (MUA) and NMR tracings for Animals 34 and 41. Column 1 shows typical raw MUA for Animal 34. A conditioned increase in neural activity can be observed for a reinforced T trial (a), and a reinforced L trial (b). Early (c) and later (d) extinction training to L shows gradual diminution of activity. Columns 2 and 3 represent integrated MUA and the NMR, respectively, for the same trials as those in column 1 (Animal 34). Columns 4 and 5 show integrated neural activity and the corresponding NMR for Animal 41. Triangles indicate CS and US onsets.

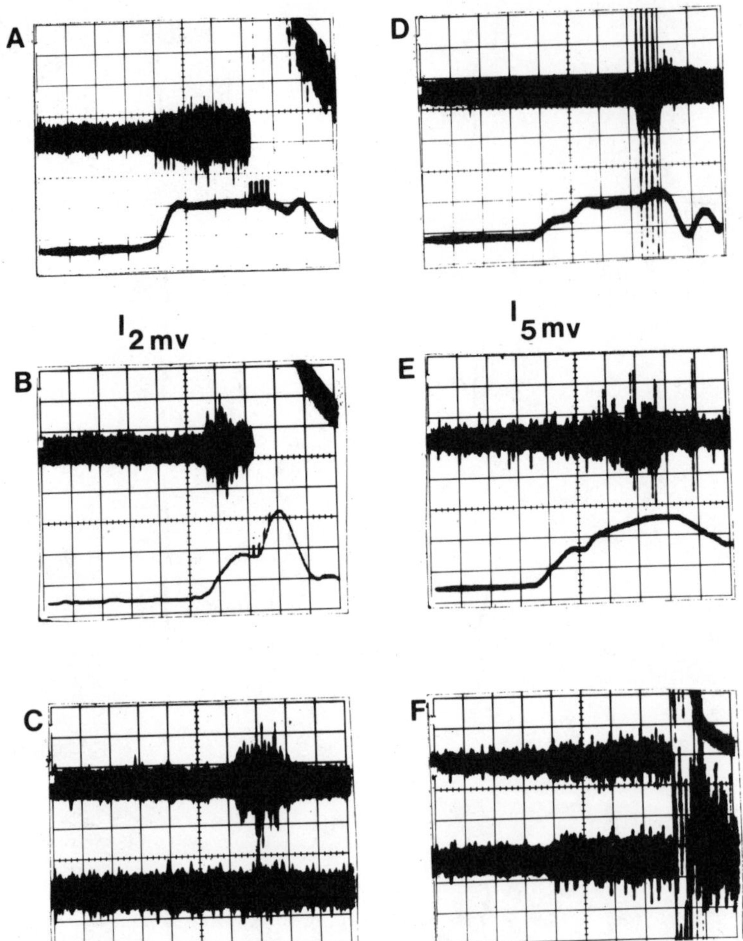

Fig. 2. Multiple-unit activity (MUA) and NMR tracings for Animals 81, 85, 86, and 94. The CS-US interval was .5 sec, and the US was a 50 msec train of dc pulses to the eye: a. Concurrent recording from the hippocampus and right NMR on a reinforced tone trial (Animal 85); b. A similar record from another animal (86); c. Concurrent recording of MUA from the hippocampus (upper trace) and brain stem (lower trace) on a nonreinforced light trial (Animal 86); d. Concurrent recording from the brain stem and right NMR on a reinforced tone trial (Animal 81); e. Similar record on a nonreinforced light-tone trial from Animal 94; f. Concurrent recording from the hippocampus (upper trace) and brain stem (lower trace) on a reinforced tone trial (Animal 94). Calibration: X 100.

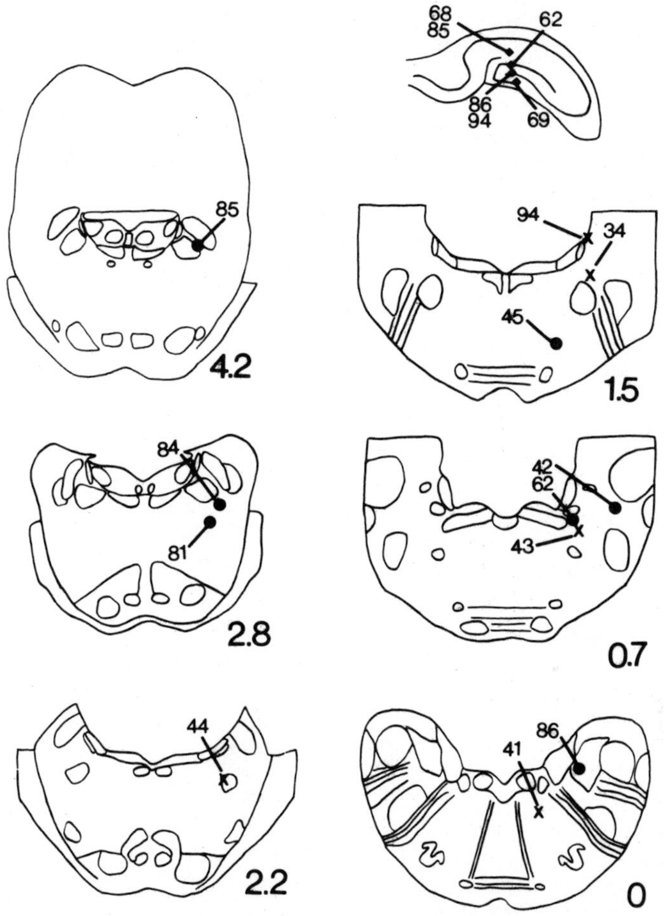

Fig. 3. Selected transverse sections through the brain stem showing location of recording electrode tips for hits (X) and misses (●). The hemi-section of the right dorsal hippocampus appears in the upper right-hand portion. Numbers to the lower right-hand corner of brain stem sections refer to distance (mm) rostral from the level of the abducens nerve. Other numbers designate individual animals.

activity and behavioral CRs for animal 41, with electrodes located within the efferent projection of accessory abducens motoneurons.

Inspection of polygraph records revealed that the maximum point of inflection of integrated activity for hits fell within ± 50 ms of that of the behavioral CR. However, there was very little consistency from session to session, or often within a session, of the one measure preceding the other. Thus, although integrated unit activity was closely coupled to the behavioral CR in latency, it has proven impossible with our methods to establish an invariant temporal sequence in which the unit activity of the brain precedes the initiation of the behavioral CR. More often it appeared as if the recording electrode was "down stream" from crucial events such as to lag slightly behind the behavioral response. Animal 94 (Fig. 2e) is a case in point. Hopefully, single-unit recordings from regions with highly-correlated activity will address the crucial issue of comparative latency between brain events and behavior with greater resolution.

The peak amplitude of integrated unit activity from hit electrodes was compared with that of the peak amplitude of the behavioral CR on a sample of nonreinforced trials during CI training. These trials are not obscured by eye shock artifact. Animal 94 is typical: a sample of 45 nonreinforced trials from one session of CI training yielded a Pearson product-moment correlation between the amplitude of integrated activity and the amplitude of the CR of $r = .52$; $t(43) = 3.99$, $p < .001$.

Evoked Responses to Eye Shocks

Brief electric shocks via eye shock electrodes elicited evoked potentials from brain stem electrodes. Shocks were dc pulses .1-.3 msec and 20-70 volts delivered via a Wagner ground circuit in parallel with the preparation to reduce recording artifact (see Becker et al., 1961). The latency of the first response to eye shock ranged from short latency response of approximately 1.5 for animal 34 to 5 ms for animal 85. Evoked responses were not observed from animals 41, 42, and 45.

Stimulation of contralateral (left) eye did not always elicit evoked responses from the brain stem, and when contralateral responses were observed, their latency was typically greater than that of the ipsilateral response by 105 msec. We suspect that secondary or higher-order afferents to the contralateral brain stem from eye shock underlies the rapid conditioning of the contralateral NMR once the ipsilateral CR has been established. It is worth noting that there is little anatomical evidence of direct primary afferentation from trigeminal sensory neurons representing the cornea and periocular region to the contralateral sensory trigeminal complex (Panneton and Burton, 1981).

Finally, there was little correlation between the latency and amplitude of evoked brain stem response and the degree to which unit activity recorded from that electrode was correlated with behavioral conditioning. Animals 81 and 85, both classified as misses in terms of conditioning, gave evoked brain stem responses to shocks to either eye with latencies in the 2-3 msec range. Animal 94, by contrast, gave evoked responses to stimulation of either eye with latencies of 4 ms.

ESB evoked NMR. At the conclusion of all experiments involving recording from the brain stem, animals were stimulated via brain stem electrodes. Current levels of dc pulses ranged from 30-600 μA in 50 msec trains of 200-500 pps and with pulse durations of .1-1.0 msec. Ipsilateral NMRs could be elicited in 9 out of 12 cases and with little or no accompanying motor involvement. There was little apparent correlation between the minimal current density needed to evoke the NMR and whether the electrode was a hit or miss as far as conditioning is concerned. Thus, animals 41, 42, 43, 62, 84, and 85 gave NMRs with current levels of 30 uA, whereas animals 34 and 44 required current levels of 600-700 uA to elicit a response. Animals 45, 81, 86, and 94 did not respond to brain stem stimulation.

Role of the Hippocampus

Berger and Thompson and their associates have performed elegant electrophysiological experiments of conditioning-dependent neural activity of the hippocampus and other limbic-system structrues during NMR conditioning (e.g., Berger et al. 1980; Thompson, et al. 1980). We have been able to replicate the basic findings of Berger and Thompson by implanting low-impedance microelectrodes like those used for brain stem recording into the ipsilateral hippocampus of 6 animals (see Fig. 3). In all cases, unit activity was coupled with the behavioral CR. Figure 2a shows concurrent oscillographic tracings to the tone CS for animal 85, with electrode tip located in the stratum radiatum of the dorsal CA1 field. Note the latency of above-noise unit activity and the CR are essentially the same on this trial. Another example is that of animal 86, with electrode tip in stratum pyramidale of CA3. Here, unit activity followed initiation of the response by 10-20 msec.

Activity recorded from the hippocampus was often correlated with conditioned responses where the brain stem was not. Figure 2c illustrates this with concurrent recording of unit activity from the hippocampus (upper trace) and the brain stem (lower trace) on an extinction trial to the light CS on which the animal made a behavioral CR. On the other hand, concurrent recording from the hippocampus and brain stem were highly correlated in the case of animal 95 (e.g., Fig. 2f). Measurement of the amplitude of integrated unit activity on 45 nonreinforced trials during CI training for this animal yield a Pearson produce-moment correlation of $r = .94$; $t(43) = 18.72$, $p < .001$. In addition, the amplitude of unit activity from the hippocampus was correlated CR amplitude on these trials. The obtained correlation of $r = .51$ is very close to that reported above for the brain stem electrode of this animal and also statistically significant, $t(43) = 3.89$, $p < .001$.

Stimulation of the brain via hippocampal electrodes failed to produce NMRs, although struggling was observed in some cases with high levels of current.

Lesion Experiments

Lesion experiments were designed to delimit the volume of brain in the metencephalon that might be crucial for performance of the conditioned response. Based on preliminary observations, and consistent with the anatomical distribution of brain stem electrodes employed in the previously described experiments of neural activity during conditioning, we anticipated that ipsilateral lesions of the dorsolateral pons might disrupt the acquisition and retention of behavioral CRs. This proved to be the case, as Fig. 4 illustrates. Rows a and b of Fig. 4 show representative polygraph tracing to a tone CS (row a) and a light CS before (PRE) and after (POST) lesioning the brain stem. The lesion was produced by RF current and resembled that shown in Fig. 5.

The encouraging aspect of these lesions is that they eliminate the CR, but left the UR to eye shock unimpaired. The tracings in rows a and b of Fig. 4 were from the animal in the lower portion of Fig. 5. This lesion involves the parabrachial region of the pons on the side ipsilateral to the eye shock.

Row c of Fig. 4 depicts representative polygraph tracings of NMRs from another lesioned animal, one that did not lose its CR following lesioning. The lesion for this animal was more medial than that of the disrupted animal (see upper portion of Fig. 5), involving central gray and locus coeruleus. Thus, Fig. 5 illustrates striking propinquity between lesions that disrupted CRs and those that did not. Row d of Fig. 4 illustrates a rare CR of low amplitude in an animal that received a disrupting lesion of the dorsolateral pons prior to conditioning. This tracing is typical of those seen on the few trials that contained a criterion CR.

Our startegy in lesion experiments was to make small lesions in the suspected critical zone and large lesions nearby. To date we have histological verification of lesions for 21 animals. Of these 9 were classified as disrupted (D) and 12 as nondisrupted

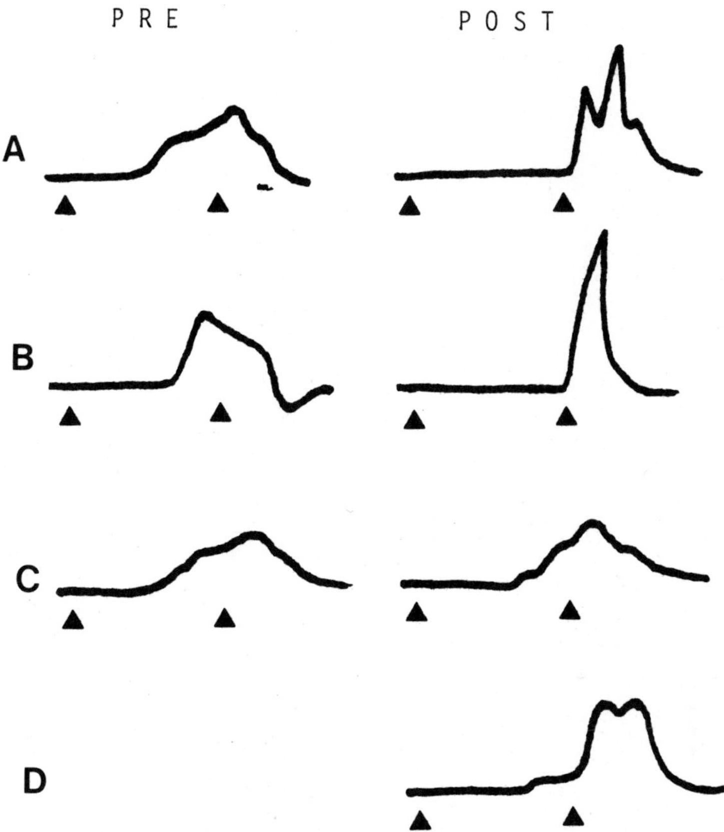

Fig. 4. Representative NMRs from lesion experiments. For each tracing the onset of the CS is marked by the left-hand triangle, and the onset of the US is marked by the right-hand triangle. Upward deflections occurring after CS onset but before US onset are CRs. Those occurring after US onset are URs. PRE refers to a pre-lesioning trial. POST refers to a post-lesioning trial. a. Representative NMRs to light CS (L) for animal in the Disrupted (D) group. b. Representative NMRs to the tone (T) CS for another animal in the D group. c. Representative NMRs to L for an animal in the Nondisrupted (ND) group. d. An NMR to T for a D animal that was lesioned prior to training. This tracing shows a rare CR on the fourth session of training.

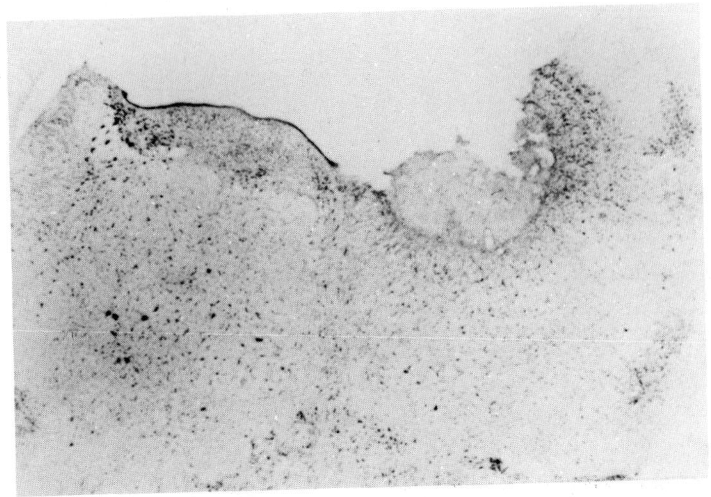

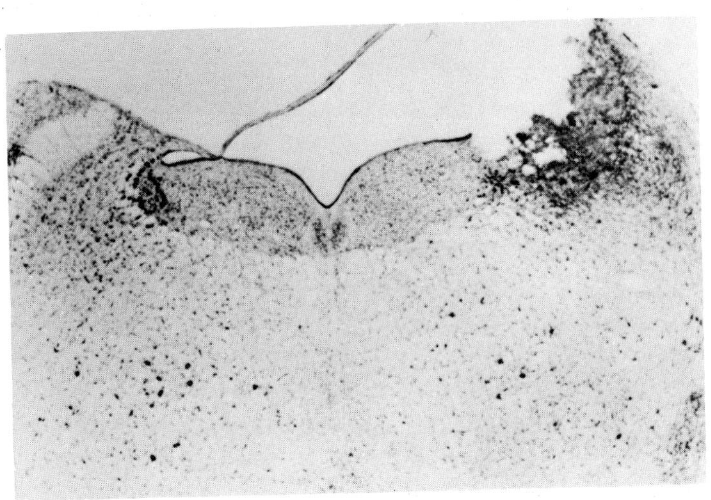

Fig. 5. Photomicrographs (X10) of Nissl-stained transverse sections. The top photograph is from an animal from the Nondisrupted (ND) group. This section is at the level of the parabrachial nuclei. The lesion (right side) includes all CG, and portions of mlf, LC, and MES 5. The bottom photograph is a section from the same level of the brainstem for an animal from the Disrupted (D) group. The lesion includes bc and parabrachial nuclei, portions of LC and most of MES. Abbreviations: CG = central gray; mlf = medial longitudinal fasiculus; LC = locus coeruleus; MES 5 = mesencephalic nucleus of the fifth nerve.

(ND). All D animals showed profound loss of CRs but no loss of URs. In addition, we ran a number of sham operated animals under conditions similar to those employed by lesioned animals.

Another aspect of our strategy for lesion experiments was to investigate the effect of lesions on acquisition of CRs by naive animals lesioned prior to training and, in addition, to assess the loss and savings of CRs on well-conditioned animals trained prior to lesioning. These were experiments on CR retention.

Yet another aspect of our strategy was to assess acquisition of CRs to the eye contralateral to the lesioned side of the brain, and therefore contralateral to the originally trained NMR. Contralateral conditioning was invariably spared in lesioned animals, even those classified as D animals.

Finally, most animals were trained to more than one CS, typically a light, an 85 dB (SPL) tone, and/or an 85 dB (SPL) burst of white noise. Training procedures were basically the same as those described above. Lesioned animals were typically given 2 days to recover from surgery (range: 1-4 days), and the average survival time before sacrifice was 24 days (range: 11-61).

The results of lesioning prior to acquisition training are summarized in Table 1. The tabled entries are the percentage of reinforced trials containing a criterion CR, and they are based on 5 sessions. Note that the 4 animals in the Disrupted category (5-7, 52, 56, 57) gave an average of only 3 per cent CRs (range: 0-8) while the control animals, Nondisrupted and Shams combined, give 20-80 per cent CRs over a comparable period of training.

Table 1. Percentage of Trials with CRs to Light (L) and Tone (T) CSs for Lesioned (Disrupted and Nondisrupted) and Sham-Operated Animals: Acquisition Training

	Disrupted		Nondisrupted		Sham	
	T	L	T	L	T	L
Mean	3	0	46	20	67	62
Range	0-8	0	--	--	59-78	32-80
N	4	4	1	1	5	5

Table 2. Percentage of Trials with CRs to Light (L) and Tone (T) for Lesioned (Disrupted and Nondisrupted) and Sham-Operated Animals: Retention Testing (Pre-Lesioning vs. Post-Lesioning)

	Disrupted		Nondisrupted		Sham	
	T	L	T	L	T	L
Pre $\overline{X}$	97	88	99	92	95	92
Range	94-100	71-97	98-100	83-99	92-100	81-99
N	3	5	5	11	6	6
Post $\overline{X}$	4	3	87	88	96	93
Range	0-10	0-8	73-100	56-99	92-99	83-98
N	3	5	5	11	6	6

Table 3. Percentage of Trials with CRs to Light (L) and Tone (T) CSs for Lesioned (Disrupted and Nondisrupted) and Sham-Operated Animals: Acquisition to Contralateral Eye

	Disrupted		Nondisrupted		Sham	
	T	L	T	L	T	L
Mean	90	83	87	83	95	93
Range	82-100	60-100	74-100	40-98	84-100	84-100
N	7	9	2	4	7	7

Table 2 shows the results of the retention experiment. Disrupted animals (4-6, 4-16, 47, 5-3, 5-5) ranged from 0-10 per cent CRs over 5 postoperative sessions with all trials reinforced. Their CR rates were profoundly below preoperative rates and the pre- and postoperative rates of controls. While lesions of Disrupted animals all but eliminated CRs of the reinforced (ipsilateral) side, contralateral CR rates for these animals, over a single test session when

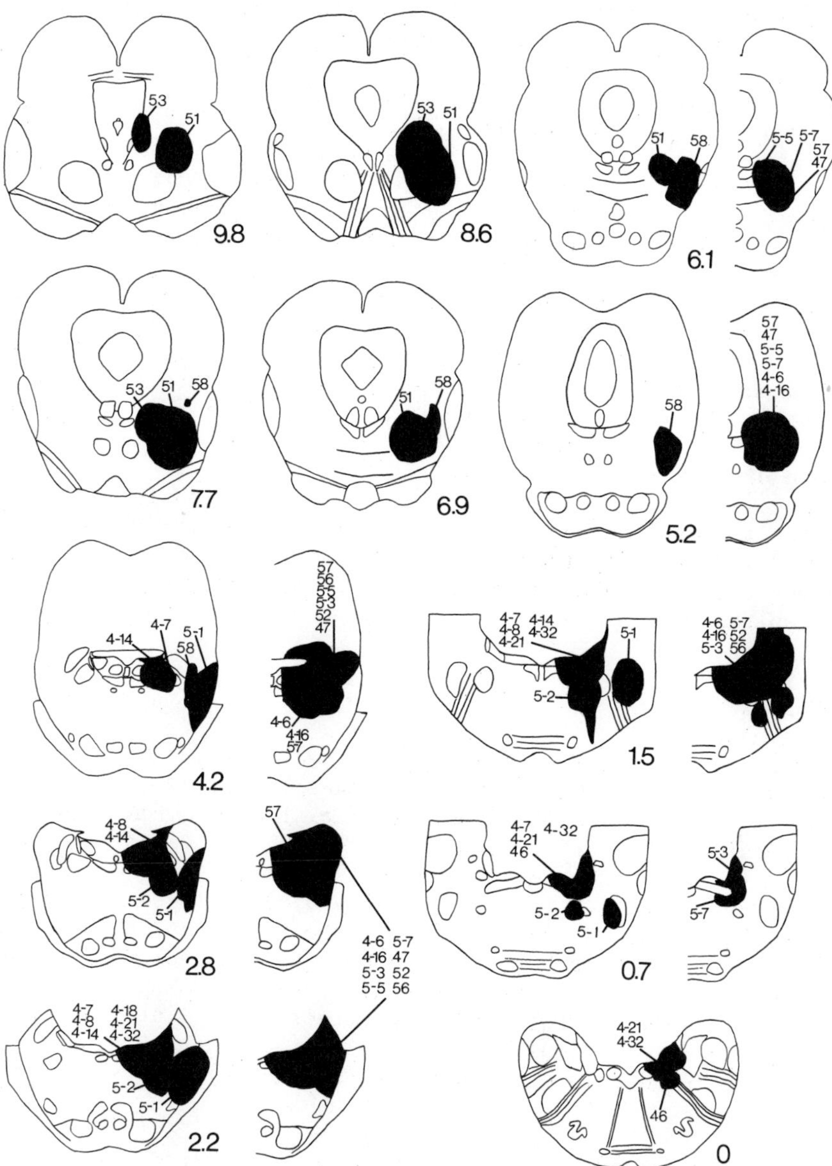

Fig. 6. Selected transverse sections through the brain stem showing the pooled area of tissue loss following lesions of the right side of the neural axis. Nondisrupted cases are depicted on whole sections; Disrupted cases are depicted on hemi-sections. Numbers to the lower right-hand portion of whole sections refer to distance (mm) rostral from the level of the abducens nerve. Other numbers designate individual animals.

the eye shock was switched to the opposite side, was quite comparable to those of controls (see Table 3).

Figure 6 depicts the histological reconstructions of tissue destroyed by lesioning for both Disrupted and Nondisrupted cases: The Disrupted cases are shown on the hemisections to the right of the corresponding complete section. The numbers in the lower left of each complete section is the distance (mm) rostral from the level of the abducens nerve (denoted 0) measured along the neural axis.

By contrasting the pooled tissue loss of Disrupted cases with that of Nondisrupted cases, one may discern tissue regions destroyed in the former group but spared in the latter. This region appears to encompass the dorsolateral pons near to the elbow of the fourth ventricle. In addition, the overall pattern of tissue critical for CRs as suggested by these data compares reasonably well with the pattern of hits and misses depicted in Fig. 3 for CR-correlated unit activity. This evidence, in short, reinforces the impression that the supratrigeminal reticular formation, extending to approximately 3 mm rostrally from the level of the abducens nerve to the level of the principle nucleus of the sensory trigeminal complex confines the crucial region.

DISCUSSION

Our approach to investigating the neural basis of the conditioned NMR in rabbit has relied on converging evidence in an attempt to ascertain the anatomical loci of crucial events responsible for the generation and performance of the CR. Early lesion studies were designed to isolate the motoneurons responsible for the unconditioned NMR (Powell et al., 1979; Berthier and Moore, 1980a). These efforts, and those of others noted in the Introduction, suggested that the primary contributor to the NMR are motoneurons of the ipsilateral accessory abducens nucleus. Powell and Moore (1980) subsequently verified the reports of other investigators in demonstrating the brain stimulation in the region of the brain elicits the NMR and is capable of supporting the acquisition and maintenance of normal appearing CRs.

Berthier's (1981) physiological investigation of the unconditioned NMR indicated that synaptic drive to accessory abducens motoneurons from eye shock stimulation involves disynaptic circuit from brain regions rostral to these motoneurons, most likely the principal nucleus of the sensory trigeminal complex and/or subnucleus oralis. Anatomical studies in rabbit of the projections of fibers in the ophthalmic and mandibular divisions of the trigeminal nerve, and two branches most likely carrying eye shock afferent information, are clarifying the locus of secondary afferent neurons potentially important in conditioned and unconditioned NMRs.

Electrophysiological recordings of multiple-unit activity correlated with conditioning, reported here, encourage the idea that crucial events for conditioning occur in or near to the reflex arc suggested by Berthier's (1981) study. Additional electrode placements are needed in order to define the extent of regions of activity highly correlated with behavioral CRs. In addition, single-unit studies are needed for resolution of questions concerning subpopulations of neurons in the critical zone--questions concerning the latency of action-potentials in relation to the behavioral response, and whether the unit shows evidence of associative learning prior to the first detectable CR.

Additional lesion data are needed in conjunction with further electrophysical mapping studies. Our approach has been to infer a critical brain region in dorsolateral pons by classifying lesioned animals as either Disrupted or Nondisrupted and by comparing histological material from these two groupings. From this point it will be desirable to investigate the quantitive relationship between the size of a lesion in the critical zone and the degree of CR disruption. It will also be desirable to produce fiber-sparing lesions in the critical zone as a means of determining whether it is a site of synaptic integration or merely a route of passage to motoneurons from some as yet untapped loci.

The existence of other brain regions more crucial for the conditioned NMR seems unlikely in view of the evidence in the literature. Oakley and Russell (e.g., 1977), and more recently Moore et al. (1980), have shown that the conditioned NMR of rabbit survives removal of up to 80 per cent of neocortex. A study of Enser, reviewed in Moore (1979a), reports at least some conditioning in decerebrate rabbits, and Norman et al. (1977) report eye blink conditioning in decerebrate cats.

The hippocampus plays a role in rabbit NMR conditioning, as the electrophysiological evidence reported here confirms, but this role appears to be one having to do with higher levels of information processing important for certain derivative learning phenomena (Cormier, 1981; Moore, 1979b; Solomon, 1979). While the hippocampus does not appear to be the locus of associative learning, disruption of hippocampal function (but not ablation) can disrupt associative learning (e.g., Berry and Thompson, 1979; Solomon, 1980).

Lesions of the brain stem at the level of oculomotor nuclei selectively disrupt conditioned inhibition of the rabbit NMR, but not conditioning (Berthier and Moore, 1980b; Mis, 1977). A number of considerations from these studies point to a descending system from the posterior hypothalamus and periaqueductal region of the mesencephalon that inhibits nociception. Ball (1967), for example, showed that rewarding electrical brain stimulation depresses the evoked response of the principal sensory trigeminal nucleus in rats. It is possible that such a descending system also suppresses the representation of the eye shock US which is evoked by a CS and in this way attenuates CRs on nonreinforced trials during CI training.

Given this downstream influence of learned inhibition on CRs, but not URs (see Desmond et al., 1980), and given the evidence that lesions which disrupt CRs do not disrupt URs, we suggest a neuronal model which treats the site of conditioning and the site where learned inhibition acts as being a circuit parallel to the unconditioned reflex arc. A simple version of such a model appears in Fig. 7.

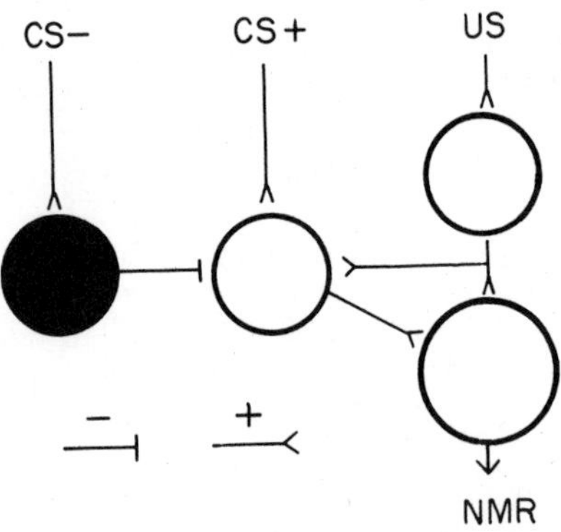

Fig. 7. Proposed neuronal organization of brain stem elements for classical conditioning on the nictitating membrane response (NMR): CS+ = reinforced CS; CS− = conditioned inhibition; US = unconditioned stimulus.

Figure 7 is useful for conceptualizing how lesions might disrupt the CR while leaving the UR intact. The model assumes that convergent inputs from CS+ and a collateral branch of the secondary afferent unit in the circuit of the UR form the basis of associative learning. This learning is mediated by a premotor element represented by the open circle at the center of the diagram. The secondary afferent element is represented by the open circle to the right and situated above the large open circle representing motoneurons controlling the NMR. A conditioned inhibitor (CS-) presumably excites some separate elements (black circle) which suppresses CRs, but not URs, by inhibiting the premotor element. The model assumes that CRs are generated by the premotor element as a consequence of pre- and/or post-synaptic facilitation such as to amplify the flow of information along a pathway from CS+ to the motoneurons. Given the model, it is evident that the lesions described in this report disrupt CRs by any or all of the following effects: 1) obliterating the premotor element 2) interrupting the input from CS+ 3) interrupting the collateral input from the UR pathway 4) interrupting the output of the premotor element to the motoneurons. If CR disruption were merely due to interrupted input from the CS, then it must occur anatomically near to the premotor element. Otherwise, it would not have been possible for conditioning of the contralateral response to proceed normally.

The model in Fig. 7 should be viewed as a collection of working hypotheses. Direct evidence of its continuing usefulness awaits anatomical studies of interconnectivity among the various elements: 1) motoneurons of the accessory abducens nucleus 2) secondary afferent neurons of the principal sensory trigeminal nucleus (and/or subnucleus) 3) premotor elements of an intercalculated reticular formation 4) elements of the mesencephalon mediating inhibition.

Such information would also aid in establishing the basis of the rapid transfer of conditioning to the contralateral NMR. For example, whether there is evidence to support the notion that collaterals from the secondary sensory elements of the US receptive field for one eye project to the contralateral receptive field in such a way as to support a weak form of associative convergence similar to that depicted in Fig. 7 and which could provide the basis for transfer of conditioning.

ACKNOWLEDGEMENTS

Preparation of this report was facilitated by ADAMHA-NIMH Grant #1 RO3 MH 33965-01 and funds provided by USPHS BRSG to the University of Massachusetts-Amherst. We also wish to thank Margaret D. Reilly for dedicated technical assistance.

REFERENCES

Baker, R., McCrea, R. A., and Spencer, R. F., 1980, Synaptic organization of the cat accessory abducens nucleus, J. Neurophysiol., 43:771.

Baldissera, F., and Broggi, G., 1968, Analysis of a trigemino-abducens reflex in a cat, Brain Res., 7:313.

Ball, G. G., 1967, Electrical self stimulation of the brain and sensory inhibition, Psychon. Sci., 8:489.

Becker, H. C., Peacock, S. M., Heath, R. C., and Mickle, W. A., 1961, Methods of stimulation control and concurrent electrographic recording, in: "Electrical Stimulation of the Brain," D. E. Sheer, Ed., University of Texas Press, Austin.

Berger, T.W., Clark, G. A., and Thompson, R. F., 1980, Learning-dependent neuronal responses recorded from limbic system brain structures during classical conditioning, Physiol. Psychol., 8:155.

Berry, S. D., and Thompson, R. F., 1979, Medial septal lesions retard classical conditioning of the nictitating membrane of rabbits, Science 205:209.

Berthier, N. E., and Moore, J. W., 1980a, Role of extraocular muscles in the rabbit (Oryctolagus cuniculus) nictitating membrane response, Physiol. Behav., 24:931.

Berthier, N. E., and Moore, J. W., 1980b, Disrupted conditioned inhibition of the rabbit nictitating membrane response following mesencephalic lesions, Physiol. Behav., 25:667.

Berthier, N. E., 1981, "The Unconditioned Nictitating Membrane Response: The Role of the Abducens Nerve and Nucleus and the Accessory Abducens Nucleus in Rabbit," Ph.D. Dissertation, University of Massachusetts, Amherst.

Cegavske, C. F., Patterson, M. M., and Thompson, R. F., 1979, Neuronal unit activity in the abducens nucleus during classical conditioning of the nictitating membrane response in the rabbit (Oryctolagus cuniculus), J. Comp. Physiol. Psychol. 95:595.

Cormier, S. M., 1981, A match-mismatch theory of limbic system function, Physiol. Psychol., 9:3.

Delgado-Garcia, J., Evinger, C., and Baker, R., 1980, Activity of identitied motoneurons in the abducens and accessory abducens nucleus of the alert cat during eye movement and retraction, Soc. Neurosci. Abstr., 6:16.

Desmond, J. E., Romano, A. C., and Moore, J. W., 1980, Amplitude of the rabbit's nictitating membrane response in the presence of a conditioned inhibitor, Animal Learn. Behav., 8:225.

Disterhoft, J. F., and Shipley, M. T., 1980, Accessory abducens nucleus innervation of rabbit retractor bulbi motoneurons localized with HRP retrograde transport, Soc. Neurosci. Abstr., 6:478.

Gray, T. S., McMaster, S. E., Harvey, J. A., and Gormezano, I., 1980, Localization of the motoneurons which innervate the retractor bulbi muscle in the rabbit, Soc. Neurosci. Abstr., 6:16.

Kraus Perkins, N., and Disterhoft, J. F., 1979, Response plasticity of auditory cortex neurons during tone-signalled conditioning, Soc. Neurosci. Abstr., 5:28.

Lashley, K. S., 1950, In search of the engram, "Experimental Biology Symposium No. 4: Physiological Mechanisms in Animal Behaviour," Cambridge University Press, Cambridge.

Martin, G. K., Land, T., and Thompson, R. F., 1980, Classical conditioning of the rabbit (Oryctolagus cuniculus) nictitating membrane response using electrical brain stimulation as the unconditioned stimulus, J. Comp. Physiol. Psychol., 94:216.

Mis, F. W., 1977, A midbrain-brain stem circuit for conditioned inhibition of the nictitating membrane response in the rabbit (Oryctolagus cuniculus), J. Comp. Physiol. Psychol., 91:975.

Mis, F. W., Gormezano, I., and Harvey, J. A., 1979, Stimulation of abducens nucleus supports classical conditioning of the nictitating membrane response, Science, 206:473.

Mizuno, N., 1970, Projection fibers from the main sensory trigeminal nucleus and the supratrigeminal region, J. Comp. Neurol., 139: 457.

Moore, J. W., 1979a, Brain processes and conditioning, in: "Mechanisms of Learning and Motivation: A Memorial Volume to Jerzy Konorski," A. Dickinson and R. A. Boakes, eds., Erlbaum: Hillsdale, N.J.

Moore, J. W., 1979b, Information processing in space-time by the hippocampus, Physiol. Psychol., 7:224.

Moore, J. W., Yeo, C. H., Oakley, D. A., and Russell, I. S., 1980, Conditioned inhibition of the nictitating membrane response in decorticate rabbits, Behav. Brain Res., 1:397.

Norman, R. J., Buchwald, J. S., and Villablanca, J. R., 1977, Classical conditioning with auditory discrimination of the eye blink in decerebrate cats, Science, 196:551.

Oakley, D. A., and Russell, I. S., 1977, Subcortical storage of Pavlovian conditioning in the rabbit, Physiol. Behav., 18:931.

O'Brien, J. H., Wilder, M. B., and Stevens, C. D., 1977, Conditioning of cortical neurons in cats with antidromic activation as the unconditioned stimulus, J. Comp. Physiol. Psychol., 91:918.

Panneton, W. M., and Burton, H., 1981, Corneal and periocular representation within the trigeminal sensory complex in the cat studied with transganglionic transport of horseradish peroxidase, J. Comp. Neurol., 199:327.

Powell, G. M., Berthier, N. E., and Moore, J. W., 1979, Efferent neuronal control of the nictitating membrane response in rabbit (Oryctolagus cuniculus): A reexamination, Physiol. Behav., 23:299.

Powell, G. M., and Moore, J. W., 1980, Conditioning of the nictitating membrane response in rabbit (*Oryctolagus cuniculus*) with electrical brain-stimulation as the unconditioned stimulus, *Physiol. Behav.*, 25:205.

Solomon, P. R., 1979, Temporal versus spatial information processing theories of hippocampal function, *Psychol. Bull.*, 86:1272.

Solomon, P.R., 1980, A time and place for everything? Temporal processing views of hippocampal function with special reference to attention, *Physiol. Psychol.*, 8:254.

Thompson, R. F., 1976, The search for the engram, *Amer. Psychol.*, 31:209.

Thompson, R. F., Berger, T. W., Berry, S. D., Hoehler, F. K., Kettner, R. E., and Weisz, D. J., 1980, Hippocampal substrate of classical conditioning, *Physiol. Psychol.*, 8:262.

Woody, C. D., Yarowsky, P., Owens, J., Black-Cleworth, P., and Crow, T., 1974, Effect of lesions of cortical motor areas on acquisition of the conditioned eye blink in the cat, *J. Neurophysiol.*, 37:385.

AUDITORY RESPONSE ENHANCEMENT DURING DIFFERENTIAL CONDITIONING IN BEHAVING RATS

Dorwin Birt and M. E. Olds

Division of Biology 216-76
California Institute of Technology
1201 E. California Boulevard, Pasadena, CA 91125

SUMMARY:

Neural unit activity has been recorded from the subcortical portions of the auditory system and surrounding structures during differential appetitive conditioning and reversal in rats. The goal has been to identify and characterize the circuitry involved in learned changes in response to auditory stimuli which are made behaviorally significant by pairing with food pellet presentation. During a single conditioning session, probes throughout the medial division of medial geniculate, the external nucleus of inferior colliculus, an anterior medial portion of inferior colliculus, and the deep portion of superior colliculus showed response enhancements which were selective for the tone paired with pellet presentation. These enhancements started as early as the first 30 ms after stimulus onset and persisted for at least 200 ms. With repeated reversal sessions the locus of points where units continued to show selective enhancement became much more restricted. Within the region of the medial geniculate, only probes in the most caudal portion showed selective enhancement throughout differential conditioning and reversal sessions. No units were found in inferior colliculus which did so. Within the deep portion of superior colliculus and subadjacent tegmentum 73% of auditory responsive units within the most posterior region showed selective enhancement throughout differential conditioning and reversal. No units in the most anterior region did so.

The known topographically organized sensory and motor relationships of neurons in some of the above regions suggest the possibility that these enhancements of response to auditory stimuli paired with food presentation may be functioning to connect the auditory stimuli with particular behavioral responses. With successive reversal sessions, as the behavioral response becomes more efficient, the number of neurons involved might become more restricted. The response enhancements are, however, much more closely time locked to stimulus onset than to behavior onset. The units are therefore not simply behaving in a pre-motor fashion. The fact that neurons in some of these regions have topographically organized relationships to both sensory stimuli and to behavior also suggests that the task of describing the sequence of changes which leads to a new behavioral response to a previously neutral stimulus may be more amenable to analysis than might have been thought.

INTRODUCTION

The response of awake, behaving animals to sensory stimuli is based not only on the physical properties of a stimulus, but also on its learned behavioral significance. Neural circuits must therefore also exist whose activity in response to sensory stimuli is modulated by the previous experience of the animal with that stimulus. We have been for some time conducting a series of experiments (Olds, et al., 1972; Olds, Nienhuis, and Olds, 1978; Birt, Nienhuis, and Olds, 1978; Birt, Nienhuis and Olds, 1979; Birt and Olds, 1981) aimed at identifying and characterizing neural circuitry involved in these changes due to learning. The experimental situation has involved freely behaving rats in a differential appetitive conditioning paradigm in which one of two tones is temporally paired with food pellet presentation while the other tone is not. The conditioned behavioral response is a rapid movement of the head and body toward the pellet dispenser following onset of the paired tone.

The experiments have had three primary goals. The first of these was to establish whether unit response changes occurred which could be shown to be a unique consequence of the pairing of tone and pellet. The second was to determine whether units exhibiting such changes could be shown to differ in anatomic locus or in response characteristics from units not showing such change. If such differences were found, then a basis would exist for identifying other portions of the circuitry involved. The third aim has been to correlate the regions where associative response changes are found with data from lesion, electrical stimulation and neuroanatomic experiments to suggest possible functions for the associative changes of sensory evoked unit responses.

METHODS:

All of the unit data for this presentation have been obtained from semi-microelectrodes chronically implanted in subcortical portions of the auditory system and surrounding structures. Multiple unit activity was recorded prior to and during the presentation of tone stimuli which lasted two seconds. The experimental setup is shown in figure 1. Auditory stimuli were delivered through a tube which was fixed in relationship to the rat's pinna.

Two types of experimental session were run. One of these consisted of 240 presentations of each auditory stimulus and 240 pellets presented in an unpaired manner. The second type of session consisted of 60 presentations of each stimulus and pellet, followed by 180 differential conditioning trials in which one of the two tones was followed at an interval of 1 second by pellet presentation.

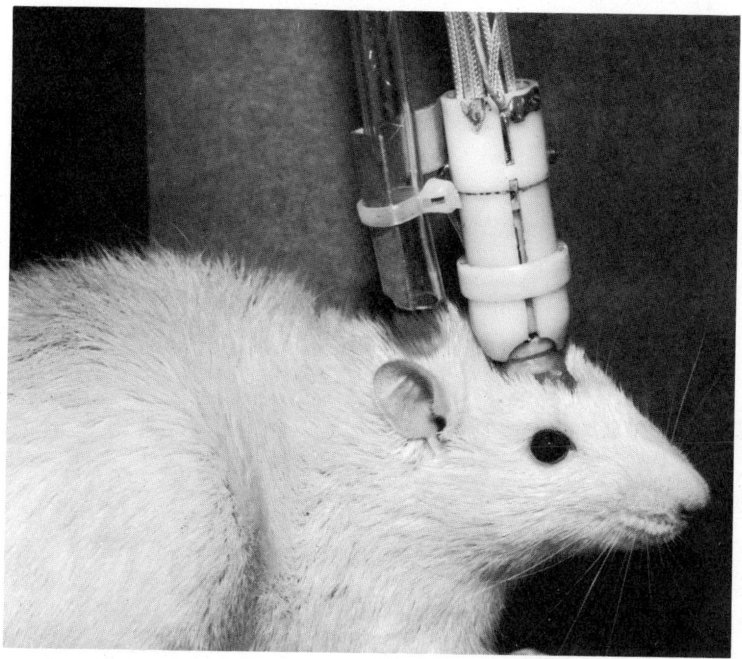

Fig. 1. Illustration of the setup for presenting tones and pellets to behaving rats and for recording unit activity and behavior. Nine fine wire probes are electrically connected to recording circuitry through a commutator system. A food magazine is available for pellet presentation. An electrostatic speaker mounted on top of the chamber produces tones which are conducted to the rat by the plastic sound tube. Not shown is the circuitry for controlling the experiments and for data collection. Head movements and locomotion produce a signal in an open ended wire which can be used to determine the latency and relative magnitude of such movements.

All measures of change occurring during conditioning sessions are based on a comparison of the response during the initial 60 unpaired trials with the response during the final 60 paired trials. In earlier experiments a single session of pseudoconditioning was followed by a single session in which the last 180 trials were differential conditioning. In all of the more recent experiments, one or more reversal sessions have also been run.

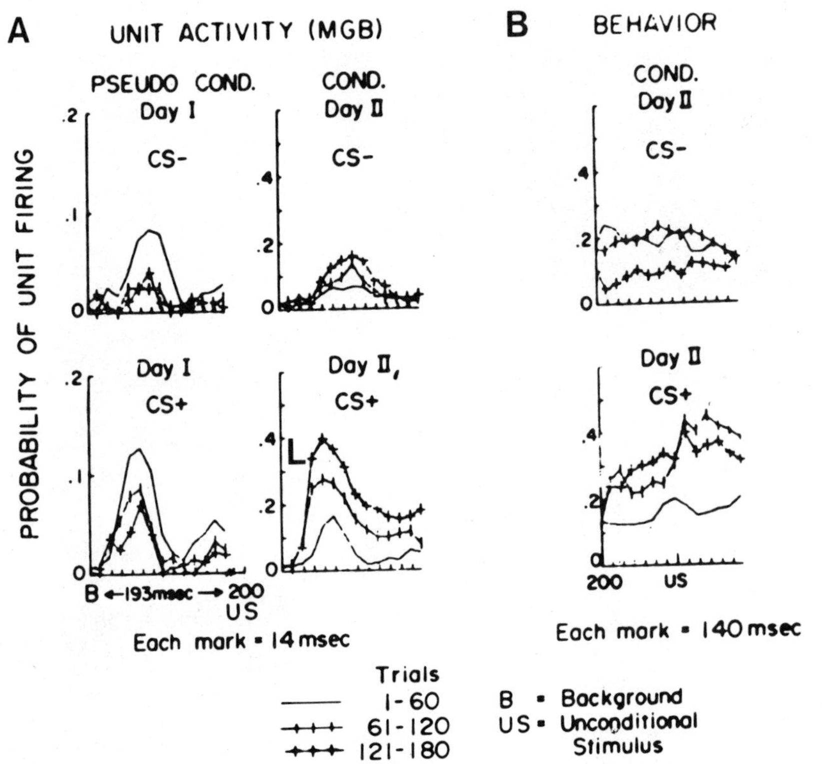

Fig. 2. Changes in response of a unit in posterior medial geniculate during a pseudoconditioning and a conditioning session. The response to each of two different tones is shown for trials early in each session, in the middle of each session, and late in each session. The tone labeled CS+ was paired with pellet presentation during the conditioning session. The latency and relative magnitude of the behavioral response is shown at three intervals during the conditioning session (Olds, Nienhuis, and Olds, 1978).

RESULTS

The basic paradigm is illustrated in figure 2 with data from a unit in the medial geniculate obtained during a pseudoconditioning session and a differential conditioning session. At the left is shown the response to each of two different frequency tones during an initial session which consisted entirely of unpaired trials. The unit was responsive to both of these tones and the response decreased with successive trials. The middle panel shows the response to the same two tones during a second session. During the first 60 trials of this session, neither tone was paired with pellet presentation. The tone designated CS+ was paired with pellet presentation during the remaining 120 trials. The curves with the vertical hatchmarks show the response during the 61st through 120th trials. The curves with the pluses shows the average response during trials 121 through 180. The response to the paired tone is enhanced starting at the second time bin, which is the period 14 to 28 ms after stimulus onset. The enhancement continues throughout the interval shown. The enhancement is selective to the paired tone, since it is much larger than the change in response to the unpaired tone. The right portion of this figure shows the magnitude of the behavioral response to each of the two tones during the conditioning session. The behavioral response occurs only to the paired tone.

One goal of these experiments was to map the distribution of points where such selective response enhancement occurred in order to see if this effect was anatomically localized. Figure 3 shows the locus of points within the region of the medial geniculate where units showing selective response enhancement were found. The top half of this figure shows the units which were responsive to the auditory stimulation. The bottom half shows the location of the units exhibiting selective enhancement. In agreement with the reports of Weinberger (Ryugo and Weinberger, 1978; Hopkins and Weinberger, 1980) and the reports of Gabriel, (Gabriel et al., 1976; Foster et al., 1980) the units showing enhancement are within a medial portion of medial geniculate. The highest proportion of enhancement units was in the caudal portion of medial geniculate and in a region just caudal to medial geniculate proper. Figure 4 similarly shows the distribution of responsive units and of units showing enhancement within the inferior colliculus. The units showing enhancement were mostly anterior and along the medial edge of the inferior colliculus. In this particular experiment, units were not recorded from the external nucleus of the inferior colliculus. Thus during a single conditioning session units within anatomically restricted portions of medial geniculate and inferior colliculus showed short latency, long duration response enhancements which were selective to the paired tone.

We were also interested in determining whether this selective

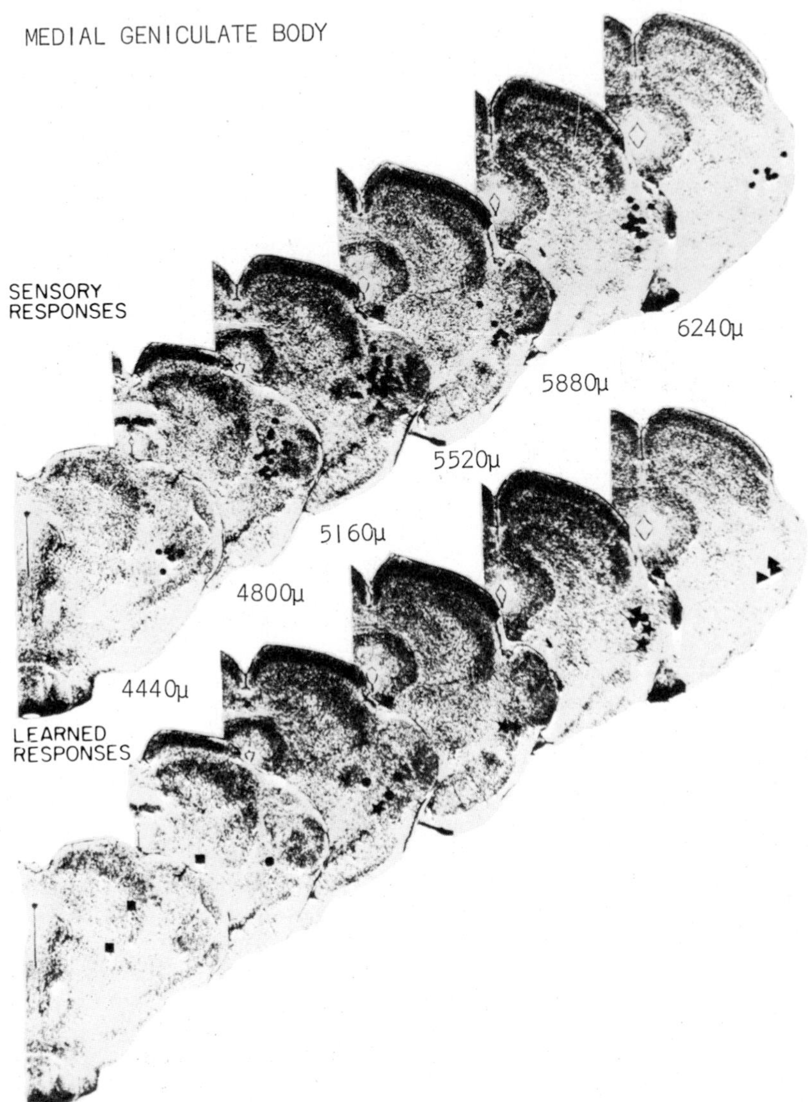

Fig. 3. The distribution of auditory responsive units in the region of the medial geniculate is shown in the top portion of this figure. The locus of units showing selective increase in response to the paired tone during conditioning is shown in the bottom portion. Units showing increase were found in the medial portion of medial geniculate and in a region immediately posterior to medial geniculate. (Olds, Nienhuis and Olds, 1978).

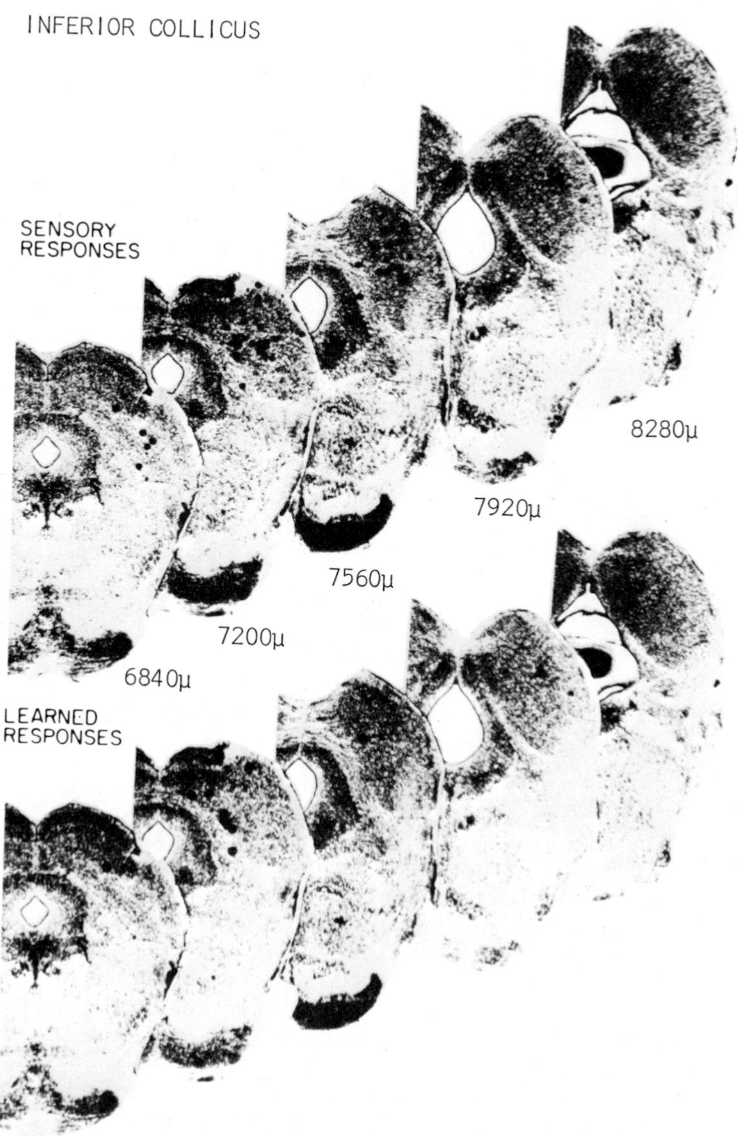

Fig. 4. The distribution of auditory responsive units in the region of the inferior colliculus is shown in the top portion of this figure. The distribution of units showing selective increase in response to the paired tone during conditioning is shown in the bottom portion. Units showing increase were found mostly anteriorly in a region near the medial border of inferior colliculus (Olds, Nienhuis and Olds, 1978).

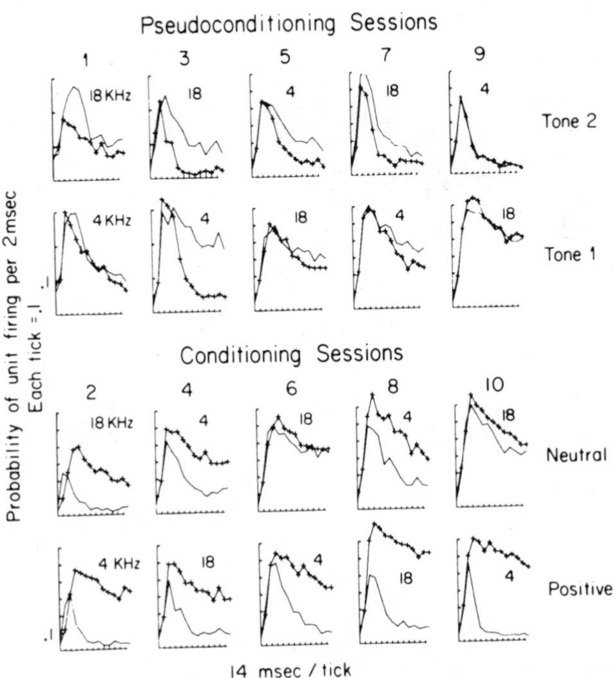

Fig. 5. Response histograms from a unit located in the caudal portion of medial geniculate during a series of pseudoconditioning, differential conditioning and reversal sessions. Unbroken lines in the post-stimulus histograms represent the average unit response to each of the two tones during the first 60 trials of each session. During these trials neither tone was paired with pellet presentation. Lines with pluses represent the unit response during the last 60 trials of each session. The tone labeled positive was paired with pellet presentation during the last 180 trials of each conditioning session. The sequence of sessions is shown by the numbers above each histogram (Birt and Olds, 1981).

enhancement was independent of the particular frequency tone which was paired with pellet presentation. For this reason and to further demonstrate that the response enhancement was a unique function of the pairing of tone and pellet we conducted another series of experiments which involved repeated reversal sessions. Figure 5 shows the results from a unit located near the caudal tip of medial geniculate which showed selective enhancement in each of five conditioning sessions. Between each differential conditioning session, a session consisting entirely of pseudoconditioning trials was run. These pseudoconditioning sessions are shown in the top half of the figure. Between each successive differential conditioning session, the paired and unpaired tones were interchanged.

As in figure 2, the unbroken lines show the response histogram to each of the two tones during the initial 60 trials of each session. The lines with plus symbols show responses to each tone during the last 60 trials of each session. During each conditioning session, shown in the bottom half, a large magnitude increase occurred in the response to the paired stimulus. This increase was always larger than any increases in response to the unpaired tone. The increase began at the 2nd or 3rd 14 ms time bin after stimulus onset and persisted at least throughout the 182 ms shown. In many cases these changes persisted throughout the 1 second interval between tone onset and pellet presentation. These changes are typical of those found in a region shown in figure 6.

Figure 6 shows the location of probes recorded in the region of the medial geniculate during differential conditioning and reversal sessions. The probes indicated with numbered squares are ones in which selective response enhancement occurred during each of 4 differential conditioning sessions. The significant difference between the distribution of these points and the points which showed selective enhancement during a single differential conditioning session is that these units occur only in a region near the caudal tip of medial geniculate. Units showing such enhancement were not observed in the rostral 2/3 of the medial division of medial geniculate.

Figure 7 shows the location of probes recorded in the inferior colliculus during successive conditioning and reversal sessions. In contrast to the results from a single session, no units in this area showed consistent response enhancement throughout conditioning and reversal sessions. Some units within the external nucleus showed selective enhancement during the first session only. This enhancement did not recur during reversals.

These experiments indicate that during differential appetitive conditioning with auditory stimuli, selective response enhancement occurs among units in the medial portion of medial geniculate, in a region just caudal to the medial geniculate, and in subdivisions

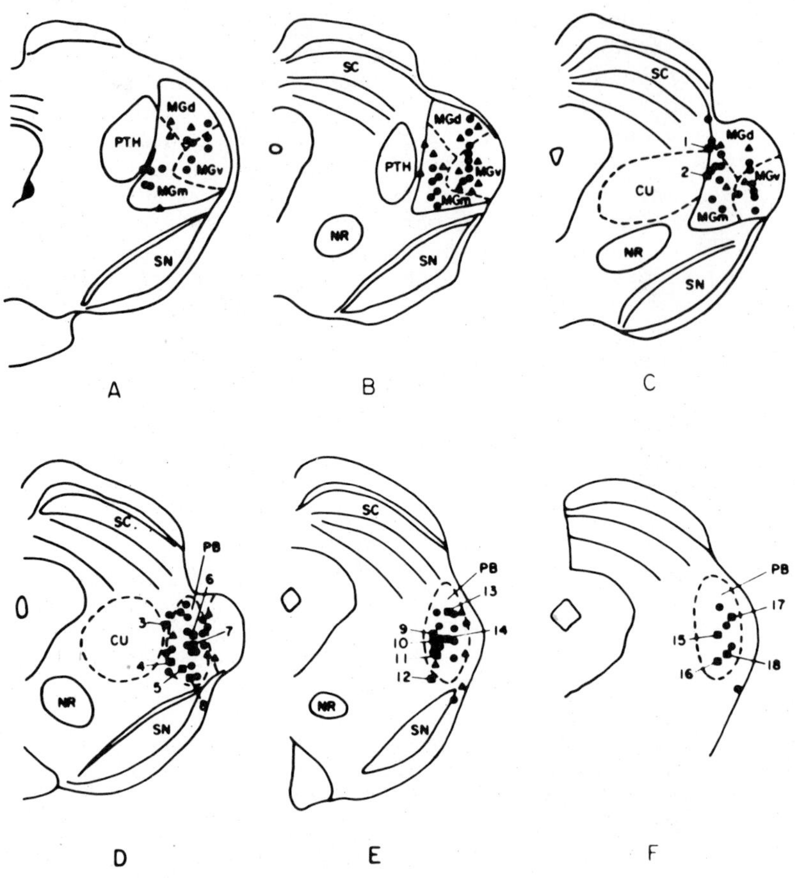

▲ No Auditory Response
● Auditory Response
■ Associative

Fig. 6. Locations of probes in MGB and in the parabrachial region. Sections A through F represent a rostral to caudal sequence (Birt and Olds, 1981).

of the inferior colliculus which surround the central nucleus.

With repeated reversal sessions the distribution of units which continue to show selective change becomes more anatomically restricted. These findings will be discussed later.

Since it was found that the units showing selective and repeatable change were localized anatomically, it was of interest to determine whether there were physiological properties which distinguished units that were likely to show selective response enhancement from

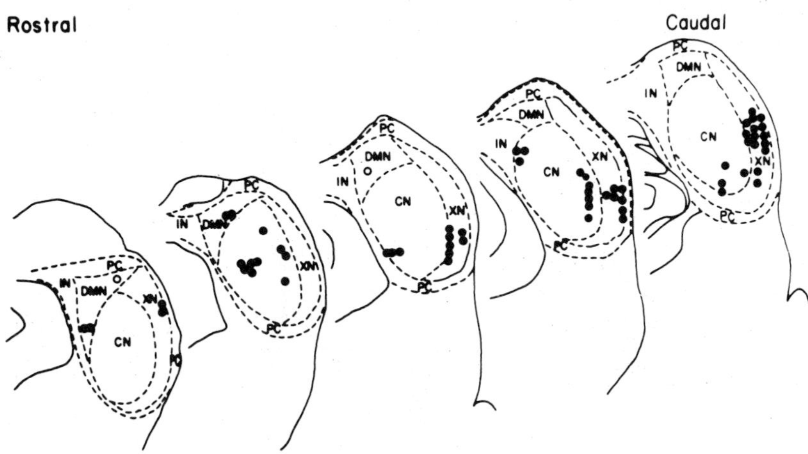

Fig. 7. Locations of responsive probes studied throughout differential conditioning and reversal in divisions of inferior colliculus. No probes in these regions showed consistent selective response enhancement (Birt and Olds, 1981).

those that were unlikely to do so. The properties we looked at were response onset latency, latency to maximum response rate, and duration of initial onset response. These properties were determined prior to conditioning sessions. The relationship of these properties to the likelihood of the units exhibiting selective enhancement is shown in figure 8. These data are taken from the sample of units in the regions of the medial geniculate and inferior colliculus which were shown in the preceding two figures. As shown here, the units which are most likely to exhibit selective response enhancement are those with the longest onset latency, those with the longest latency to maximum response rate and those with the longest duration of response prior to conditioning. Thus it appears that units likely to show repeated, selective enhancement are both anatomically and physiologically distinct from those unlikely to show such enhancement.

The next goal in these experiments was to identify other portions of the circuitry which might be involved in these response enhancements. There were several reasons for believing that the deep portions of the superior colliculus might be involved. First, neuroanatomic experiments have shown connections between the deep portion of the superior colliculus and the medial division of the medial geniculate. (Altman and Carpenter, 1961; Graham, 1977; Rafols and Matzke, 1970; Tarlov and Moore, 1966). Secondly, the principal movement which the rats make in response to the onset of the paired tone is a rapid movement of the head and/or body toward the pellet dispenser. A variety of recording, stimulation, lesion, and neuroanatomic experiments have indicated that the deep portion of the superior colliculus is involved in processes

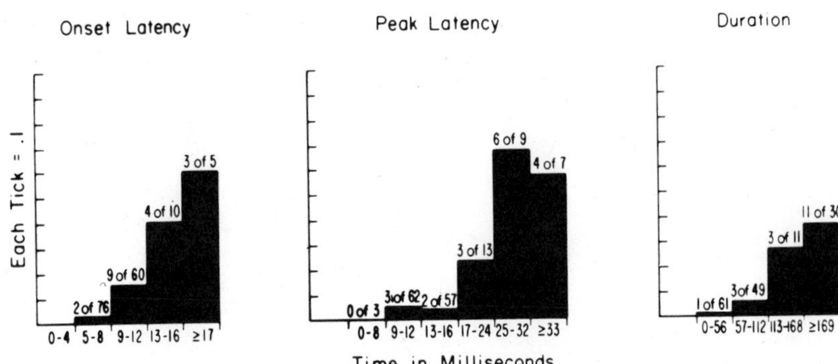

Fig. 8. Proportion of units changing associatively as a function of the pre-conditioning onset latency, latency to peak of response, and duration of initial excitatory response. Numbers above bars represent the number of associative units out of the total number of units in the category (Birt and Olds, 1981).

of orienting toward novel or behaviorally significant stimuli (Wurtz and Albano, 1980). We have therefore conducted a series of differential conditioning and reversal sessions while recording unit activity in the deep layers of the superior colliculus and the underlying tegmentum.

The anatomic locus of all units recorded in this experiment is shown in figure 9. Triangles indicate units unresponsive to tonal stimuli, circles indicate units responsive but not showing selective enhancement, squares indicate selective enhancement units. There were three important findings from the recordings in this region. First, as in previous experiments, we found that the distribution of units which showed selective enhancement throughout differential conditioning and reversal was more anatomically restricted than that of the units which showed selective enhancement during initial conditioning. Secondly, the locus of units showing selective enhancement throughout differential conditioning and reversal was localized. Such units were not found in the most rostral section of SC (Fig. 9A). Seventy three percent of all recorded units in the most posterior section of SC (Fig. 9E) were enhancement units. The proportion of recorded units which showed selective enhancement was 19%, 15% and 32% for the sections shown in fig. 9B, 9C, and 9D respectively. This distribution of enhancement units was significantly different from that expected by chance (Chi square test, p <.001). This was not simply due to the fact that the percentage of responsive units was greater in more posterior penetrations. The distribution of enhancement units is also different from that expected by chance even if the sample is limited to responsive units. (Chi square test, p <.01). The third important finding is that as in previous experiments, the response characteristics of the units in regions of response enhancement are different from those in regions where response enhancement was not found. The onset latency, the latency to peak and the duration of response of units in SC and underlying tegmentum were all significantly greater than those of units in IC (T test, p <.01 in each case). Within SC and underlying tegmentum, however, only duration of response was different

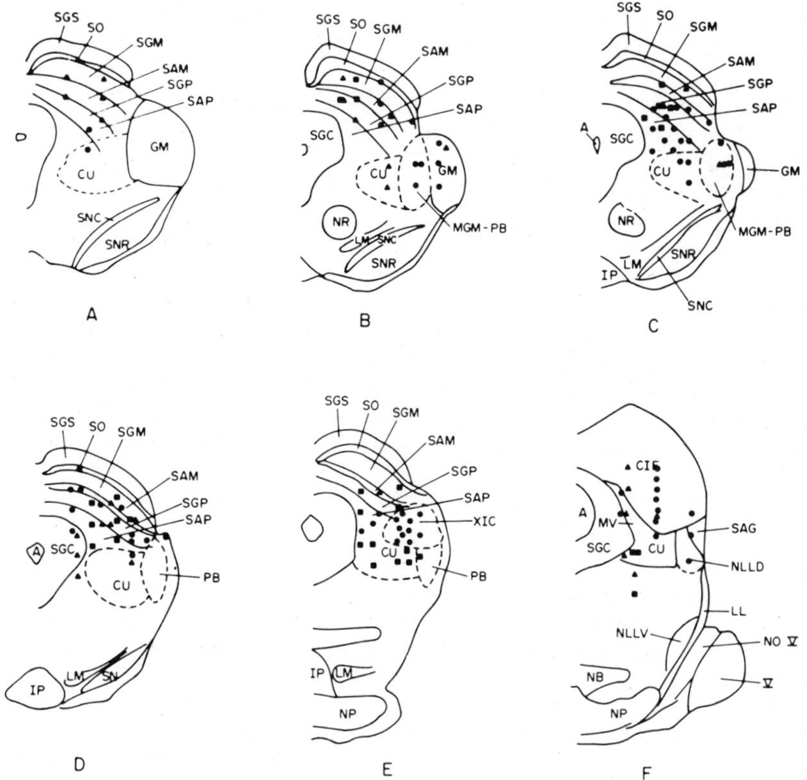

▲ No Auditory Response

● Auditory Response

■ Enhancement

Fig. 9. Locus of units recorded in the intermediate and deep-layers of the superior colliculus, the subadjacent tegmentum and in the inferior colliculus. Symbols are the same as those in figure 6.

between the units showing selective enhancement and those not showing selective enhancement. There is thus no indication that within this region a class of units with particular onset latencies or latencies to peak response is more likely to show response enhancement than another class. There may be a class of units with a sustained response which are more likely to show response enhancement.

The major features of the selective response enhancement occurring during differential conditioning and reversal are illustrated in figure 10. The upper half of this figure shows the histograms obtained from one multiple unit probe during the early part of each session (unbroken lines) and during the late part of each session (plus symbols) in response to two different frequency tones. The first session was a pseudoconditioning session in which neither the 2 khz tone nor the 16 khz tone was ever temporally paired with pellet presentation. Over the course of this session there was a small decrease in the response to each tone. The early trials of the second session (unbroken line) were also unpaired. During the remainder of trials for this session the 2 khz tone was always followed after an interval of one second by pellet presentation. The histograms obtained in the late portion of this session show that the response to the paired tone was profoundly enhanced, starting at a latency in the period 28 to 42 ms and continuing throughout the extent of the histogram. The response to the unpaired tone is essentially unchanged. The histograms in the bottom half of figure 10 show the level of behavioral response to each of the two tones under the different conditions of pairing. Two points should be noted. The first is that the enhancement of the unit response precedes by at least 132 ms the beginning of the behavioral response. During session number 2 the unit response enhancement began at the period 28 to 42 ms. The behavioral measure does not show activity until the period 240 to 320 ms. During session #4 the unit response enhancement begins during the period 14 to 28 ms after stimulus onset. The behavioral response begins during the period 160 to 240 ms. The second point to notice is that the latency and the temporal pattern of the response enhancement are not closely related to the latency and temporal pattern of the behavioral response. The behavioral response in session 4 begins at least 80 ms earlier than it did in session 2. There is no similar shift in the latency of the unit response enhancement. The temporal pattern of the behavioral response in session 2 is one of gradually increasing movement, while that in session 4 is one which quickly reaches a peak, then declines. Neither of these patterns is seen in the corresponding unit response histograms.

The changes shown in figure 10 are typical of most of those seen among units in SC and dorsal tegmentum. In most cases the selective response enhancement begins in the latency period 14 to 28 ms or 28 to 42 ms, is of large magnitude relative to the response during pseudoconditioning and persists at least up to the end of the 182 ms period portrayed in the histograms. The actual distribution of onset of selective response enhancement was 10 units with enhancement starting at 14-28 ms, 16 units at 28-42 ms, 2 units at 42-56 ms and 1 unit at 56-72 ms.

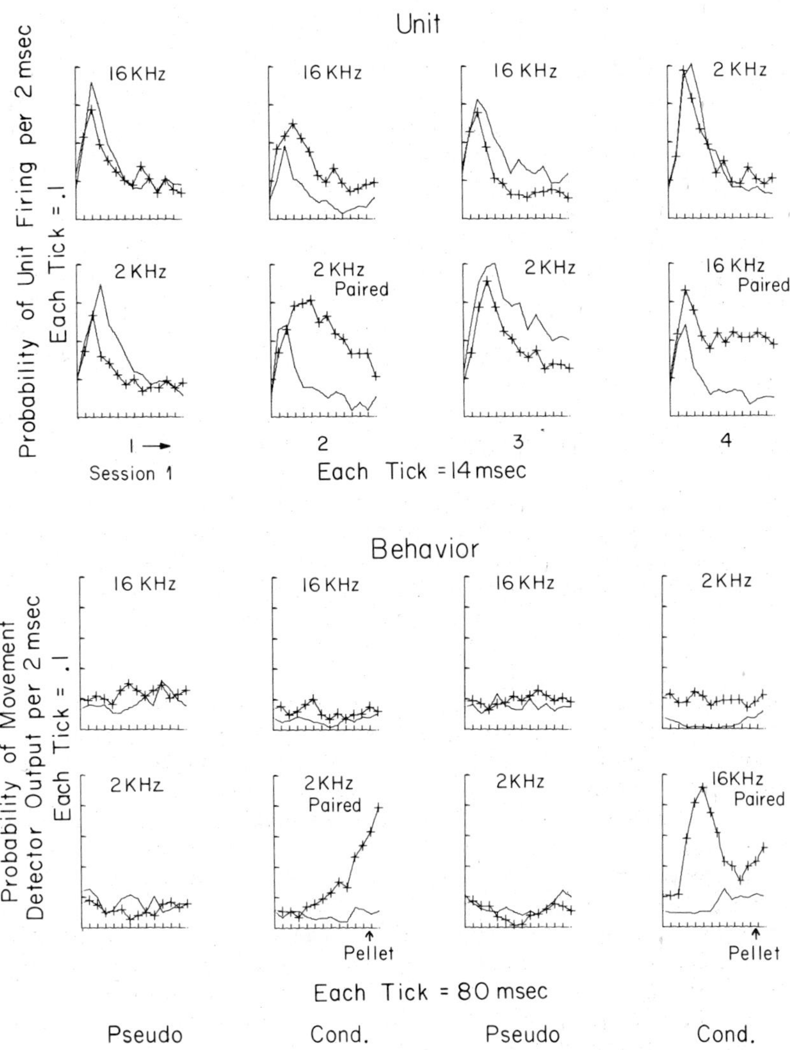

Fig. 10. The response of a unit in superior colliculus during a pseudoconditioning session, a differential conditioning session, a second pseudoconditioning session, and a reversal session. The symbols are the same as those in figure 5.

DISCUSSION

The effects of these conditioning procedures on neural responses to tone stimuli can be divided into three distinct classes. Some neurons seem essentially unaffected by learned changes of stimulus significance. Neurons in the central nucleus of the inferior colliculus (ICc) and the ventral nucleus of the medial geniculate (MGv) have responses of this type. Another group of neurons shows large magnitude, relatively short latency selective response enhancements of auditory evoked response which occur reliably throughout differential conditioning and reversal sessions. Neurons in this category were found in the intermediate and deep layers of superior colliculus (SC), in a posterior portion of the cuneiform nucleus (CU), and the parabrachial region near the caudal tip of MG. A third group of neurons also showed large magnitude selective response enhancements during some conditioning sessions, usually the first, but completely failed to show such effects during repeated sessions. Neurons in this category were found in an anterior portion of the cuneiform nucleus, in the external nucleus of IC and in the medial division of MG. It was also found that neurons in the regions where selective, repeatable change was found had temporal characteristics of their responses which differentiated them from neurons in regions where these changes were not found.

Two interpretations might account for these results. One of these is that neurons in these different regions are involved in processes of associative pairing in fundamentally different ways. Thus, some neurons might be fairly rigidly encoding the physical parameters of stimuli, others might be associatively changed by initial conditioning but not by reversals, while the response of still others would follow changes in the behavioral significance of stimuli.

A second interpretation is suggested when account is taken of a variety of data which shows that neurons in some of these regions, particularly the superior colliculus and dorsal tegmentum have topographically organized relationships to sensory stimuli and to particular motor behaviors. These studies have shown that cells respond maximally to visual, auditory, and somatosensory stimuli at particular locations. (Drager and Hubel, 1975; Gordon, 1973; Stein, 1978; Wurtz, Goldberg, and Robinson, 1980; Peck, Schlag-Rey, and Schlag, 1980; Mays and Sparks, 1980). They have also shown that locally applied electrical stimulation leads to movements of the eyes, the head, or the pinna. The direction and magnitude of movement is dependent upon the locus of stimulation. (Schiller and Stryker, 1972; Blakemore and Donaghy, 1980). Lesions of this region have been shown to result in deficits in orienting behavior. Stimulation within the same portion of dorsal tegmentum where we have found the highest proportion of enhancement units has been shown to result in forward locomotion (Parker, Russo, Mink, and

Sinnamon, 1981) and lesions of this region have been shown to interfere with striatally elicited turning (Mulas et al., 1981). All of these findings which demonstrate motor as well as sensory relationships of cells in these regions raise a crucial question. To what extent should short latency enhancements in response to particular auditory stimuli be considered modulations of sensory response due to learning about the significance of the stimulus or to what extent may they be precursors to specific movements which the animal learns to make in response to the stimulus? If they are precursors to specific movements, then as the range of movements becomes more restricted during successive reversal sessions, the distribution of units showing enhancement would also become more restricted. Thus the observation that units in some regions show enhancement only during the first conditioning session might be due to the fact that unit activity in these regions is a precursor to movements which occur only during the first session in freely behaving rats. Units in regions where enhancement reliably occurs during repeated reversals may have activity which is a precursor to conditioned movements which occur reliably throughout conditioning and reversals. There are several reasons, however, for thinking that such a fixed relationship to movement does not entirely account for our results. First, the response enhancement was highly time locked to stimulus onset but not time locked to the onset of the behavioral response. Secondly, the unit response enhancement continued to occur during blocks of trials when the animal ceased to respond behaviorally. Thirdly, the magnitude of the response enhancement was not highly correlated across trials with the magnitude of the behavioral response.

We are currently considering the hypothesis that these auditory response enhancements are at an early stage in the processing chain which connects particular behaviors of locomotion or orienting to particular stimuli. This hypothesis would predict that the distribution of units showing enhancement would be determined both by the type of stimuli used and the nature of the behavioral response, but that unit activity would not be necessarily closely related to the final behavioral output. The extensive literature which is becoming available concerning the connectivity of these regions and their ordered relationships to sensory and motor domains make it feasible to begin to describe the sequence of changes which result in these new behavioral responses to auditory stimuli. The findings that these changes are both highly localized into anatomically distinct regions and that units within these regions have distinctive response properties will further facilitate this attempt.

ACKNOWLEDGMENTS

This research was supported by PHS grant MH-16978 and NSF grant BNS 77-22289.

REFERENCES

Altman, J., and Carpenter, M., 1961, Fiber projections of the superior colliculus in the cat, J. Comp. Neurol., 116:157-166.

Birt, D., and Olds, M. E., 1981, Associative response changes in lateral midbrain tegmentum and medial geniculate during differential appetitive conditioning. J. Neurophysiol., 46:1039-1055.

Birt, D., Nienhuis, R., and Olds, J., 1978, Effects of bilateral auditory cortex ablation on behavior and unit activity in rat inferior colliculus during differential conditioning, J. Neurophysiol., 41:705-715.

Birt, D., Nienhuis, R. and Olds, M., 1979, Separation of associative from non-associative short latency changes in medial geniculate and inferior colliculus during differential conditioning and reversal in rats., Brain Res., 167:129-138.

Blakemore, C. and Donaghy, M. J., 1980, Coordination of head and eyes in the gaze changing behaviour of cats, J. Physiol., 300:317-335.

Drager, U. C., and Hubel, D. H., 1975, Responses to visual stimulation and relationship between visual, auditory, and somatosensory inputs in mouse superior colliculus, J. Neurophysiol., 38:690-713.

Foster, K., Orona, E., Lambert, R., and Gabriel, M., 1980, Neuronal activity in the auditory system during differential conditioning in rabbits, Soc. Neurosci. Abstr., 6:424.

Gabriel, M., Miller, J. D.,and Saltwick, S. E., 1976, Multiple-activity of the rabbit medial geniculate nucleus in conditioning, extinction, and reversal, Physiol. Psychol., 4:124-134, 1976.

Gordon, B., 1973, Receptive fields in deep layers of cat superior colliculus, J. Neurophysiol., 36:157-178.

Graham, J., 1977, An autoradiographic study of the efferent connections of the superior colliculus in the cat, J. Comp. Neurol., 173:629-654.

Hopkins, W., and Weinberger, N. M., 1980, Modification of auditory cortex single unit activity during pupillary conditioning, Soc. Neurosci. Absts., 6:424.

Mays, L. E., and Sparks, D. L., 1980, Dissociation of visual and saccade-related responses in superior colliculus neurons, J. Neurophysiol., 43:207-232.

Mulas, A., Longoni, R., Spina, L., Del Fiacco M., and DiChiara, G., 1981, Ipsiversive turning behaviour after discrete lesions of the dorsal mesencephalic reticular formation by kainic acid, Brain Res., 208:468-473.

Olds, J., Disterhoft, J., Segal, M., Kornblith, C., and Hirsh, R., 1972, Learning centers of the rat brain mapped by measuring latencies of conditioned unit responses, J. Neurophysiol., 35:202-219.

Olds, J., Nienhuis, R., and Olds, M. E., 1978, Patterns of conditioned unit responses in the auditory system of the rat, 59:209-228.

Parker, S. M., Russo, R. C., Mink, J. W., and Sinnamon, H. M., 1981, Forward locomotion in the diencephalon and mesencephalon mapped by electrical stimulation, Soc. Neurosci. Absts., 7:753.

Peck, C. K., Schlag-Rey, and Schlag, J., 1980, Visuo-oculomotor properties of cells in the superior colliculus of the alert cat, J. Comp. Neurol., 194:97-116.

Rafols, J., and Matzke, H., 1970, Efferent projections of the superior colliculus in the opossum, J. Comp. Neurol., 138:147-160.

Ryugo, D. K., and Weinberger, N. M., 1978, Differential plasticity of morphologically distinct neuron populations in the medial geniculate body of the cat during classical conditioning, Behav. Biol., 22:275-301.

Schiller, P. H., and Stryker, M., 1972, Single-unit recording and stimulation in superior colliculus of the alert rhesus monkey, J. Neurophysiol., 41:55-64.

Tarlov, E. C., and Moore, R. Y., 1966, The tecto-thalamic connections in the brain of the rabbit, J. Comp. Neurol., 126:403-422.

Wurtz, R. H., and Albano, J. E., 1980, Visual-motor function of the primate superior colliculus, Ann. Rev. Neurosci., 3:189-226.

Wurtz, R. H., Goldberg, M. E., and Robinson, D. L., 1980, Behavioral modulation of visual responses in the monkey: Stimulus selection for attention and movement, Prog. Psychobiol. Physiol. Psychol., 9:44-86.

ENDOGENOUS AUDITORY POTENTIALS IN THE CAT: A P300 MODEL

Jennifer S. Buchwald and Nancy S. Squires

Mental Retardation Research Center, Brain Research Institute and Department of Physiology, University of California Medical Center, Los Angeles, California 90024

INTRODUCTION

Endogenous evoked potentials are those whose characteristics are determined by the psychological context in which a stimulus occurs, rather than by the physical parameters of the stimulus itself (Donchin et al., 1978; Hillyard et al., in press). Such potentials are produced by unexpected stimuli within a sequence of expected stimuli in any stimulus modality (Simson et al., 1977; Squires et al., 1977; Desmedt and Debecker, 1979), or by the omission of an expected stimulus (Picton et al., 1974; Simson et al., 1976; Sutton et al., 1967). For example, if a subject is asked to count a click of one intensity which occurs only infrequently during a series of clicks of another intensity, only the rare, unexpected click produces endogenous wave forms (Fig. 1) (Ritter et al., 1972; Squires et al., 1975; Roth et al., 1976). These potentials have been associated with sequential processing and short-term memory functions (Squires et al., 1976), and have been shown to be abnormal in various clinical populations (Goodin et al., 1978; Squires et al., 1979, Pfefferbaum et al., 1979). Thus, experimental analyses and identification of the generator sources of endogenous potentials would be of clinical importance as well as of basic neurophysiological interest.

Animal models of human electrophysiological events provide a means of determining brain substrates essential for particular evoked potential components and of delineating underlying neural mechanisms. The effectiveness of this approach has been demonstrated in the case of the auditory brain stem responses (ABRs), whose neural sources have been extensively studied in animal preparations (Buchwald, 1981). Such experimental data have, in part,

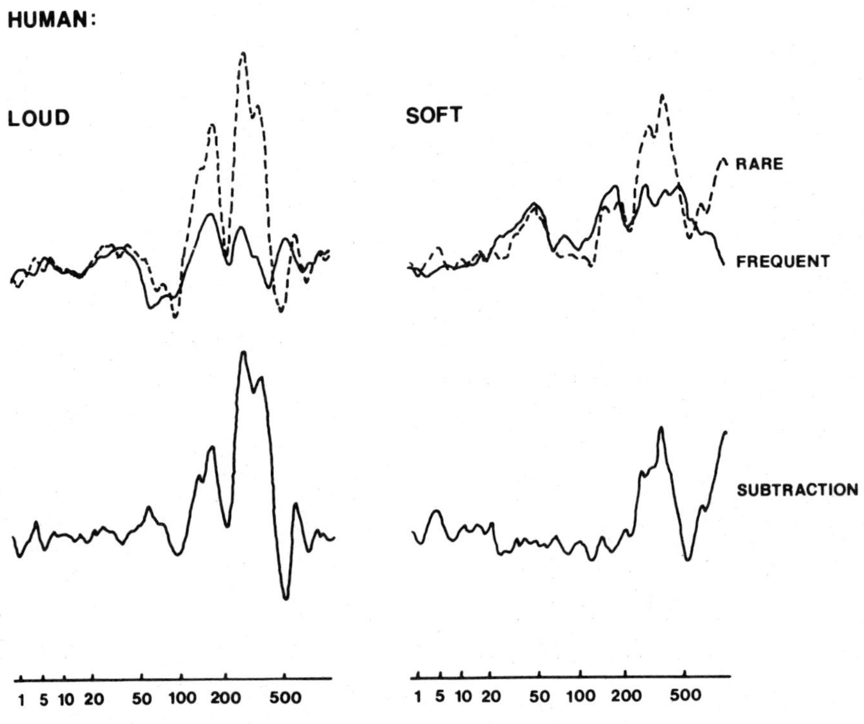

Fig. 1. Endogenous P3 potentials recorded and averaged from a human subject during presentations of frequent (80%) soft clicks and rare (20%) loud clicks (left traces) or of frequent loud and rare soft clicks (right traces). The difference potentials obtained by subtraction of the frequent click response from the rare stimulus response is shown in the bottom traces.

led to the correlation of ABR abnormalities in the human with levels or regions of brainstem pathology (Nodar et al., 1980; Starr and Hamilton, 1976; Stockard et al., 1977). The purpose of the present study was to determine whether endogenous potentials can be reliably obtained in the cat with procedures similar to those which produce endogenous potentials in humans. Demonstration of such potentials would provide an experimental model in which generator systems could subsequently be investigated.

METHODS

Five adult cats have been studied from which generally similar results were obtained. Under pentobarbital anesthesia, stainless steel screw electrodes were implanted just off the midline on the inter-aural plane, 1cm anterior and posterior, and in the frontal sinus, with leads connected to a head plug imbedded in acrylic. During testing the animal was awake and restrained in a canvas bag with its head held in a fixed position by bars extending from the stereotaxic frame to stainless steel tubes cemented in the head mount. Acoustic stimuli were presented free-field through a speaker placed at a constant location in the sound isolation chamber, 15cm in front of the cat's nose. Hearing level (HL) was based on threshold for normal hearing adults. Three types of stimuli were presented in random order with a fixed ISI of 1.5 sec: a 4 KHz tone (1 sec duration, 50 dBHL), a loud click (.1 ms duration, 70 dBHL), and a soft click (.1 ms duration, 40 dBHL). The tone occurred with a probability of .05 and served as an eyeblink conditioning stimulus (CS). At the termination of the tone a 50 ms train of five .1 ms duration shocks was delivered as the unconditioned stimulus (UCS) through bipolar subcutaneous electrodes dorsal to the left supraorbital margin. Each session consisted of four runs of 500 stimulus presentations. In two runs the loud click occurred frequently (P = .80) and the soft click rarely (P = .15). In the other two runs the probabilities of the two clicks were reversed. EEG from the skull electrode was referenced either to the frontal sinus electrode or to a subcutaneous needle electrode on the bulla, amplified with a gain of 20,000 and a bandpass of .3 Hz to 3 KHz, and averaged on-line with a PDP 11-10 computer. The recording was digitized with a non-linear time base from 0-1500 ms. The non-linear time base permitted clear visualization of all auditory evoked response components, which increase in duration with increasing peak latency (Picton et al., 1974). Eye movements and orbicularis oculi EMG were monitored from subcutaneous electrodes above and at the outer canthus of the left eye.

RESULTS

Presentation of the click stimuli to the awake naive cat,

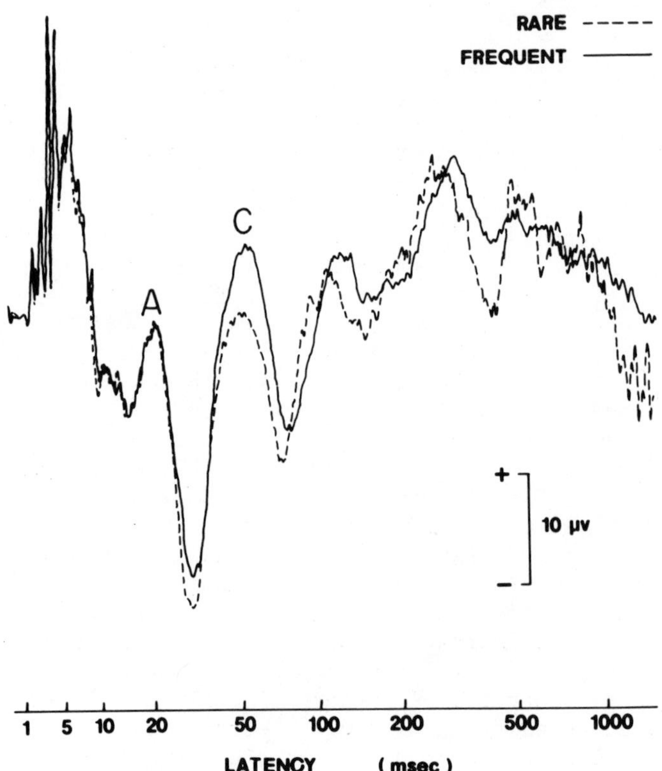

Fig. 2. Evoked potentials of naive cat TG to the loud click in the rare and in the frequent stimulus condition. Traces represent grand averages across 4 recording sessions.

without CS reinforcements, resulted in a prolonged series of evoked potentials (Buchwald et al., 1981) (Fig. 2). The short latency ABRs were clearly visible and differentiated the loud and soft clicks but remained constant across sessions and stimulus probability. In contrast, the longer latency responses were highly variable. A positive component with peak latency of 17-25 ms (wave A) was generally present, followed by a large negative trough and a subsequent positivity with a peak at 50-75 ms (wave C) (Fig. 2). Potentials subsequent to wave C were not consistently recorded from the naive cat. In Figure 2, one cat's responses to the loud click, presented in either the rare or the frequent stimulus configuation, are illustrated. In general, the long latency potentials tended to become smaller during and across recording sessions. None was consistently larger to the rare than to the frequent stimulus, as evidenced by peak-to-peak amplitude comparisons. In cat TG, for example (Fig. 2), from the 30 ms negative trough to the peak of wave C, the rare/frequent ratios were .97 (loud) and 1.02 (soft); from the peak of wave C to the subsequent negativity, the ratios were .97 (loud) and .79 (soft).

The CS-UCS pairings served to focus the animal's attention to the auditory modality. Conditioned eyeblink responses occurred with latencies greater than 100 ms and were confined to the tone (Fig. 3). Short-latency (15-30 ms) reflex eyeblinks were sometimes elicited by the loud clicks; these did not covary with stimulus probability (Norman et al., 1974; Norman et al., 1977). After CS-UCS training commenced, an eyeblink conditioned response quickly developed which was specific to the CS and did not accompany the loud or soft click stimuli. In contrast to the habituation sessions, under these conditions attention was clearly focused to the auditory modality as indicated by the discriminative conditioned response. When responses to the click stimuli were compared, the rare stimulus was found to produce a differential enhancement of the 30 ms negative trough preceding wave C, of wave C, and of a positive component in the 200-500 ms latency range. This effect is shown for one cat in Fig. 4. The concurrently recorded EMG and oculogram showed no consistent activity in these time periods.

When the frequent-click response was subtracted from the rare-click response, a difference potential was observed for within-session and across-session recordings for a single cat as well as when grand averages across cats were subtracted. Difference potentials for three cats are summarized in Figs. 5 and 6. Considerable variability in waveform occurred across cats, but enhancements of the negative component preceding wave C, of wave C (or a coincident positive component in the 50-100 ms range), and of a positivity in the 200-500 ms range were generally observed in the difference potentials. Rare loud clicks usually induced larger difference potentials than the rare soft clicks. However, the evoked potentials to loud and soft rare clicks showed essentially equivalent percent-

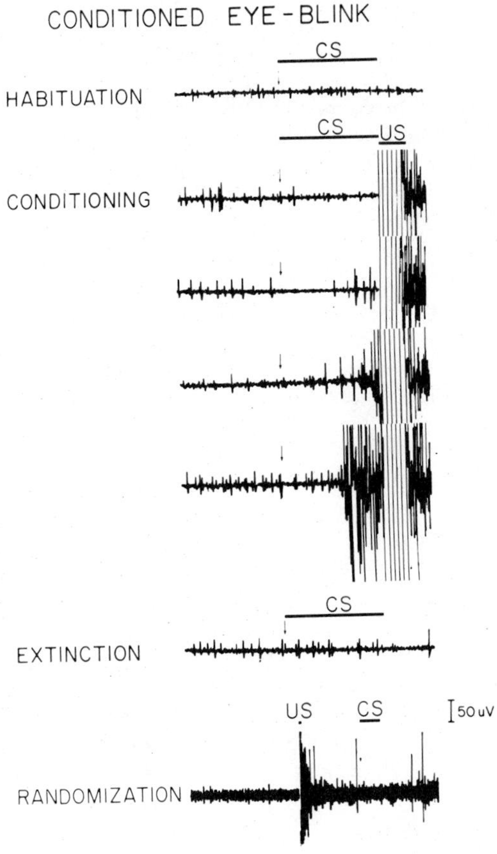

Fig. 3. Typical development of a conditioned blink response in one cat. CRs were characterized by a long-latency (greater than 100 msec) burst of EMG activity which developed after CS and US pairings. Traces A through D represent changes in EMG responsiveness to the CS which typically occurred over one to two training sessions. (From Norman et al., 1974)

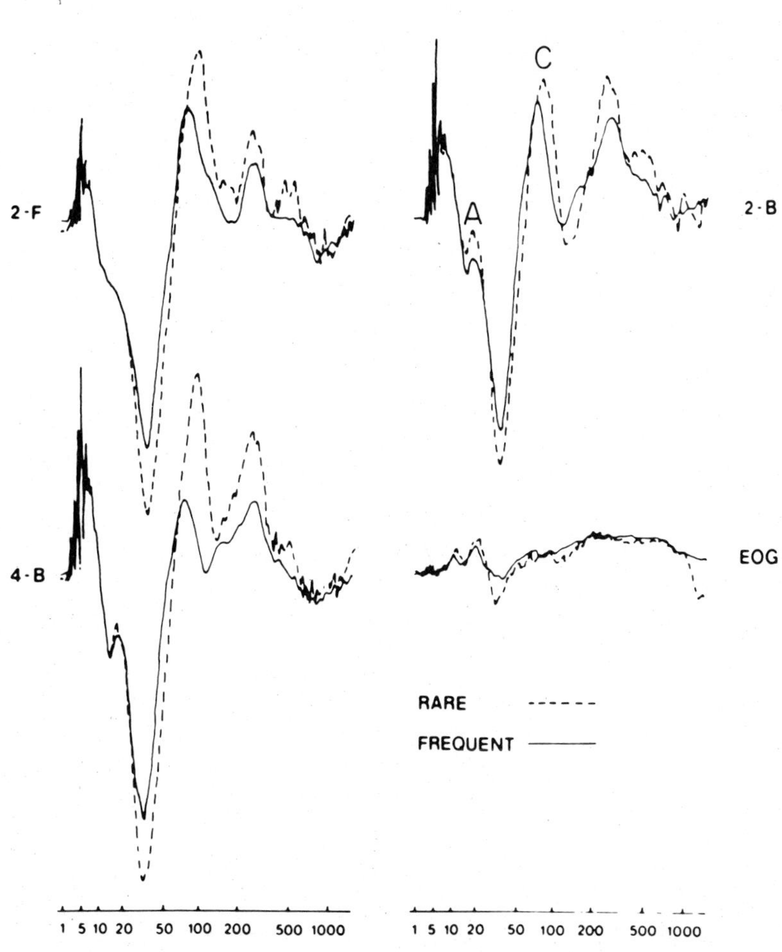

Fig. 4. Evoked potentials of cat FC during a session with well discriminated conditioned eyeblinks. The rare stimulus was the loud click. Recordings are from a rostral electrode referenced to frontal sinus (2F) or bulla (2B) and from a positive electrode referenced to bulla (4B). The oculogram (EOG) was recorded from the conditioned eye.

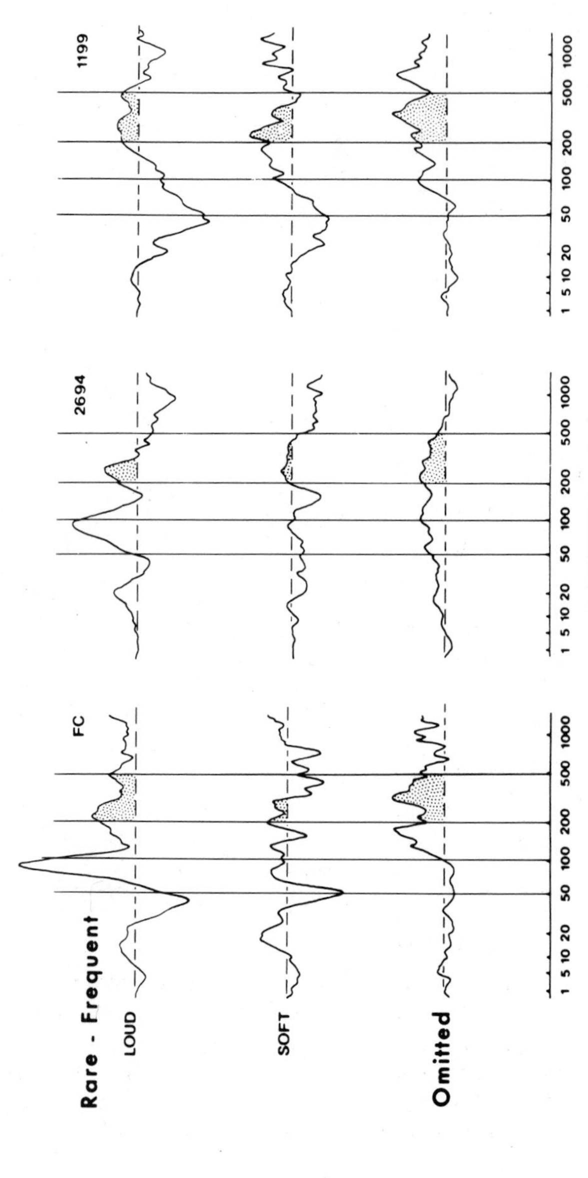

Fig. 5. Difference potentials obtained by subtraction of the grand averages across four sessions for cats FC, 2694 and 1199. The rare stimulus was loud (top) or soft (middle). Potentials resulting from stimulus omission (bottom) are averaged across 3 to 6 sessions. The waveforms associated with the loud clicks are plotted at half scale in order to facilitate comparisons of morphology.

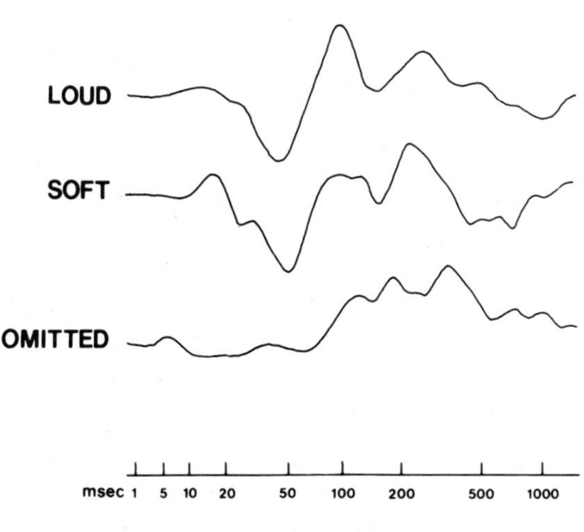

Fig. 6. Grand averages across three cats of the difference potentials, rare minus frequent, for the loud and soft click stimuli. The third waveform is the response to omitted rare stimuli averaged across the same three cats. The evoked potential difference associated with the loud stimulus is plotted at half the vertical gain of the other two waveforms.

age enhancements. Peak-to-peak measurements (mean of 3 cats) between the 30 ms negative trough and wave C showed a rare/frequent enhancement of 1.51 (loud) and 1.20 (soft); between wave C and the subsequent negativity around 150 ms of 1.75 (loud) and 2.54 (soft); and between this 150 ms negativity and the 200-500 ms positivity of 1.76 (loud) and 1.77 (soft). Two-way analyses of variance were performed on these peak-to-peak amplitudes, for each stimulus type, as a function of component and probability. For both the loud and soft click the main effect of component was significant. The main effect of probability was significant ($p < .05$) for the loud click but not for the soft click. However, the probability by component interaction was significant for both stimuli ($p < .01$), indicating a variable magnitude of the effect of probability across components.

In order to determine whether the difference potential was simply a function of startle or arousal to an unexpected stimulus, additional sessions were carried out in which stimulus-omission was substituted for the rare stimulus. Consistent enhancement of the positivity between 200 and 500 ms resulted from this procedure, as illustrated by the omitted-stimulus potentials in Fig. 5 and 6. Although the morphology varied somewhat between cats it was replicable within cats. In one cat (FC), omitted-stimulus potentials were observed in 11 of 12 sessions, with approximately 6 months intervening between the first 6 sessions and the last 6 sessions.

DISCUSSION

The electrophysiological responses described here for cats resemble human endogenous potentials in several respects. They occur only when the stimuli are task relevant, they depend upon the improbability of the stimuli, they are not dependent upon a particular stimulus parameter, e.g., intensity, and at least some subset of the potentials is produced by stimulus omissions. In the human a negativity at 200 ms (N_2) and a positivity at 300 msec (P_3) are the endogenous potentials that have been emphasized, although the endogenous activity may begin somewhat earlier (Goodin et al., 1978). In the cat, endogenous activity appears to commence with a 30-40 ms negativity followed by a 50-100 ms positivity, a small negativity at 150 ms, and a 200-500 ms broad positivity.

The 50-100 ms positivity, which is enhanced under the procedures of this experiment, coincides with wave C. Wave C disappears after bilateral hemispherectomy, during rapid (10/sec) rates of stimulation, and under conditions of barbiturate anesthesia (Buchwald et al., 1981). To the extent that the endogenous wave enhancement is, at least in part, channeled through the generator system of wave C, this requires the cerebral hemispheres. The later 200-500 ms positivity has not yet been related to any brain region or possible neural generator in the cat. Along parametric dimensions it appears similar to the positivity reported to accompany conditioned pupillary dilation responses in the paralyzed cat (Wilder et al., 1981). In the human, the surface recorded P_3 potential has been correlated with potentials with similar parametric characteristics recorded from the hippocampus and amygdala (Wood et al., 1980; Halgren et al., 1980).

In conclusion, we suggest that the current procedure is an animal analog of procedures used to study endogenous activity in the human. The resultant potentials in the cat are more accessible to neurophysiological analysis than those in the human so that generator systems of the endogenous potential components may be experimentally explored and their neural mechanisms described.

SUMMARY

Surface recordings in the awake cat were carried out under conditions similar to those which produce endogenous brain activity in human subjects. Only during procedures in which the cat was conditioned to attend to the auditory modality were responses dependent upon stimulus probability. In such cats, rare click stimuli, which differed in intensity from the frequent click stimuli, produced a series of unique evoked potentials across the 30 to 500 ms latency range. These responses resemble human endogenous potentials in that they depend on the task-relevance and improbability of the stimulus, they do not depend on a particular stimulus parameter, and at least some subset of the potentials is produced by unexpected stimulus omissions.

REFERENCES

Buchwald, J.S., 1981, Generators of auditory evoked potentials, _in_: "Handbook of Electrocochleography and Brain Stem Electrical Responses," E. Moore, ed., Grune & Stratton, Inc., New York.

Buchwald, J.S., Hinman, C., Norman, R.J., Huang, C.-M., and Brown, K., 1981, Middle- and long-latency auditory evoked responses recorded from the vertex of normal and chronically lesioned cats, _Brain Res._ 205 :91.

Desmedt, J.E. and Debecker, J., 1979, Wave form and neural mechanism of the decision P350 elicited without pre-stimulus CNV or readiness potential or random sequences of near-threshold auditory clicks and finger stimuli, _Electroenceph. clin. Neurophysiol._, 47 :671.

Donchin, E., Ritter, W. and McCallum, W.C., 1978, Cognitive psychophysiology: The endogenous components of the ERP, _in_: "Event-Related Brain Potentials in Man," E. Callaway, P. Tueting and S.H. Koslow, eds., Academic Press, New York.

Goodin, D.S., Squires, K.C., Henderson, B.H. and Starr, A., 1978,

An early event-related cortical potential, Psychophysiol., 15: 360.

Goodin, D., Squires, K. and Starr, A., 1978, Long latency event related components of the auditory evoked potential in dimentia, Brain, 101:635.

Halgren, E., Squires, N.K., Wilson, C.L., Rohrbaugh, J.R., Babb, T.L. and Crandall, P.H., 1980, Endogenous potentials generated in the human hippocampus and amygdala by unexpected events, Science, 210:803.

Hillyard, S., Squires, K.C. and Squires, N.K., in press, The psychophysiology of attention, in: "Attention: Theory, Brain Functions, and Applications, D. Sheer, ed., Erlbaum, Hillsdale, New Jersey.

Nodar, R.H., Hahn, J. and Levine, H.L., 1980, Brain stem auditory evoked potentials in determining site of lesion of brain stem gliomas in children, Laryngoscope, 90:258.

Norman, R., Buchwald, J.S. and Villablanca, J., 1977, Classical conditioning with auditory discrimination of the eyeblink in the chronic decerebrate cat, Science, 196:551.

Norman, R.J., Villablanca, J.R., Brown, K.A., Schwafel, J.A. and Buchwald, J.S., 1974, Classical eyeblink conditioning in the bilaterally hemispherectomized animal., Exp. Neurol., 44:363.

Pfefferbaum, A., Horvath, T.B., Roth, W.T. and Kopell, B.S., 1979, Event-related potential changes in chronic alcoholics, Electroenceph. clin. Neurophysiol., 47:637.

Picton, T.W., Hillyard, S.A. and Galambos, R., 1974, Evoked responses to omitted stimuli, in: "Major Problems of Brain Electrophysiology," M.N. Livanov, ed., Academy of Sciences, USSR.

Picton, T.W., Hillyard, S.A., Krausz, H.I. and Galambos, R., 1974, Human auditory evoked potentials. I. Evaluation of components, Electroenceph. clin. Neurophysiol., 36:179.

Ritter, W., Simson, R. and Vaughan, H.G., Jr., 1972, Association cortex potentials and reaction time in auditory discrimination, Electroenceph. clin. Neurophysiol., 33:547.

Roth, W.T., Ford, J.M., Lewis, S.J. and Kopell, B.S., 1976, Effects of stimulus probability and task-relevance on event-related potentials, Psychophysiol., 13:311.

Simson, R., Vaughan, H.G., Jr. and Ritter, W., 1976, The scalp topography of potentials associated with missing visual or auditory stimuli, Electroenceph. clin. Neurophysiol., 40:33.

Simson, R., Vaughan, H.G., Jr. and Ritter, W., 1977, The scalp topography of potentials associated with missing visual or audi-tasks, Electroenceph. clin. Neurophysiol., 42:528.

Squires, K.C., Wickens, C., Squires, N.K. and Donchin, E., 1976, Effect of stimulus sequence on the waveform of the cortical event-related potential, Science, 193:1142.

Squires, N., Donchin, E., Squires, K. and Grossberg, S., 1977, Bisensory stimulation: inferring decision-related processes from the P300 component, J. Exp. Psychol, Human Percept. Perform., 3:299.

Squires, N.K., Galbraith, G.C. and Aine, C.J., 1979, Event-related potential assessment of sensory and cognitive deficits in the mentally retarded, in: "Human Evoked Potentials: Applications and Problems," D. Lehman and E. Callaway, eds., Plenum Press, New York.

Squires, N.K., Squires, K.C. and Hillyard, S.A., 1975, Two varieties of long-latency positive waves evoked by unpredictable auditory stimuli in man, Electroenceph. clin. Neurophysiol., 38: 387.

Starr, A. and Hamilton, A., 1976, Correlation between confirmed site of neurological lesions and abnormalities of far-field auditory brainstem responses, Electroenceph. clin. Neurophysiol., 41:595.

Stockard, J.J., Stockard, J.E. and Sharbrough, F.W., 1977, Detection and localization of occult lesions with brainstem auditory evoked responses, Mayo Clin. Proc., 52:761.

Sutton, S., Tueting, P., Zubin, J. and John, E.R., 1967, Information delivery and the sensory evokedpotential, Science, 155: 1436.

Wilder, M.B., Farley, G.R. and Starr, A., 1981, Endogenous late positive component of the evoked potential in cats corresponding to P300 in humans, Science, 211:605.

Wood, C.C., Allison, T., Goff, W.R., Williamson, P.D. and Spencer, D.B., 1980, On the neural origin of P300 in man, Progress in Brain Research, 54.

ACKNOWLEDGMENTS

This research was supported by USPHS Grants HD 05958, 04612, AG 01754 and NS 5725.

CENTRAL PROCESSING TIME FOR A CONDITIONED RESPONSE IN A VERTEBRATE MODEL SYSTEM

David H. Cohen

Department of Neurobiology and Behavior
State University of New York at Stony Brook
Stony Brook, N.Y.

SUMMARY

For some years we have been developing visually conditioned heart rate change in the pigeon as a vertebrate model system for cellular analyses of associative learning. The behavioral model is now well-established, and substantial progress has been realized in delineating the neuronal circuitry mediating the conditioned response. With this information as a foundation we have been able to initiate cellular neurophysiological studies to (a) describe the temporal properties of the information flow along the identified pathways during conditioned responding, and (b) identify sites of training-induced modification. This report deals with the temporal properties of the information flow, and the results indicate that central latencies and processing time are surprisingly short. Thus, the system may be considerably more "analyzable" than might have been anticipated.

INTRODUCTION

Over the past fifteen years we have been engaged in a long-term effort to develop a vertebrate model system for rigorous cellular analyses of associative learning (Cohen, 1969, 1974a, 1980). This system involves visually conditioned heart rate change in the pigeon, and the sequence of our analytic efforts has been as follows. First, we developed the behavioral model which required establishing a standardized paradigm to produce rapid acquisition of a quantifiable conditioned response in a pharmacologically immobilized preparation. Second, and of paramount importance, we undertook to delineate the neuronal pathways that must be intact for normal acquisition of this response. Third, as sufficient information regarding this circuitry was obtained, we were able to initiate cellular neurophysiological studies of the more peripheral segments of the implicated pathways in order to specify the temporal properties of the information flow through the system. Fourth, this in turn has permitted us most recently to initiate studies directed toward identifying specific synaptic fields that undergo training-induced modification, a prelude to exploring the mechanisms of such long-term information storage during associative learning.

The objective of this report is to focus upon what we have learned regarding the temporal properties of the neuronal activity that mediates the conditioned response. However, appreciation of these data requires brief summaries of certain properties of the behavioral model and of some features of the functional neuroanatomy of the conditioned response.

BEHAVIORAL MODEL

The behavioral model is now well-developed and is proving remarkably effective for cellular neurophysiological studies during conditioning (see Cohen and Goff, 1978). The standardized paradigm involves the repeated presentation of a 6-sec pulse of whole field retinal illumination, the conditioned stimulus (CS), immediately followed by a 500-msec foot-shock, the unconditioned stimulus (US). The US elicits marked cardioacceleration as an unconditioned response (UR), and after a sufficient number of CS-US pairings the light alone reliably elicits a conditioned cardioacceleratory response of predictable dynamics. A stable CR develops within 10 such pairings, and asymptotic performance obtains in 30-40 pairings (Fig. 1). The CR is highly resistant to extinction, and we have shown that orienting and sensitization responses account for but a small proportion of the overall response.

Regarding the specific response characteristics (see Cohen and Goff, 1978), early light presentations, independent of foot-shock, elicit a small cardioacceleration (the orienting response) that habituates rapidly. Introducing foot-shock then transforms this small rate increase into a sensitization response of different dynamics, but this too extinguishes rapidly. The CR is a monotonic cardioacceleration with a latency of approximately 1 sec and with maximal values in the fifth or sixth seconds of the CS period; the properties of this response have now been specified in considerable quantitative detail.

Through various investigations (summarized in Cohen and Goff, 1978) we have evaluated a number of experimental variables with

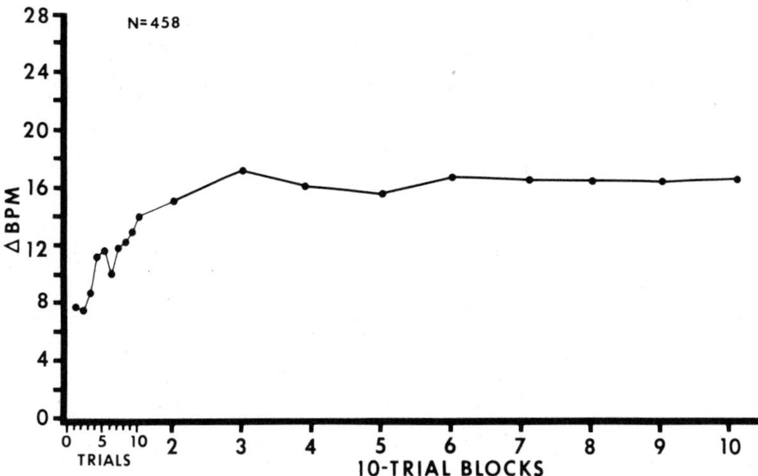

Fig. 1. Acquisition of conditioned heart rate change in the pigeon. The curve represents mean heart rate changes in beats/min (BPM) between the 6-sec CS and the immediately preceding 6-sec control periods. Each point represents a group mean for a block of 10 training trials, with the exception of the first block for which individual trial means are shown. (Adapted from Cohen and Goff, 1978.)

respect to their roles in affecting the acquisition, asymptotic level, and dynamics of the CR. We have shown that conditioned heart rate change interacts minimally, if at all, with concomitantly developing CRs, and we have developed an immobilized preparation allowing precise stimulus control and training to asymptotic CR levels in a single session of approximately 2 hrs (Gold and Cohen, 1981). Moreover, in this immobilized preparation the quantitative properties of the CR do not differ from those of non-immobilized animals.

In summary, the behavioral model is a robust and effective system for cellular neurophysiological studies of associative learning. It has numerous technical advantages such as rapid acquisition, consistent response dynamics among animals, and pharmacological immobilization. Furthermore, it potentially allows study of a broad range of learning phenomena in a single system, including habituation, sensitization, conditioning and differentiation. Finally, it might be noted that use of an avian model could ultimately facilitate investigations of a developmental nature.

RELEVANT NEURONAL CIRCUITRY

Given an effective behavioral model, identification of the pathways mediating development of the CR is the most essential and challenging criterion the model system must satisfy (Cohen, 1969; Kandel and Spencer, 1968). We began this effort by defining four segments of the system: (a) the visual pathways transmitting the CS information, (b) the somatosensory pathways transmitting the US information, (c) the descending pathways mediating expression of the CR, and (d) the efferent pathways mediating the UR. Our approach has entailed beginning at the periphery of each of these segments and tracing them systematically centrally. Thus, for the CS and US pathways analysis was initiated at the sensory periphery while for the efferent segments it began at the extrinsic cardiac nerves. We have assumed that such an analysis of the input and output segments of the system would ultimately lead to the identification of sites of convergence of the CS and US pathways, as well as of their sites of coupling to the CR pathways. Recent data tend to justify such an assumption (e.g. Ritchie, 1979; Gibbs et al., in press).

For the purposes of this report only two segments of the system need be reviewed, namely the visual pathways transmitting the CS information and the descending pathways mediating expression of the CR.

Pathways Transmitting the Conditioned Stimulus Information

Beginning our analysis at the visual periphery, we established that bilateral enucleation prevents CR development, excluding participation of any non-retinal photoreception (Cohen, 1974a, 1980, in preparation) (see Fig. 3). Next, we evaluated the possible involvement of cell groups receiving a direct retinal projection, the distribution of such projections being remarkably similar in avian and mammalian brains (Cohen and Karten, 1974). As might be expected, we found no deficits in conditioning consequent to destruction of any single optic tract target (Cohen, 1974a, 1980, in preparation). This, perhaps, is not surprising, since each of these cell groups is responsive to whole field illumination, such that considerable opportunity is available for parallel transmission of the CS information.

Since in mammals severe deficits in visual learning follow interruption of visual pathways to the cortex, we turned to an examination of the possible involvement in conditioning of the homologous pathways of the avian brain. Two such systems have been described, the thalamofugal and tectofugal pathways (Fig. 2), which are homologous respectively to the mammalian geniculostriate and tecto-thalamo-extrastriate pathways (see Cohen and Karten, 1974). Our initial question was whether interrupting either of these

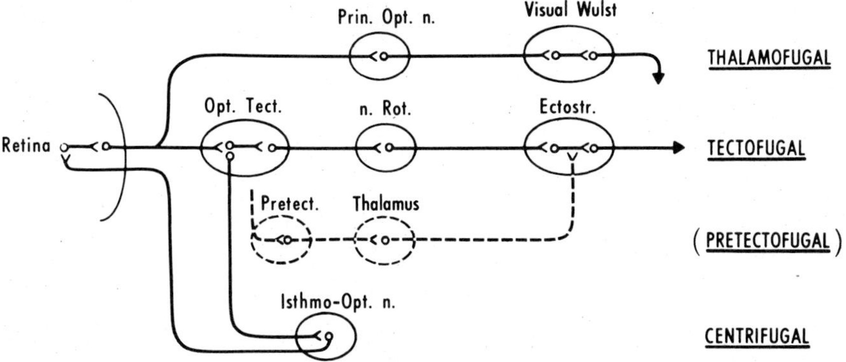

Fig. 2. Schematic illustration of the major ascending visual pathways of the bird. The broken lines indicating the pretectofugal pathway reflect its speculative nature, and the hypothesized pretectofugal projection from the thalamus to the ectostriatum is intended to suggest a termination either upon or in the immediate region of the ectostriatum. Abbreviations: Ectostr. = ectostriatum; Isthmo-Opt. n. = isthmo-optic nucleus; n. Rot. = nucleus rotundus; Opt. Tect. = optic tectum; Prectect. = pretectal region; Princ. Opt. n. = principal optic nucleus of the thalamus. (From Cohen, 1974a.)

systems would affect CR acquisition. The results were negative. However, we did find that the combined interruption of the two pathways by a lesion including both the visual Wulst and ectostriatum prevented CR development (Cohen, 1974a, 1980, in preparation) (Fig. 3). However, an attempt to cross-validate this finding by combined interruption of the two pathways at the thalamic level produced only a transient deficit. This, in conjunction with various electrophysiological observations in our laboratory, suggested the existence of a third ascending pathway that either converges with the tectofugal pathway upon the ectostriatum or terminates in its immediate vicinity. Given the similarity of avian and mammalian visual pathways, we hypothesized that this pathway may be of pretectal origin (Fig. 2) and conducted an experiment in which the principal optic nucleus, nucleus rotundus and the pretectal terminal field of the optic tract were destroyed. This produced acquisition deficits comparable to those following the combined lesion of the visual Wulst and ectostriatum (Fig. 3); lesions of the pretectal region alone produced no deficit (Cohen, 1974a, 1980, in preparation).

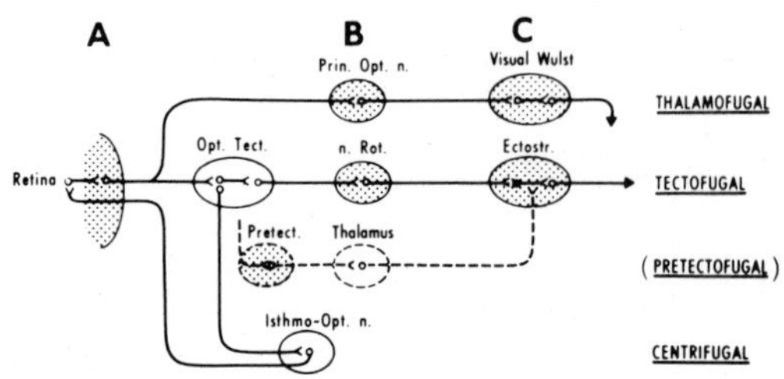

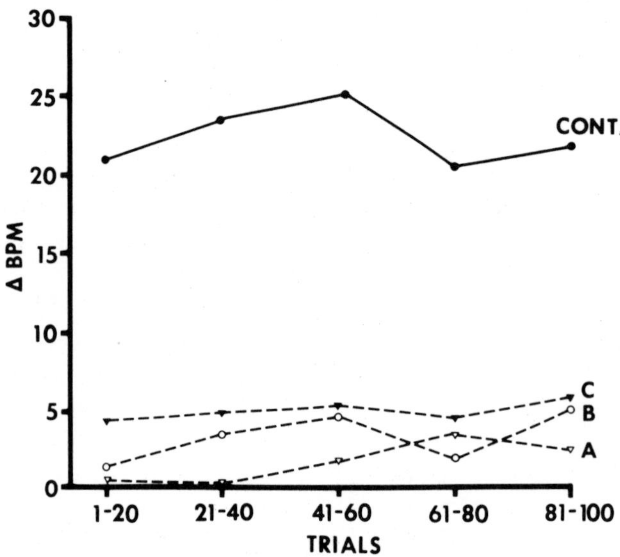

Fig. 3. Visual system lesions that prevent CR acquisition. Each broken line represents an experimental group, while the solid line shows the performance of control birds (CONT.). Curve A illustrates the performance of animals with bilateral enucleation (A in upper panel). Curve B illustrates the performance of animals with a combined lesion of the principal optic nucleus, nucleus rotundus and the pretectal terminal field of the optic tract (B in upper panel). Curve C illustrates the performance of animals with a combined lesion of the visual Wulst and ectostriatum (C in upper panel). For all curves, each point represents the mean heart rate change in beats/min (BPM)

between the 6-sec CS period and an immediately preceding 6-sec control period. See Fig. 2 for abbreviations in upper panel.

Thus, it appears that each of the ascending visual pathways is capable of transmitting effective CS information, and it is only with their combined destruction that CR development is precluded. This provides, then, a first-approximation to the pathways transmitting the CS information, and while it cannot be definitively argued that these pathways are necessary _and_ sufficient, our results are certainly suggestive of this.

Descending Pathways Mediating Expression of the Conditioned Response

In accordance with our strategy of beginning the analysis of each segment of the system at its periphery, our initial efforts to describe the CR pathways were initiated at the final common path for heart rate change (Cohen, 1974b). A behavioral study involving various combinations of cardiac denervation and pharmacological blockade demonstrated that the CR is mediated entirely by the extrinsic cardiac nerves, that both the vagi and sympathetics contribute to the CR, and that the sympathetic innervation provides the major contribution to CR magnitude (Cohen and Pitts, 1968). Subsequent anatomical study of the pre- and postganglionic cardiac innervation indicated that (a) the right sympathetic cardiac nerve exerts the primary chronotropic influence; (b) the cells of origin of this nerve are restricted to the sympathetic ganglia associated with the last three cervical segments (ganglia 12-14), with a large majority in ganglion 14; (c) the preganglionic projections upon these cells arise from the last cervical and upper three thoracic segments; and (d) the preganglionic cells of origin are located in the column of Terni, a well-defined cell group just dorsal to the central canal (Macdonald and Cohen, 1970) (Fig. 4). More recently, the fiber spectrum of the right cardiac sympathetic nerve has been quantitatively described with electron microscopy; the fiber group associated with cardioacceleration has been determined; and criteria have been established for electrophysiologically identifying postganglionic cardiac neurons in the unanesthetized bird (Cabot and Cohen, 1977).

Concomitant with these studies, the parasympathetic cardiac innervation was also investigated. In that regard, the cells of origin of the vagal cardiac fibers were anatomically localized to a limited region of the dorsal motor nucleus (Cohen et al., 1970; Cohen and Schnall, 1970). Subsequently, we have described quantitatively the fiber spectrum of the vagus and of various of its branches, determined the vagal compound action potential components associated with bradycardia, and established criteria for

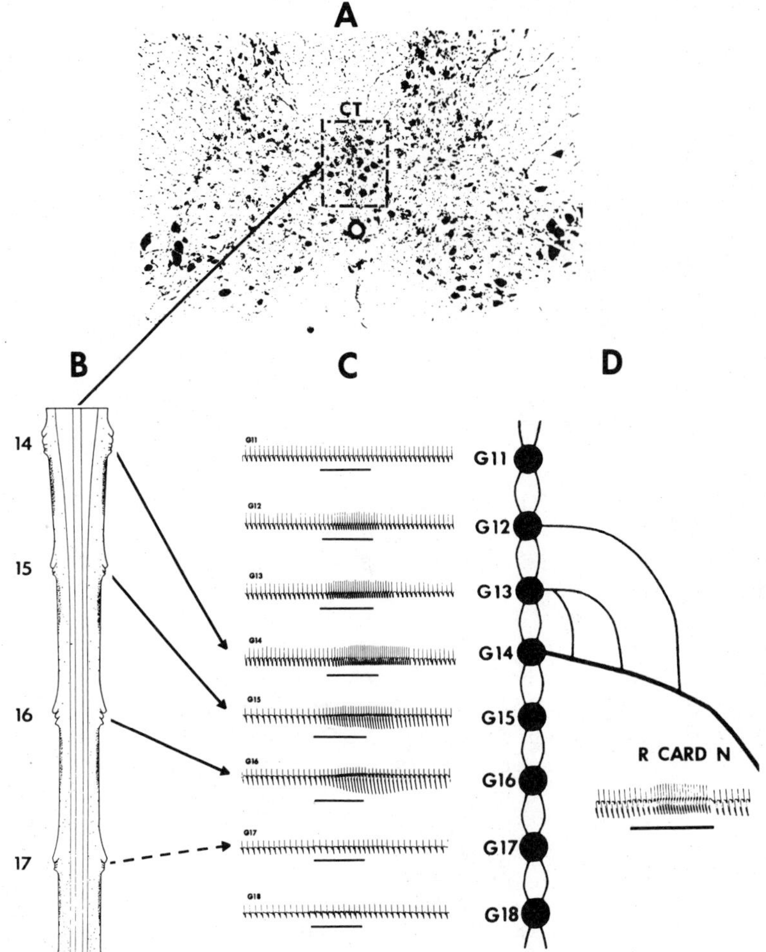

Fig. 4. Schematic illustration of the sympathetic component of the final common path. Panel A, adapted from Macdonald and Cohen (1970), shows a photomicrograph of a transverse section through segment 15 of the pigeon spinal cord. The outlined cell group dorsal to the central canal is the sympathetic preganglionic column, the column of Terni (CT). Panel B illustrates schematically a horizontal view of the pigeon spinal cord from segments 14-17. Preganglionic fibers from the column of Terni that influence heart rate emerge from segments 14-16 and sometimes 17. Panel C shows the heart rate change following stimulation of sympathetic ganglia G11-G18. (From Macdonald and Cohen, 1970.)

Horizontal bars indicate stimulation periods. Panel D illustrates sympathetic ganglia 11-18 with the branches of the right cardioaccelerator nerve (R CARD N) emerging from ganglia 12-14. (From Macdonald and Cohen, 1970.) Also shown is the effect of stimulating the right cardioaccelerator nerve. (Composite figure from Cohen, 1974a.)

electrophysiologically identifying vagal cardiac cells in the unanesthetized bird (Schwaber and Cohen, 1978a,b).

Thus, the final common path of our model system is well-described, and criteria for identifying the cardiac motoneurons in cellular neurophysiological conditioning studies have been established. The next question then concerns the central pathways that converge upon these motoneurons, and considerable progress has been made in that regard. However, this information is not necessary for the principal focus of this report, and the reader is referred to a recent review by Cohen (1980).

TEMPORAL PROPERTIES OF THE INFORMATION FLOW

Returning to the major theme of this report, the remaining sections will address the temporal properties of the neuronal activity that mediates the conditioned heart rate response. While we know that the heart rate CR has a latency of approximately 1 sec and persists for 6 sec, this does not necessarily imply that the central processing time is of the same order of magnitude. By characterizing the discharge of the cardiac motoneurons during conditioned responding, it should be possible to transform the temporal characteristics of the behavioral CR into a "neurophysiological time domain" that excludes delay time at the motor periphery. If, in addition, one can determine the temporal properties of the retinal output, then an estimate of central processing time could be obtained. Finally, information on the response latencies of neurons along the central pathways could be utilized to cross-validate such estimates.

In a broader context, determining the temporal properties of the information flow through system is basic to gaining some sense of its "analyzability." Moreover, it would establish the temporal boundary conditions for analyzing and interpreting cellular neurophysiological data from central structures along the implicated pathways.

Discharge Properties of the Cardiac Motoneurons

With respect to the cardiac sympathetic postganglionic neurons, we have extensively studied the discharge properties of such cells in right ganglion 14 (Cabot and Cohen, in preparation) (Fig. 4). Recall that this ganglion, which is perhaps homologous to the mammalian stellate ganglion, contains the great majority of the cells of origin of the right cardiac nerve (Cabot and Cohen, 1977; Macdonald and Cohen, 1970) and exerts the primary chronotropic effect on the heart (Macdonald and Cohen, 1970). Furthermore, on the basis of quantitative electron microscopic study of the cardiac nerve branch arising from right ganglion 14 we are able to estimate that there is a maximum of 1500 cardiac neurons that are localized in small clusters in the rostroventral aspect of the ganglion. These cells have soma diameters of 15-30 μ and unmyelinated axons 0.2-1.2 μ in diameter that conduct at 0.4-2.0 m/sec (Cabot and Cohen, 1977).

In recording from these neurons, an initial important observation was that they are responsive to the visual stimulus prior to any training. The latency of this "orienting" response is approximately 100 msec, and the response itself consists of a short burst of action potentials, followed by a brief depression of discharge, and a subsequent return to maintained activity levels or slightly higher before light termination.

If one continues to present the light unpaired with foot-shock, then this orienting response habituates. However, the effect of conditioning training is the opposite, increasing both the probability of occurrence and magnitude of the initial light-evoked response. As shown in Fig. 5, conditioning does not alter the 100-msec latency or alter the conformation of the response pattern. A striking feature of this discharge pattern is that it consists primarily of a phasic component, followed by a minimal tonic component. Indeed, many cells show no tonic component whatsoever. It may be noted that the phasic response has a duration of only 300-400 msec. This suggests that the central processing time is $\lesssim$ 400 msec and that the maintenance of the 6-sec heart rate response occurs at the periphery and reflects a non-linear input-output relation between the sympathetic innervation and the heart. Supporting this contention is our finding that simulating the discharge of the cardiac sympathetic postganglionics with electrical stimulation of the right cardiac nerve for 100 msec evokes a tachycardia of 4-6 sec duration that closely resembles the conditioned heart rate response (Cabot and Cohen, in preparation).

In an analogous study of the vagal cardiac neurons (Gold and Cohen, 1979, in press) we have found that, similar to the sympathetic innervation, these cells also respond to the visual stimulus prior to training (Fig. 6). However, in this case the response consists of a decrease in discharge. Also similar to the sympathetics, the vagal cardiac neurons show both phasic and tonic components of their light-evoked discharge change, although in the vagal cells the tonic component is considerably more prominent than in

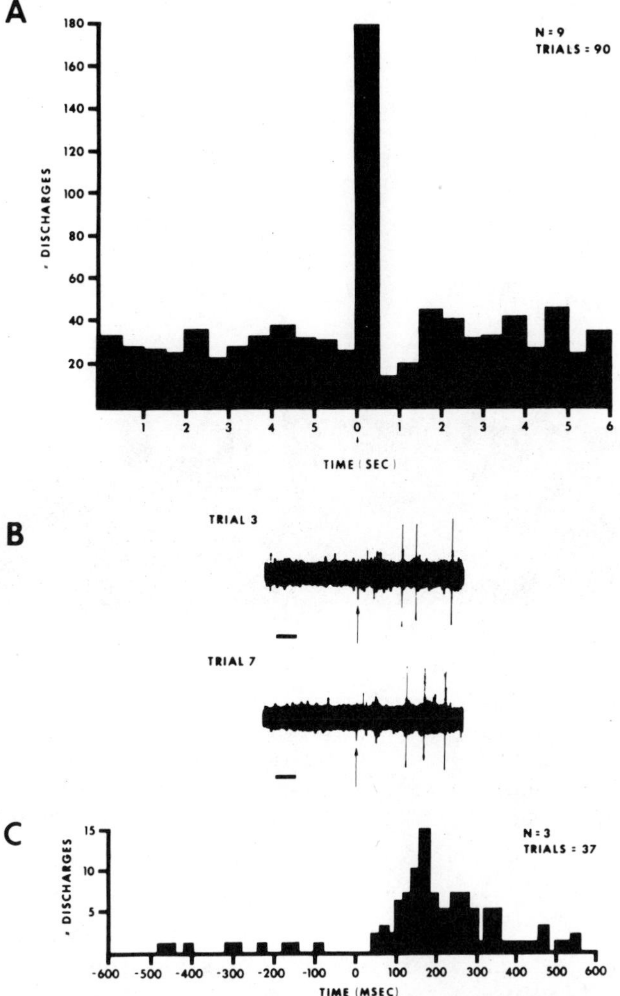

Fig. 5. Discharge of cardiac sympathetic postganglionic neurons during conditioned responding. Panel A shows a summary peristimulus time histogram of the responses of 9 cardiac postganglionic neurons to 10 CS presentations. The arrow indicates onset of the 6-sec CS; bin width is 500 msec. Note that the phasic response is confined to the first 500-msec bin. Panel B shows representative responses of one of these units on 2 of the 10 CS presentations. The arrows indicate CS onset, and the calibration bar represents 50 msec. Panel C shows a peristimulus time histogram of the discharges of 3 units for the 600 msec

immediately before and after CS onset. Note that the phasic component of the response has a latency of approximately 100 msec (first significant deviation from maintained activity) and a duration of 300-400 msec. (From Cohen, 1980.)

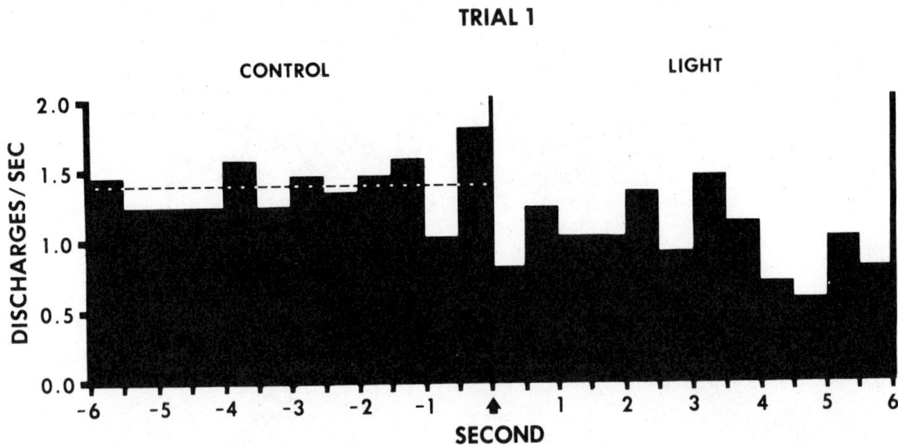

Fig. 6. Peristimulus time histogram of vagal cardiac neurons during a light presentation before training. The arrow indicates CS onset, and the broken line indicates the mean discharge rate during the 6-sec control period preceding the light. (From Gold and Cohen, in preparation.)

the sympathetic neurons. The effect of associative training is to amplify this stimulus-evoked discharge reduction. However, unlike the cardiac sympathetics, the latency of the vagal response decreases over training. Early in conditioning the response latency is approximately 100 msec, and this decreases to 60-80 msec at asymptotic performance (Gold and Cohen, in press) (Fig. 7).

These data for the motoneurons mediating the conditioned heart rate change lead to a number of conclusions. First, as suggested some time ago by denervation experiments (Cohen and Pitts, 1968), both the sympathetic and vagal cardiac innervations contribute to the CR in a synergistic manner. Second, the latencies of these motoneuronal responses are considerably shorter than might have been predicted from the latency of the heart rate change. (It might be noted that the difference between the vagal and sympathetic

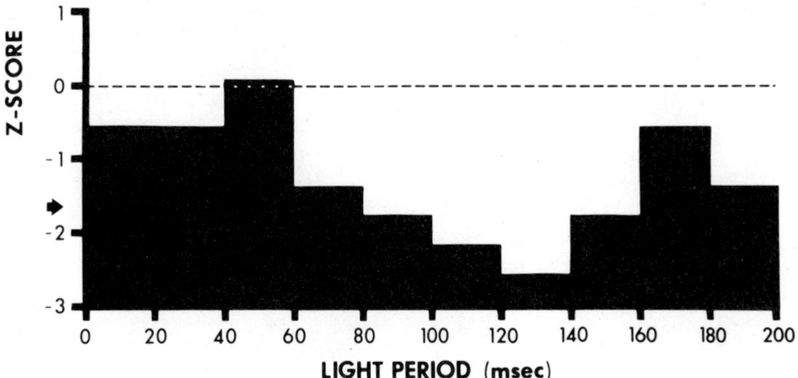

Fig. 7. Poststimulus histogram showing the latency of the discharge change of vagal cardiac neurons in response to the CS during asymptotic performance. The ordinate indicates the standardized score for each 20-msec bin relative to the baseline distribution, and the arrow indicates the standardized score (z = -1.65) below which values differ significantly from baseline at the .05 level. (From Gold and Cohen, in preparation.)

response latencies to the CS is consistent with the time required for conduction from the medulla to the preganglionic cell column plus the relay time from the pre- to the postganglionic neurons (Leonard and Cohen, 1975).) Third, the increase in the sympathetic outflow to the heart is by far the primary contributor to the conditioned cardioacceleration (Cohen and Pitts, 1968), and this consists primarily of a phasic response of 300-400-msec duration. Thus, the CR is largely mediated by a short duration burst of sympathetic activity with a latency of approximately 100 msec. Finally, the effect of associative training is to increase both the probability of occurrence and the magnitude of the unconditioned responses to the light in both sympathetic and vagal cardiac innervations, while non-associative treatment produces an attenuation of these initial light-evoked responses.

The Retinal Output

With respect to the retinal ganglion cells, we have previously established that they behave as a largely homogeneous population in response to whole field illumination and that their response consists of a short burst at light onset, followed by cessation of discharge during sustained illumination, and a more labile burst at stimulus termination (Duff and Cohen, 1975a,b). From experiments where we recorded from single optic tract fibers during conditioning (Wall et al., 1980; Wild and Cohen, in preparation) we were able to generate a population histogram that reliably characterizes the retinal output during CS presentation (Fig. 8). These data indicate that the discharge at CS onset has a minimum latency of 18 msec and persists for a maximum of 80 msec. It might be noted that the retinal output shows no training-induced modification (Wall et al., 1980; Wild and Cohen, in preparation), and therefore this latency range remains invariant over conditioning.

Central Processing Time

If one assumes that the shortest latency retinal ganglion cell responses are associated with the shortest latency responses of the cardiac motoneurons, then an estimate of central processing time would be approximately 40 msec for the most rapid vagal response and 80 msec for the earliest sympathetic response (cf. Figs. 5, 7 and 8). A somewhat more conservative estimate is derived by comparing the shortest latency retinal ganglion cell responses to the maxima of the phasic vagal and sympathetic responses. This approach gives central processing time values of approximately 110 msec and 140 msec for the vagal and sympathetic responses respectively (cf. Figs. 5, 7 and 8).

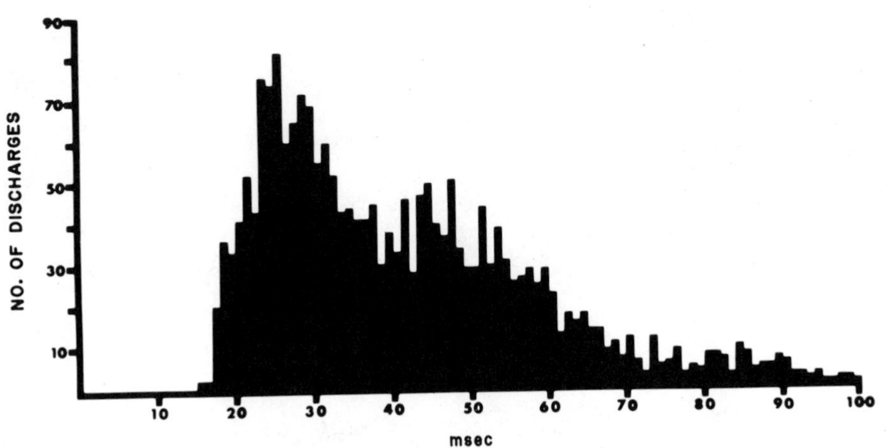

Fig. 8. Poststimulus histogram of the response of retinal ganglion cells (optic tract fibers) at CS onset. (From Wild and Cohen, in preparation.)

Beyond latency considerations, these data for the CS periphery and final common path have further implications for the organization of the neuronal activity mediating the CR. One can view the retinal output in response to the CS as an excitatory wave at simulus onset that has a duration of approximately 80 msec. In all likelihood this wave represents the initial "trigger" for the phasic components of the motoneuronal responses. For the vagal cardiac neurons this phasic component has a duration of approximately 80-100 msec (Fig. 7), while for the cardiac sympathetics the duration of the phasic component is 300-400 msec (Fig. 5). Thus, one might view the information flow through the system as initiating with an 80-msec wave at the retinal output that is then transmitted along the identified pathways to be expressed ultimately as an 80-100-msec wave (reflected as decreased discharge) at the vagal cardiac neurons and as a 300-400-msec wave (reflected as increased discharge) at the cardiac sympathetic postganglionic neurons. Consequently, the maximal temporal dispersion of the CS-evoked activity would be no greater than a factor of five. Furthermore, since the effect of associative training is to augment the initial light-evoked response along the pathway, one might hypothesize a mechanism as straightforward as the facilitation of synaptic transmission at one or more sites along the identified pathways.

Are Responses of More Central Structures Consistent with the Boundary Conditions Established at the Sensory and Motor Peripheries?

An important motivation for studying the temporal response characteristics at the sensory and motor peripheries was to establish temporal boundary conditions that would assist in the interpretation of responses of more central structures along the identified pathways. In turn, the responses of neurons in such structures provide a means of evaluating the validity of the estimated temporal boundary conditions.

It is only recently that we have had the opportunity to begin analysis of structures beyond the periphery, and these efforts have focussed upon a systematic investigation of the visual pathways transmitting the CS information. The rationale is that this approach is the most likely to identify sites of information storage associated with conditioning (Cohen, 1980). In any case, we have obtained data from the thalamic relays of both the thalamofugal and tectofugal visual pathways (see Fig. 2) that are germane to the present temporal considerations.

Analogous to the retinal ganglion cells and cardiac motoneurons, cells in the principal optic nucleus and nucleus rotundus show prominent phasic responses (Gibbs and Cohen, 1980; Wall et al., 1980). (These, incidentally, are differentially modified by associative training, while the tonic components are not.) The minimum response latency of the principal optic nucleus cells at CS onset is 20-25 msec, and the peak of the population response (reconstructed from single unit data) is 30-35 msec. These are retino-recipient neurons that constitute the thalamic relay of the avian geniculo-striate homologue, and thus, while not surprising, it is reassuring that the temporal characteristics of their discharge at CS onset are consistent with those of the retinal ganglion cell discharge (Fig. 8). Analogous data for the nucleus rotundus indicate a minimum latency of approximately 30 msec with a modal response to the CS at approximately 35 msec. Since at least one, and in all likelihood two, tectal neurons probably intervene between the optic tract and nucleus rotundus (Fig. 2), these values are also consistent with the retinal ganglion cell data.

Thus, while the temporal properties of neurons along the implicated visual pathways are not particularly challenging with respect to validating the temporal boundary conditions established at the sensory and motor peripheries, it is essential that they be consistent with the overall input-output time across the system. Fortunately, this first opportunity to assess the validity of our estimate of input-output time, albeit undemanding, maintains this estimate intact.

CONCLUDING COMMENTS

In summary, the above findings with respect to the temporal properties of the information flow through our model system suggest that it may be considerably more "analyzable" than our initial expectations. Although in no sense a "simple" system, our model might be viewed as a "relatively simple" system, and there are promising possibilities for simplifying it yet further by studying subsystems of the identified circuitry. It is quite encouraging that the model has now developed to a point where we can ask basic questions regarding the organization of the relevant circuitry, and we have recently succeeded in identifying the most peripheral sites of training-induced modification (Gibbs and Cohen, 1980; Gibbs et al., in press). This, in turn, is now permitting us to initiate investigations directed toward describing the cellular mechanisms of such modification.

REFERENCES

Cabot, J.B., and Cohen, D.H., 1977, Avian sympathetic cardiac fibers and their cells of cell origin: Anatomical and electrophysiological characteristics, Brain Research, 131:73-87.

Cabot, J.B., and Cohen, D.H., in preparation, Discharge patterns of cardiac sympathetic postganglionic neurons during development of a conditioned heart rate response.

Cohen, D.H., 1969, Development of a vertebrate experimental model for cellular neurophysiologic studies of learning, Cond. Ref., 4: 61-80.

Cohen, D.H., 1974a, The neural pathways and informational flow mediating a conditioned autonomic response, in: "Limbic and Autonomic Nervous System Research," L.V. DiCara, ed., Plenum Press, New York.

Cohen, D.H., 1974b, Analysis of the final common path for heart rate conditioning, in: "Cardiovascular Psychophysiology," P.A. Obrist, A.H. Black, J. Brener, and L.V. DiCara, eds., Aldine Publishing Co., Chicago.

Cohen, D.H., 1980, The functional neuroanatomy of a conditioned response, in: "Neural Mechanisms of Goal-Directed Behavior and Learning," R.F. Thompson, L.H. Hicks, and V.B. Shvyrkov, eds., Academic Press, New York.

Cohen, D.H., in preparation, Avian visual pathways involved in conditioned heart rate change to whole field retinal illumination.

Cohen, D.H., and Goff, D.G., 1978, Conditioned heart rate change in the pigeon: Analysis of acquisition patterns, Physiol. Psychol., 6:127-141.

Cohen, D.H., and Karten, H.J., 1974, The structural organization of the avian brain: An overview, in: "Birds: Brain and Behavior," I.J. Goodman and M.W. Schein, eds., Academic Press, New York.

Cohen, D.H., and Pitts, L.H., 1968, Vagal and sympathetic components of conditioned cardioacceleration in the pigeon, Brain Res., 9:15-31.

Cohen, D.H., and Schnall, A.M., 1970, Medullary cells of origin of vagal cardioinhibitory fibers in the pigeon. II. Electrical stimulation of the dorsal motor nucleus, J. Comp. Neurol., 140:321-342.

Cohen, D.H., Schnall, A.M., Macdonald, R.L., and Pitts, L.H., 1970, Medullary cells of origin of vagal cardioinhibitory fibers in the pigeon. I. Anatomical studies of peripheral vagus nerve and the dorsal motor nucleus, J. Comp. Neurol., 140:299-320.

Duff, T.A., and Cohen, D.H., 1975a, Retinal afferents to the pigeon optic tectum: Discharge characteristics in response to whole field illumination, Brain Res., 92:1-19.

Duff, T.A., and Cohen, D.H., 1975b, Optic chiasm fibers of the pigeon: Discharge characteristics in response to whole field illumination, Brain Res., 92:145-148.

Gibbs, C.M., and Cohen, D.H., 1980, Plasticity of the thalamofugal pathway during visual conditioning, Neurosci. Abstr., 6:424.

Gibbs, C.M., Cohen, D.H., Broyles, J., and Solina, A., in press, Conditioned modification of avian dorsal semiculate neurons is a function of their response to the unconditioned stimulus, Neurosci. Abstr.

Gold, M.R., and Cohen, D.H., 1979, Discharge properties of vagal cardiac neurons during conditioned heart rate change, Neurosci. Abstr., 5:43.

Gold, M.R., and Cohen, D.H., 1981, Heart rate conditioning in the pigeon immobilized with α-bungarotoxin, Brain Res., 216:163-172.

Gold, M.R., and Cohen, D.H., in preparation, Discharge patterns of vagal cardiac neurons during the development of a conditioned heart rate response.

Kandel, E.R., and Spencer, W.A., 1968, Cellular neurophysiological approaches to learning, Physiol. Rev., 48:65-134.

Leonard, R.B., and Cohen, D.H., 1975, Responses of postganglionic sympathetic neurons in the pigeon to peripheral nerve stimulation, Exper. Neurol., 49:466-486.

Macdonald, R.L., and Cohen, D.H., 1970, Cells of origin of sympathetic pre- and postganglionic cardioacceleratory fibers in the pigeon, J. Comp. Neurol., 140:343-358.

Ritchie, T.C., 1979, Intratelencephalic visual connections and their relationship to the archistriatum in the pigeon (Columba livia), Doctoral Dissertation, University of Virginia.

Schwaber, J.S., and Cohen, D.H., 1978a, Electrophysiological and electron microscopic analysis of the vagus nerve of the pigeon, with particular reference to the cardiac innervation, Brain Res., 147:65-78.

Schwaber, J.S., and Cohen, D.H., 1978b, Field potential and single unit analysis of the avian dorsal motor nucleus of the vagus and criteria for identifying vagal cardiac cells of origin, Brain Res., 147:79-90.

Wall, J., Wild, J.M., Broyles, J., Gibbs, C.M., and Cohen, D.H., 1980, Plasticity of the tectofugal pathway during visual conditioning, Neurosci. Abstr., 6:424.

Wild, J.M., and Cohen, in preparation, Responses of single optic tract fibers during development of visually conditioned heart rate change.

MECHANISM AND GENERALITY OF STIMULUS SIGNIFICANCE CODING IN A MAMMALIAN MODEL SYSTEM

Michael Gabriel, Edward Orona, Kent Foster
and Richard W. Lambert
Department of Psychology
University of Texas at Austin
Austin, TX 78712

SUMMARY

Electrolytic lesions of the anteroventral (AV) nucleus of the thalamus impaired significantly retention performance of rabbits in a discriminative avoidance task. In addition the lesions abolished the excitatory, discriminative neuronal discharges which had developed in the cingulate cortex during the course of behavioral acquisition, prior to the induction of the lesions. These results are discussed in relation to a model of cingulate cortical and anterior thalamic functioning, derived from past studies. Two additional studies are presented, which had the objective of determining whether the neuronal encoding processes previously observed in the cingulate cortex and in the AV nucleus occur as well in other linked cortical and thalamic systems (the prefrontal cortex and mediodorsal nucleus of thalamus, and the auditory cortex and medial geniculate nucleus of thalamus). The overall pattern of results suggested a sequential involvement of these major brain systems in associative processes during the course of behavioral acquisition. Certain components of the systems studied (e.g., the ventral division of the medial geniculate nucleus and the medial division of the mediodorsal nucleus) did not manifest neuronal encoding processes related to the discriminative task.

INTRODUCTION

The work in our laboratory has been directed toward identifying the neural substrates of behavioral learning through the study of the neuronal (multiple-, and single-unit) correlates of discriminative avoidance conditioning in rabbits. Past studies with this model system have focussed on the neuronal activity in the cingulate area of the cerebral cortex, and the reciprocally interconnected anteroventral (AV) thalamic nucleus. The results showed that neurons in the deep laminae (V, VI) of the cingulate cortex develop differential responsiveness to the positive and negative conditional stimuli (the CS+ and CS-, respectively) shortly after the onset of training. In contrast, differential neuronal activity developed in the AV nucleus and in the superficial cortical laminae (I-IV) in a late stage of training, concurrently with the advent of asymptotic discriminative behavior. During the same late training stage, many of the deep laminar records that had manifested rapid discriminative acquisition showed fading and/or loss of the neuronal discrimination (Gabriel, Foster & Orona, 1980a; Foster, Orona, Lambert & Gabriel, 1980).

These results led to the hypothesis that the early-forming discriminative neuronal activity in the deep laminae represented the initial neuronal encoding of the associative significance of the conditional stimuli. The encoding was proposed to be a causal precursor of the discriminative behavior. With continued training, the neuronal code is <u>relegated</u> to the AV nucleus, by way of the corticothalamic pathway. Thus the neurons in the AV nucleus are "taught" via cortical "instructions" to produce their own discriminative activity. When the AV nuclear neurons begin to produce discriminative activity, that activity is relayed via the thalamocortical axons to the superficial laminae of the cingulate cortex, accounting for the late-developing discriminative activity in those laminae. It was hypothesized that the late discriminative activity relayed to the cingulate cortex is a signal informing cortex that thalamus has acquired the neuronal code, promoting <u>disengagement</u> of the cortex from further coding of stimulus significance. Thus, initial acquisition of the significance code occurs in the deep cingulate laminae, but with continuing training, coding is taken over by the AV nucleus, and the cortex disengages from the process. These arguments are developed in more detail in a review by Gabriel, Foster, Orona, Saltwick and Stanton (1980b).

The most recent work in our laboratory, reported here, has concerned two general issues which have emerged from the past results. The first involves testing the hypothetical causal mechanism derived from our model of cingulate cortical and anterior thalamic functioning. Specifically, Experiment 1 was designed to determine whether activity which develops in a late training stage within the superficial laminae of the cingulate cortex is driven by the late-developing activity in the AV nucleus. In this same experiment we also sought to determine whether the integrity of the AV nucleus is essential for normal retention of the discriminative behavior.

The second major issue addressed here concerns the generality of the early cortical and later thalamic encoding processes. That is, does discriminative neuronal activity develop in a sequential fashion first in cortex, and later in thalamus, for systems other than the cingulate cortex and the AV nucleus? Knowledge of the configuration of systems which do manifest this pattern and those which do not, as well as the detailed similarities and differences between various systems, could provide important insight into the telodiencephalic mechanisms underlying behavioral acquisition.

Experiment 2 represents our attempt to answer the question of generality with regard the prefrontal area of the rabbit cortex and the thalamic nucleus (medialis dorsalis: MD) with which the prefrontal area is reciprocally interconnected (Benjamin, Jackson and Golden, 1978). The prefrontal cortex (PFC) and the MD nucleus were selected for study because of their close neuroanatomical relationship to the cingulate cortex and because of the considerable experimental literature implicating these structures in learning processes (see reviews by Warren and Akert, 1964; Rosenkilde, 1979; Fuster, 1980).

The CS+ and CS- used in our studies have been auditory stimuli. In experiment 3, we addressed the issue of generality by studying the neuronal activity in the auditory cortex and the medial geniculate nucleus (MGN) of the thalamus, i.e., the structures involved in modality-specific processing of CS information. In addition, experiment 3 was designed to provide information on the possibility that the neuronal encoding previously studied in the limbic cortical and thalamic structures may be secondary to events occurring further "upstream" within the sensory pathway.

The data presented here on the PFC system and the auditory projection system are portions of larger studies by Orona (1981) and by Foster (1981), respectively.

METHODS

General Procedure for all Experiments

The details of procedure have been presented in other reports (e.g., Foster et al., 1980). The subjects were 73 male rabbits of the New Zealand White strain, weighing 1.5-2.0 Kg at the time of their delivery to the laboratory. The learning task was differential avoidance conditioning. Training involved successive presentation of two tone stimuli in a random order, the positive conditional stimulus (CS+) and the negative conditional stimulus (CS-). For each rabbit, the CS+ was 1 kHz or 8 kHz, 80 dB relative to 0.0002 dyne/cm^2, with a rise time of 3 msec. The CS- was the other (1 kHz or 8 kHz) tone. The assignment of frequencies to rabbits was counterbalanced. Onset of the CS+ was followed after 5 sec by a constant-current footshock (1.5 mA) delivered through the grid floor of a rotating wheel apparatus (Brogen & Culler, 1936), and terminated by the footshock-produced locomotion. Locomotion during the CS+ terminated it and prevented footshock. The CS- was never followed by footshock. Thus, the rabbits learned to avoid footshock by locomoting to the CS+, and they learned non-response to the CS-. The rabbits received 120 trials daily (60 with each stimulus) until a criterion of behavioral discrimination was attained. The criterion required that the percentage of conditioned responses to the CS+ exceed the percentage to the CS- by 60 or more, in two consecutive sessions. Following criterion 65 of the rabbits received 3 overtraining sessions. Prior to training each rabbit received a pretraining (PT) session in which the tones to be used as CSs, and the footshock (UCS) were presented in a noncontingent (explicitly unpaired) manner. This procedure provided a way to assess the behavioral and neuronal responses to the tones before training, under stress comparable to training.

Each rabbit was anesthetized with sodium pentobarbital for surgical implantation of three chronically indwelling stainless-

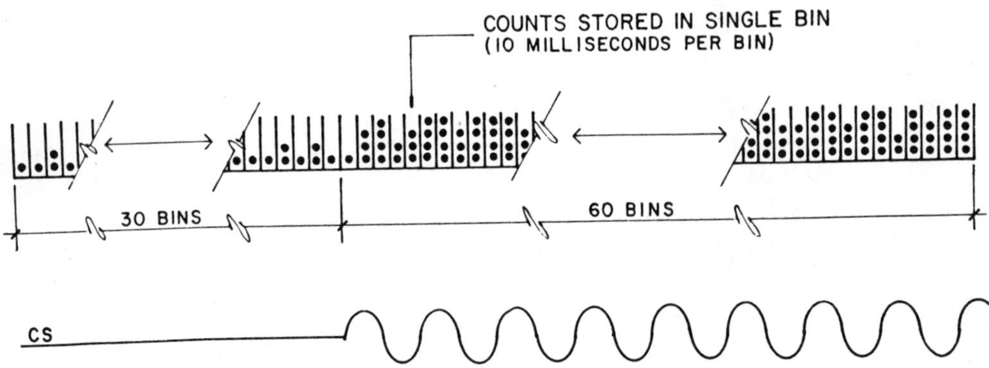

Fig. 1. Construction of peristimulus neuronal histograms for quantification of the neuronal responses to the CS+ and CS- during training. Neuronal spikes exceeding a preset Schmitt trigger level were stored and cumulated as counts (dots, in the figure) in consecutive 10-msec bins prior to and after CS-onset. Separate histograms were constructed for the CS+ and the CS-, each based on the 60 trials given in each session. The frequency of counts in each of the first 20 bins after CS-onset was subtracted from the mean of the 30 pre-CS bins. The difference in each case was divided by the standard deviation of the pre-CS bins, yielding a single score (z-score) for each bin. Also, the mean frequencies in consecutive blocks of 10 bins each were subtracted from the mean of the pre-CS bins, and these differences were divided by the pre-CS standard error, yielding T-scores for the neuronal response in 100 msec periods after CS-onset.

steel semi-microelectrodes (range of tip lengths: 10-60 um, see Foster et al., 1980, for the details of the implantation procedure).

Behavioral training was begun 7-10 days following the surgery. Throughout training, unit activity was fed from the rabbit through a shielded low-noise cable into high-pass active filters (bandwidth = 500-10,000 Hz) and subsequently into pulse height discriminators. The outputs of the discriminators were fed into a computer, programmed to process the neuronal data and to control the behavioral training, on-line. The computer calculated numerical scores for each session, representing the average frequency of neuronal firing in consecutive 10-, and 100-msec periods after CS- onset (see Figure 1).

After behavioral testing each rabbit was given an overdose of sodium pentobarbital, and transcardiac perfusion with normal saline followed by formalin. Each brain was frozen and sectioned at 40 microns and the sections containing the electrode tracks were photographed while still wet. After photography, the sections were subjected to a metachromatic stain for nissl substance and myelinated axons using formol-thionin (see Donovick, 1974).

Procedure for Experiment 1

We have proposed that late-developing discriminative activity of the superficial laminae of the cingulate cortex represents activity projected to those laminae from the AV nucleus, and that retention of the behavioral discrimination depends on the integrity of the AV nucleus. To test these ideas, bilateral electrolytic lesions were made in the AV nucleus after completion of behavioral acquisition. The effects of the lesions on behavior and neuronal activity in the cingulate cortex were assessed during a subsequent retention test.

Nineteen rabbits received training and overtraining using our standard procedures. Prior to behavioral training three recording electrodes were implanted in the cingulate cortex. In addition, stainless-steel lesioning electrodes (tip lengths: 500 microns) were placed bilaterally in the AV nuclei. On the day after the completion of overtraining 10 of the rabbits received bilateral electrolytic lesions (1.5 ma. for 30 or 45 seconds) of the AV nuclei. Control subjects (*N* = 7) had lesioning electrodes implanted but they did not receive lesions. On the eight day after the completion of overtraining all rabbits received a test for retention of the avoidance habit, consisting of extinction to a criterion followed by reacquisition. The criterion for reacquisition was the same as that used during original acquisition.

Subjects (*N* = 7) that had a minimum of 1/3 of the AV nucleus destroyed in each hemisphere were considered to have AV nuclear lesions. Lesioned subjects with less than 1/3 of the nuclei destroyed (N = 5) were placed into a partial lesion group.

RESULTS

Experiment 1: Lesions of the AV nucleus, Behavior and Cingulate Cortical Neuronal Activity

There were no significant differences prior to the lesion between the three groups (lesion, partial lesion and control) in the mean frequencies and latencies of conditioned responses during, acquisition and overtraining, or in the mean numbers of trial-blocks to the acquisition criterion (see above). However, there were group differences in the performance of conditioned responses after the lesion, during the extinction and subsequent reacquisition tests (Figure 2). The mean frequency of conditioned responses of control

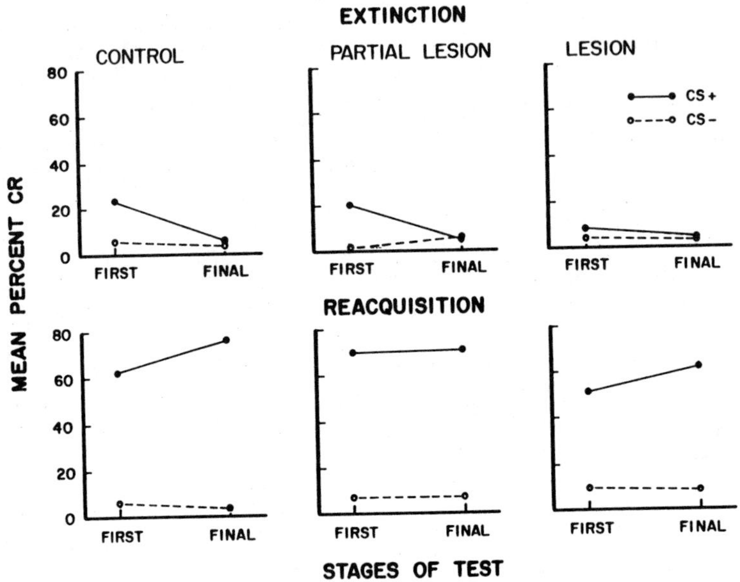

Fig. 2. The mean percent CR (conditioned response) to the CS+ and CS- during extinction and during reacquisition for the control, partial lesion and lesion groups. (Reprinted with permission, 1981).

subjects to the CS+ significantly exceeded the mean to the CS- ($p < .05$). This result also occurred in the partial lesion group ($p < .05$) but the CS+ did not evoke a significantly greater frequency of behavioral responses than did the CS- in the lesion group ($p > .3$). These effects are evident from inspection of the left hand plotted pairs of mean values in the upper panels of Figure 2. The right hand plotted values in each panel illustrate the absence of significant differences in conditioned responding to the CS+ and CS- in the final stage of the extinction test, this due to the essential cessation of all behavioral responding, by virtue of the extinction process, during the final stage.

Group differences were also observed during the reacquisition test (Figure 2, lower panels). The mean frequency of conditioned responses to the CS+ in the lesion group was significantly reduced relative to the control group mean ($p < .01$) and relative to the mean of the partial lesion group ($p < .01$). This pattern of differences held for both the initial and final stages of the reacquisition test.

Because of a relatively great variability in the criterial measures of behavioral performance, there were no significant group differences in the numbers of trial blocks to the extinction and reacquisition criteria. However the differences that did occur were in the expected direction given the significantly reduced frequency of behavioral responding manifested by the lesioned subjects, relative to the controls and partially lesioned subjects.

In summary, there was a significant attenuation in the frequency of behavioral responses of the lesioned subjects to the CS+, during extinction and reacquisition. The attenuation occurred relative to the responses of the controls and the subjects with partial lesions. There were no significant differences between the controls and the partially lesioned subjects. These results give rise to an interesting comparison between the effects of the lesions on behavior, and the neuronal activity in the intact AV nucleus. The lesions attenuated exclusively the behavioral responses to the CS+, and they produced no alteration of the behavioral response to the CS-. The discriminative neuronal discharge acquired by neurons of the AV nucleus was exclusively an increment in response to the CS+ and no change in response to the CS- (e.g., Gabriel, et al., 1980a).

The analysis of the neuronal activity in the cingulate cortex during behavioral acquisition provided replication of our past results indicating distinctive acquisition of discriminative neuronal activity at different depths within the cingulate cortex (Gabriel, et al., 1980a; Foster et al., 1980). During pretraining, the cingulate cortical neuronal response to the tone to be used as CS+ did not differ significantly from the response to the CS-

(Figure 3, upper left panel). However, significant discriminative neuronal activity in the form of a greater neuronal response

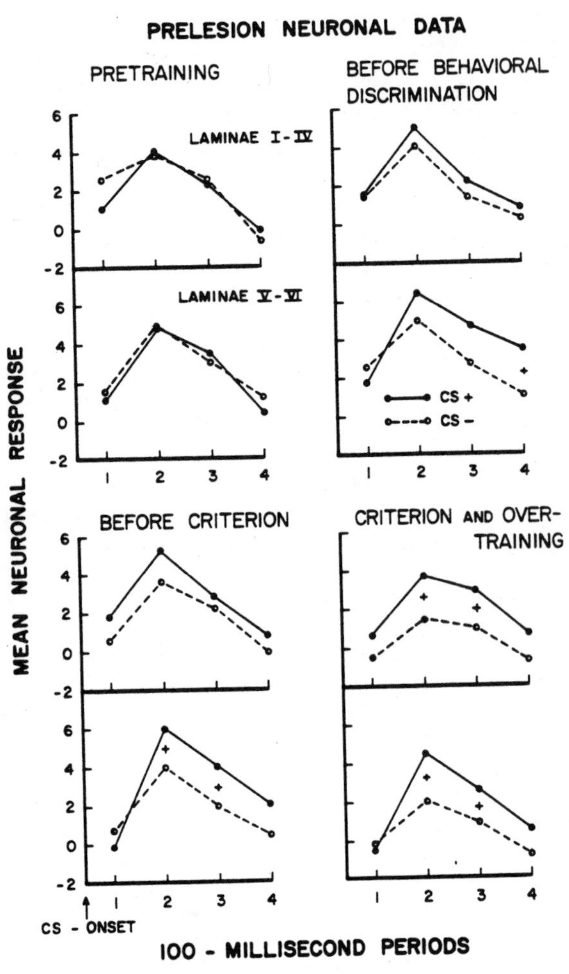

Fig. 3. Average discharges in neurons of the cingulate cortex in consecutive periods of 100 msec following onset of the CS+ and CS-. Data are shown for pretraining and for three stages of behavioral acquisition. The upper half of each graph shows the results obtained from the superficial laminae of the cingulate cortex and the lower half shows the results obtained from the deep laminae. The cross-marks indicate 100-msec periods at which significantly greater neuronal discharges occurred to the CS+ than to the CS-. (Reprinted with permission, 1981).

to the CS+ than to the CS- developed in the deep laminae (V, VI) of the cingulate cortex during the initial stages of behavioral acquisition, prior to the criterion of discriminative behavioral performance (Figure 3, upper right and lower left panels). Also,

CINGULATE CORTICAL DISCRIMINATIVE DISCHARGE

A. BEFORE LESION OF THE AV NUCLEUS

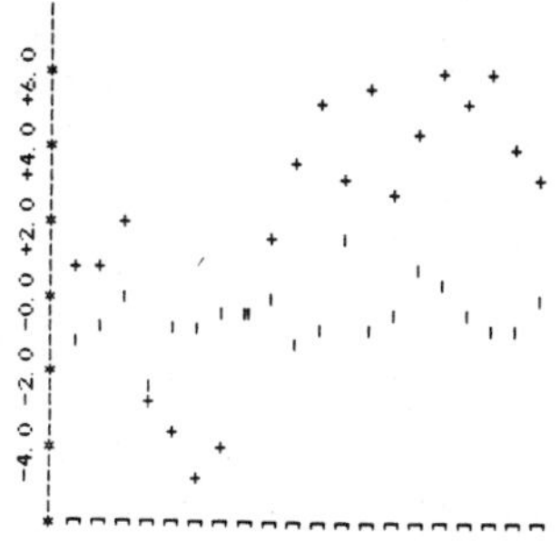

B. AFTER LESION OF THE AV NUCLEUS

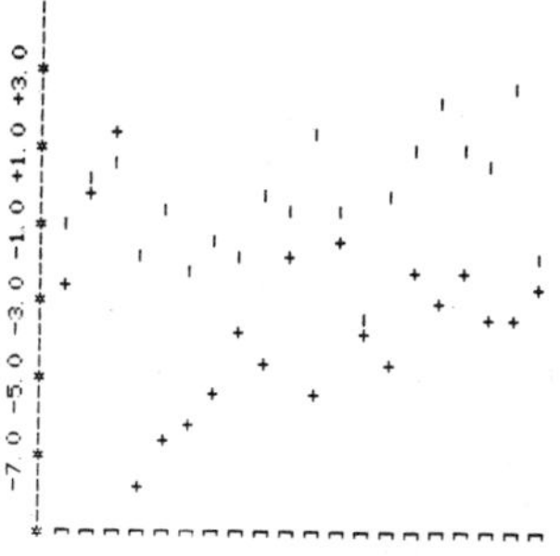

Fig. 4. The effect of a lesion in the anteroventral (AV) thalamic nucleus on average CS-evoked neuronal discharges in the cingulate cortex. The figure portrays the data of a representative subject, with a recording electrode in Lamina I. Each plotted point represents the average magnitude of the neuronal discharge, either to the CS+ (plus signs) or to the CS- (minus signs) in the form of _z_-scores (see Figure 1). Data are shown for the first 20 consecutive 10-millisecond periods after CS-onset. The upper panel shows the data obtained during the final overtraining session prior to the lesion. The lower panel shows the data obtained after the lesion, during the criterial session of reacquisition. (Reprinted with permission, 1981).

as in the past studies, significant discriminative activity developed in the superficial laminae (I-IV) preferentially in the late stage of acquisition, during criterion attainment and overtraining (Figure 3, lower right panel).

The lesions of the AV nucleus had a pronounced effect on the neuronal activity of the cingulate cortex during extinction testing and reacquisition. Generally, the excitatory and discriminative neuronal discharge in the control group was replaced by a below-baseline "off" response in the lesioned subjects (Figure 4).

During the initial stage of extinction (Figure 5, upper panels) the average overall (nondiscriminative) magnitude of the neuronal discharge at 100-200 milliseconds after CS-onset in the lesioned and partially lesioned subjects was significantly reduced relative to the average in the control group ($\underline{p} < .01$ and $\underline{p} < .05$ for the lesioned and partially lesioned subjects, respectively). Absence of any significant effect involving the stimulus factor (CS+/CS-) from this analysis suggested that discriminative neuronal discharges did not occur in any group during the initial stage of extinction.

Nevertheless, the lesion factor did interact with the stimulus factor during the final stage of extinction (Figure 5, lower panels) and during the final reacquisition stage (Figure 6, lower panels). In these instances, the lesion transformed the neuronal discharge to the CS+ from one that was excitatory and discriminative (i.e., significantly greater than the discharge to the CS- in the control group) to a below-baseline "off" response that was not significantly different from the discharge to the CS-.

The analysis of the data in the final extinction stage for both the control and the partially lesioned groups yielded significantly greater mean neuronal discharges to the CS+ than to the CS- in the third and fourth periods of 100-milliseconds after CS-onset ($\underline{p} < .05$ in both instances). There were no significant discriminative effects however, for the lesion group.

Essentially the same results occurred during the final reacquisition stage. In this instance the mean neuronal discharge to the CS+ in the control group exceeded significantly the mean discharge to the CS- ($\underline{p} < .05$), but the stimuli did not produce significant differences in the lesion groups. Also, the mean discharge to the CS+ in the control group significantly exceeded the means for the partial lesion group ($\underline{p} < .05$) and for the lesion group ($\underline{p} < .01$). The two groups with lesions were not significantly different, and there were no significant group differences in discharges to the CS-. The 100-millisecond period after CS-onset did not contribute significantly to these effects, thus the results

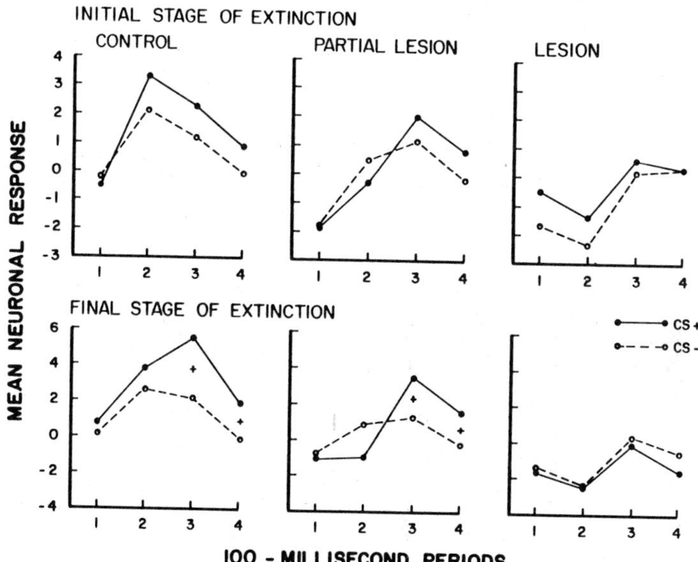

Fig. 5. Average discharges in neurons of the cingulate cortex in consecutive periods of 100 milliseconds following onset of CS+ and CS-. Data are shown for the initial (upper panels) and final (lower panels) stages of extinction defined respectively as the first session and the session in which the extinction criterion was attained (Reprinted with permission, 1981).

given above refer to the overall mean obtained by summing over periods.

It was not possible to obtain data for an initial (precriterial) reacquisition stage for the partial lesion group due to the very rapid behavioral reacquisition in this group. Thus, the comparison conducted at this stage involved only the lesion and control groups (Figure 6, upper panels). Again, the lesion factor yielded a significant result ($p < .033$) indicating a reduced cingulate cortical neuronal discharge in the lesioned subjects as compared to

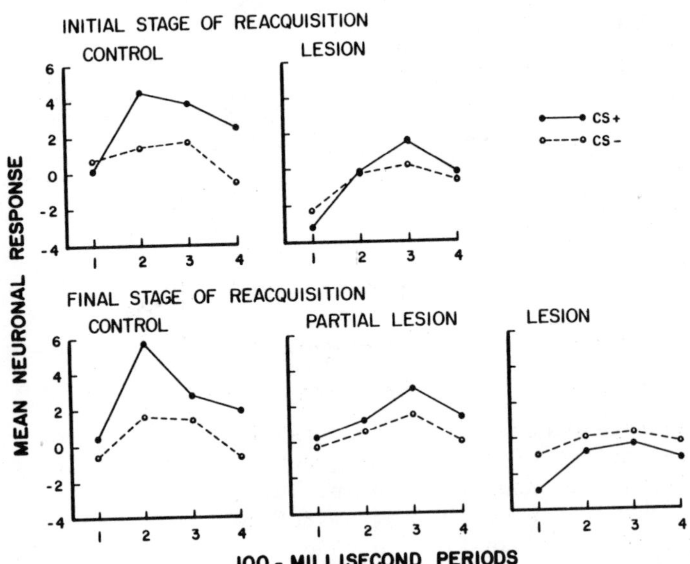

Fig. 6. Average discharges in neurons of the cingulate cortex in consecutive periods of 100 milliseconds following onset of the CS+ and CS-. Data are shown for the initial and final stages of reacquisition, defined respectively as all precriterial sessions, and the two consecutive sessions in which the behavioral criterion was attained (see Methods, reprinted with permission, 1981).

the controls. In this instance, the overall stimulus factor was significant ($p < .013$) but the interaction of stimulus with lesion condition was only marginally so ($p < .07$). Nevertheless inspection of the interaction means (Figure 6, upper half) suggests the presence of a discriminative neuronal discharge in the control subjects and its absence in the lesioned subjects.

Discussion

Lesions of the AV nucleus abolished the CS+-driven excitatory (above baseline) neuronal activity in the rabbit cingulate cortex, during retention of active avoidance behavior. Instead of the excitatory and discriminative neuronal activity, the lesioned rabbits manifested nondiscriminative and largely inhibitory (below baseline) responses to the CSs. Moreover, the overall pattern of the data suggested that the effect of the lesion was a graded one. There was invariably a greater inhibitory response and a more total abolition of neuronal discrimination in the group composed of subjects who sustained virtually total destruction of the AV nucleus, compared with subjects that sustained only partial destruction.

These results indicate that discriminative neuronal activity in the cingulate cortex is critically dependent upon the integrity of its connections with the AV nucleus. Thus, our hypothetical model of the interactive functioning of those two structures (see INTRODUCTION) is supported.

The axon terminals of neurons of the AV nucleus occur specifically in superficial laminae (I-IV) of the cingulate cortex. This relationship led to the suggestion (Gabriel et al., 1980a; Foster et al., 1980) that the late-developing discriminative neuronal activity in the superficial laminae reflected the driving action being exerted by the AV nuclear neurons, which also manifest late-developing discriminative activity. But even though the neurons in the superficial laminae manifested development of discriminative activity at a later stage of acquisition than did the deep laminar neurons, in the present as well as in our past studies, our analyses provided no indication of a selective effect of the lesion within the superficial laminae. Instead the lesions seemed to block neuronal excitation and discrimination in both superficial and deep laminae. Thus, although the thalamocortical axons terminate in the superficial laminae, removal of their influence abolished discriminative activity at all cortical depths.

Destruction of the AV nucleus amounts to removal of an prominent excitatory influence in cingulate cortex. What is left over seems to be a predominance of inhibitory responsiveness on the part of neurons in this region. The question then becomes, what is the

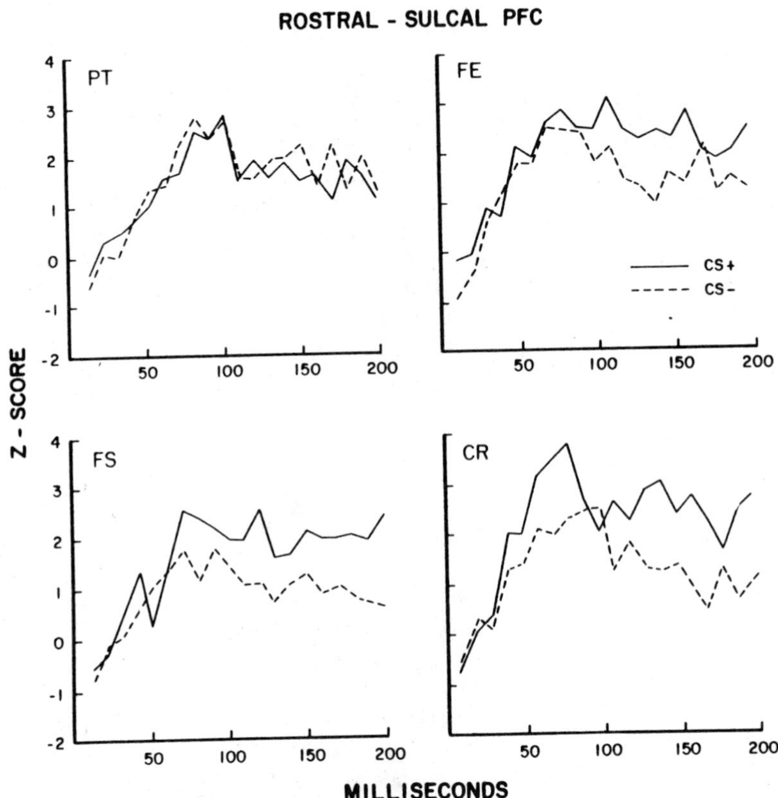

Fig. 7. Average neuronal discharges in neurons of the rostral/sulcal prefrontal cortex (PFC) in consecutive periods of 10 milliseconds following the onsets of the CS+ and CS-. Data are shown in the separate panels for pretraining (PT), the session of first exposure (FE) to the conditioning procedure, the session in which the first significant (FS) behavioral discrimination occurred, and the session in which the criterion (CR) of behavioral performance was attained. (Reprinted with permission, 1981).

origin of the inhibitory influence?

We have argued elsewhere (Gabriel et al., 1980b) that the hippocampal formation exerts inhibitory control over discriminative neuronal activity (significance code) in the cingulate cortex. The effect of presenting the CS+ is to remove the inhibitory influence from the hippocampal formation, permitting the significance code to flow freely to the response priming center (i.e., the neostriatum) and to release the primed behavioral response (Gabriel et al., 1980b, Pp. 185-200). It would be compatible with this hypothesis to suggest that the fibres which project from the hippocampal formation (i.e., the subiculum) to the cingulate and retrosplenial cortices (e.g., Sorensen, 1980; Meibach & Siegel, 1977) may be the ones which mediate the inhibitory effects in the cortex. This hypothesis will be tested by examining associative neuronal activity in the cingulate cortex in subjects with hippocampal lesions. It is expected that such lesions will produce a predominance of excitatory neuronal activity in the cingulate cortex instead of the predominance of inhibitory effects seen in the present study. We would also suggest that the extra excitatory activity may be involved in mediating the behavioral over-responding so frequently manifested by hippocampectomized animals (see Gabriel et al., 1980b, Pp. 200-204).

Experiment 2: Neuronal Significance Coding in the Prefrontal Cortex and MD Thalamic Nucleus

The prefrontal cortex (PFC) is the cortical projection zone of the MD nucleus, occupying the anterior portion of the hemispheric medial wall to a midcallosal section. Recent neuroanatomical studies have indicated that subdivisions exist for the PFC in rabbits and other animals: approximately the caudal two-thirds of this region intercommunicates via reciprocal axonal projections with the lateral (non-olfactory) component of the MD nucleus; the rostral one-third of the PFC as well as a lateroventral region surrounding the rhinal sulcus, have reciprocal interconnection with the medial (olfactory) component of the MD nucleus (see Benjamin, Jackson & Golden, 1978). The data of Experiment 2 were obtained from a total of 42 recording loci distributed in the two subdivisions of PFC (12 in the rostral/sulcal area and 12 in the caudal area) and in the MD nucleus (9 in the medial division and 9 in the lateral division).

The average magnitudes of nueronal discharges to the CS+ and CS-, in the PFC and the MD nucleus, are shown for the various stages of behavioral acquisition in Figures 7-10. The data at brief latency with fine temporal grain (i.e., 10-millisecond resolution) are shown in Figures 6 and 8 for the rostral and caudal

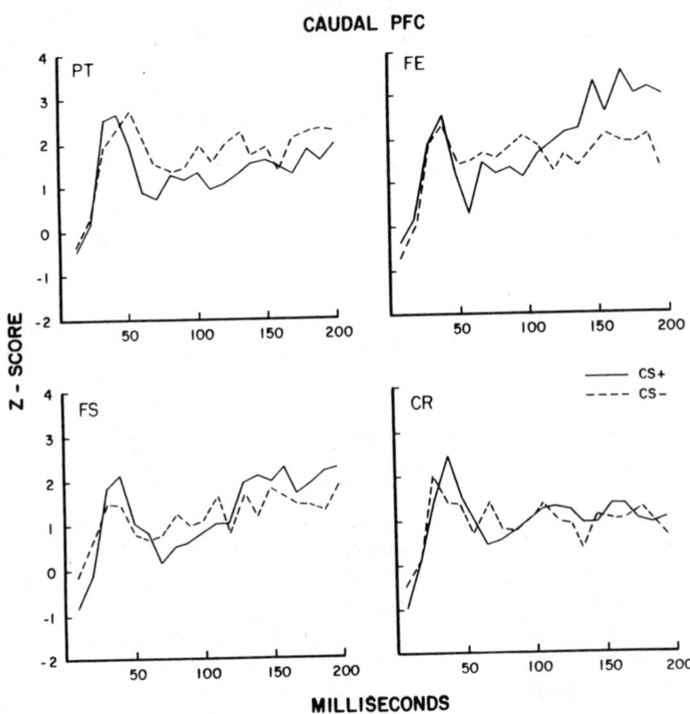

Fig. 8. Average neuronal discharges in neurons of the caudal prefrontal cortex (PFC) in consecutive periods of 10 milliseconds following the onsets of the CS+ and CS-. Data are shown for pre-training (PT) and the stages of behavioral acquisition, as indicated in the legend of Figure 7 (Reprinted with permission, 1981).

subdivisions, respectively. The remaining figures show the average discharges at longer latencies (for the four consecutive 100-millisecond periods after CS-onset) in both of the subdivisions of the PFC and the MD nucleus.

Analysis of variance indicated no significant differences in the average neuronal discharges to the CSs during pretraining (PT) when they were presented noncontingently with the footshock UCS. However significant discriminative discharges, greater to the CS+ than to the CS–, occurred during acquisition. In addition, there were differences between the various subdivisions of the PFC and the MD nucleus in the development of the discriminative discharges. Neurons in the rostral/sulcal subdivision of PFC manifested significant discriminative neuronal activity in the first exposure (FE) to the training procedure. This discriminative effect continued to occur during the remaining stages of acquisition through the session of criterion-attainment (see Figures 7 and 9). However the medial division of the MD nucleus, with which the rostral/sulcal PFC is reciprocally interconnected, did not manifest significant discriminative neuronal activity in any stage of training (Figure 10, upper half).

In contrast to the rostral/sulcal PFC the caudal subdivision of the PFC manifested a significant discriminative neuronal discharge in the first stage of conditioning, but not in the subsequent conditioning stages (Figure 8 and lower half of 9). Moreover the lateral division of the MD nucleus, with which the caudal PFC is reciprocally interconnected manifested significant discriminative activity in the later stages of acquisition (FS, CR, Figure 10, lower half). All of the regions studied showed the same results during the three postcriterial (overtraining) sessions as were manifested during the criterial session.

Discussion

The present results indicated that the past demonstrations of development of discriminative neuronal activity in cingulate cortex at an early stage of acquisition, and its development at a later stage in the AV nucleus, may be generalized to the caudal PFC and the lateral division of the MD nucleus. Thus, the cortical-to-thalamic relegation of the discriminative neuronal code for stimulus significance occurs in at least these two limbic configurations. Nevertheless, differences in the form of the discriminative encoding between the cingulate cortical-AV nuclear system and the caudal PFC-lateral MD nuclear system raise interesting possibilities for future elaboration of the present model system. The greatest magnitude of discriminative neuronal activity to occur in the caudal PFC occurred in the session of first exposure to conditioning, and its latency in that session was quite brief,

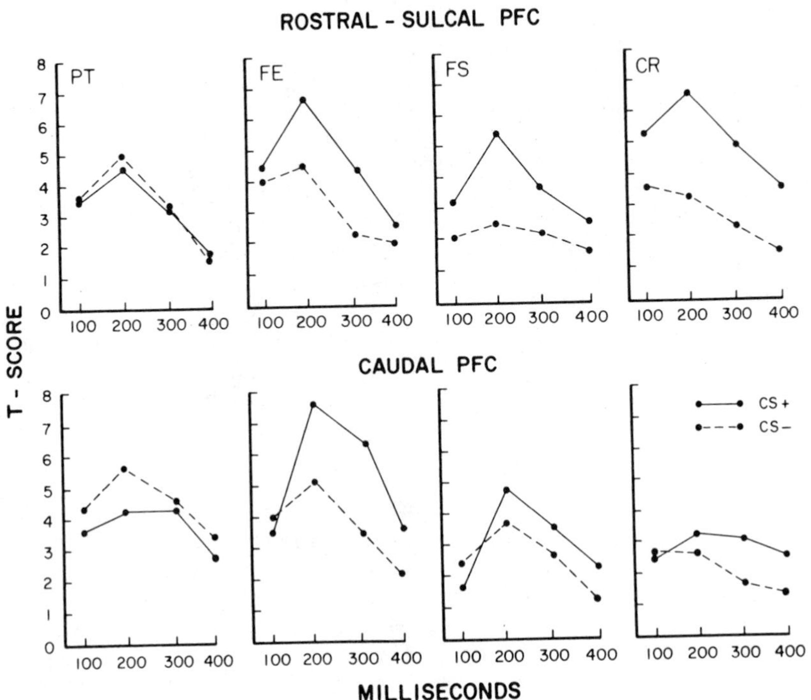

Fig. 9. Average neuronal discharges in neurons of the rostral/ sulcal subdivision of the prefrontal cortex (PFC, upper panels) and for the caudal subdivision of the PFC (lower panels) in consecutive 100-millisecond periods after the onsets of the CS+ and CS−. Data are shown for pretraining and for the various stages of behavioral acquisition as indicated in the legend of Figure 7. (Reprinted with permission, 1981).

occurring in the interval from 100 to 200 milliseconds. In contrast, the cingulate cortex manifested its discriminative effect only marginally in the first conditioning session, and only at relatively great latencies (300 milliseconds) during that initial session. Discriminative activity in the cingulate cortex occurred at briefer latencies and larger

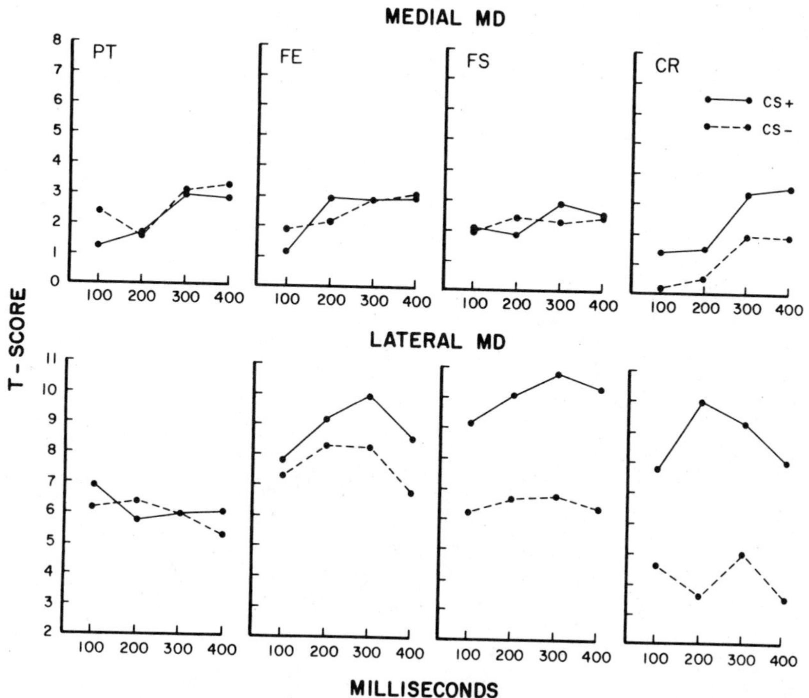

Fig. 10. Average neuronal discharges in neurons of the medial subdivision of n. medialis dorsalis (MD, upper panels) and for the lateral subdivision of the MD nucleus (lower panels) in consecutive 100-millisecond periods after the onsets of the CS+ amd CS-. Data are shown for pretraining (PT) and for the various stages of behavioral acquisition, as indicated in the legend of Figure 7. (Reprinted with permission, 1981).

magnitudes, in later stages of behavioral acquisition, such as the session of first significant behavioral discrimination, and the session of criterion attainment. These results suggest that discriminative neuronal activity in the caudal PFC developed earlier in the sequence of conditioning trials than does activity in the cingulate cortex. Similarly, the discriminative activity in the lateral division of the MD nculeus developed at an earlier stage of training (during the session of first significant behavioral discrimination) than did the activity in the AV nucleus, which did not appear until the criterial session. In short, the PFC-MD nuclear system acquired discriminative activity after fewer trials than the cingulate cortical-AV nuclear system. These results considered in conjunction with the demonstration of a direct reciprocal axonal interconnection of the PFC and the cingulate cortex (Bassett & Berger, 1980) suggest that the earlier-developing discriminative code in the PFC-MD system may be causally relevant to the later-developing cingulate cortical-AV nuclear code.

An additional point to be stressed from the present results is the idea that the principal of cortical-to-thalamic relegation of significance code is not inviolable for all corticothalamic systems of the brain. The rostral/sulcal PFC acquired robust discriminative activity in the first exposure to conditioning, as in the caudal PFC. However the activity in the rostral/sulcal PFC did not decline during the later training stages, as did the activity in the caudal PFC. Moreover the medial division of the MD nucleus, reciprocally interconnected with the rostral/sulcal PFC, <u>never</u> developed discriminative activity during the course of training. Thus whereas the cingulate cortex and AV nucleus, and the caudal PFC and lateral MD nucleus both constitute corticothalamic systems which manifest relegation of discriminative activity, the rostral/sulcal cortex linked with the medial MD nucleus would appear to be a non-relegating corticothalamic system.

It is interesting to consider the behavioral relevance of the distinction between relegating and non-relegating systems. Perhaps relegating systems are involved in the coding of stimuli whose associative significance endures from trial-to-trial and from day-to-day. Because of this endurance, it may be beneficial for the sake of their memorial preservation, to relegate the codes for stimulus significance to a subcortical locus such as the MD or AV nuclei. In contrast, the non-relegating code of the rostral/sulcal PFC may reflect the process of "working memory" (see Honig, 1978) which applies to cues whose associative significance undergoes moment-by-moment or day-by-day variation. Of course, a working memory system would also be expected to contribute to performance of tasks such as the present one (in which cue significance has endurance) even though such a contribution may not be its principal function. This assumption is consistent with our observation of non-relegating discriminative activity in the rostral/sulcal PFC. It also provides an account of the relatively mild behavioral and retentive effects of AV nuclear lesions (Experiment 1). Thus, lesions may have produced mild behavioral effects because the behavior is subserved redundantly by the rostral PFC encoding processes.

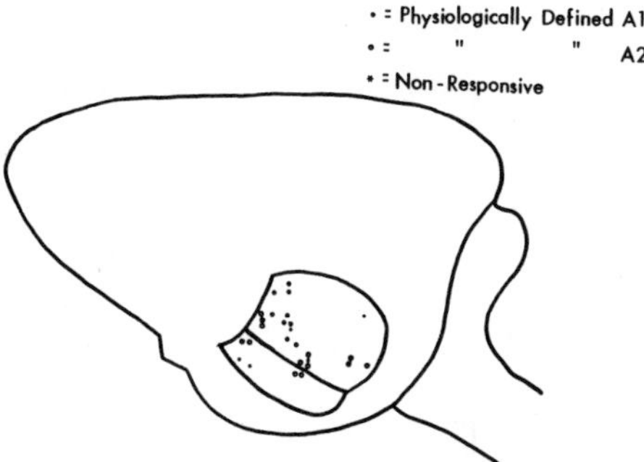

Fig. 11. A schematic lateral view of the rabbit cerebral hemisphere with the primary and secondary auditory cortices (AI and AII) outlined. The depiction is based on that presented by Monnier and Gangloff (1961). The filled and open dots represent loci of neuronal records manifesting respectively static and labile physiological response properties characteristic of AI and AII (see Foster, 1981). (Reprinted with permission, 1981).

Experiment 3: Discriminative Neuronal Activity in the Auditory Cortex and Medial Geniculate Nucleus

The idea that the cortical-to-thalamic relegation of neuronal significance code for discriminative avoidance conditioning does not occur in all systems received further support from our studies of the neuronal activity in the auditory system. Instead of a cortical-to-thalamic sequential progression, the auditory system manifested late-developing discriminative neuronal activity in restricted components, both at the cortical and thalamic levels. Only one component of the system (the medial division of the MGN) manifested early developing discriminative neuronal activity. The detailed presentation of these results follows.

The topographic distribution of recording loci in the primary and secondary auditory cortices is portrayed in Figure 11. The primary auditory cortex (AI) developed a discriminative neuronal

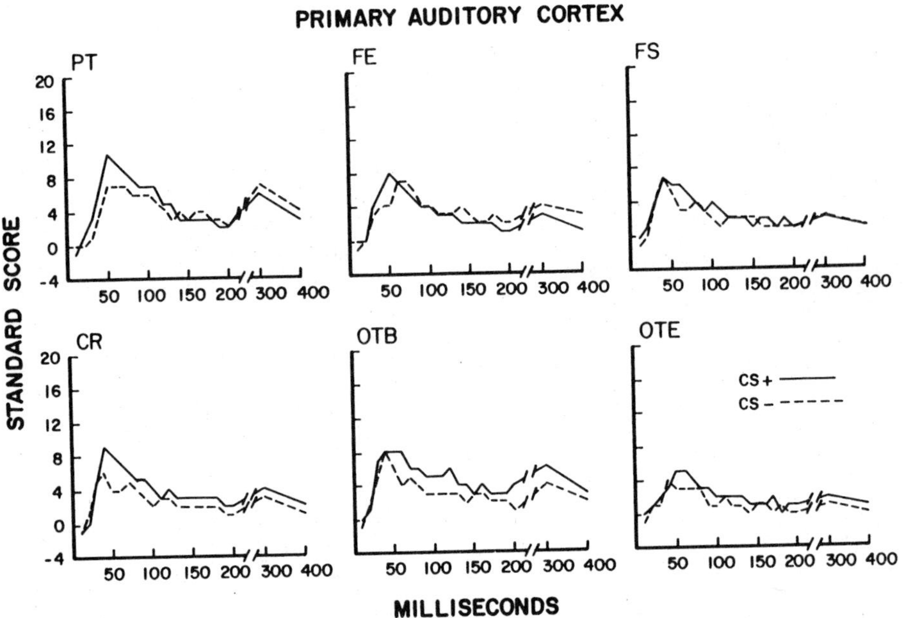

Fig. 12. Average neuronal discharges in neurons of the primary auditory cortex (AI) in 20 consecutive periods of 10 milliseconds, and in two consecutive periods of 100 milliseconds each, following the onsets of the CS+ and the CS-. The data are shown in the separate panels for the stages of precriterial behavioral acquisition (PT = pretraining; FE = session of first exposure to conditioning, FS = session of the first significant behavioral discrimination; CR = session in which the behavioral criterion was attained). Also shown are data of two postcriterial overtraining (OT) sessions, the beginning session (OTB) and the ending session (OTE). (Reprinted with permission, 1981).

discharge during the overtraining sessions as indicated by the occurrence of a significantly greater neuronal response to the CS+ relative to the CS- during the second period of 100 milliseconds

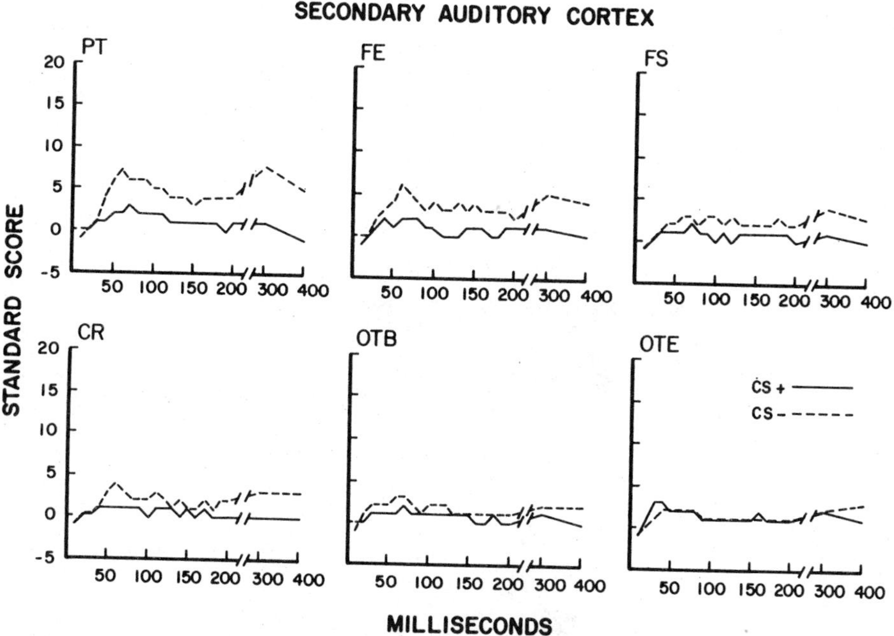

Fig. 13. Average neuronal discharges in neurons of the secondary auditory cortex (AII) in 20 consecutive periods of 10 milliseconds, and in two consecutive periods of 100 milliseconds each, following the onsets of the CS+ and the CS-. The data are shown in the separate panels for the stages of precriterial behavioral acquisition (PT = pretraining; FE = session of first exposure to conditioning; FS = session of the first significant behavioral discrimination; CR = session in which the behavioral criterion was attained). Also shown are data of two postcriterial overtraining (OT) sessions, the beginning session (OTB) and the ending session (OTE). (Reprinted with permission, 1981).

after CS onset, in all three of the overtraining sessions ($p < .05$ in all cases; see Figure 12). There were no significant discriminative effects prior to overtraining in AI.

The average neuronal discharge in the secondary auditory cortex (A2, Figure 13) manifested a significant bias during pretraining to the tones subsequently to be used as CS-. This bias was not due to the particular frequency of the CS-, as both of the tones (1kHz and 8kHz) served as CS- equally often. Because of this prewired differential effect in A2, the "discriminative discharge" which developed was one of an unusual sort. It took the form of a

RABBIT MEDIAL GENICULATE NUCLEUS

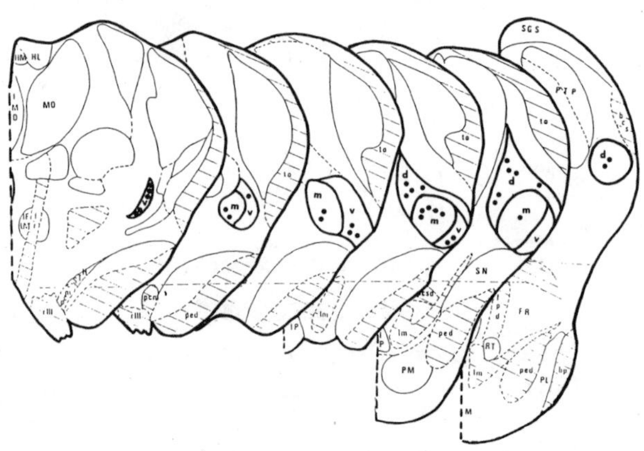

Fig. 14. Successive coronal views of the rabbit diencephalon derived from the atlas of Urban and Richard (1972). Added to the atlas diagram are outlines, depicting the cytoarchitectural subdivisions (v = ventral; m = medial; d = dorsal) of the rabbit medial geniculate nucleus, following Morest (1964) and Gerhard (1968). The dots depict the histologically verified loci of the electrodes for unit recording. (Reprinted with permission, 1981).

disappearance of prewired effect. As in the case of the associative change in the AI the disappearance of the prewired effect in A2 occurred in a very late stage of training (during but not prior to the postcriterial overtraining sessions).

Neuroanatomical and neurophysiological studies have indicated that the MGN in cats and other mammals is composed of a dorsal, a ventral and a medial subdivision (see Morest, 1964). By using the data presented by Morest for cats, and available information on the cytoarchitecture of the rabbit MGN (Gehard, 1968) we classified

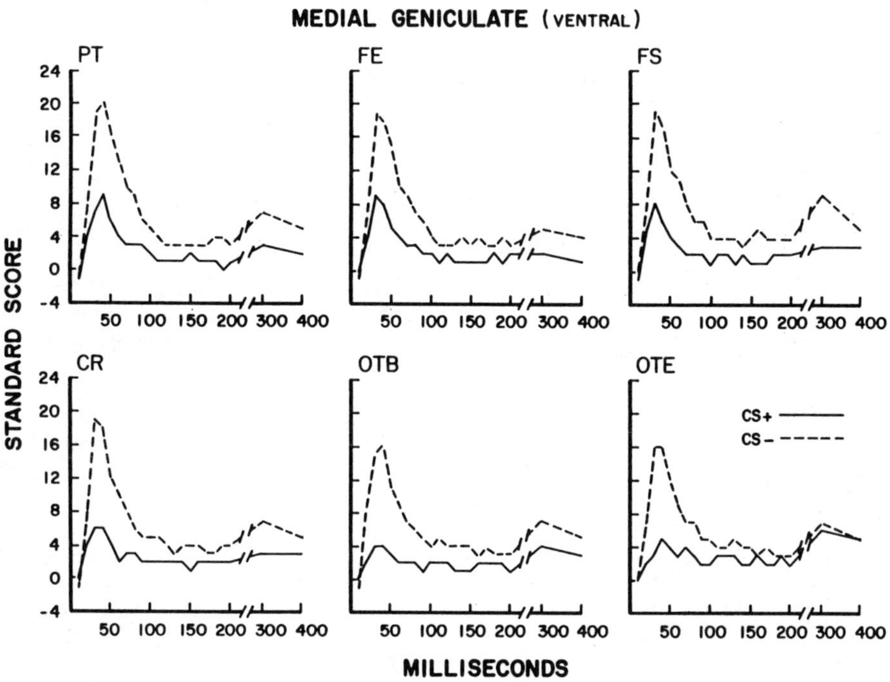

Fig. 15. Average neuronal discharges in neurons of the ventral subdivision of the MGN in 20 consecutive periods of 10 milliseconds, and in two consecutive periods of 100 milliseconds each, following the onsets of the CS+ and the CS-. The data are shown in the separate panels for the stages of precriterial behavioral acquisition (PT = pretraining; FE = session of first exposure to conditioning; FS = session of the first significant behavioral discrimination; CR = session in which the behavioral criterion was attained). Also shown are data of two postcriterial overtraining (OT) sessions, the beginning session (OTB) and the ending session (OTE). (Reprinted with permission, 1981).

each electrode track with regard to the nuclear subdivision. The distribution of recording sites is shown in Figure 14.

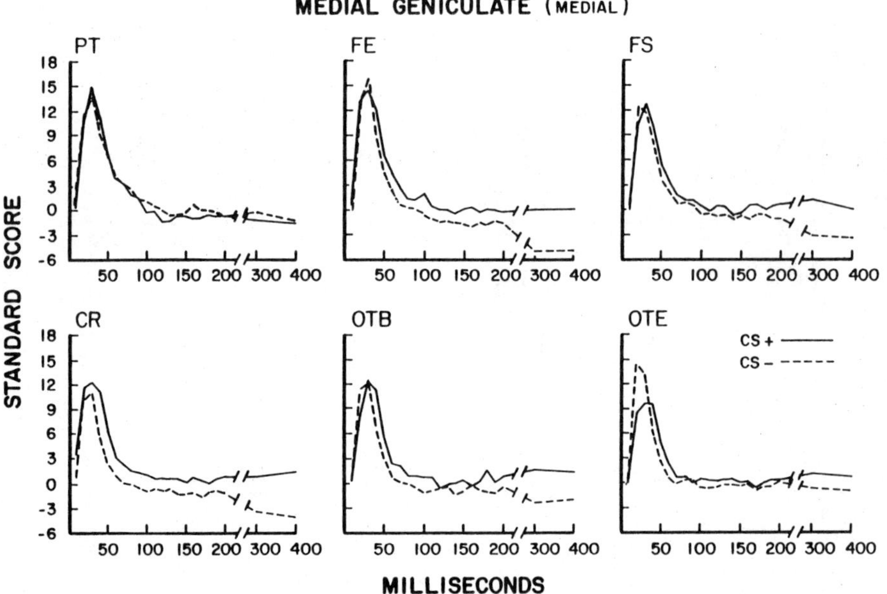

Fig. 16. Average neuronal discharges in neurons of the medial subdivision of the MGN in 20 consecutive periods of 10 milliseconds, and in two consecutive periods of 100 milliseconds, following the onsets of the CS+ and the CS- . The data are shown in the separate panels for the stages of precriterial behavioral acquisition (PT = pretraining; FE = session of first exposure to conditioning; FS = session of the first significant behavioral discrimination; CR = session in which the behavioral criterion was attained). Also shown are data of two postcriterial overtraining (OT) sessions, the beginning session (OTB) and the ending session (OTE). (Reprinted with permission, 1981).

The ventral division of the MGN represents the relay nucleus of the classical auditory projection pathway. The analyses indicated that there were no significant alterations of neuronal activity in this subdivision during the course of acquisition and overtraining (Figure 15). Rather, the neuronal records manifested substantial biases to one or the other of the two auditory CSs during the pretraining session. As in A2, the average bias favored the CS-, accounting for the significantly greater neuronal response to that stimulus relative to the CS+ during pretraining (compare the dotted-line function to the solid line function in the upper left panel of Figure 15). Note in the remainder of Figure 15, that a similar "prewired" differential neuronal response continued to occur during the course of acquisition and overtraining. Thus, the ventral subdivision of the MGN would appear to be a region in which the neuronal analysis is concerned quite exclusively with the acoustic parameters of the incoming stimuli, not their associative significance. Prior results from our laboratory (Gabriel, Saltwick & Miller, 1976) and from other laboratories (Ryugo & Weinberger, 1978; Birt & Olds, 1981) have been in essential agreement with this conclusion.

The average activity for the records from the dorsal and medial subdivisions of the MGN did not manifest systematic prewired differential discharges to the CSs (see the data of pretraining, upper left panels in Figures 16 and 17). However, significant discriminative discharges developed in both of these subdivisions during the course of behavioral acquisition. The discriminative effect in the medial subdivision occurred during the second period of 100 milliseconds and at all subsequent periods, in the very first session of training. The effect continued to occur during the remaining stages of acquisition, but it was not present during the final overtraining session (Figure 16).

In contrast, the significant discriminative effect in the dorsal subdivision did not first occur until the criterial session, and it continued to occur during the postcriterial (overtraining) sessions (Figure 17).

It should be mentioned that the discriminative effects just reported carried over into subsequent testing sessions which for the sake of brevity are not reported upon here. Thus, extinction training and reacquisition of the original problem were given after overtraining. The medial subdivision which during overtraining had lost its previously acquired discriminative discharge did not reacquire the effect during behavioral reacquisition. However, the discriminative activity in the dorsal division, which was clearly present at the end of overtraining, declined during extinction, and was reinstated during reacquisition. These results are reported fully in a separate paper (Foster, 1981).

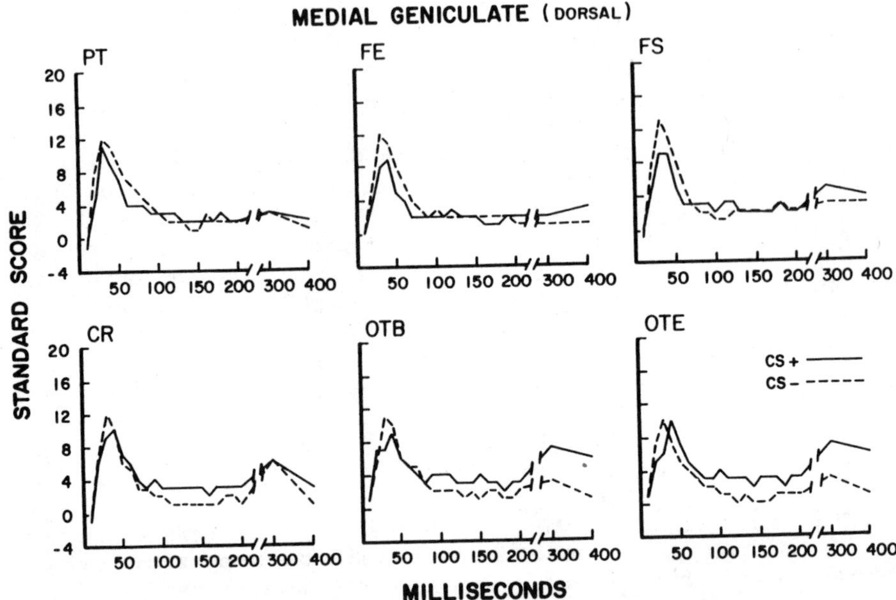

Fig. 17. Average neuronal discharges in neurons of the dorsal subdivision of the medial geniculate nucleus in 20 consecutive periods of 10 milliseconds, and in two consecutive periods of 100 milliseconds each, following the onsets of the CS+ and the CS-. The data are shown in the separate panels for the stages of precriterial behavioral acquisition (PT = pretraining; FE = session of first exposure to conditioning, FS = session of the first significant behavioral discrimination; CR = session in which the behavioral criterion was attained). Also shown are data of two postcriterial overtraining (OT) sessions, the beginning session (OTB) and the ending session (OTE). (Reprinted with permission, 1981).

Discussion

Neuronal activity in the auditory cortex and MGN did not manifest a sequential progression of discriminative activity from cortex to thalamus as seen in the limbic structures. Instead, the predominant outcome for the auditory structures was the development of discriminative neuronal activity in a late stage of acquisition (as in the auditory cortex and the dorsal subdivision of the MGN), or no discriminative activity (as in the ventral subdivision of the MGN). Only the medial subdivision of the MGN manifested discriminative activity at an early stage of training (the first exposure to conditioning).

The occurrence of early-developing discriminative neuronal activity in the medial subdivision raises the possibility of a direct causal relationship between that activity and the early-developing activity in the PFC (Experiment 2) and cingulate cortex (Gabriel, et al., 1980a). Thus perhaps the discriminative activity in the PFC and cingulate cortices is projected directly to those loci from the medial subdivision or perhaps the medial subdivision receives direct influence from the PFC and cingulate cortices.

This interpretation is plausible and it will be checked in future studies, although it is somewhat mitigated by the observation of rather striking differences between the discriminative activity in the medial division and the PFC and cingulate cortices during reversal training. The discriminative activity appropriate to original acquisition persisted in the PFC and cingulate cortices during several of the initial reversal training sessions (Gabriel et al., 1980b; Orona, 1981), but there was not significant manifestation of the original discriminative response in the medial subdivision of MGN during reversal training (Foster, 1981). Given these results it seems certain that if a direct causal linkage does exist between these two regions it is not a completely fixed linkage. Rather it is one that can be interrupted by such things as new CS-UCS contingencies which occur at the outset of reversal learning problems.

Consideration of the results from Experiments 2 and 3 together with past data from our laboratory suggest the existence of two fundamental classes of brain substrate for discriminative avoidance conditioning. The members of one class (PFC, deep cingulate laminae, medial subdivision of MGN, brainstem reticular formation) all have in common the manifestation discriminative neuronal activity at an early training stage, before the inception of discriminative behavior or before the completion of acquisition to the behavioral asymptote. The members of the second class (AV nucleus, superficial cingulate laminae, lateral subdivision of the MD nucleus, dorsal subdivision of the MGN, auditory cortex) manifest discriminative behavior coincidentally with the advent of asymptotic discriminative behavior, or after the advent of such behavior.

These results may have an important implication for the general question of the functional neuroanatomy of the learning process. It is the idea that neural processes relevant to the acquisition of new behavior, and neural processes relevant to the performance of already acquired behavior, occur in substantially distinct neuroanatomical substrates.

ACKNOWLEDGEMENTS

The work presented here was supported by the University of Texas Research Institute, The Spencer Foundation, and NIMH Grants 26276 and 31351 to MG.

The data presented in Experiments 3 and 4 represented portions of the results from the doctoral theses of Dr. Edward Orona and Dr. Kent Foster, respectively. Dr. Orona's current address is: Yerkes Primate Laboratory, Atlanta, Georgia 30322. Dr. Foster's current address is: Barrow Neurological Institute, Phoenix, Arizona 85013.

REFERENCES

Akert, K., 1964, Comparative anatomy of frontal cortex and thalamofrontal connections in: "The Frontal Granular Cortex and Behavior," J. M. Warren and K. Akert, eds., McGraw-Hill, New York.

Bassett, J. L., Berger, T. W., 1980, Association connections between anterior and posterior limbic cortices in the rabbit, Soc. Neurosci. Abstr. Bull., 31.2.

Benjamin, R. M., Jackson, J. C., and Golden, G. T., 1978, Cortical projections of the thalamic mediodorsal nucleus in the rabbit, Brain Res., 141:251-265.

Birt, D., and Olds, M. E., 1981, Associative response changes in lateral midbrain tegmentum and medial geniculate during differential appetitive conditioning, J. Neurophysiol. (in press).

Brogden, W. J., and Culler, F. A., 1936, A device for motor conditioning of small animals, Science, 83:269.

Donovick, P. J., 1973, A metachromatic stain for neural tissue, Stain Technology, 49:49-51.

Foster, K., Orona, E., Lambert, R., and Gabriel, M., 1980. Early and late acquisition of discriminative neuronal activity during differential conditioning in rabbits: Specificity within the laminae of cingulate cortex and the anteroventral thalamus, J. Comp. Physiol. Psychol., 94:1069-1086.

Foster, K., 1981, Unit activity in the auditory system of rabbit during differential conditioning, reversal, and extinction. Doctoral dissertation, University of Texas at Austin.

Fuster, J. M., 1980,"The prefrontal cortex: Anatomy, physiology, and neuropsychology of the frontal lobe,"Raven Press, New York.

Gabriel, M., Foster, K., and Orona, E., 1980a, Interaction of the laminae of cingulate cortex and the anteroventral thalamus during behavioral learning, Science, 208:1050-1052.

Gabriel, M., Foster, K., Orona, E., Saltwick, S. E., and Stanton, M., 1980b, Neuronal activity of cingulate cortex, anteroventral thalamus and hippocampal formation in discriminative conditioning: Encoding and extraction of the significance of conditional stimuli, in: "Progress in Psychobiology and Physiological Psychology" (Vol. 9), J. M. Sprague, and A. N. Epstein, eds., Academic Press, New York.

Gabriel, M., Saltwick, S. E., and Miller, J. D., 1975, Conditioning and reversal of short-latency multiple-unit responses in the rabbit medial geniculate nucleus, Science, 189:1108-1109.

Gabriel, M., Miller, J.D., and Saltwick, S.E., 1976, Muliple unit activity of the rabbit medial geniculate nucleus in conditioning, extinction and reversal, Physiol. Psychol., 4:124-134.

Gerhard, L., 1968,"Atlas des mittle-und zeischenhirns des kaninchens,"Springer-Verlag, New York.

Honig, W. K., 1978, Studies of working memory in the pigeon, in: "Cognitive Processes in Animal Behavior", S. H. Hulse, H. Fowler, and W. K. Honig, eds., Lawrence Erlbaum, Hillsdale, New Jersey, 211-248.

Meibach, R. C., and Siegel, A., 1977, Subicular projection to the posterior cingulate cortex in rats. Exp. Neurol., 57:264-274.

Monnier, M., and Gangloff, H., 1961,"Atlas for stereotoxic brain research on the conscious rabbit." Elsevier, Amsterdam.

Morest, D. K., 1964, The neuronal architecture of the medial geniculate body of the cat, J. Anatom., 98:611-630.

Orona, E., 1981, Unit activity of the prefrontal cortex and the mediodorsal thalamic nucleus during discriminative avoidance conditioning and reversal in rabbits. Doctoral Dissertation, University of Texas at Austin.

Rosenkilde, C. E., 1979, Functional heterogeneity of the prefrontal cortex in the monkey: a review, Behav. Neurol. Biol. 25:301-345.

Ryugo, D. K., and Weinberger, N. M., 1978, Differential plasticity of morphologically distinct neuron populations in the medial geniculate body of the cat during classical conditioning, Behav. Biol., 22:275-301.

Sorensen, K. E., 1980, Ipsilateral projection from the subiculum to the retrosplenial cortex in the guinea pig, J. Comp. Neurol., 193:893-911.

Urban, I., and Richard, P., 1972,"A stereotaxic atlas of the New Zealand rabbit's brain,"C. C. Thomas, ed., Springfield, Illinois.

THE NEURAL INTEGRATION OF FEEDING AND DRINKING HABITS

John Garcia, Kenneth W. Rusiniak, Stephen W. Kiefer
and Federico Bermudez-Rattoni
Department of Psychology and Mental Retardation Research
Center, University of California Los Angeles, CA 90024

SOME "ANCIENT HISTORY" ON CONDITIONED FLAVOR AVERSIONS

For the rat, the interaction of food-related cues and the visceral feedback following ingestion largely determines future consummatory behavior. In early work (Garcia & Koelling, 1966), it was shown that taste cues were most readily associated with illness; conditioned taste aversions were formed after only a single taste-illness experience. Unlike most other demonstrations of classical conditioning, the delay between the taste conditioned stimulus (CS) and the illness unconditioned stimulus (US) could be an hour or more and strong taste aversions still would be formed. In contrast to tastes, an audio-visual signal was a poor CS for illness conditioning, acquiring little or no aversive properties following a single toxic US. If footshock was used as a US, the converse obtained. An audio-visual CS was readily associated with footshock US whereas taste was a poor CS in shock avoidance conditioning.

Garcia and Ervin (1968) have hypothesized that the affinity of the taste CS for association with the illness US was reflected in the anatomical organization of the central nervous system. First order CS taste afferents and US afferents from the gastrointestinal tract converge in the brainstem in the nucleus solitarius. Furthermore, the "emetic center" (Borison & Wang, 1953) is located nearby, just lateral to the nucleus solitarius in the lateral reticular formation. These close anatomical relationships provide at least a convenient feedback loop for the processing of information regarding gustatory qualities of food and subsequent visceral effects following ingestion of poison.

The taste-visceral feedback loop works in both directions, positively to increase consumption of beneficial foods as well as negatively to decrease consumption of dangerous substances. When an arbitrary taste CS is followed by recuperation from toxicosis or repletion of vitamin deficits, the palatability of that taste is increased so the animal consumes greater quantities in the future (Garcia et al., 1967; Green & Garcia, 1971). The propensity to associate taste with visceral feedback has been demonstrated in a wide variety of vertebrate species (Garcia et al., 1977) reflecting the common properties of brainstem and midbrain mechanisms of animals feeding upon the vegetable kingdom which is replete with nutrients and toxins. Invertebrate feeders also exhibit the food-poison affinity (e.g. Gelperin, 1975).

Besides having taste properties potential foods also have other sensory qualities such as odors. In general, odor is treated like an external CS, resembling the audio-visual CS in terms of its associative affinities. Odor alone is a weak CS for a toxic US but it is an effective CS for footshock US, again paralleling the conditioning results found with the audio-visual CS.

Although odors are weak cues for illness-induced aversions, when presented in compound with a taste, an odor becomes a strong associative cue if the compound is followed by illness. A demonstration of these results by Rusiniak et al. (1979) showed the following pattern: (a) taste alone was a strong CS for a toxin US, (b) odor alone was a weak CS for the same toxin US, but (c) when taste and odor were presented as a compound CS, the odor became a strong CS when tested alone in extinction. This effect was termed _potentiation_ to reflect the fact that a previously weak odor cue became a strong associative cue simply by presenting it in conjunction with a taste.

The potentiation of a weak odor CS by a strong taste CS has considerable theoretical value for those interested in conditioning and learning. Normally, in classical or instrumental conditioning a stronger, more informative component of a compound CS or signal tends to "overshadow" or "block" conditioning to the weaker components (Mackintosh, 1974).

Taste potentiation of food-related cues is not limited to odor stimuli. It has been shown in birds that the concomitant presentation of taste and color cues, when followed by illness, result in color aversions which are stronger than if the color was conditioned alone. For example, Brett et al. (1976) found that a red-tailed hawk fed normally on white mice would not acquire a discriminatively specific aversion for black mice followed by poison, presumably because black and white laboratory mice taste alike. But when a distinctive bitter taste was imparted to the black mouse and this color-taste compound was followed by illness, a robust visual aversion to black mice was formed. Taste potentiated color aversions have also been demonstrated in pigeons by Clark et al. (1979) using similar procedures; (a) when presented alone, taste was a strong CS for a toxic US, (b) color was a weak CS for the same toxic US, but (c) when color was combined with taste as a compound CS, color proved to be a strong CS when tested alone in extinction.

RECENT STUDIES ON THE ROLE OF ODOR IN TOXIPHOBIC CONDITIONING

Since the original demonstration of odor potentiation by taste, we have examined the limits and specificity of the phenomenon in more detail. In a recent set of experiments (Rusiniak et al., 1981), the interactions of taste and odor components in a compound flavor CS were examined as a function of specific nature of the US. Briefly, rats were exposed to an odor which was either presented with plain water or saccharin water. The location of the odor component was varied; food flavors were placed either on a disc surrounding the spout where it could only be sniffed by the rat, or placed directly in the water where it was licked as well as sniffed. Presentation of these various stimulus configurations was followed by illness in one experiment and footshock in a second experiment.

Some of the results from these experiments are shown in Figure 1 where the mean suppression of fluid consumption (calculated as a percentage of a water baseline) is shown for a pretest and subsequent extinction test of odor alone. When the US was toxin-induced illness, odor alone on the disc was a weak CS (Group O_D). Odor on the disc was potentiated by adding saccharin to the water (Group O_DT). Mixing the odorant in the distilled water was more effective (Group O_W) and scented water was further potentiated by saccharin (Group O_WT). The opposite array of results was obtained when footshock was used as a US. As seen on the right side of Figure 1, odor alone on the disc (Group O_D) was a strong CS for footshock. As the odor became tied more closely to the fluid itself and its concomitant taste properties, conditioning to the odor became weaker; Group O_W which had the odor in the distilled water showed weaker conditioning, and Group O_WT was weaker yet. The addition of taste to an odor-shock situation had the same "interference" effect found in traditional studies in classical conditioning. Therefore the potentiation of odor CS is apparently specific to those situations which involve a visceral feedback US.

The potentiation of odor by taste, besides being relatively specific to illness conditioning, also depends upon the specific arrangement of stimuli <u>at the time of conditioning</u>. In a study by Palmerino et al. (1980), various preexposure manipulations and training combinations of odor and taste cues were paired with illness. Potentiation of odor aversions was found only

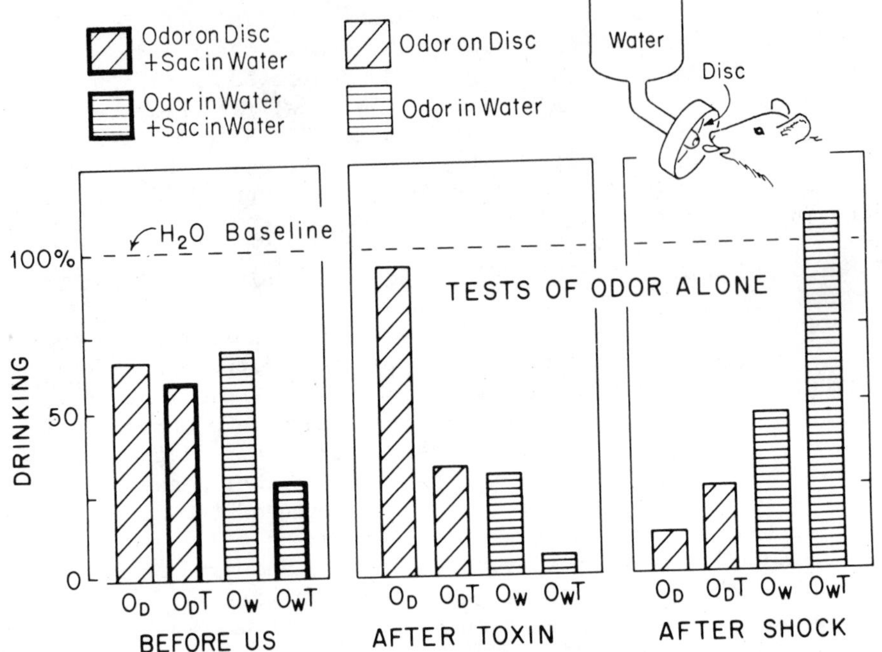

Figure 1. Summary of results indicating that when odor is associated with a food related cue (taste) and followed by delayed illness, potentiated odor aversions were formed which are stronger than odor-illness conditioning. Conversely, if a shock US is used, odor alone is a strong CS which actually becomes degraded if presented together with taste. Subscripted letters indicate whether the odorant was on a disc (D) surrounding the water spout or in the water (W). "T" means that the water contained saccharin. (Redrawn from Rusiniak et al., 1981).

in those conditions where taste and odor were presented as a compound CS on the poison trial. Association of odor and taste on a trial prior to the taste-poison trial (sensory preconditioning) or after the taste-poison trial (second order conditioning) produced weak odor aversions at best. A second experiment by Palmerino et al. tested the effect of temporal delay of the poison US on potentiated odor aversions. As mentioned previously, taste-illness associations can be formed even with long delays. The effect of delayed illness was tested for both odor alone conditioning and taste-potentiated odor conditioning. Groups of rats were given a single exposure to either the taste of saccharin, the odor of almond on the disc, or the compound odor-taste CS; these were followed at various intervals by intubation of a toxic lithium chloride (LiCl) solution. Figure 2 presents the results of the experiment and confirms that taste aversions can be formed with illness delays up to 4 hours. Odor alone conditioning, on the other hand, has a steep delay gradient. A CS-US delay of 30 minutes produced virtually no conditioning, indicating that odor is a poor signal for slow acting poisons. Groups of rats given compound odor-taste conditioning displayed delay gradients for the odor aversion which were essentially the same as that found for taste. Significant odor aversions were found even with a 6 hour CS-US delay.

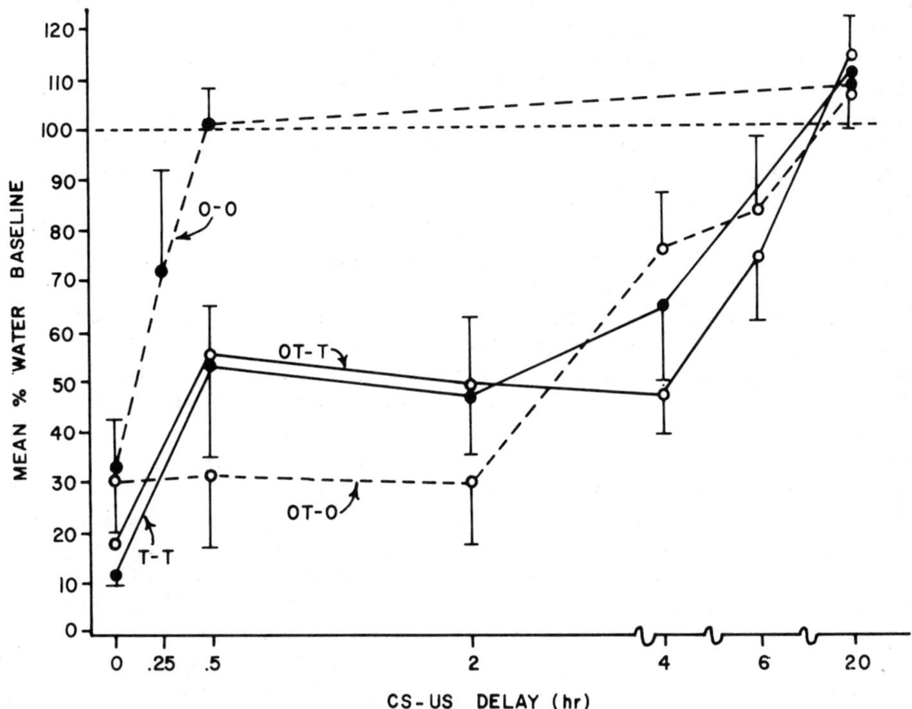

Figure 2. Delay of poison gradients for almond odor (O) and saccharin taste (T). Groups were poisoned after various CS-US delays. The first letter or letters prior to the hyphen refers to the CS paired with poison in acquisition: O = odor, T = taste, OT = odor taste compound. The letter after the hyphen indicates the stimulus tested following training. (Replotted from Palmerino et al., 1980).

The potentiation mechanism in the animal kingdom is matched by a corresponding phenomena in the vegetable kingdom. Most natural plant poisons are bitter substances which are not volatile. Therefore, the poison itself offers an excellent taste CS and a toxic US, but the poison has no odor CS to prevent herbivores from biting the plant. However, most poisonous plants have an associated odor stemming from an independent volatile substance which is not poisonous in itself. Apparently, through co-evolution, plants have developed an odor-taste-poison association which provides protection from herbivores which possess the odor-taste-illness potentiation mechanism (Eisner & Grant, 1981).

THE "GATING" OF ODOR BY TASTE INTO THE FEEDING SYSTEM

The strong synergism found in toxiphobia conditioning between tastes and odors probably reflects an adaptive specialization in mammalian evolution. For the rat, constant sniffing produces a myriad of odor sensations that could be related to food, potential sexual partners, predators, or any number of other environmental stimuli. Because processing of odor information is so continuously variable, many odors could intervene between an odor and delayed illness; thus, any one odor must have a steep associative gradient if that channel is to be cleared for other odors, as was shown in Figure 2. Taste, on the other hand, tends to be restricted to episodes of actual food consumption. Meals are typically eaten in discrete bouts so that few tastes intervene between a taste CS and delayed illness. Unlike odor, taste is specific to food ingestion. In a similar sense, any experience of illness (or a poison US) would typically be related to actual ingestion of a meal. The experience of gastrointestinal distress, because it is food related, necessitates a memory search for the previous food-related CS, specifically taste. The retrieval and association of taste with illness are mediated by the similarity of neural mechanisms rather than by the classic association by similarity of sensations of taste and illness. The odor associated by contiguity with the taste CS also becomes a strong associative cue for the illness because it is indexed as a food-related cue by the specific taste stimulus. Conceptually, taste operates an "and gate" by which odor becomes a food-related cue. Once the odor is indexed as food related it becomes more accessible to the conditioning effects of a food-related visceral US but less accessible to the conditioning effects of a painful peripheral US (Fig. 1). Also, the odor indexed to food acquires the same prolonged delay of reinforcement gradient as taste (Fig. 2).

We have commenced a research program to explore the neural mechanism underlying the toxiphobia conditioning phenomena outlined above. One major consideration was the nature of the toxic US. As outlined by Borison and Wang (1953), there are two major routes of stimulation that produce nausea. One route is by gastric irritation, information of which is carried principally by the vagus (X) nerve. A second route is the circulatory system. Blood-borne chemicals are monitored and detected by specialized receptor cells in the area postrema, a region also located in the brainstem. The toxin types and their routes have been manipulated experimentally (Wang & Borison, 1951), demonstrating that severing the vagus nerve blocked the vomiting in dogs normally produced by gastric irritation yet the same dogs were capable of vomiting if they were given a blood-borne toxin.

A parallel situation in rats has been obtained in our laboratory and in other's using conditioned taste aversions rather than vomiting as the dependent variable (Coil et al., 1978; Coil & Norgren, in press; Kiefer et al., 1980; Kiefer et al., 1981). The results from the experiments are summarized in Figure 3. Normal rats develop conditioned taste aversions if the toxin is the local gastric irritant copper sulfate ($CuSO_4$) or a blood-borne toxin such as apomorphine or alcohol. Taste aversion conditioning in vagotomized rats is almost completely blocked when $CuSO_4$ is given intragastrically as the US. Vagotomized rats acquire normal taste aversions with blood-borne toxins. Area postrema lesions, on the other hand, result in the opposite effects from vagotomies: intragastric irritation produces normal taste aversions but a blood-borne toxin is no longer an effective aversive US.

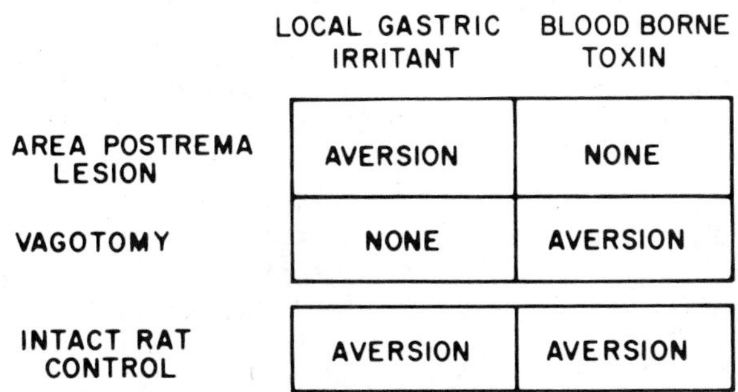

LOCAL GASTRIC IRRITANT
BLOOD BORNE TOXIN
AREA POSTREMA LESION
AVERSION
NONE
VAGOTOMY
NONE
AVERSION
INTACT RAT CONTROL
AVERSION
AVERSION

Figure 3. Summary of experiments (see text) which tested aversion learning in vagotomized rats and rats with area postrema lesions utilizing the two main types of nausea-inducing US: local gastric irritation or toxin injected into the blood.

IN SEARCH OF THE "AND-GATE"

A second major endeavor in our laboratory has been to determine the neural mechanisms involved in the potentiation of odor by taste during toxiphobia conditioning. Assuming the existence of a neural "and-gate" which would switch odor into food-related systems, we have examined two regions of the central nervous system where odor-taste interactions could possibly occur.

One region hypothesized to be crucial for taste potentiation of odor stimuli was the gustatory neocortex, a small region on the anterolateral part of the rat brain (Benjamin & Akert, 1959). Ablations of this region disrupt taste-illness conditioning (Braun et al., 1972; Hankins et al., 1974), and because odor potentiation was shown to be dependent upon taste, the gustatory neocortex appeared to be a potentially important region for odor potentiation. To determine the role of the taste cortex in potentiation, intact rats and rats lacking gustatory neocortex were given either a taste, an odor, or an odor-taste compound followed by intragastric intubation of LiCl (Kiefer & Rusiniak, 1979). After two training trials, tests with odor alone and taste alone were given to all rats. The results from the first acquisition trial and the subsequent odor and taste tests are shown in Figure 4. On the first exposure to the stimuli, rats lacking gustatory neocortex failed to display normal neophobia for the odor-taste compound (compare responses to OT by controls and lesioned rats in the upper half of Fig. 4). After two acquisition trials, the test trials with the odor and taste components revealed relatively specific effects of the lesions. Taste conditioning was disrupted completely by the ablations. In contrast, the ablations did not affect odor conditioning or the potentiation of an odor aversion (lower right quadrant, Fig. 4). Despite the fact that no operated rat trained with the odor-taste compound (OT) formed any aversion to the taste, these rats still displayed potentiated odor aversions relative to the odor-alone group. Apparently, integrity of the gustatory neocortex is not necessary for the acquisition of a potentiated odor aversion. The "and-gate" function must be carried on elsewhere.

A preliminary series of studies conducted in our laboratory examined the role of the amygdala in potentiation (Bermudez-Rattoni et al., 1981). It has been shown that the amygdala receives both gustatory and olfactory afferents (Norgren, 1974; White, 1965) making this structure a likely candidate for odor-taste interactions. In each experiment rats were implanted with bilateral cannulae aimed at the amygdala. To produce "reversible" amygdala lesions, infusions of procaine were used. Such infusions suppress normal electrophysiological activity for about 2 hours. In an initial experiment, four groups of rats were given a single exposure to an odor-taste

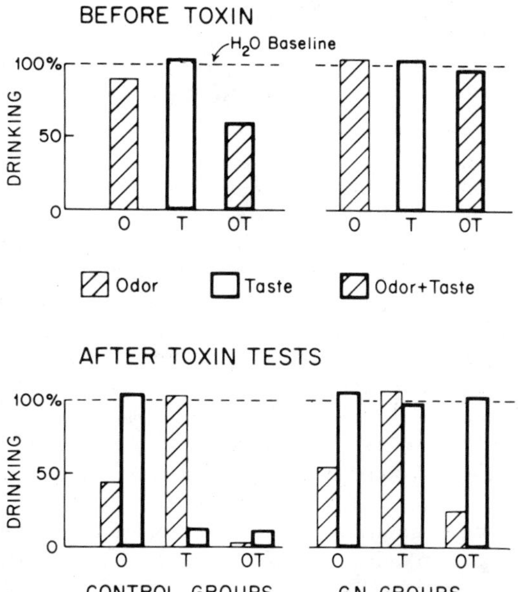

Figure 4. Mean percent consumption by normal rats and rats lacking gustatory neocortex during acquisition and testing using a toxiphobia conditioning paradigm. Group designations indicate whether rats received odor-illness (O), taste-illness (T), or odor plus taste-illness (OT) conditioning on the acquisition trial. Note that the gustatory group given OT failed to display normal neophobia for the flavor. Odor and taste were tested separately (panel B). Gustatory neocortex ablations specifically disrupted taste conditioning. However, rats lacking gustatory neocortex still developed taste potentiated odor aversions. (Redrawn from Kiefer & Rusiniak, 1979).

(OT) compound. One group was a normal control, a second group was given procaine just prior to presentation of the compound CS, a third group was given procaine following OT exposure, and a fourth group received the procaine just before LiCl intubation. Intubation of LiCl was administered to all rats 30 minutes after exposure to the odor and taste. The results of the experiment are shown in panel A of Figure 5. Following OT-illness, all groups displayed approximately equivalent taste aversions, reducing consumption by 70-80%. But the group given procaine prior to the OT exposure (Pre-CS) displayed attenuated odor aversions relative to the other three groups. These data suggest that disruption of odor potentiation could be produced by disrupting amygdala functioning just prior to the CS experience.

The deficits in odor potentiation found with procaine-treated rats could be related to disruptions of the integration of odor and taste information. It is also possible that pre-CS infusion of procaine in the amygdala disrupts simple odor detection or odor-illness associations. To test if odor perception was affected by procaine treatment, three groups of rats (normal, procaine pre-CS, and handled control) were given a single exposure to almond odor while drinking familiar tap water. After a minute exposure the rats were given 1 mA, 1 sec footshock. The results from the subsequent odor test, shown in Figure 5B, indicated that all three groups showed significant suppression of consumption in the presence of the odor. These data indicate that procaine treated rats were not anosmic because they could develop normal associations between an odor and footshock.

A third experiment tested whether amygdala dysfunction produced by procaine infusion would disrupt odor-illness conditioning. Control rats (both saline infused and handled) and rats given procaine prior to odor exposure were given a single odor-illness training trial using immediate administration of the poison so that direct odor-illness learning could be obtained. The results of the subsequent odor test (Figure 5C) indicated that pretreatment with procaine disrupted conditioning. These results suggest that the disruptions in potentiation of odor aversions described above can be attributed to a deficit in the formation of odor-illness associations, and that the amygdala dysfunctions may not have been related to odor-taste integration but rather odor-illness associative learning. The effect was specific to toxiphobia conditioning because odor-shock learning was not affected significantly by procaine treatment.

These preliminary results indicate that the amygdala may be involved in the "and-gate" function, but much more research is needed before a definitive answer can be given. In the near

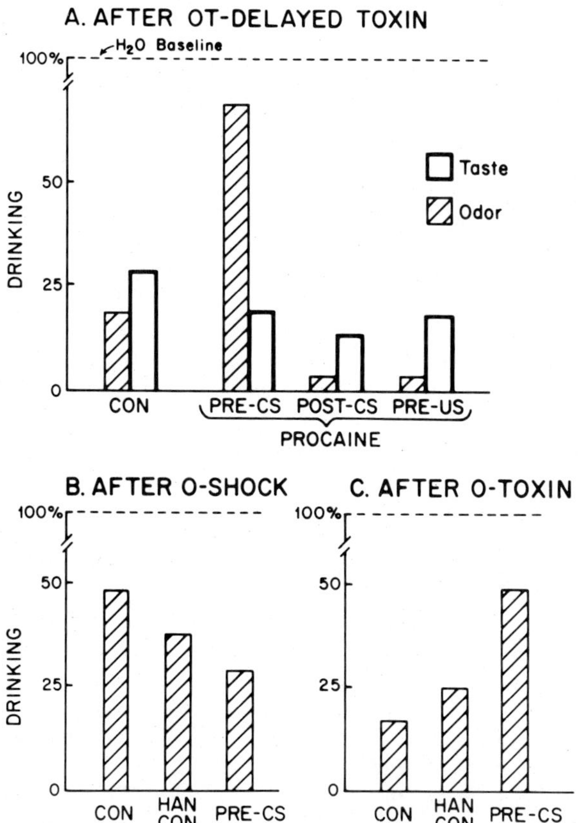

Figure 5. Summary of three experiments which tested the effects of temporary amygdala dysfunction induced by procaine infusion. In A, rats were given procaine infusions before flavor experience (pre-CS), after flavor experience (post-CS), or before illness experience (pre-US) and all rats were then tested with the odor and taste components. Note that procaine given before flavor presentation specifically disrupted odor associations. In B, three groups of rats (control group, handled control group, and procaine group which was infused prior to odor experience) were given odor-shock training and then tested with odor alone. Procaine infusion had no significant effect on odor-shock learning. In the last experiment (C) three groups of rats were given odor-illness conditioning. Disruptions in odor conditioning were found in the procaine treated rats. (Redrawn for Bermudez-Rattoni et al., 1981).

future we intend to follow up our lesion work with microelectrical recordings to make a more definitive search for the site of possible "and-gate" action. Odor potentiation by taste is the key to our strategy and the behavioral response of the rat to aversive tastes and odors (i.e. gaping, see Grill & Norgren, 1979) is an important end point. The rat gapes and thrusts out its tongue to the taste of poison as if to eject it from the mouth. This is the final common pathway for the conditioned aversion. An arbitrary odor does not elicit this response, but after potentiation by taste and illness, the odor elicits a strong gaping reaction indicating that the odor has acquired control of the final common pathway of the toxiphobic system. Therefore, it must have entered that system via a putative "and-gate." With high hopes, we will work our way up this final common efferent pathway and down the afferent streams of odor, taste and visceral feedback to search for the elusive and perhaps mythical "and-gate" in the memory stores of the poisoned rat.

REFERENCES

Benjamin, R.M. and Akert, K. 1959. Cortical and thalamic areas involved in taste discrimination in the albino rat. J. Comp. Neur. 111: 231.

Bermudez-Rattoni, F., Rusiniak, K.W. and Garcia, J. 1981. Conditioned flavor aversion: Disruption of odor-taste potentiation by reversible amygdala lesion. Paper presented at the 11th Annual Society for Neuroscience, Abs., Los Angeles.

Borison, H.L. and Wang, S.C. 1953. Physiology and pharmacology of vomiting. Pharmacol. Rev. 5: 193.

Braun, J.J., Slick, T.B. and Lorden, J.F. 1972. Involvement of gustatory neocortex in the learning of taste aversions. Physiol. Behav. 9: 637.

Brett, L.P., Hankins, W.G. and Garcia, J. 1976. Prey-lithium aversions III: Buteo hawks. Behav. Biol. 17: 87.

Clarke, J.C., Westbrook, R.F. and Irwin, J. 1979. Potentiation instead of overshadowing in the pigeon. Behav. Neur. Biol. 25: 18.

Eisner, T. and Grant R.P. 1981. Toxicity, odor aversion, and "olfactory aposematism." Sci. 213: 476.

Garcia, J. and Ervin, F.R. 1968. Gustatory-visceral and telereceptor-cutaneous conditioning--adaptation in internal and external milieus. Comm. Behav. Biol. 1: 389.

Garcia, J., Ervin, F.R., Yorke, C.H. and Koelling, R.A. 1967. Conditioning with delayed vitamin injections. Sci. 155: 716.

Garcia, J. and Koelling, R.A. 1966. Relation of cue to consequence in avoidance learning. Psychon. Sci. 4: 123.

Garcia, J., Rusiniak, K.W. and Brett, L.P. 1977. Conditioning food-illness aversions in wild animals: Caveant Cononici, In Operant-Pavlovian Interactions (H. David and H.M.B. Hurwitz, Eds.), pp. 273-316, Lawrence Erlbaum Press, New Jersey.

Gelperin, A. 1975. Rapid food aversion learning by a terrestrial mollusk. Sci. 189: 567.

Green, K.F. and Garcia, J. 1971. Recuperation from illness: Flavor enhancement for rats. Sci. 173: 749.

Grill, H.J. and Norgren, R. 1978. The taste reactivity test. I Mimetic responses to gustatory stimuli in neurologically normal rats. Brain Res. 143: 263.

Hankins, W.G., Garcia, J. and Rusiniak, K.W. 1974. Cortical lesions: Flavor illness and noise-chock conditioning. Behav. Biol. 10: 173.

Kiefer, S.W., Cabral, R.J., Rusiniak, K.W. and Garcia, J. 1980. Ethanol-induced aversions in rats with subdiaphargmatic vagotomies. Behav. Neur. Biol. 29: 246.

Kiefer, S.W. and Rusiniak, K.W. 1979. Involvement of gustatory neocortex in the rat's neophobic and associative responses to taste and odor stimuli. Paper presented at the 9th Annual Society for Neuroscience Meeting, Abs. pg. 129, Atlanta.

Mackintosh, N.J. 1974. The Psychology of Animal Learning, Academic Press, New York.

Norgren, R. 1974. Gustatory afferents to ventral forebrain. Brain Res. 81: 285.

Palmerino, C.C., Rusiniak, K.W. and Garcia, J. 1980. Flavor-illness aversions: The peculiar roles of odor and taste in memory for poison. Sci. 208: 753.

Rusiniak, K.W., Hankins, W.G. and Garcia, J. and Brett, L.P. 1979.. Flavor-illness aversions: Potentiation of odor by taste in rats. Behav. Neur. Biol. 25: 1.

Rusiniak, K.W., Palmerino, C.C. and Forthman, D. 1981. Odor and taste: Effects of odor location on synergistic interactions during illness and shock paradigms. Paper presented at the 61st Annual Western Psychological Association Meeting, Abs. pg. 217, Los Angeles.

Wang, S.C. and Borison, H.L. 1951. The vomiting center: A critical experimental analysis. Arch. Neur. Psych. 63: 928.

White, L. 1965. Olfactory bulb projections of the rat. Anat. Rec. 152: 465.

ACKNOWLEDGEMENTS

Supported by the following grants: National Institute of Health Research Grant NS 11618 and Program Project Grants HD 05958 and NIAAA AA 03513.

THE AMYGDALA CENTRAL NUCLEUS: CONTRIBUTIONS TO CONDITIONED CARDIOVASCULAR RESPONDING DURING AVERSIVE PAVLOVIAN CONDITIONING IN THE RABBIT

Bruce S. Kapp,[1] Michela Gallagher,[2] Craig D. Applegate,[1] and Robert C. Frysinger[1]
[1]Department of Psychology, University of Vermont
Burlington, Vt.
[2]Department of Psychology, University of North Carolina
Chapel Hill, N.C.

SUMMARY

The research described represents an attempt to determine the exact amygdala components which contribute to the acquisition of conditioned responding during aversive conditioning. Our initial analysis focuses on the amygdala central nucleus and its contribution to the acquisition of conditioned bradycardia during Pavlovian fear conditioning in the rabbit. The results demonstrate that (a) lesions of the central nucleus attenuate the magnitude of the conditioned bradycardia response, (b) the administration of β-adrenergic antagonists and opiate agonists into the region of the central nucleus also attenuate the magnitude of the conditioned bradycardia response, (c) the medial component of the central nucleus projects directly to cardioregulatory nuclei in the dorsal medulla including the site of origin of cardioinhibitory neurons in the rabbit, (d) electrical stimulation of the central nucleus in rabbit produces profound, short-latency bradycardia and depressor responses, with maximum bradycardia elicited from the site of origin of the central nucleus-dorsal medulla projection, and (e) during the course of the conditioning procedure increases in central nucleus neuronal activity develop to the conditioned stimulus (CS) at the time when the conditioned bradycardia response develops. In some cases the magnitude of the increase in neuronal activity to the CS was significantly correlated with the magnitude of the bradycardia response to the CS over the course of the conditioning session.

The results are consistent with the hypothesis that at least one function of the amygdala central nucleus in the acquisition of conditioned bradycardia may be in the motoric expression of the conditioned response to the CS by modulation of vagal preganglionic cardioinhibitory neurons within the dorsal medulla.

INTRODUCTION

It is now well documented that the amygdala complex contributes to the acquisition and retention of aversively conditioned responses. Indeed, numerous studies have demonstrated that lesions of the amygdala interfere with the ability of a variety of species to acquire a variety of conditioned responses in a number of aversive conditioning paradigms.[1] These response acquisition deficits are generally reflected in lower frequencies of conditioned response emission in active avoidance paradigms, reduced freezing behavior and thereby greater frequencies of baseline responding in CER paradigms, and reduced suppression of punished responses in punishment paradigms.

Since animals with amygdala lesions demonstrate relatively normal (a) sensitivity thresholds to aversive stimuli,[2] (b) unconditioned orienting responses to the presentation of a novel stimulus subsequently used as a CS in aversive conditioning,[3] and (c) acquisition of simple operant responses for positive reinforcement,[3,4] the lesion-induced acquisition deficits cannot readily be accounted for by gross sensory or motor abnormalities. However, since amygdala lesions reduce the frequency of a variety of unconditioned responses to threatening or fear arousing stimuli,[5] it has been proposed that such lesions interfere with the arousal of fear motivation and that this general impairment may underlie the lesion-induced conditioned response acquisition deficits during aversive conditioning.[3,5,6] If this is a valid hypothesis, then an analysis of the functional role of the amygdala in aversive conditioning must incorporate an analysis of the role of the amygdala in fear motivation and, in turn, the involvement of fear in aversive conditioning, the latter an analysis which has formed the basis for continuing controversy among learning theorists.

The emergence of the new anatomical techniques demonstrate that the amygdala is a complex, heterogeneous group of nuclei, each possessing its own unique afferent and efferent projection systems. Given this complexity, an obvious approach to a better understanding of the contribution of the amygdala to aversive conditioning and fear motivation is to first determine the specific amygdala components which contribute to these processes using a simple fear conditioning procedure. Recently, we have adopted such an approach and have initially focused upon the amygdala central nucleus and its contribution to the acquisition of conditioned heart rate responding in the rabbit during Pavlovian fear conditioning. While it is recognized that interactions among several amygdala nuclei are of probable importance, the central nucleus appeared particularly suited for our initial analysis for the reasons outlined below.

THE AMYGDALA CENTRAL NUCLEUS: A FOCAL POINT FOR INVESTIGATION

Our choice of the central nucleus was guided by several lines of evidence. First, two studies had demonstrated that lesions primarily confined to the central nucleus in rat produced marked deficits in the acquisition of conditioned responding in passive avoidance conditioning paradigms,[7,8] a finding similar to that observed following large amygdala lesions. Since conditioned responding in these paradigms typically involves species-typical fear responses (i.e., freezing) to conditioned threatening stimuli, the results were consistent with the interpretation based on the findings from larger lesions that such lesions interfere with the arousal of fear. Second, those investigators studying stimulation-induced somatic and autonomic components of affective behaviors, including those described as fear-like, consistently reported that such responses were elicited from sites within the central nucleus,[9-12] a finding consistent with the data and interpretation from lesion studies. Although other nuclei in addition to the central nucleus were suggested in the production of these responses, the central nucleus was consistently implicated. Third, it had been demonstrated in the cat that the central nucleus possessed a heavy projection to a variety of brainstem areas extending as far caudal as the medulla.[13] The remarkable feature of this projection system was that it appeared to overlap considerably with regions which, when electrically stimulated, resulted in both somatic and autonomic components of affective behavior.[14,15] This correspondence suggested that the central nucleus and its descending projection systems may play a functional role in the elicitation of emotional responses.

CARDIOVASCULAR RESPONDING DURING PAVLOVIAN FEAR CONDITIONING IN THE RABBIT: A BEHAVIORAL PARADIGM

Given the above evidence, the central nucleus appeared to be an important focal point for investigation. However, the evidence was collectively composed of data gathered across different species using different behavioral response measures and techniques. It was apparent, therefore, that to more accurately determine if and how the central nucleus contributed to aversive conditioning, an analysis confined to a single species and initially to a single response system was a necessity. Our choice of the conditioned bradycardia response system in the rabbit during Pavlovian fear conditioning was for several reasons.

First, the parameters of this response system using aversive Pavlovian procedures have been well-defined in the rabbit,[16-18] making it an attractive model response system for investigations into the neural substrates of autonomic conditioning. Second, stimulation of the central nucleus in the cat produces a pattern of species-typical defensive responses including profound cardiovascular alterations,[9-12] suggesting a central nucleus contribution to cardiovascular adjustments in response to threatening stimuli. These findings were consistent with more recent evidence demonstrating a direct projection from the region of the central nucleus to cardioregulatory nuclei in the dorsal medulla of cat,[13] providing an anatomical substrate for a central nucleus influence on the cardiovascular system. Third, lesions of the avian amygdalar homologue produce marked deficits in conditioned heart rate responding during aversive Pavlovian conditioning,[19] suggesting a function for this homologue in conditioned heart rate responding, a function which may generalize to the mammalian amygdala. Fourth, since heart rate in the rabbit decelerates in the presence of a predator,[20] this bradycardia response may represent one of a constellation of species-typical fear responses in the rabbit which, through Pavlovian conditioning procedures, can be conditioned to neutral stimuli. In this context, this response system may be analogous to the species-typical fear response of freezing in the rat, a response which is readily conditioned to neutral stimuli and which is reduced by amygdala lesions.[5]

AMYGDALA CENTRAL NUCLEUS LESIONS: EFFECTS ON THE ACQUISITION OF CONDITIONED HEART RATE RESPONDING DURING PAVLOVIAN FEAR CONDITIONING

Initially, we examined the effects of lesions of the central nucleus on the acquisition of conditioned bradycardia in loosely restrained rabbits using a Pavlovian conditioning procedure.[21] A five second tone (CS) is initially presented for 15 trials to habituate the bradycardia orienting response to the introduction of a novel stimulus. Immediately following these trials, 45 conditioning trials are presented in which the offset of the CS is coincident with the onset of a 2.0 ma, 500 msec eyelid shock (US). Heart rate is recorded for the five seconds immediately preceding the presentation of the CS and for the duration of the five second CS period.

Figure 1 shows the effects of lesions confined primarily to the central nucleus on the acquisition of conditioned bradycardia to the CS, expressed as the percent change in heart rate to the CS from the immediately preceding five second pre-CS period. First, note the decelerative conditioned response in unoperated animals (UNOP COND) and surgical control animals (SURG COND) when compared to a pseudoconditioning group (UNOP PSEUDO) receiving 45 unpaired presentations of both the CS and US. Second, note that either bilateral lesions damaging approximately 50% or less (Small Ace) or those damaging greater than 50% (Large Ace) of each central nucleus produced a statistically significant impairment in the acquisition of the conditioned response reflected in a decreased magnitude of deceleration in response to the CS (p's < .002). These lesion effects occurred in the absence of statistically significant effects on baseline (pre-CS) heart rate or on the heart rate orienting response and its habituation to tone alone.

The results of this experiment are similar to those reported by Cohen[19] in which lesions of the avian amygdala homologue produced a marked attenuation of the magnitude of the conditioned tachycardia response in pigeon during aversive Pavlovian conditioning. The results are also consistent with the many reports demonstrating that amygdala lesions produce deficits in the acquisition of a variety of conditioned responses during aversive conditioning. Furthermore, assuming that bradycardia represents one of a constellation of species-typical fear responses to threatening stimuli in the rabbit, the results are consistent with the recent conclusions of Werka, Skär and Ursin[6] who, in examining the effects of central nucleus lesions on a variety of responses in the rat, concluded that such lesions reduce fear. While the mechanism(s) by which these lesions produce such an interference have yet to be determined, the results of additional experiments, to be described in the following sections, yield important insights.

PHARMACOLOGICAL MANIPULATIONS OF THE CENTRAL NUCLEUS: EFFECTS ON THE ACQUISITION OF CONDITIONED HEART RATE RESPONDING

While the results from our lesion study suggested a contribution of the central nucleus to the acquisition of conditioned bradycardia, the possibility exists that the deficits reflect damage to fibers of passage rather than to the central nucleus *per se*. This limitation of the lesion technique can be circumvented by the use of specific receptor agonists and antagonists applied to the region of the central nucleus. Furthermore, with the use of specific pharmacological agents affecting specific neural systems, additional information can be gained concerning the afferent and efferent connections by which the central nucleus influences the acquisition of conditioned bradycardia. Since (a) the noradrenergic afferentation to the amygdala is unevenly distributed with the central nucleus receiving a particularly rich innervation,[22,23] and (b) β-adrenergic blockade within the amygdala impairs retention of aversive conditioning in rats,[24] we investigated the effects of β-adrenergic receptor blockade in the region of the central nucleus on the acquisition of conditioned bradycardia.[25]

Using a conditioning procedure identical to that described for

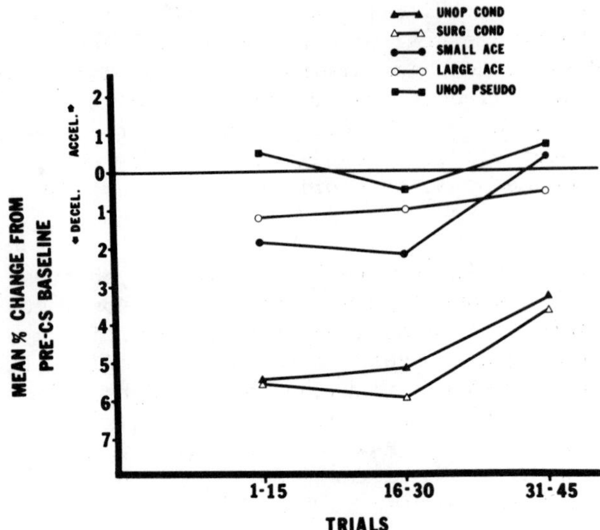

Fig. 1. Mean percent change in heart rate to the CS from pre-CS baseline for 45 conditioning trials for groups (n's=8) receiving lesions of the central nucleus. Data points represent means for 15 trial blocks. See text for details.

our lesion study, rabbits were prepared with cannulae aimed at the dorsal surface of the central nucleus and, following 10-14 days of surgical recovery, were injected with 40 nmole (1.0 μl) of dl-propranolol or vehicle two minutes prior to the conditioning session. Figure 2 demonstrates that dl-propranolol (DL-P COND) significantly attenuated the magnitude of the conditioned bradycardia response when compared with a vehicle-injected (VEHICLE) control group ($p < .02$). Dl-propranolol exerted no significant effects on baseline (pre-CS) heart rate, the heart rate orienting response, or on responding in a pseudoconditioning group (DL-P PSEUDO vs. UNOP PSEUDO). Furthermore, injections of either d-propranolol (40 nmole), the dextro isomer of propranolol with relatively weak β-blocking activity (Fig. 3; Group D-P COND), as well as injections of the β-agonist, l-isoproterenol (20 nmole) in combination with dl-propranolol (40 nmole), yielded no significant effects (Fig. 3; Group DL-P + L-ISO). These results provide support for the interpretation that dl-propranolol alters heart rate conditioning by interfering with β-adrenergic activity. Finally, to determine if the effects of dl-propranolol were specific to the region of the central nucleus, injections were made from 1.0-2.0 mm dorsal to the central nucleus (Fig. 3; Group DL-P DORSAL). No significant

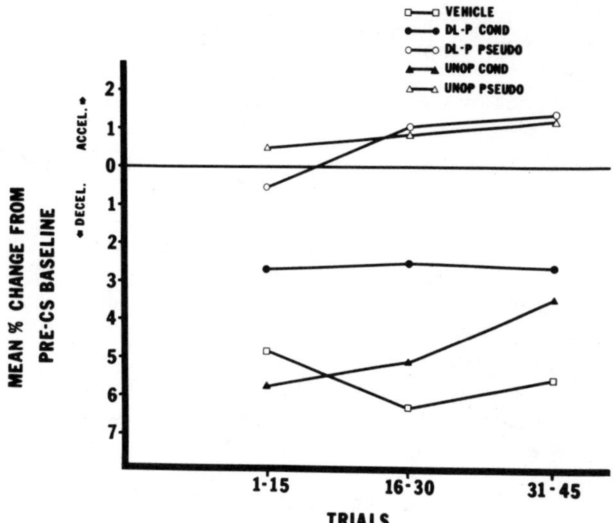

Fig. 2. Mean percent change in heart rate to the CS from pre-CS baseline for groups (n's=8) UNOP COND, VEHICLE, DL-P COND, DL-P PSEUDO, and UNOP PSEUDO. Data points represent means for 15 trial blocks.

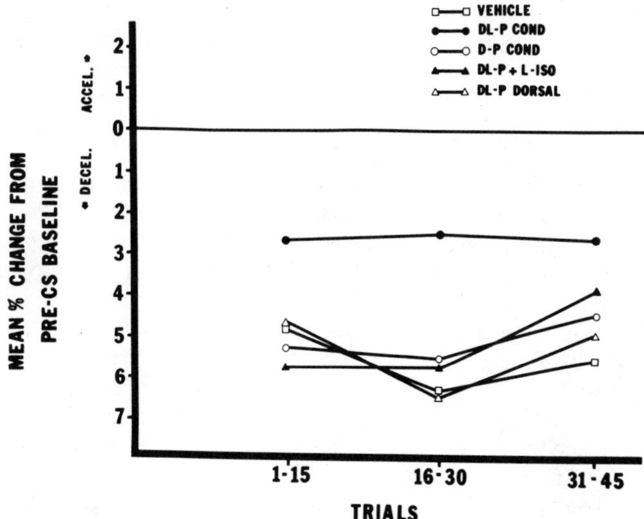

Fig. 3. Mean percent change in heart rate to the CS from pre-CS baseline for groups (n's=8) VEHICLE, DL-P COND, D-P COND, DL-P + L-ISO and DL-P DORSAL.

effects on heart rate conditioning were produced by these injections. Histological analyses also revealed that conditioned responses in animals injected with dl-propranolol with cannula placements at the level of the central nucleus were generally of lower magnitude than those of animals with cannulae positioned either anterior or posterior to the central nucleus.

Several important findings emerge from this experiment. First, the results are similar to those following lesions of the central nucleus. Second, the attenuation in the magnitude of the conditioned bradycardia appears to be due to the β-adrenergic antagonist property of dl-propranolol since the effect was stereospecific and blocked by a combined injection of a β-adrenergic agonist and antagonist. Third, the results suggest that dl-propranolol exerts its effects in the region of the central nucleus. Taken together with the rich noradrenergic afferentation of the central nucleus[22,23] and the presence of β-receptors in the amygdala,[26] the results support the interpretation that (a) damage to the central nucleus per se, rather than fibers of passage, contributed to the effects observed in our lesion study and (b) activity at β-adrenergic synapses within the region of the central nucleus contributes to the acquisition of the conditioned bradycardia response. Whether or not dl-propranolol produces its effects by affecting catecholamine projections originating from the locus coeruleus or from medullary catecholamine systems is an interesting focus for future research which should aid to our understanding of the contribution of central nucleus afferent systems to the acquisition of conditioned bradycardia.

Recently, several reports have suggested the involvement of opioid peptides in learning and memory processes.[27] Our previous research demonstrating that opiate manipulations within the amygdala complex alter retention of aversive conditioning in rats,[28] and the demonstration of high concentrations of opioid peptides and receptors within the central nucleus region,[29,30,31] prompted us to examine the effects of opiate manipulations within the central nucleus region on the acquisition of conditioned bradycardia.[32] Using our standard injection and conditioning procedure, with the exception that 20 rather than 45 paired conditioning trials were administered, animals injected with the opiate agonist levorphanol (5.0 nmole in 1.0 μl) into the region of the central nucleus (Fig. 4; Group LEV COND) demonstrated significant attenuation of the conditioned bradycardia response when compared to animals receiving vehicle injections. Conversely, injections of naloxone (2.5 nmole) significantly enhanced the magnitude of the conditioned response. These drugs exerted no significant effects on baseline (pre-CS) heart rate, the heart rate orienting response, or on responding in pseudoconditioning groups. Support for the interpretation that the effects of levorphanol and naloxone were due to specific effects on opiate receptors was found in two additional groups, one given injections of the inactive enantiomer of levorphanol, dextrorphan (5.0 nmole), and the other given combined injections of levorphanol (5.0 nmole) and naloxone (2.5 nmole). Both groups did not differ statistically from the vehicle-injected control group. Finally, injections of levorphanol from 1.0-2.0 mm dorsal to the central nucleus were without effect, and in a limited number of animals with cannulae positioned anterior, lateral and posterior to the central nucleus, the response magnitudes were similar to those of the vehicle-injected group.

The results of this experiment, similar to those of the lesion and noradrenergic blockade experiments, suggest a contribution for the central nucleus, and in particular a central nucleus opiate system, in the acquisition of the conditioned bradycardia response. While the precise role which this system plays in the acquisition of the response has not been established, it is of interest that neither administration of opiate agonists into the central nucleus of rats,[33] nor systemic administration of opiate antagonists[34] alters shock sensitivity. Hence, it is unlikely that the effects of levorphanol and naloxone were due to alterations in shock sensitivity. Recently, however, it has been reported that opiate administration into the central nucleus decreases emotional reactivity in rats,[35] a finding consistent with the findings that central nucleus lesions

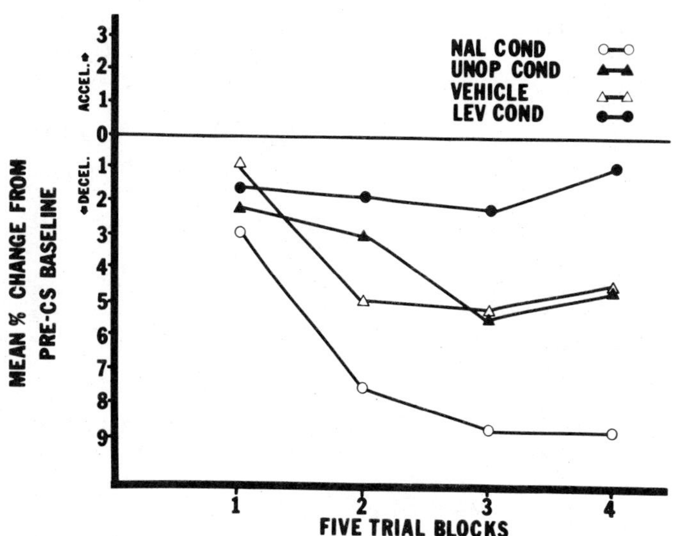

Fig. 4. Mean percent change in heart rate to the CS from pre-CS baseline for groups (n's=8) receiving central nucleus injections of levorphanol or naloxone. Data points represent means for 5 trial blocks.

decrease emotional reactivity and fear-like behavior in rats.[6] As discussed previously, if bradycardia represents a species-typical fear response to a threatening stimulus in the rabbit, then the results of our opiate study are consistent with the findings in rats.

CENTRAL NUCLEUS PROJECTIONS TO CARDIOVASCULAR REGULATORY NUCLEI IN THE RABBIT

The results demonstrating the effects of central nucleus manipulations on the acquisition of conditioned bradycardia, taken together with (a) the finding of a direct projection from the region of the central nucleus to the dorsal motor nucleus of the vagus (DMN) and the nucleus of the solitary tract (NTS) in the cat,[13] (b) the evidence demonstrating that conditioned bradycardia in the rabbit is mediated primarily by the vagus nerves,[18] and (c) the evidence that the DMN of the rabbit contains preganglionic cardioinhibitory neurons[36] that could serve as the origin of the final pathway for the expression of the conditioned bradycardia, led to a determination of a direct central nucleus projection to the NTS/DMN complex in the rabbit.[37,38] Such an analysis was of the utmost importance in an attempt to assess the functional contribution of this nucleus to the acquisition of the bradycardia response.

Unilateral injections of various volumes (15-100nl) of horseradish peroxidase (HRP) were injected into rabbits at the border of the NTS and DMN. Figure 5 presents sections through the amygdala of a representative case. Within the amygdala large numbers of labeled neurons were found ipsilaterally primarily within the large-celled, medial component of the central nucleus, with highly concentrated numbers located anteriorly in this component (Fig. 5D). The labeled cells extended anteriorly into the sublenticular substantia innominata, and at more anterior levels labeled cells were located within the lateral component of the bed nucleus of the stria terminalis. In no case were labeled cells observed within other amygdala nuclei.

In a second experiment injections of equal parts of ^{3}H-proline and leucine into the central nucleus produced terminal labeling within the nucleus ambiguus, the NTS and the DMN.[38] Label was observed to both encapsulate and distribute within the DMN but varied in concentration depending on the anterior-posterior level. Within the NTS label was distributed in areas demonstrated to receive cardiovascular afferents in the rabbit.[38] In summary, a direct projection exists in the rabbit from the medial central nucleus to cardiovascular regulatory nuclei, a finding which offers the central nucleus the potential to directly influence the cardiovascular system in this species, and in particular cardioinhibitory neurons within the DMN.

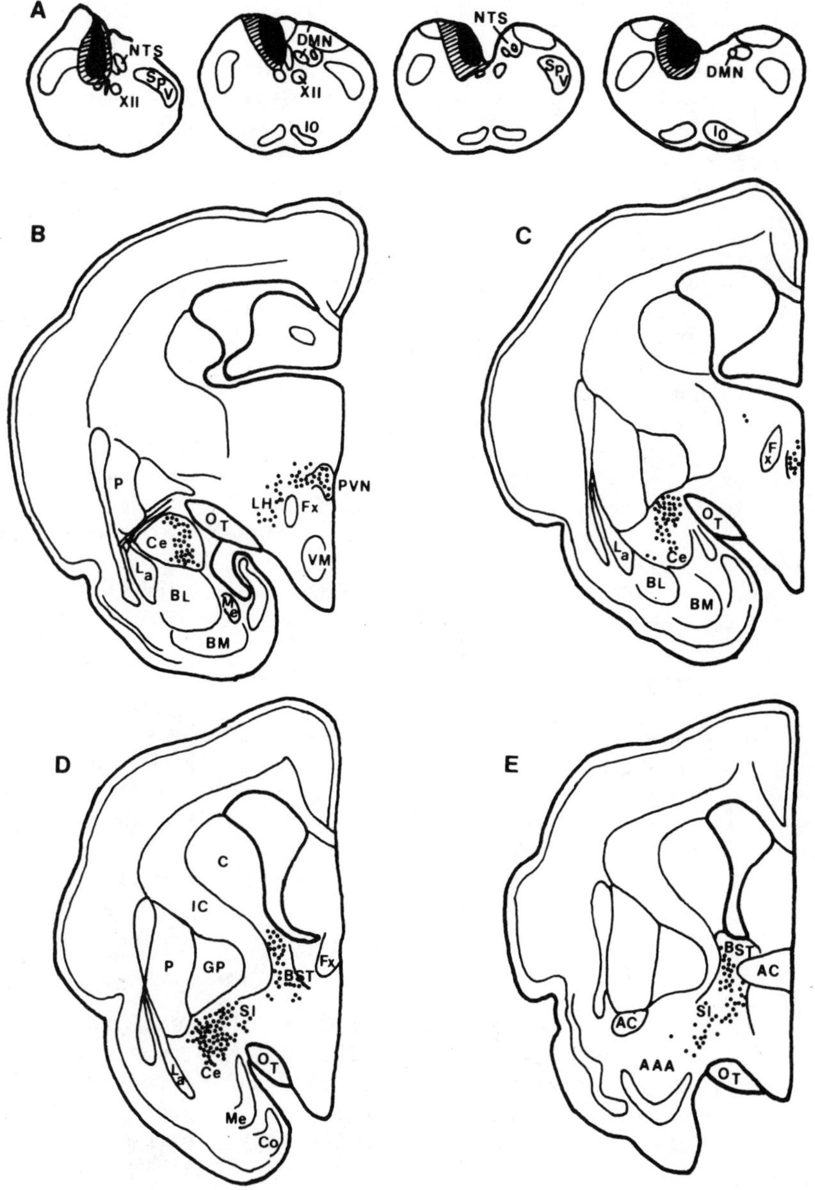

Fig. 5. Labeled neurons in the amygdala of a representative case following four injections of HRP at different rostral-caudal levels of the NTS/DMN complex (A). Each dot represents one labeled neuron from that section alone. B-E, caudal to rostral, respectively. Ce, central nucleus; SI, substantia innominata; BST, bed nucleus of the stria terminalis.

STIMULATION OF THE AMYGDALA CENTRAL NUCLEUS: EFFECTS ON HEART RATE, BLOOD PRESSURE, AND SOMATOMOTOR BEHAVIOR IN THE RABBIT

The attenuation of the magnitude of the conditioned bradycardia from manipulations of the central nucleus, and the existence of direct central nucleus projections to cardioregulatory nuclei suggest the working hypothesis that this nucleus may function in the morotic expression of the conditioned bradycardia response by a direct or indirect (e.g., via the NTS) modulation of vagal preganglionic cardioinhibitory neurons within the DMN. In this respect the central nucleus may possess, *at least in part*, a cardiomotor function. If this interpretation is valid, then electrical stimulation of the central nucleus might be predicted to produce vagally-mediated bradycardia in the rabbit. That this is the case has recently been demonstrated in anesthetized and awake rabbits in our laboratory.[39,40]

In our first experiment stimulation at sites within the central nucleus of rabbits anesthetized with α-chloralose produced bradycardia and depressor responses, with maximum bradycardia elicited from sites within the anterior, medial component of the nucleus. The bradycardia (a) commenced within one second of stimulation, (b) persisted under artificial ventilation and immobilization with Flaxedil and (c) was attenuated or abolished by I.V. injections of atropine methylnitrate. A representative case demonstrating the anatomical specificity for the anterior, medial central nucleus in the production of bradycardia in an anesthetized rabbit is shown in Figure 6. Note that bradycardia is produced by stimulation at sites within the globus pallidus but that sites immediately dorsal or ventral to the medial central nucleus (sites 2,3,7,8) yield greatly reduced or negligible bradycardia compared to sites within the medial central nucleus (sites 4-6). In additional cases, sites located lateral to the medial central nucleus and within the ventral putamen and lateral central nucleus yielded either negligible bradycardia or bradycardia of far less magnitude than that elicited from the medial central nucleus.

Stimulation of the central nucleus in the awake animal resulted in a similar short-latency bradycardia response, most frequently accompanied by increased respiratory rate and decreased amplitude to stimulation onset. Current intensities up to threefold those which elicited a 10% bradycardia response invariably produced an arrest of ongoing motoric behavior of varying duration which commenced immediately upon stimulation onset.

In summary, stimulation at sites yielding maximum bradycardia and depressor responses were located at the site of origin of the central nucleus descending projection to cardioregulatory nuclei. It is not unreasonable to assume, therefore, that these responses may be due to stimulation of the cells of origin of this projection which in turn may either directly or indirectly activate vagal preganglionic cardioinhibitory neurons within the DMN. Finally, and perhaps most important in the context of aversive conditioning, it has been demonstrated in the rabbit that the conditioned cardiovascular response pattern to a conditioned stimulus during the initial stages of Pavlovian fear conditioning is characterized by vagally-mediated bradycardia and depressor responses,[17] responses similar in direction to those elicited by stimulation of the central nucleus. Hence, the results are consistent with the notion that the central nucleus may play a rather direct role in the expression of cardiovascular and perhaps other autonomic (e.g., respiratory) and somatic (e.g., behavioral arrest) responses to conditioned stimuli during Pavlovian fear conditioning.

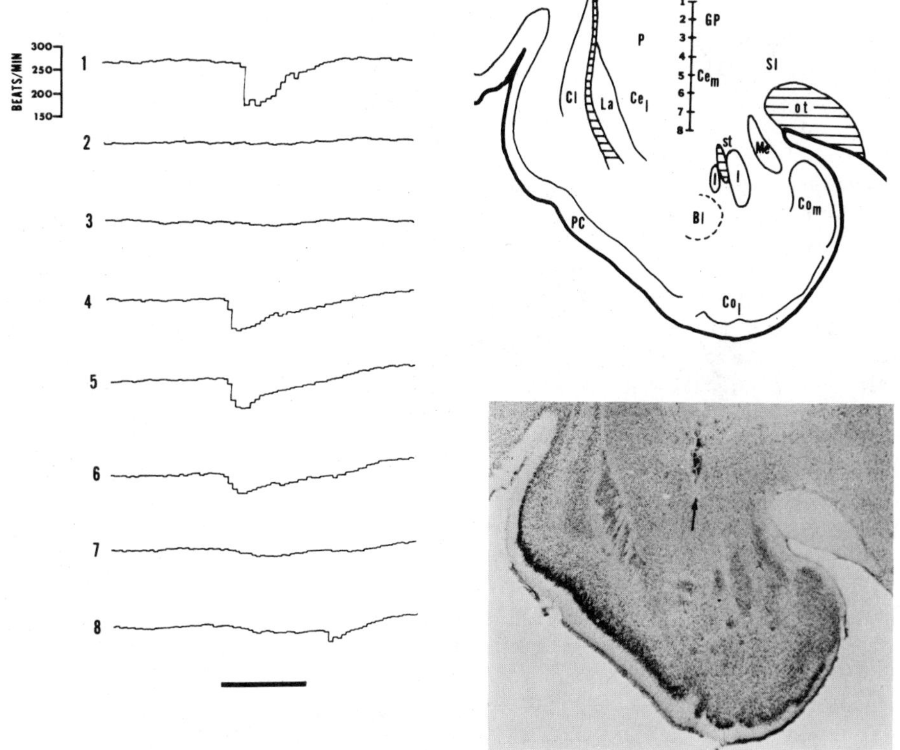

Fig. 6. Heart rate cardiotachograph responses produced by 5.0 second stimulation (500 μA, 100 Hz, 0.5 msec pulse duration) of sites adjacent to and within the medial central nucleus. Each site is separated by 500 μm. The arrow points to a portion of the electrode track as it penetrates the medial central nucleus. Ce_m, medial central nucleus; Ce_l, lateral central nucleus; GP, globus pallidus; P, putamen.

NEURONAL ACTIVITY OF THE CENTRAL NUCLEUS DURING PAVLOVIAN FEAR CONDITIONING

If the central nucleus functions in the motoric expression of the conditioned bradycardia response, then it might be expected that changes in central nucleus neuronal activity should develop to the CS during our Pavlovian conditioning procedure and that these changes should occur at the time when conditioned bradycardia responses develop to the CS. In recent experiments in which we have recorded multiple unit activity from the central nucleus during Pavlovian conditioning we have found cases which satisfy these expectations.[41] The data from one such case is presented in Figure 7. Presented are the mean heart rate change and mean neuronal change from a central nucleus placement in response to the five second tone CS for five trial blocks across three phases of the Pavlovian fear conditioning paradigm; a twenty trial orienting phase in which the CS was presented alone, a twenty trial conditioning phase in which the CS and US were paired, and a twenty trial extinction phase in which the CS was presented alone. A significant increase in multiple unit activity to the CS emerged during the conditioning phase of the procedure, and the development of this activity to the CS over trials paralleled the development of the conditioned bradycardia response to the CS. Of particular significance was the finding that the magnitude of the change in neuronal activity to the CS was significantly correlated with the magnitude of the bradycardia response to the CS over the course of the session ($p < .02$; $r = -0.42$). The neuronal activity was characterized by low levels of spontaneous, pre-CS activity, and the short-latency (40 msec) increases in activity to the CS which emerged (Figure 8) were sustained for the five second duration of the CS but at a lower level than during the first 100 msec.

It is important to note that multiple unit activity from only 12 of 34 placements within the central nucleus demonstrated significant short latency increases to the CS which emerged during the conditioning phase, and significant correlations between neuronal and heart rate response magnitudes were found in only three of these cases. This suggests that not all neuronal elements of the central nucleus were responding in a unitary fashion under the experimental conditions and may point to heterogeneity of function for this nucleus.[42] Nevertheless, the emergence of short-latency increases in neuronal activity to the CS and the fact that the magnitude of the neuronal response in some cases correlates significantly with the magnitude of the bradycardia response to the CS is consistent with the hypothesis that the central nucleus functions in the motoric expression of the conditioned bradycardia response to the CS. However, whether such neuronal activity reflects the activity of projection neurons to the dorsal medulla has yet to be determined.

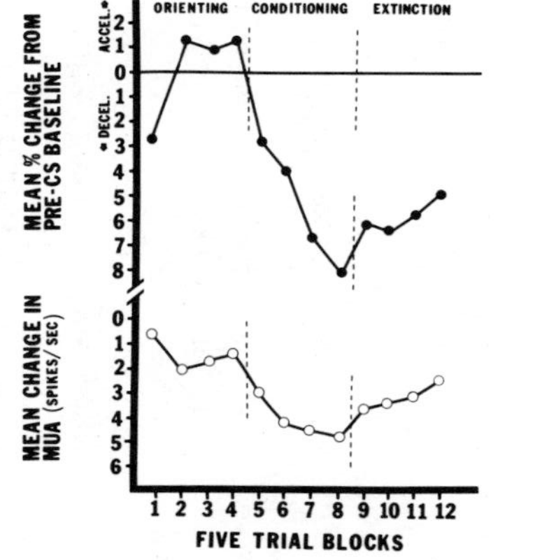

Fig. 7. Changes in heart rate and central nucleus multiple unit activity (MUA) to the CS during orienting, conditioning and extinction components of a conditioning session. See text for details.

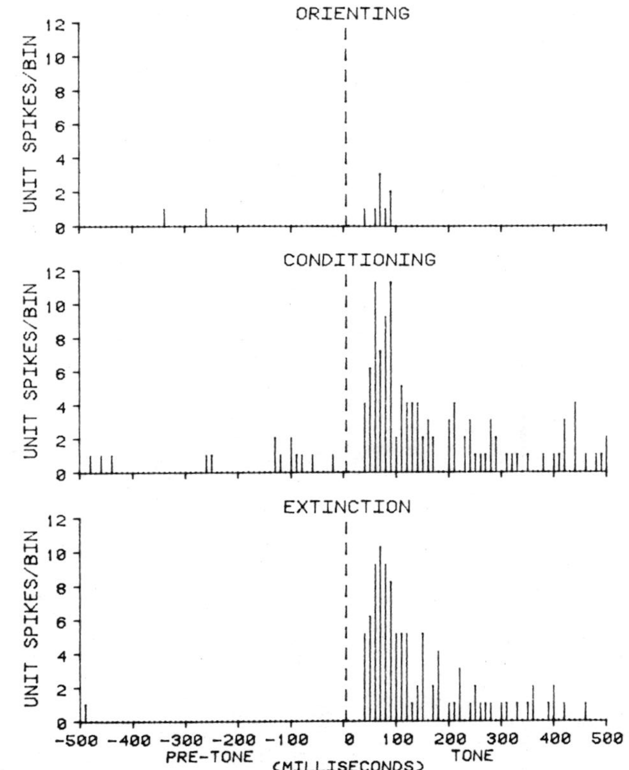

Fig. 8. Histograms of multiple unit activity for the case depicted in Fig. 7. Shown are unit spikes/10 msec bin, summed across each of the 20 trials of orienting, conditioning and extinction, for the 500 msec preceding and the first 500 msec of the CS.

CONCLUSIONS

Returning to our initial discussion pertaining to the contribution of the amygdala to aversive conditioning and fear motivation, the data gathered from our own efforts, as well as those of others, suggest that at least one function of one component of the amygdala, the central nucleus, may be in the motoric expression of conditioned heart rate and perhaps other conditioned autonomic (e.g., respiratory) and somatic (e.g., behavioral arrest) responses during Pavlovian fear conditioning. Obviously, more research will be necessary to further test the validity of this hypothesis, as well as to determine the existence of additional functions (e.g., associative) for the central nucleus in aversive conditioning. Of equal importance will be an analysis of the manner in which this nucleus interacts with other intra- and extra-amygdala structures, not only in its contribution to aversive conditioning, but also to other behaviors.[42] Indeed, given the complex nature of the central nucleus afferent and efferent projections which is emerging, further research may well reveal such a multifunctional role.

ACKNOWLEDGEMENTS

The research and preparation of this manuscript was supported by USPHS grants MH 31811, MH 32292, NS 16107, and RCDA award KO2 MH 00118 to B.S.K.

REFERENCES

1. G. Goddard, Functions of the amygdala, Psychol. Bull. 62:89 (1964).
2. N. J. Russo, B. S. Kapp, B. K. Holmquist, and R. E. Musty, Passive avoidance and amygdala lesions: Relationship with pituitary-adrenal system, Physiol. Behav. 16:191 (1976).
3. A. A. Spevack, C. T. Campbell, and L. Drake, Effect of amygdalectomy on habituation and CER in rats, Physiol. Behav. 15:199 (1975).
4. P. G. Henke, Effects of reinforcement omission on rats with lesions in the amygdala, J. Comp. Physiol. Psych. 84:187 (1973).
5. D. C. Blanchard and R. J. Blanchard, Innate and conditioned reactions to threat in rats with amygdaloid lesions, J. Comp. Physiol. Psych. 81:281 (1972).
6. T. Werka, J. Skär, and H. Ursin, Exploration and avoidance in rats with lesions in amygdala and piriform cortex, J. Comp. Physiol. Psych. 92:672 (1978).

7. M. McIntyre and D. G. Stein, Differential effects of one vs. two stage amygdaloid lesions on activity, exploratory and avoidance behavior in the albino rat, Behav. Biol. 9:451 (1973).
8. S. P. Grossman, L. Grossman, and L. Walsh, Functional organization of the rat amygdala with respect to avoidance behavior, J. Comp. Physiol. Psych. 88:829 (1975).
9. S. M. Hilton and A. W. Zbrozyna, Amygdaloid region for defense reactions and its efferent pathway to the brain stem, J. Physiol. 165:160 (1963).
10. E. Roldan, R. Alvarez-Pelaez, and A. Fernandez deMolina, Electrographic study of the amygdaloid defense response, Physiol. Behav. 13:779 (1974).
11. G. Stock, K. H. Schlör, H. Heidt, and J. Buss, Psychomotor behaviour and cardiovascular patterns during stimulation of the amygdala, Pflügers Archiv. 376:177 (1978).
12. H. Ursin and B. R. Kaada, Functional localization within the amygdaloid complex in the cat, EEG Clin. Neurophysiol. 12:1 (1960).
13. D. A. Hopkins and G. Holstege, Amygdaloid projections to the mesencephalon, pons and medulla oblongata in the cat, Exp. Brain Res., 32:529 (1978).
14. V. C. Abrahams, S. M. Hilton, and A. Zbrozyna, Active muscle vasodilation produced by stimulation of the brain stem. Its significance in the defense reaction, J. Physiol., 154:491 (1960).
15. J. H. Coote, S. M. Hilton, and A. W. Zbrozyna, The ponto-medullary area integrating the defense reaction in the cat and its influence on muscle blood flow, J. Physiol. 229:257 (1973).
16. A. Fredericks, J. W. Moore, F. U. Metcalf, J. S. Schwaber, and N. Schneiderman, Selective autonomic blockade of conditioned and unconditioned heart rate changes in rabbits, Pharm. Biochem. Behav. 2:493 (1974).
17. D. A. Powell and E. Kazis, Blood pressure and heart rate changes accompanying classical eyeblink conditioning in the rabbit (Oryctolagus Cuniculus), Psychophysiol. 13:441 (1976).
18. N. Schneiderman, D. H. VanDercar, A. L. Yehle, A. A. Manning, T. Golden, and E. Schneiderman, Vagal compensatory adjustment: Relationship to heart rate classical conditioning in rabbits, J. Comp. Physiol. Psych. 68:175 (1969).
19. D. H. Cohen, Involvement of avian amygdala homolog (archistriatum posterior and mediale) in defensively conditioned heart rate change, J. Comp. Neurol. 160:13 (1975).
20. O. V. Frisch, HerzFrequenzänderung bei Drückreaktion junger Nestflücher, Z. Tierpsychol. 23:497 (1966).

21. B. S. Kapp, R. C. Frysinger, M. Gallagher, and J. Haselton, Amygdala central nucleus lesions: Effects on heart rate conditioning in the rabbit, Physiol. Behav. 23:1109 (1979).
22. J. H. Fallon, D. A. Koziell, and R. Y. Moore, Catecholamine innervation of the basal forebrain. II. Amygdala, suprahinal cortex and entorhinal cortex, J. Comp. Neurol. 180:509 (1978).
23. V. M. Pickel, M. Segal, and F. E. Bloom, A radiographic study of the efferent pathways of the nucleus locus coeruleus, J. Comp. Neurol. 155:15 (1974).
24. M. Gallagher, B. S. Kapp, R. E. Musty, and P. A. Driscoll, Memory formation: Evidence for a specific neurochemical system in the amygdala, Science 198:423 (1977).
25. M. Gallagher, B. S. Kapp, R. C. Frysinger, and P. R. Rapp, β-adrenergic manipulation in amygdala central nucleus alters rabbit heart rate conditioning, Pharm. Biochem. Behav. 12:419 (1980).
26. D. B. Bylund and S. H. Snyder, Biochemical identification of the β-adrenergic receptor in mammalian brain, Mol. Pharm. 12:1279 (1976).
27. J. L. Martinez, Jr., R. A. Jenson, R. B. Messing, H. Rigter, and J. L. McGaugh (Eds.), Endogenous Peptides and Learning and Memory Processes, Academic Press, New York (1981).
28. M. Gallagher and B. S. Kapp, Manipulation of opiate activity in the amygdala alters memory processes, Life Sci. 23:1973 (1978).
29. C. Gros, P. Pradelles, J. Humbert, F. Dray, G. Le Gal La Salle, and Y. Ben-Ari, Regional distribution of met-enkephalin within the amygdaloid complex and bed nucleus of the stria terminalis, Neuro. Lett. 10:193 (1978).
30. R. Simantov, M. G. Kuhar, G. R. Uhl, and S. H. Snyder, Opioid peptide enkephalin: Immunohistochemical mapping in rat central nervous system, Proc. Natl. Acad. Sci. U.S.A. 74:2167 (1977).
31. R. R. Goodman, S. H. Snyder, M. J. Kuhar, and W. S. Young III, Differentiation of delta and mu opiate receptor localizations by light microscopic autoradiography, Proc. Natl. Acad. Sci. U.S.A. 77:6239 (1980)
32. M. Gallagher, B. S. Kapp, C. L. McNall, and J. P. Pascoe, Opiate effects in the amygdala central nucleus on heart rate conditioning in rabbits, Pharm. Biochem. Behav. 14:497 (1981).
33. R. J. Rodgers, Influence of intra-amygdaloid opiate injection on shock thresholds, tail flick latencies and open field behavior in rats, Brain Res. 153:211 (1978).
34. A. Goldstein, G. T. Pryor, L. S. Otis, and F. Larsen, On the role of endogenous opioid peptides: Failure of naloxone to influence shock escape threshold in the rat, Life Sci. 18:599 (1976).

35. S. E. File and R. J. Rodgers, Partial anxiolytic action of morphine sulfate following microinjection into the central nucleus of the amygdala in rats, Pharm. Biochem. Behav. 11:313 (1979).

36. J. S. Schwaber, and N. Schneiderman, Aortic nerve activated cardioinhibitory neurons and interneurons, A. J. Physiol. 299:783 (1975).

37. J. S. Schwaber, B. S. Kapp, and G. Higgins, The origin and extent of direct amygdala projections to the region of the dorsal motor nucleus of the vagus and the nucleus of the solitary tract, Neuro. Lett. 20:15 (1980).

38. J. S. Schwaber, B. S. Kapp, G. A. Higgins, and P. R. Rapp, The origin, extent and terminal distribution of direct amygdala central nucleus projections to the dorsal motor nucleus and nucleus of the solitary tract, Neuro. Abs. 6:816 (1980).

39. B. S. Kapp, M. Gallagher, M. D. Underwood, C. L. McNall, and D. Whitehorn, Cardiovascular responses elicited by electrical stimulation of the amygdala central nucleus in the rabbit, Submitted, Brain Res. (1981).

40. B. S. Kapp, C. D. Applegate, M. D. Underwood, and C. L. McNall, Electrical stimulation of the amygdala central nucleus in the awake rabbit: Effects on heart rate, respiration and somatomotor behavior, Neuro. Abs. 7 (1981).

41. C. D. Applegate, R. C. Frysinger, B. S. Kapp, and M. Gallagher, Neuronal activity recorded from the amygdala central nucleus during aversive Pavlovian heart rate conditioning in the rabbit, Neuro. Abs. 7 (1981).

42. J. S. Schwartzbaum and J. R. Morse, Taste responsivity of amygdaloid units in behaving rabbits: A methodological report, Brain Res. Bull. 3:131 (1978).

CONDITIONING: MODIFICATION BY PERIPHERAL MECHANISMS*

Joe L. Martinez, Jr.

Psychobiology Department
School of Biological Sciences
University of California
Irvine, CA 92717

ABSTRACT

This paper examines the idea that peripheral hormones, particularly those of the sympatho-adrenal system, are part of the normal machinery of learning and memory. Blood-borne hormones, although widely distributed in the body have very specific actions because of the nature and location of their receptive sites.

Evidence was presented that the adrenal medullary systems are important for 4-OH amphetamine and Met- and Leu-enkephalin effects on avoidance conditioning, because their actions are dependent on the integrity of the adrenal medulla.

Also examined was the question of whether 4-OH amphetamine, Met- and Leu-enkephalin affect avoidance conditioning by acting directly on the brain or at some peripheral site. It was suggested that even though 4-OH amphetamine may be measured in brain following i.p. injection that its action to enhance retention of an inhibitory avoidance response was mediated peripherally. This suggestion was based on a comparison of dose-response effectiveness of amphetamine

---

*This research was supported by Research Grants MH 12526 (to James L. McGaugh and Joe L. Martinez, Jr.) from the U.S. Public Health Service and BNS 76-17370 (to James L. McGaugh) from the National Science Foundation. Most of the research reported in this paper was conducted in the laboratories of James L. McGaugh and Henk Rigter. I gratefully acknowledge their collaboration, advice and support. Also, the collaborative work of K. Ishikawa, R. A. Jensen, R. B. Messing, and B. J. Vasquez contributed significantly to this research.

and 4-OH amphetamine on intracranial self-stimulation behavior and avoidance conditioning and the fact that the effèct of 4-OH amphetamine is abolished by adrenal medullectomy. Similarly, it is likely that both Met- and Leu-enkephalin have a primary site of action in the periphery in impairing acquisition of a one-way active avoidance task, because adrenal medullectomy appears to completely abolish the actions of Met-enkephalin and shifts the effective dose of Leu-enkephalin to higher doses. However, Leu-enkephalin, which apparently has a site of action distant from the adrenal medulla, did not alter EEG activity at a dose 50 times greater than its behaviorally effective dose also suggesting that Leu-enkephalin has a primary site of action in the periphery.

INTRODUCTION

Changes in the nervous system that result from conditioning are usually described in terms of central processes such as anatomical, biochemical, or neurophysiological changes in regional brain areas [11,14,56]. However, it is becoming apparent that changes in peripheral nervous or endocrine function may also be correlated with performance of conditioned avoidance behaviors[13,33,34]. The importance of these peripheral systems to conditioning was pointed out in 1968 by Levine[21]. More recent findings that the memory enhancing properties of amphetamine seem to depend on the integrity of the adrenal medulla[32], that the monoamine inhibitor, reserpine or a peripherally acting analog of reserpine, syrosingopine, prevent learning[41,59], that phentolamine, an α-adrenergic antagonist drug with a limited ability to cross the blood-brain barrier attenuates amnesia induced by frontal cortex stimulation[54], and finally that adrenal medullectomy abolishes the amnestic effects of amygdala stimulation[36], all underscore the importance of peripheral systems. Also, the findings of numerous studies have shown that learning and memory are affected by adrenocorticotropic hormone (ACTH), peptide fragments of ACTH, and corticosteroids (see[5,10,20]).

Thus, most would agree, that peripheral mechanisms, particularly the pituitary-adrenal and sympatho-adrenal systems influence the strength of a learned response. Taking this logic one step further, this may mean that peripheral mechanisms are part of the normal machinery of information storage in mammalian species. This conclusion is not surprising if one considers the fact that both the peripheral nervous and endocrine systems are interconnected and for the most part contiguous with the central nervous system.

The study of the influence of peripheral systems on learning and memory, at first glance, lacks the aesthetically pleasing specificity of knowing that each neuron is synaptically connected to other neurons, in an organized way. However, hormonal responses have high specificity because of the nature and location of their receptors[55]. Certain amino acid sequences of some hormones, such as $ACTH_{4-10}$, are known to affect a variety of conditioned behaviors[5] and neuronal membranes in very specific ways[62]. Thus, if one follows the practice of naming hormones for their most prominent action, then $ACTH_{4-10}$ may be a learning modulatory hormone[35].

On the other hand, if one considers the fact that in the CNS many monoaminergic neurons lack postsynaptic densities, and that neurotransmitter or neuromodulator substances released from these synapses might act at distant receptors[4] the situation is quite comparable to studying the effects of peripheral hormones on the brain. In any case, peripherally released hormones might affect the brain in rather specific ways. For example, hormones could act at peripheral receptors and affect CNS functioning through afferent feedback. Since most peripheral hormones such as ACTH, norepinephrine and epinephrine do not readily pass the blood-brain barrier[1,2], it is possible that they affect brain regions lying outside the blood-brain barrier. Others have postulated that pituitary hormones may flow retrogradely up the pituitary stalk to affect the brain[62]. Finally, peptide hormones may be locally concentrated in the brain at specialized sites, such as circumventricular organs[60]. Therefore, it is likely that hormones do affect the brain in specific ways and that an increased understanding of these processes in relation to the neural events that occur during conditioning will shed light on the neurobiology of learning and memory.

PERIPHERAL CATECHOLAMINES AND MEMORY

My own interest in this approach began with a study in which it was found that a large dose range of d-amphetamine given intraventricularly following training in an inhibitory avoidance task did not alter later retention performance[26]. Of course, it is possible that the amphetamine was not in the right place, at the right time, at the appropriate concentration to affect retention, but these results led to further studies suggesting that the effect of amphetamine on memory is related to adrenal medullary function. We found that posttrial peripheral administration of d-amphetamine, which crosses freely into the brain, and 4-OH amphetamine, which supposedly does not, enhanced retention of an inhibitory avoidance response at similar doses[26,32]. The dose response curve of 4-OH amphetamine may be found in Figure 1.

In order to determine which peripheral adrenergic system was involved in the amphetamine-induced enhancement of retention, further experiments were conducted using 6-hydroxydopamine which produces a chemical sympathectomy, or adrenal medullectomy to remove important peripheral stores of catecholamines. Sympathectomy shifted the effective dose of both amphetamine and 4-OH amphetamine to lower doses, while adrenal medullectomy abolished the enhancing actions

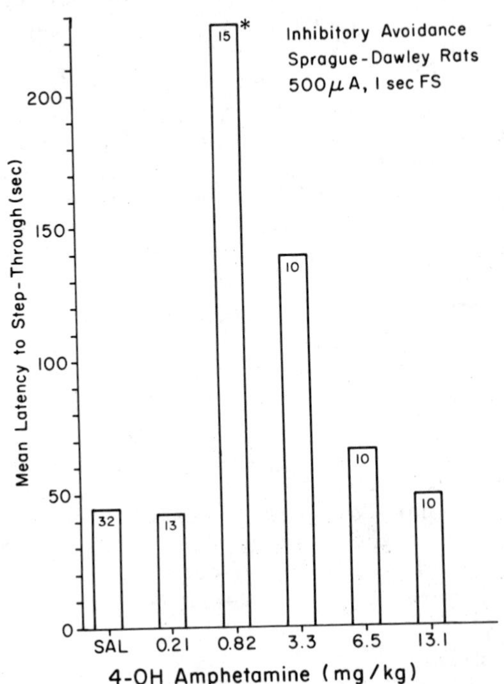

Figure 1. Immediate posttrial treatment (i.p.) with a 0.82 mg/kg dose of DL-4-OH-amphetamine significantly ($p < 0.01$) enhances retention performance tested 72 hr following training. The number of animals used in each dose condition is shown in the bars. [from Martinez et al.[32]].

of both amphetamines[26,32]. These studies indicated that amphetamine may affect memory by acting on the adrenal medulla, presumably by initiating release of the contents of chromaffin cells.

GENERALITY OF THE EFFECT OF 4-OH AMPHETAMINE ON MEMORY

The action of 4-OH amphetamine on retention of a one-way active avoidance and swim-escape response was studied in sham-operated (SHAM) and adrenal medullectomized (ADXM) rats. The details of the procedures have been published elsewhere[28,45]. Briefly, for active avoidance training, a rat was placed into a dark compartment of a two-compartment box. The door was opened partway forming a hurdle. The animal had 10 sec to shuttle to the safe white compartment, or a 640 μA footshock was administered which was terminated by the animal escaping to the white compartment. Eight training trials were given on Day 1, and immediately following training the animals were injected i.p. with one of several doses of 4-OH amphetamine (0.41, 0.82 or 8.2 mg/kg). On Day 2, 24 hr later, the animals were given 8 additional training trials.

Figure 2 shows that a 0.82 mg/kg dose of 4-OH amphetamine significantly increased the number of avoidance responses the SHAM animals made on DAY 2. However, adrenal medullectomy abolished

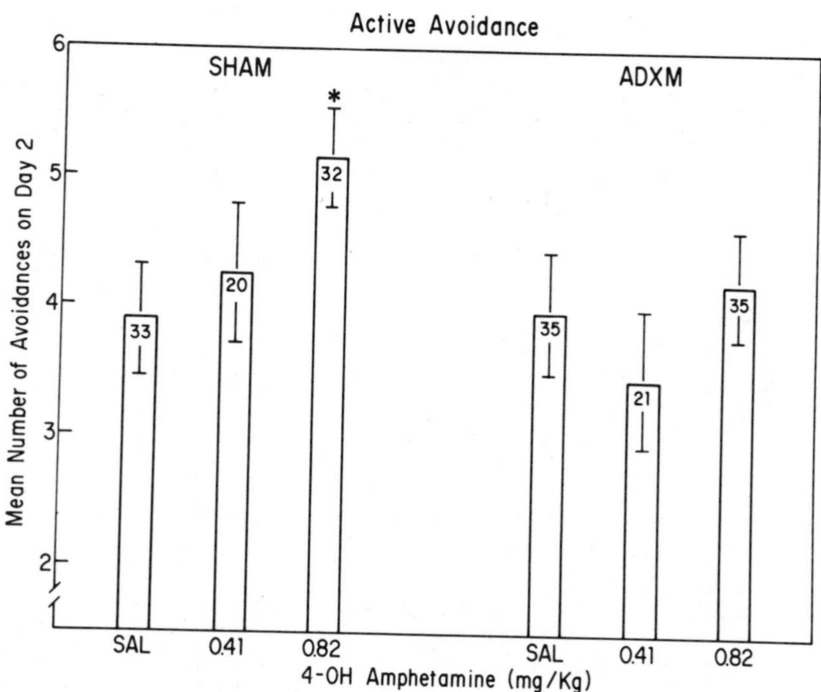

Figure 2. Avoidance scores on Day 2 of conditioning of both sham-operated (left panel) and adrenal demedullated (right panel) rats receiving intraperitoneal injections of either saline or 0.41 or 0.82 mg/kg dl-4-OH amphetamine immediately after training on Day 1. The sham-operated animals that received 0.82 mg/kg 4-OH amphetamine made significantly ($p < 0.5$) more avoidances than did the animals that received saline, demonstrating that 4-OH amphetamine enhances retention of an active avoidance response in these animals. The number of animals in each dose condition is shown in the bars. [From Martinez et al.[23]].

the actions of 4-OH amphetamine in ADXM rats. Thus, the integrity of the adrenal medulla is necessary for the actions of 4-OH amphetamine in active avoidance as it is in inhibitory avoidance conditioning[26,32].

The swim escape task consists of placing rats in one corner of a large rectangular plastic tub that is filled partway with water. The time taken by each rat to find a pole in the opposite corner and grasp it with at least two paws was recorded. After the animal climbed out of the water it was injected with either saline, 0.41, 0.82, or 1.64 mg/kg 4-OH amphetamine. For the retention test 24 hr later, each rat was given a second trial exactly as in training. Both SHAM and ADXM rats evidenced learning by escaping from the water significantly faster on the second day than they did on the first. However, 4-OH amphetamine was without effect in both groups[24].

Taken together, the results of these studies suggest that the effect of 4-OH amphetamine on memory may not generalize to all tasks, and is restricted at the present time to shock-motivated avoidance tasks. The fact that opposite locomotor responses are required to perform the inhibitory and active avoidance responses makes it unlikely that any effect of 4-OH amphetamine on general activity levels contributed to the observed results.

DOES 4-OH AMPHETAMINE DIRECTLY AFFECT THE BRAIN?

The rationale for this study was two-fold. First, it is possible that central and peripheral catecholamine systems interact. Many years ago Javoy et al.[18] reported that adrenalectomy increased the turnover of central catecholamines. Ogren and Fuxe[40] and Roberts and Fibiger[47] found that destroying projections of the nucleus locus coeruleus did not impair acquisition or retention of a shuttle or inhibitory avoidance task. However, if destruction of the locus coeruleus was combined with adrenalectomy, then acquisition and retention was severly impaired. Second, it is possible that significant quantities of 4-OH amphetamine do cross into the brain to affect catecholamine systems. Thus, it was determined whether peripheral administration of 4-OH amphetamine affects concentrations of norepinephrine and dopamine in regional brain areas, concentrations of norepinephrine and epinephrine in the adrenal glands, and whether 4-OH amphetamine could be detected in the brain[32,34].

Naive untrained rats were injected i.p. with either saline, 0.82 or 8.2 mg/kg 4-OH amphetamine. Ten, 30, or 60 minutes following injection the rats were decapitated and their brains were dissected according to a modified procedure of Shellenberger and Gordon[48] (see [38]) into amygdala, hypothalamus, hippocampus, midbrain, striatum, and the cortex overlying the striatum. The animals' adrenal glands were also removed.

All catecholamine determinations were performed using a procedure that has been described[17]. The procedure consisted of n-butanol extraction and detection by means of high performance liquid chromatography combined with electrochemical detection.

The high dose of 8.2 mg/kg 4-OH amphetamine significantly reduced concentrations of norepinephrine in all of the brain areas measured and similarly reduced concentrations of dopamine in all areas except the hypothalamus and midbrain. On the other hand, the behaviorally active dose of 0.82 mg/kg 4-OH amphetamine in the avoidance conditioning paradigms significantly reduced dopamine concentrations in the amygdala and hippocampus. These data may be found in Figures 3 and 4 (right two panels).

Surprisingly, we were able to detect significant quantities of 4-OH amphetamine in the brain. Inspection of Figures 3 and 4 (left panels) shows that the clearance rate of 4-OH amphetamine was not coincident with the decreases in catecholamine concentrations. In

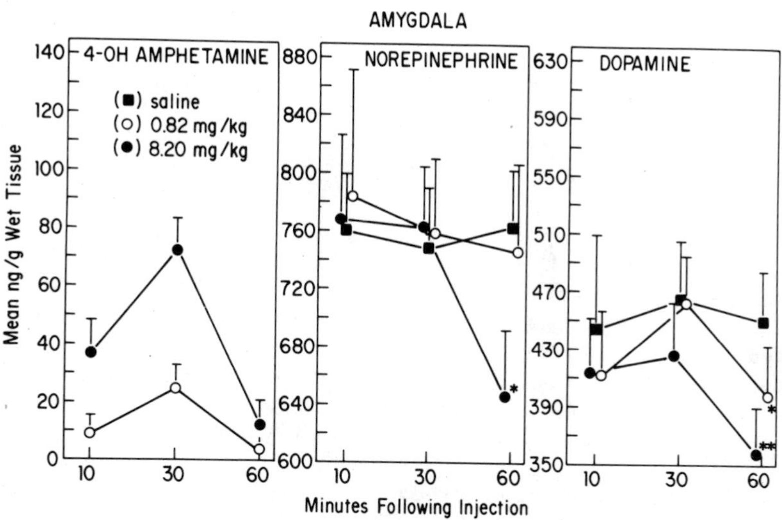

Figure 3. Concentrations of 4-OH amphetamine, norepinephrine, and dopamine measured in amygdala 10, 30 or 60 minutes following an i.p. injection of 4-OH amphetamine. Norepinephrine concentrations were reduced by the larger dose of 8.2 mg/kg ($p < .05$), whereas dopamine was reduced by both the 0.82 ($p < .05$) and 8.2 mg/kg dose ($p < .01$) in comparison to the saline control group ($n = 5$, at each dose level).

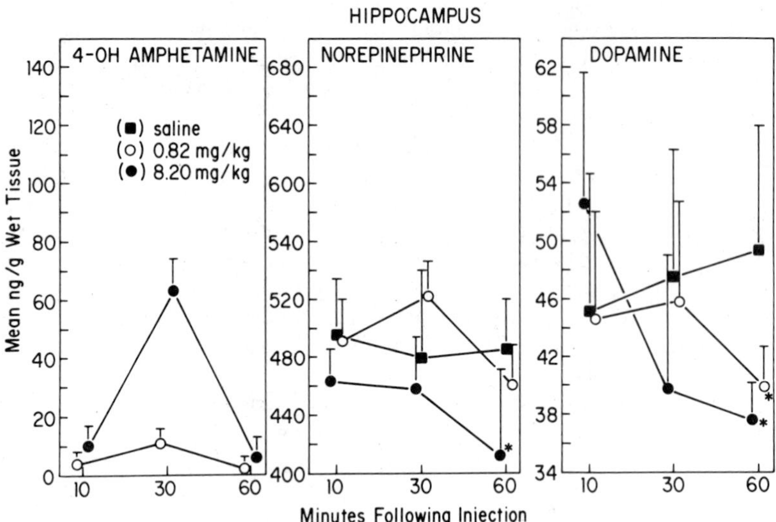

Figure 4. Concentrations of 4-OH amphetamine, norepinephrine, and dopamine measured in hippocampus 10, 30 or 60 minutes following an i.p. injection with 4-OH amphetamine. Norepinephrine concentrations were reduced by the larger dose of 8.2 mg/kg ($p < .05$), whereas dopamine was reduced by both the 0.82 ($p < .05$) and 8.2 mg/kg dose ($p < .05$) in comparison to the saline control group ($n = 5$, at each dose level).

all cases, significant decreases in catecholamine concentrations were only observed at the 60 min timepoint, whereas in all cases the peak concentrations of 4-OH amphetamine in the brain were observed at 30 min. However, these data agree with the generally accepted principle that amphetamines cause a net increase in the release of norepinephrine and dopamine, probably by blocking the presynaptic reuptake mechanism of these neurotransmitters[9].

4-OH amphetamine also produces a dose-dependent decrease in the concentrations of norepinephrine and epinephrine in the adrenal gland. Figure 5 shows that significant reductions of these hormones were only observed with the 8.2 mg/kg dose 60 min following injection. However, the magnitude of the decrease was quite impressive. Compared to the saline controls, it was 1.30 μg for norepinephrine and 3.50 μg for epinephrine.

It should be kept in mind that these were untrained animals and

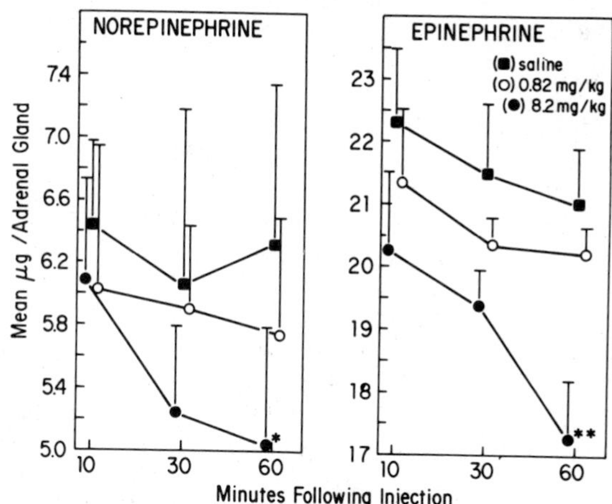

Figure 5. Concentrations of norepinephrine and epinephrine measured in adrenal gland 10, 30 or 60 minutes following an i.p. injection with 4-OH amphetamine. Norepinephrine ($p < .05$) and epinephrine ($p < .02$) were reduced by the larger dose of 8.2 mg/kg in comparison to their saline control group 60 min following injection.

the contribution of the stress of the training experience to decreases in catecholamine concentrations observed in the brain and adrenal glands is not known at this time. Nevertheless, these data raise the possibility that the effect of 4-OH amphetamine in enhancing memory may be due, at least partially, to a direct action on the brain.

In a somewhat different way, we attempted to determine whether 4-OH amphetamine directly affects the brain by determining whether it influences intracranial self-stimulation[6]. The reason for doing this is that there are many parallels between the effects of drugs on memory and ICSS behavior[52]. For example, d-amphetamine facilitates retention of an inhibitory avoidance task[26] and ICSS[51]. Further, Wise and Stein[61] reported that inhibition of norepinephrine biosynthesis by diethyldithiocarbamate abolished ICSS while replacement of norepinephrine directly into the brain reinstated the ICSS behavior. Similar effects have been reported for inhibitory avoidance conditioning[37,53]. Thus, if 4-OH amphetamine were crossing into the brain to directly affect the brain and hence avoidance conditioning, then it should affect ICSS behavior in much the same way as d-amphetamine.

The methods and procedures for implanting electrodes into the lateral hypothalmic area to induce ICSS behavior have been described [61]. In this study the effects on ICSS behavior of 0.5 mg/kg of dl-amphetamine and dl-4-OH amphetamine given i.p. were compared. It may be seen in Figure 6 that amphetamine, but not 4-OH amphetamine, facilitates the rate of ICSS.

In a second phase of this study some of the rats tested with amphetamine or saline were either adrenal demedullated or sham-operated and tested for ICSS behavior. Interestingly, adrenal medullectomy decreased the rate of ICSS from a mean of 3768.57 (SEM ± 738.11) before surgery to 2675.00 (± 566.36) (n = 7) following surgery. However, for the sham-operated rats there was no difference in the rate of ICSS behavior before ($\overline{X}$ = 3100.50 ± 698.46) (n = 7) or after surgery ($\overline{X}$ = 3141.00 ± 677.18).

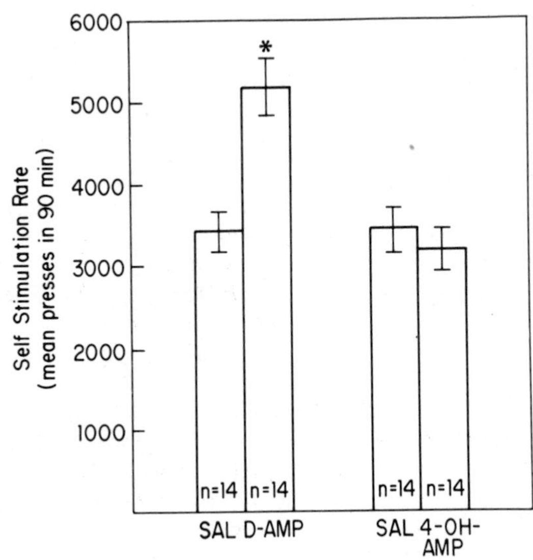

Figure 6. A dose of 0.5 mg/kg (i.p.) dl-amphetamine significantly ($p < .001$) enhances the rate of intracranial self-stimulation behavior induced by stimulation of the lateral hypothalamus. A dose of 0.5 mg/kg dl-4-OH amphetamine has no effect on self-stimulation behavior.

The results of this study show that 4-OH amphetamine at a dose of 0.5 mg/kg does not alter the rate of ICSS behavior while the same dose of d-amphetamine enhances the rate of ICSS. Even though a complete dose response was not determined, it may be concluded that 4-OH amphetamine is less potent than d-amphetamine in affecting ICSS behavior. However, in the case of inhibitory avoidance conditioning this is not the case. Martinez et al.[26,32] showed that under identical experimental conditions that 0.82 mg/kg of dl-4-OH amphetamine enhanced retention if given following training, whereas a 1.0 mg/kg dose of d-amphetamine was necessary to produce an equivalent effect. While a 0.82 mg/kg dose of 4-OH amphetamine is equimolar to a 1.0 mg/kg dose of amphetamine, the fact that a racemic form of 4-OH amphetamine was used suggests that it may be more potent than d-amphetamine in its ability to enhance retention of an inhibitory avoidance response. This suggests that the primary action of 4-OH amphetamine may be in the periphery.

Interestingly, the finding that adrenal medullectomy reduces the rate of ICSS behavior may mean that the maintenance of ICSS is mediated, at least in part, through peripheral mechanisms. This agrees with earlier work of Ball[3] who reported that vagotomy also reduced the rate of ICSS behavior.

CONCLUSIONS

Taken together the data indicate that 4-OH amphetamine enhances retention of conditioned avoidance responses motivated by shock. The enhancing action of 4-OH amphetamine may not be generally applicable to all aversively motivated learning situations since it had no effect on retention of a swim escape response. The integrity of the adrenal medulla is necessary for the enhancing action of 4-OH amphetamine and the drug produces a dose dependent decrease in the concentrations of norepinephrine and epinephrine in the adrenal medulla. However, 4-OH amphetamine may be measured in brain and is related in a general way to decreases in regional brain concentrations of norepinephrine and dopamine. This suggests that 4-OH amphetamine may affect memory by a dual action on the brain and adrenal medulla. However, a comparison of the effect of comparable doses of amphetamine and 4-OH amphetamine on ICSS behavior showed that amphetamine facilitated whereas 4-OH amphetamine had no effect on the rate of ICSS. This is what would be expected if amphetamine entered the brain with more facility than 4-OH amphetamine. Yet, in inhibitory avoidance conditioning 4-OH amphetamine may be more potent than amphetamine in enhancing retention performance. Thus, even though 4-OH amphetamine may be measured in brain its primary action in affecting avoidance conditioning may be in the periphery.

PERIPHERAL ENKEPHALINS AND AVOIDANCE CONDITIONING

Previously, we reported that microgram amounts of peripherally administered Met- or Leu-enkephalin, or D-Ala-D-Leu-enkephalin (DADLE) impaired acquisition of a step-through one-way active avoidance response[45,46]. Subsequently, we replicated and extended these findings for Met-and Leu-enkephalin to a step-up active avoidance task in another strain of rats[31,44]. We also determined that the impairment in acquisition by Met-enkephalin was naloxone reversible, whereas for Leu-enkephalin it was not. Also, the enkephalin actions on avoidance conditioning were probably not due to any analgesic effect of the peptides or due to non-specific effects on performance of the avoidance response[45] (reviewed in [30]).

The low doses of enkephalin needed to produce these behavioral effects and the current controversy of whether enkephalins cross into the brain in sufficient quantities to be of physiological significance[7,42] led us to consider the possibility that enkephalin effects on avoidance conditioning may be related to peripheral mechanisms. Since the existence of enkephalin-like peptides in the sympathetic nervous system including the adrenal medulla is well-established (for review see [63]) and chromaffin cells of the adrenal medulla have been shown to have opiate receptors[19], and enkephalin-like materials are released by the same stimuli that produce secretions of catecholamines[58], it seemed possible that the adrenal medulla might be important for enkephalin actions on avoidance conditioning. To investigate this question, adrenal medullectomized rats were given doses of enkephalin that are known to impair acquisition of avoidance conditioning in normal Wistar rats (10 μg/kg, i.p.). The step-up active avoidance task has been described[31,44] and is similar to the step-through procedure already described. Animals were injected 5 min before training, placed in the avoidance box, and given 10 sec to avoid a footshock (0.3 mA) by stepping up onto a small platform. Eight trials were run, and the number of avoidance responses the animal made was taken as the measure of acquisition performance. In these studies, the adrenal demedullations and sham operations were performed 2 weeks prior to training. Post mortem analysis of plasma corticosterone showed no differences between the sham-operated and ADXM groups, but plasma epinephrine was significantly decreased[29,31].

Figure 7 shows that adrenal medullectomy abolishes the impairing actions of both Met- and Leu-enkephalin on active avoidance conditioning. Adrenal demedullation by itself had no significant effect on acquisition of the response, which agrees with previous research [39,50]. Interestingly, increasing the dose of Leu-enkephalin by 10-100 fold in adrenal medullectomized rats restores its behavioral action, whereas increasing the dose of Met-enkephalin (10 or 100 fold) or decreasing it (10 fold) does not. Adrenal medullectomy apparently abolishes the impairing action of Met-enkephalin

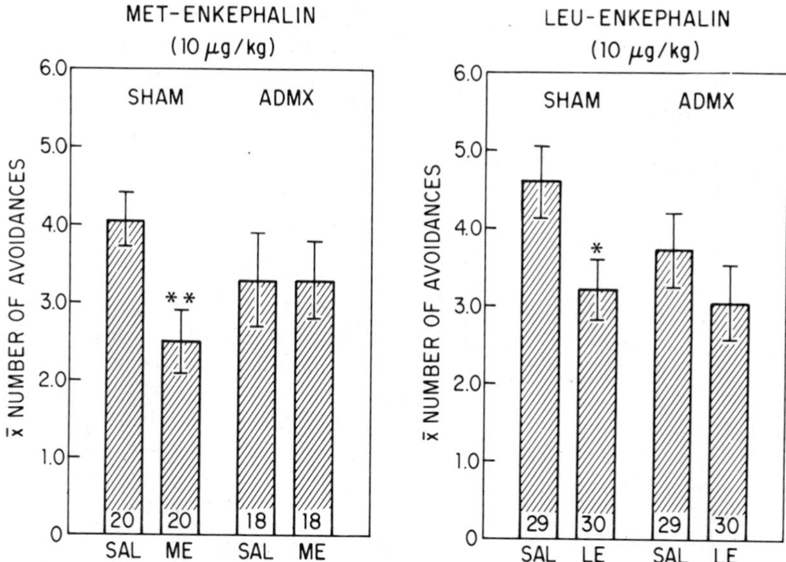

Figure 7. Met-enkephalin (left panel) at a dose of 10.0 μg/kg administered to rats i.p. 5 min before training impairs acquisition of an active avoidance response in sham-operated (SHAM) ($p < .02$) rats, whereas adrenal medullectomy (ADXM) abolishes the effect ($p > .05$). Leu-enkephalin (right panel) at a dose of 10.0 μg/kg also impairs acquisition of the response in SHAM controls ($p < .02$) but was ineffective in ADXM rats ($p > .05$). The number of animals used in each dose condition is shown in the bars. Adrenal medullectomy by itself had no significant effect on acquisition of the active avoidance response in either group.

on acquisition of this particular one-way active avoidance response [29]. The results suggest that the adrenal medulla is an important site of action for Met-enkephalin since its removal abolishes its actions.

On the other hand, adrenal medullectomy shifts the dose response function for Leu-enkephalin to higher doses suggesting that the adrenal medulla is an important source of enkephalins. If this interpretation is correct, then the behavioral effect of Leu-enkephalin is produced by a combination of endogenous Leu-enkephalin released from the adrenal medulla and exogenous Leu-enkephalin administered through injection. However, this interpretation seems unlikely in view of the small quantities of opiate-like peptides measured in rat adrenal medulla (0.29 nmol/g wet wt)[58] (see also

15), and the fact that adrenal medullectomy in the absence of drug treatment had no effect on avoidance conditioning. Taken together, the results do support the interpretation that exogenously administered Met-enkephalin acts on the adrenal medulla in some way, while Leu-enkephalin acts at a distant site to impair acquisition of the avoidance response.

DOES LEU-ENKEPHALIN DIRECTLY AFFECT THE BRAIN?

The results of studies reviewed in the previous section, that Leu-enkephalin affects conditioning at a site remote from the adrenal medulla, suggested that Leu-enkephalin might be directly affecting CNS function in some way. Rapoport et al.[42] showed that some peptides derived from β-lipotropin have sufficient cerebrovascular permeability to produce measurable brain uptake in 3-11 minutes. Others have shown that enkephalins produce eliptiform EEG activity when administered directly into the brain[57]. The rationale for the following studies was to determine whether neurophysiological responses of the *in vitro* hippocampal slice preparation are sensitive to superfusion of Leu-enkephalin and whether intrahippocampally recorded EEG would be altered by systemically administered Leu-enkephalin.

The methods of hippocampal slice preparation and maintenance have been described[12]. In this study it was found that concentrations of DADLE as low as 10 nM dramatically increased the magnitude of the population spike response of pyramidal cell neurons to stimulation of their Schaffer-commissural afferents. This effect had a rapid onset and was quickly eliminated when the peptide was removed from the perfusion medium. Figure 8 shows that enhancement of the population spike was blocked by the opiate receptor antagonist naloxone, which by itself, had no effect. Thus, the hippocampus is very responsive to enkephalin[25].

Given the sensitivity of the hippocampus to DADLE, it seemed possible that systemically administered Leu-enkephalin should alter the electrical activity of the hippocampus, if it passes directly into the brain to affect ongoing CNS function. The methods of implantation of chronic cortical and hippocampal electrodes, EEG recording, and computer-based analysis of the EEG used in the present study (Martinez & de Neef, unpublished observations) have been described[27,28]. Untrained naive rats were given six 2-minute preinjection baseline recording sessions and all postinjection changes in the EEG in both cortex and hippocampus are expressed as percent changes from the preinjection baseline. Rats were injected with either saline, 50 or 500 μg/kg Leu-enkephalin, i.p. and the EEG was recorded for 29 minutes following the injection.

No overt changes in the EEG were observed such as epileptiform

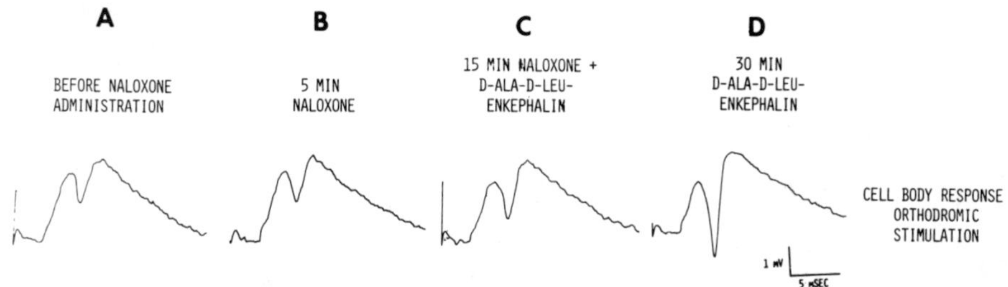

Figure 8. The effects of 0.5 μM naloxone and 50 nM enkephalin on the response recorded at the cell body layer of the regio superior to stimulation of the Schaffer-commissural projection. The naloxone, applied for 5 min before and for the first 15 min of enkephalin infusion, had no detectable effects by itself (B) but did largely, though not completely, block the usual enkephalin-produced enhancement of the population spike (C). For the last 30 min of the experiment, enkephalin infusion was continued but without simultaneous treatment with naloxone and, as is evident from the last panel of the figure, enkephalin produced its typical effects on the population spike (D). [From Martinez et al.[25]].

activity following systemic administration of Leu-enkephalin, as are observed following intraventricular administration[57]. Computer-based analysis of the EEG showed that Leu-enkephalin did not alter the EEG recorded from the hippocampus. However, Figure 9 shows that the percentage of time occupied by 18-20 Hz EEG activity and the amplitude of these waves recorded from the cortex was increased by 500 μg/kg Leu-enkephalin in comparison to 50 μg/kg Leu-enkephalin, but not to the saline control group (except for a decrease as compared to saline recorded 19 min following injections). Interestingly, the onset of these effects was 3-7 minutes following injection in agreement with Rapoport et al.[42] who measured significant uptake of opioid peptides in brain 3-11 minutes following injections. However, the lack of effect of Leu-enkephalin on the hippocampus, which is very sensitive <u>in vitro</u> to the actions of DADLE, and the fact that in general the EEG changes observed in the cortex following 500 μg/kg Leu-enkephalin did not differ from the saline control groups suggests that Leu-enkephalin given systemically does not pass directly into the brain to affect ongoing EEG activity.

CONCLUSIONS

Systemically administered Met- and Leu-enkephalin impair acquisition of an active avoidance response at similar doses. Their

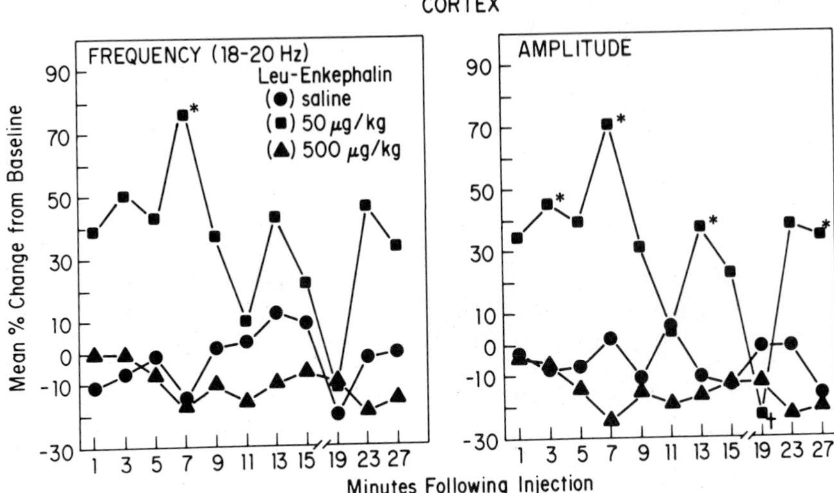

Figure 9. Changes in 18-20 Hz EEG activity recorded in cortex in comparison to preinjection baseline following injection of saline (n = 7), 50.0 µg/kg (n = 6) or 500.0 µg/kg (n = 7) Leu-enkephalin (i.p.). Significant changes were observed between the 500 and 50 µg/kg doses in the amount of time occupied by 18-20 Hz activity and the relative amplitude of these waves at various time points beginning 3-7 min after injection (*). In one case there was a significant difference between 500 µg/kg and saline (†), for amplitude 19 min following drug treatment.

actions on behavior are probably not mediated by the same mechanisms since the action of Met- but not Leu-enkephalin is blocked by the opiate antagonist naloxone[31,44]. Also, adrenal medullectomy apparently abolishes the impairing effect of Met- but not Leu-enkephalin, suggesting that Met-enkephalin acts on the adrenal medulla while Leu-enkephalin acts at a distant site. Even though the adrenal medulla contains enkephalin-like peptides[63], it is not likely that endogenous release of these substances contributes to the observed effects of exogenous enkephalins because of the small quantities of enkephalin-like peptides found in the rat adrenal medulla[58] and the fact that adrenal medullectomy which removes an endogenous store of enkephalins does not affect acquisition of the one-way active avoidance response. These findings agree with other data demonstrating that the two peptides have different behavioral actions[43].

It seems likely that, with regard to their impairing action on avoidance conditioning, the primary action of both Met- and Leu-enkephalin is in the periphery. This suggestion is supported by the finding that adrenal medullectomy abolished the actions of Met-enkephalin. In the case of Leu-enkephalin, adrenal medullectomy shifts the effective dose to higher doses suggesting that Leu-enkephalin acts at a site distant from the adrenal medulla. However, in view of the fact that peripherally administered Leu-enkephalin at a dose that is 50 times greater than the behaviorally active dose, does not significantly alter brain EEG activity, particularly in the hippocampus, also suggests that the primary action of Leu-enkephalin is in the periphery.

GENERAL DISCUSSION

Figure 10 below presents a schematic diagram of the pituitary-adrenal and sympatho-adrenal systems. Enkephalin-like peptides may be considered an integral part of the sympatho-adrenal system since they are found in the adrenal medulla[63] and the sympathetic chain[16], whose postganglionic efferent nerves are adrenergic. It has been suggested[30] that there may be an interrelationship between these two systems and that an understanding of the importance of this relationship for behavior depends on gaining more knowledge of opioid systems.

The data reported in this paper provide evidence that stimulating the sympatho-adrenal system with exogenously administered agents influences avoidance conditioning. It was suggested that the functioning of this system during a learning experience may be a normal part of the machinery of learning and memory. Indeed, the fact that altering the function of the sympatho-adrenal system affects the strength of a learned response is evidence for this view.

However, the sympatho-adrenal system is not necessary for learning, since avoidance conditioning may be observed in the absence of an adrenal medulla, the sympathetic nervous system or both[26,32]. A possible explanation for the lack of an effect on avoidance conditioning in adrenal demedullated animals may relate to the stressfulness of the task. Thus, adrenal demedullation does not impair inhibitory[32,49] or one-way active avoidance conditioning [23,39,50], but does impair acquisition of a two-way avoidance response[8,22]. Adrenal demedullation which removes most chromaffin tissue reduces the capacity of the organism to respond to stress and the system fails only under conditions of high stress of pharmacological challenge.

A most interesting question raised by these studies is how do exogenously administered 4-OH amphetamine and the enkephalins affect the storage of information in the brain. As outlined in the Introduction, there are several possible ways. These include passing directly into the brain through the blood circulating

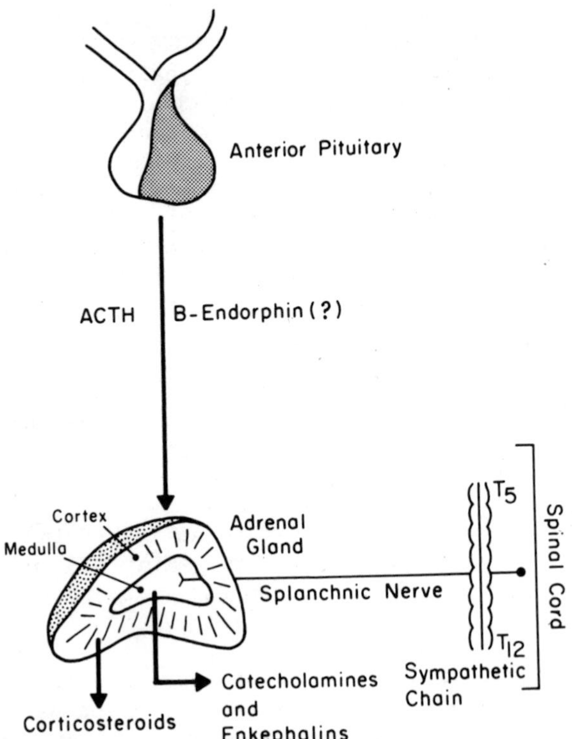

Figure 10. Schematic diagram of the major components of the pituitary-adrenal axis. The adrenal gland is composed of two major parts, the adrenal cortex and the adrenal medulla. The adrenal cortex releases corticosteroids in response to adrenocorticotropic hormone (ACTH) from the pituitary gland. The adrenal medulla releases the catecholamines norepinephrine and epinephrine and possibly the enkephalin-like peptides in response to stimulation from the splanchnic nerve. [From Martinez et al.[30]].

system, affecting regions lying outside the blood brain barrier, local concentration by specialized brain organs, or by acting on peripheral receptors which promote neuronal afferent feedback. At present, there is no way to choose among these possibilities. Yet, as noted earlier, a blood-borne hormone has a unique action because of the specificity and location of its receptive site. Thus, an understanding of how these agents affect CNS function and learning and memory is dependent on the characterization and localization of these receptive sites.

REFERENCES

1. Allen, J. P., Kendall, J. W., McGilvra R., and Vancura, C., Immunoreactive ACTH in cerebrospinal fluid, J. Clin. Endocrinol. Metab., 38:586 (1974).
2. Axelrod, J., Weil-Malberbe, H., and Tomchick, R., The physiological disposition of ^{3}H-epinephrine and its metabolite metanephrine, J. Pharm. Exp. Ther., 127:251 (1959).
3. Ball, G. G., Vagotomy: effect of electrically elicited eating and self-stimulation in the lateral hypothalamus, Science, 184:484 (1974).
4. Beaudet, A. and Descarries, L., The monoamine innervation of rat cerebral cortex: synaptic and nonsynaptic axon terminals, Neuroscience, 3:851 (1978).
5. Beckwith, B. E. and Sandman, C. A., Behavioral influences of the neuropeptides ACTH and MSH: a methodological review, Neurosci. Biobeh. Rev., 2:311 (1978).
6. Belluzzi, J. and Martinez, Jr., J. L., Differential actions of dl-amphetamine and dl-4-OH amphetamine on intracranial self-stimulation behavior, in preparation.
7. Conford, E. M., Braun, L. D., Crane, P. D., and Olendorf, H., Blood-brain barrier restriction of peptides and the low uptake of enkephalins, Endocrinology, 103:1297 (1978).
8. Conner, R. L. and Levine, S., The effects of adrenal hormones on the acquisition of signaled avoidance behavior, Hor. Behav., 1:73 (1969).
9. Cooper, J. R., Bloom, F. E., and Roth, R. H., "The Biochemical Basis of Neuropharmacology," Oxford University Press, New York (1978).
10. de Wied, D., Peptides and behavior, Life Sci., 20:195 (1977).
11. Dunn, A., Biochemical correlates of training experiences: A discussion of the evidence, in: "Neural Mechanisms of Learning and Memory," M. R. Rosenzweiz and E. L. Bennett, eds., The MIT Press, Cambridge (1976).
12. Dunwiddie, T., Madison, V., and Lynch, G., Synaptic transmission is required for initiation of long-term potentiation, Brain Res., 150:413 (1978).
13. Gold, P. E. and McCarty, R., Plasma catecholamines: changes after footshock and seizure-producing frontal cortex stimulation, Behav. Neur. Biol., 31:247 (1981).
14. Greenough, W. T., Development and memory: the synaptic connection, in: "Brain and Learning," T. Teyler, ed., Greylock, Stamford (1978).
15. Hexum, T. D., Yang, Y.-Y. T., and Costa, E., Biochemical characterization of enkephalin-like immunoreactive peptides of adrenal glands, Life Sci., 27:1211 (1980).
16. Hughes, J., Kosterlitz, H. W., and Smith, T. W., The distribution of methionine-enkephalin and leucine-enkephalin in the brain and peripheral tissues, Brit. J. Pharmacol., 61:639 (1977).

17. Ishikawa, K. and McGaugh, J. L., Simultaneous determination of monoamine transmitters, precursors and metabolites in a single mouse brain, J. Chromatogr., in press.
18. Javoy, F., Klowinski, J., and Kordon, C., Effects of adrenalectomy on the turnover of norepinephrine in the rat brain, Eur. J. Pharmacol., 4:103 (1968).
19. Kumakura, K., Karoum, F., Guidotti, A., and Costa, E., Modulation of nicotinic receptors by opiate receptor agonists in cultured adrenal chromaffin cells, Nature, 283:489 (1980).
20. Leshner, A. I., "An Introduction to Behavioral Endocrinology," Oxford University Press, New York (1978).
21. Levine, S., Hormones and conditioning, in: "Nebraska Symposium on Motivation," W. J. Arnold, ed., University of Nebraska Press, Lincoln (1968).
22. Levine, S. and Soliday, S., An effect of adrenal demedullation on the acquisition of a conditioned avoidance response, J. Comp. Physiol. Psychol., 55:214 (1962).
23. Martinez, Jr., J. L., Ishikawa, K., Hannan, T., Liang, K. C., Vasquez, B. J., Jensen, R. A., Sternberg, D., Brewton, C., and McGaugh, J. L., Actions of 4 OH-amphetamine on active avoidance conditioning and regional brain concentrations of norepinephrine and dopamine, Soc. Neurosci. Abst., 7 (1981).
24. Martinez, Jr., J. L., Ishikawa, K., Liang, K. C., Jensen, R. A., Brewton, C., Sternberg, D., Messing, R. B., and McGaugh, J. L., 4-OH amphetamine enhances retention of an active avoidance response in rats and decreases regional brain concentrations of norepinephrine and dopamine, in preparation.
25. Martinez, Jr., J. L., Jensen, R. A., Creager, R., Veliquette, J. Messing, R. B., McGaugh, J. L., and Lynch G., Selective effects of enkephalin on electrical activity of the *in vitro* hippocampal slice, Behav. Neur. Biol., 26:128 (1979).
26. Martinez, Jr., J. L., Jensen, R. A., Messing, R. B., Vasquez, B. J., Soumireu-Mourat, B., Geddes, D., Liang, K. C., and McGaugh, J. L., Central and peripheral actions of amphetamine on memory storage, Brain Res., 182:157 (1980).
27. Martinez, Jr., J. L., Jensen, R. A., Vasquez, B. J., Lacob, J. S., McGaugh, J. L., and Purdy, R. E., Acquisition deficits induced by sodium nitrite in rats and mice, Psychopharmcol., 60:221 (1979).
28. Martinez, Jr., J. L., McGaugh, J. L., Hanes, C.L., and Lacob, J. S., Modulation of memory processes induced by stimulation of the entorhinal cortex, Physiol. Behav., 19:139 (1977).
29. Martinez, Jr., J. L. and Rigter, H., Enkephalin actions on avoidance conditioning may be related to adrenal medullary function, in preparation.

30. Martinez, Jr., J. L., Rigter, H., Jensen, R. A., Messing, R. B., Vasquez, B. J., and McGaugh, J. L. Endorphin and enkephalin effects on avoidance conditioning: the other side of the pituitary-adrenal axis, in: "Endogenous Peptides and Learning and Memory Processes," J.L. Martinez, Jr., R. A. Jensen, R. B. Messing, H. Rigter, and J. L. McGaugh, eds. Academic Press, New York (1981).

31. Martinez, Jr., J. L., Rigter, H., and van der Gugten, J., Enkephalin effects on avoidance conditioning are dependent on the adrenal glands, in: "Endocrinology, Neuroendocrinology, Neuropeptides I.," E. Stark, G. B. Makara, Zs. Ács, and E. Endröczi, eds., Pergamon Press, London (1981).

32. Martinez, Jr., J. L., Vasquez, B. J., Rigter, H., Messing, R. B., Jensen, R. A., Liang, K. C., and McGaugh, J. L., Attenuation of amphetamine-induced enhancement of learning by adrenal demedullation, Brain Res., 195:433 (1980).

33. Mason, J. W., Organization of the multiple endocrine responses to avoidance in the monkey, Psychosom. Med. 30:774 (1968).

34. Mason, J. W., The integrative approach in medicine - implications of neuroendocrine mechanisms, Perspect. Biol. Med., 17:333 (1974).

35. McGaugh, J. L. and Martinez, Jr., J. L., Learning modulatory hormones: an introduction to endogenous peptides and learning and memory processes, in: "Endogenous Peptides and Learning and Memory Processes," J. L. Martinez, Jr., R. A. Jensen, R. B. Messing, H. Rigter, and J. L. McGaugh, eds., Academic Press, New York (1981).

36. McGaugh, J. L., Martinez, Jr., J. L., Jensen, R. A., Hannan, T. J., Vasquez, B. J., Messing, R. B., Liang, K. C., Brewton, C. B., and Spiehler, V. R., Modulation of memory storage by treatments affecting peripheral catecholamines, in: "Neurobiology of Learning and Memory," H. Matthies, ed., Raven Press, New York, in press.

37. Meligeni, J. A., Ledergerber, S. A., and McGaugh, J. L., Norepinephrine attenuation of amnesia produced by diethyldithiocarbamate, Brain Res., 149:155 (1978).

38. Messing, R. B., Vasquez, B. J., Spiehler, V. R., Martinez, Jr., J. L., Jensen, R. A., Rigter, H., and McGaugh, J. L., ^{3}H-Dihydromorphine binding in brain regions of young and aged rats, Life Sci., 26:921 (1980).

39. Moyer, K. E. and Bunnell, B. N., Effect of adrenal demedullation on an avoidance response in the rat, J. Comp. Physiol. Psychol., 52:215 (1959).

40. Ogren, S. and Fuxe, K., Learning, brain noradrenaline and the pituitary-adrenal axis, Med. Biol., 52:399 (1974).

41. Palfai, T. and Walsh, T. J., The role of peripheral catecholamines in reserpine-induced amnesia, Behav. Neur. Biol., 27:423 (1979).

42. Rapoport, S. I., Klee, W. A., Pettigrew, K. D., and Ohno, K. Entry of opioid peptides into the central nervous system, Science, 207:84 (1980).

43. Rigter, H., Attenuation of amnesia in rats by systemically administered enkephalins, Science, 200:83 (1978).

44. Rigter, H., Dekker, I., and Martinez, Jr., J. L., A comparison of the ability of opioid peptides and opiates to affect active avoidance conditioning in rats, Regul. Pept., in press.

45. Rigter, H., Jensen, R. A., Martinez, Jr., J. L., Messing, R. B., Vasquez, B. J., Liang, K. C., and McGaugh, J. L., Enkephalin and fear-motivated behavior, Proc. Nat. Acad. Sci. USA, 77:3729 (1980).

46. Rigter, H., Hannan, T. J., Messing, R. B., Martinez, Jr., J. L., Vasquez, B. J., Jensen, R. A., Veliquette, J., and McGaugh, J. L., Enkephalins interfere with acquisition of an active avoidance response, Life Sci., 26:337 (1980).

47. Roberts, D. S. C. and Fibiger, H. C., Evidence for interactions between central noradrenergic neurons and adrenal hormones in learning and memory, Pharmacol. Biochem. Behav., 7:191 (1977).

48. Shellenberger, M. K. and Gordon, J. H., A rapid, simplified procedure for simultaneous assay of norepinephrine, dopamine, and 5-hydroxy-tryptamine from discrete brain areas. Analytical Biochemistry, 39:356 (1971).

49. Silva, M. T. A., Extinction of a passive avoidance response in adrenalectomized and demedullated rats, Behav. Biol., 9:553 (1973).

50. Silva, M. T. A., Effects of adrenal demedullation and adrenalectomy on an active avoidance response of rats, Physiol. Psychol., 2:171 (1974).

51. Stein, L., Effects and interactions of imipramine, chlorpromazine, reserpine and amphetamine on self-stimulation: possible neurophysiological basis of depression, in: "Recent Advances in Biological Psychiatry," Vol. 4, J. Wortis, ed., Plenum Press, New York (1962).

52. Stein, L., Norepinephrine reward pathways: role in self-stimulation, memory consolidation, and schizophrenia, University of Nebraska Press, Lincoln (1974).

53. Stein, L., Belluzzi, J. D., and Wise, C. D., Memory enhancement by central administration of norepinephrine, Brain Res., 84:329 (1975).

54. Sternberg, D. B. and Gold, P. E., Effects of α- and β-adrenergic receptor antagonists on retrograde amnesia produced by frontal cortex stimulation, Behav. Neur. Biol., 29:289 (1980).

55. Sutherland, E. W., Studies on the mechanism of hormone action, Science, 177:401 (1972).

56. Thompson, R. F., Patterson, M. M., and Berger T., Associative learning in the mammalian nervous system, in: "Brain and Learning," T. Teylor, ed., Greylock, Stamford (1978).
57. Urca, G., Frenk, H., Liebeskind, J. C., and Taylor, A. N., Morphine and enkephalin: analgesic and epileptic properties, Science, 197:83 (1977).
58. Viveros, O. H., Diliberto, Jr., E. J., Hazum, E., and Chang, K.-J., Opiate-like meterials in the adrenal medulla: evidence for storage and secretion with catecholamines, Molec. Pharmacol., 16:1101 (1979).
59. Walsh, T. J. and Palfai, T., Peripheral catecholamines and memory: characteristics of syrosingopine-induced amnesia, Pharmacol. Biochem. Behav., 11:449 (1979).
60. Weindl, A. and Sofroniew, M. V., Relation of neuropeptides to mammalian circumventricular organs, in: "Neurosecretion and Brain Peptides," J. B. Martin, S. Reichin, and K. L. Bick, eds., Raven Press, New York (1981).
61. Wise, C. D. and Stein, L., Facilitation of brain self-stimulation by central administration of norepinephrine, Science, 163:299 (1969).
62. Witter, A., Gispen, W. H., and de Wied, D., Mechanisms of action of behaviorally active ACTH-like peptides, in: "Endogenous Peptides and Learning and Memory Processes," J. L. Martinez, Jr., R. A. Jensen, R. B. Messing, H. Rigter, and J. L. McGaugh, eds., Academic Press, New York (1981).
63. Yang, H.-Y. T., Hexum, T., and Costa, E. Opioid peptides in adrenal gland, Life Sci., 27:1119 (1980).

CENTRAL MECHANISMS RESPONSIBLE FOR CLASSICALLY CONDITIONED CHANGES IN NEURONAL ACTIVITY

James H. O'Brien and Kevin J. Quinn

Department of Medical Psychology
The Oregon Health Sciences University
Portland, Oregon

SUMMARY

Data relevant to a model of cortical single neuron conditioning from two related studies are presented and the results compared with those in the current literature in this field. Although peripheral stimulation can serve as an effective CS in a neural classical conditioning paradigm, central stimulation of major thalamocortical input systems cannot. These results raise problems for theories of neural learning. Evidently the patterned activation of different types of input systems is necessary for associative conditioning in pyramidal tract neurons in the motor cortex of cats.

INTRODUCTION

Studies of single neuron changes during conditioning have been of increasing interest in recent years in an attempt to understand the physiological basis of learning. Furthermore, the need for precise control over the conditions under which learning takes place has led to the use of model systems for investigation at both the behavioral and neural level. Classical conditioning is one such general paradigm that has proved to be a useful tool because it enables one to define experimentally, with great precision, the necessary elements for learning to occur. Thus, in classical conditioning, there is a change in the response of the organism to the CS as a function of the pairing of the CS with a following US.

A key problem for the neurophysiological analysis of learning has been expressed by Robert Doty[1] as the "temporal paradox of conditioning." The paradox arises because it is the preceding stimulus, the CS, whose effectiveness is altered rather than that of the subsequent stimulus, the US. These two points, the necessity for pairing of events and the "temporal paradox" of this pairing form two of the basic questions for research in the neurophysiology of learning.

Cohen (2), Thompson (3), and Woody (4) have all advocated the use of classical conditioning of specific response systems as model systems ideal for the analysis of neural events underlying observed changes in behavioral output. An important consideration in this analysis has been determining whether the modifications in neural activity recorded in a particular experiment represent local or projected changes. That is, change in response by a neuron could be the passive result of changes in activity occurring elsewhere which are then relayed through the neuron being monitored or this change in response could be an active process occurring locally at the post- or pre-synaptic membrane. This latter alternative offers the greatest opportunity for gaining additional insight into the basic mechanisms underlying changes in CNS activity during conditioning.

The work of both Olds and Woody and their associates (5,6,7, 8,9) have offered important insights on this issue. Work in our laboratory has also been aimed at the local learning issue for many years. One technique for pinpointing sites of local learning involves truncating the neural system being studied. Thus, O'Brien and Fox (10,11) demonstrated that cells in the motor cortex of the cat undergo changes in firing pattern during a sensory classical conditioning paradigm which exhibit the major characteristics of learning (habituation, conditioning, and extinction). O'Brien, Wilder and Stevens (12) have shown more recently that pyramidal tract (PT) cells in the postcruciate cortex of the cat show changes in firing rate attributable to a differential classical conditioning paradigm when the US was antidromic activation of the PT cell. This and other evidence (13) indicated that PT cells in the motor cortex were indeed sites of local learning. Quinn and O'Brien (14) and Quinn (15) further truncated this system by using antidromic activation of PT cells as the US and thalamic stimulation as the CS in the hope of being able to further delineate the specific pathways functioning as CS input to the cells.

The purpose of the present report is to review the results of the O'Brien, Wilder, and Stevens paper and the Quinn and O'Brien paper in the context of some of the current literature in this field (7,16,17,18,19,20,21,22,23) and discuss the implications of this work for theories concerning CNS plasticity.

METHODS

Experiment 1 (12)

Preparation. Surgery was performed on cats under ether anesthesia. The saphenous vein was cannulated, an endotracheal tube was inserted and the animal then was placed in a stereotaxic instrument. The temporal muscles were reflected and small burr holes were made in the skull to permit insertion of the microelectrode and the PT stimulation electrode. All exposed tissue and stereotaxic pressure points then were infused with xylocaine (repeated every 3 hr). A microelectrode, glass-coated wire (25 um) or etched stainless steel insect pin (2-5 um), was placed in the postcruciate cortex (approximately 1.5 mm posterior to the suclus and 1.5 mm lateral from the midline). A concentric macroelectrode (.25 mm-diam. stainless steel wire in hypodermic stock) was placed in the PT at the level of the brain stem (P 8.0, L 1.0). The final vertical placement of the PT electrode was determined by the antidromic response in the cortex. Ether anesthesia was terminated, gallamine triethiodide (Flaxedil) was infused and artificial respiration was begun. The stroke volume was adjusted to maintain tracheal CO_2 levels at 3.6-4.0% as monitored on a Godart capnograph.

Experimental design. A classical conditining paradigm was used, with pyramidal stimulation as the US. Electrical stimulation through subcutaneous needles in the left and right hind paws was used for the conditioned stimuli, with the CS+ to one paw paired with the US and the CS- to the other paw unpaired; hind paw assignment for CS+ and CS- was the same for all the neurons recorded from an individual cat but was randomized among cats. This balanced the groups for any possible differences between contralateral and ipsilateral paws. The sequence of CS+ and CS- presentation was randomized within a block of 25 trials and the intertrial interval was randomized around a mean of 12 sec (range of 6-18 sec). A differential conditioning paradigm was used because it controls not only for sensitization and pseudoconditioning but also for momentary changes in the state of the animal, such as blood pressure, CO_2 level, electrode movement, and other factors affecting neuronal spike activity. The total series consisted of 150 trials without the US but with both the CS+ and CS-, 450 trials containing 225 CS+ paired with the US and 225 CS- unpaired, and again 150 trials without the US. This corresponds to habituation, conditioning, and extinction, respectively. The CS-US interval was 550 msec.

For the experimental group of 20 cats, the pyramidal stimulation voltage was set so that each stimulus produced an antidromic spike in the recorded cortical neuron. For the control group of 22 cats, the pyramidal stimulation voltage was first determined for antidromic firing and then set just below threshold so that no antidromic spikes were produced in the recorded cortical neuron. A similarity of stimulus voltage for the two groups was achieved by choosing neurons for the control group that required slightly higher stimulus voltages to produce an antidromic spike. We assumed the voltage required reflected the distance of the axon from the stimulating electrode. The purpose of the control group was to determine whether the antidromic activation in the experimental group was sufficient to produce conditioning or whether regular orthodromic pathways were contributing to the conditioning.

The CSs were three .2-ms pulses at a frequency of 250 Hz, and a voltage adjusted to just above threshold for a unit response (generally 5-10 V). On the basis of results of a behavioral experiment (24) these stimuli do not appear to have any aversive character. The US for the experimental group was a 100-ms train of twenty-five .1-ms pulses at a voltage just above the threshold to elicit an antidromic response in the recorded neuron. The usual antidromic response showed a latency of 1-2 ms and followed to stimulation around 200-300/sec. The parameters for pyramidal stimulation in the control group were the same except the voltage was set below the threshold to elicit an antidromic spike in the cortical neuron. No differences were found for the latencies of antidromic spikes in the control and experimental groups. The average stimulus voltage was 15 V in the experimental group and 18 V in the control group. The experiment and unit data collection were controlled on-line by a PDP-12 computer. The unit data were recorded through a Bak cathode follower and modified Tektronix 122 preamplifier (filter 500 Hz-3 kHz) and were continuously monitored on an oscilloscope to assure that the Schmitt trigger setting reliably excluded noise.

Basic quantification of data. Twenty-five trial blocks of unit data were accumulated in the form of a peristimulus histogram and the response represented as a difference score between the mean rate of a selected portion of the CS-US interval and the mean rate of the 1-sec pre-CS period.

Experiment 2 (14,15)

The procedures for Experiment 2 were similar to those for Experiment 1 with the following exceptions. The cats were prepared surgically under halothane anesthesia approximately one week before running of the experiment. At this time, plastic tubes were attached to the skull which enabled the animal to be mounted in a Kopf semi-chronic headholder during the experimental phase. The PT electrode was placed at a thalamic level (AP +6.0, L 5.5). Bipolar electrodes were placed in the ventral posterolateral (VPL) (AP +9.0, L 6.5, V +1.5) and the ventral lateral (VL) (AP 11.0, L 4.5, V 2.0) nuclei of the thalamus. Final vertical placement of these electrodes was determined by monitoring evoked activity in the thalamus to peripheral limb stimulation and in the cortex to thalamic stimulation. Stimulation of VPL and VL served as the CSs in Experiment 2 as opposed to stimulation of the right and left hind limbs which served as the CSs in Experiment 1. Thalamic stimulation parameters were one 0.1 ms pulse at about 14 volts. The experimental design was identical to that used in Experiment 1 and neuronal data were grouped and analyzed in a similar fashion.

RESULTS

Figure 1 shows the principal results of Experiment 1. In this experiment, stimulation of the right and left hindpaws served as the CSs. The top graph shows the responses of those neurons in which the PT stimulus was above threshold for producing antidromic spikes. The bottom graph shows the responses of those neurons in which the PT stimulus was just below threshold for antidromic activation.

In the top graph, stimulation of the hindpaw which was consistently paired (CS+) with the US (suprathreshold PT stimulation) resulted in a neuronal response which incremented over conditioning trials and dropped off during extinction trials when the CS+ was again presented alone. Stimulation of the hind limb which was not paired (CS-) with the US resulted in a neuronal response which showed a gradual increment for the initial 100 conditioning trials and then slowly leveled off. The development of a differential response of neurons over trials to the CS+ versus the CS- was statistically significant ($\underline{F}[8, 527] = 4.45$, $\underline{p} < .001$).

In the bottom graph, although there was a gradual increment in response to both the CS+ and CS- over trials, a differential increase to the CS+ versus the CS- did not occur. The experiment displayed in the bottom graph was run to assess the importance of afferent systems activated by the US in the development of conditioning. Together, the top and bottom graphs demonstrate that the antidromic activation of the neuron is necessary in order to show development of differential conditioning. Neurons selected for the experimental results displayed in the top and bottom graphs were always PT neurons; however, for the group in the top graph the stimulus level for the PT electrode was set just above threshold for producing antidromic spikes while for the group in the bottom graph the PT stimulus was set just subthreshold for producing antidromic spikes. The average voltage levels used in these experiments for PT stimulation were quite similar (in fact, the voltage level used for neurons in the bottom graph was slightly higher).

Together the results in Figure 1 indicate that the antidromic activation of the PT neuron can function as an effective US in a differential conditioning paradigm in which the CSs are peripheral limb stimulation.

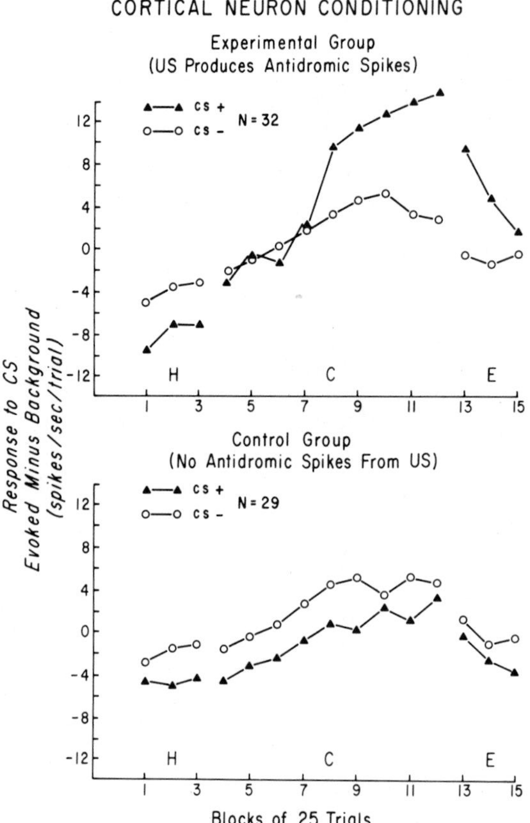

Figure 1. Differential conditioning of cortical neurons with paw stimulation as the CS. Top: Pyramidal tract stimulation (US) set to produce antidromic activation of the recorded neuron; note that a differential response change develops between the CS+ and CS-. Bottom: Pyramidal tract stimulation set below threshold to produce antidromic activation of the recorded neuron; note that no differential conditioned response occurs.

Figure 2 shows the principal results of Experiment 2. In this experiment, stimulation of VPL and VL served as the CSs (as opposed to stimulation of the hindlimbs in Experiment 1). As for Experiment 1, the US was stimulation of the PT. For Experiment 2, the US was always set just above threshold for producing antidromic spikes. Thalamic stimulation produces a stereotyped response pattern in PT cells (14,15) consisting of an early latency (< 10 ms) and a longer latency, rebound (100-200 ms) excitatory response.

Figure 2 shows the results for both the early (top graph) and rebound (bottom graph) excitatory response periods. The smaller N for the early response period is due to the fact that fewer cells showed a tendency to respond to both VPL and VL stimulation at this latency. All cells studied showed the longer latency response to both VPL and VL stimulation.

As can be seen in Figure 2, there was no evidence of differential conditioning to the CS+ versus the CS- for either the early or the rebound excitatory response periods. In addition, there was no evidence of a general increment in response to either the CS+ or CS- which was seen in both the top and bottom graphs of Figure 1. These results indicated that simple activation of discrete thalamic nuclei could not function as effective CSs when paired with antidromic activation of the neuron as the US.

DISCUSSION

The negative results of Experiment 2, when combined with the positive results of Experiment 1, present a dilemma. Presumably a major pathway by which the peripheral CR input reached the PT cells in Experiment 1 was via thalamocortical afferents to which VPL and VL fibers would make a significant contribution. Thus, there would not seem to be any reason why VPL or VL fibers, per se, would be unable to support conditioning. Thus, the negative results of Experiment 2 present a problem of interpretation.

The results of Experiment 1 support the concept that antidromic activation of the neuron can serve as an effective US. A number of other studies also support this conclusion. Black-Cleworth, et al. (7) were able to condition a behavioral response (eye blink) using electrical stimulation of the motor branch of the facial nerve as the US. In related work, Mis, Gormezano, and Harvey, (21) Martin, Land and Thompson, (2) and Powell and Moore (22) all reported some measure of success in obtaining conditioning of nictitating membrane extension using electrical stimulation of the abducens nucleus as the US. In work closely related to the present study, Baranyi and Feher (16,17,18) have reported some measure of success in obtaining conditioning of PT cell activity

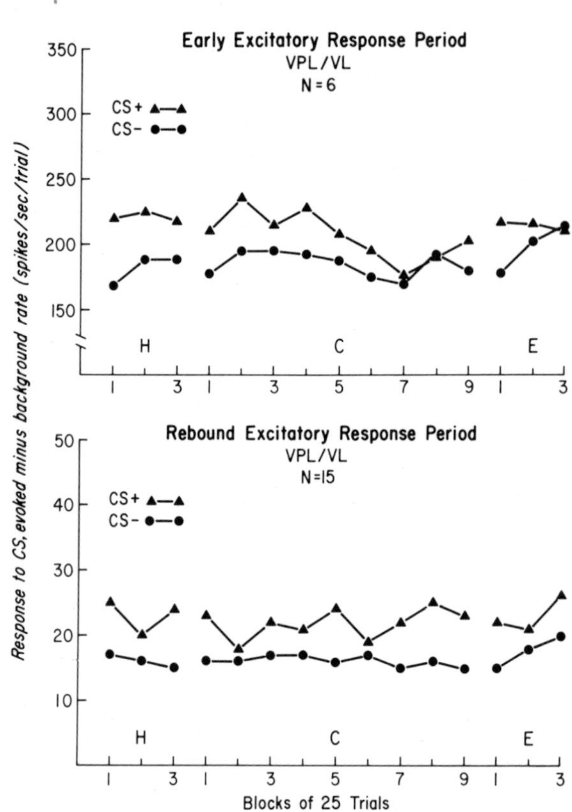

Figure 2. Response of PT cells to thalamic stimulation during administration of conditioning paradigm. Upper graph - early excitatory response period. Lower graph - rebound excitatory response period. H = blocks of habituation trials, C = blocks of conditioning trials, E = blocks of extinction trials.

using antidromic stimulation as the US. Furthermore, Bindman et al. (19) have shown long lasting potentiation of PT activity following antidromic activation. Taken as a whole, these data weigh heavily in favor of the ability of central stimulation of motor output systems to serve as effective USs.

Comparisons of Figures 1 and 2 show that the overall magnitude of response of cells in Experiment 2 was much higher than in Experiment 1. Direct thalamic stimulation is much more effective in driving PT cell activity than peripheral stimulation. It is possible that the failure to obtain a conditioned increase in activity in Experiment 2 was due to the fact that the neurons were already being driven at 100% effectiveness and no further increase was possible. However, further data of Quinn and O'Brien (14) and Quinn (15) indicate that it is possible to produce increased rates of firing in PT cells in response to stimulation of VPL under special circumstances (coactivation of the nonspecific thalamus).

A third possibility for the negative results concerns the selection of an inappropriate CS-US interval. Baranyi and Feher (17) using stimulation of VL as the CS and PT stimulation as the US found that CS-US intervals of less than 100 ms duration were necessary in order to obtain positive results. Thus, there is a large discrepancy between the interval selected for use in Experiment 2 (550 ms) and the "optimal" interval as defined by Baranyi and Feher (17). It should be noted, however, that their intertrial interval (ITI) was only 1 sec. Others (23) have found that ITIs this short tend to produce nonassociative changes in neuronal firing. Although they used appropriate controls for pseudoconditioning, the shortness of their ITI makes the results of Baranyi and Feher (17) difficult to interpret.

In addition, it should be noted that the behavioral literature has by and large supported the contention that optimal conditioning is obtained with CS-US intervals of .5 sec or greater, depending on the response system studied. Furthermore, positive results were obtained in Experiment 1 with a 550 ms CS-US interval.

Thus, in terms of the parameters selected for use in Experiment 2, there does not seem to be a good explanation for the negative results. This points to the conclusion that a simple hypothesis of pairing of neural events as the underlying mechanism for neuronal associative conditioning may be inaccurate. The major difference between Experiments 1 and 2 would appear to be the manner in which the cells were activated by the CS. In the former case, the CS was a complex patterned activation of a variety of pathways whereas in the latter the CS was a relatively discrete and homogeneous activation of one class of input fibers.

At least for the case of associative conditioning in the motor cortex, the effective CS would not appear to be the simple activation of a particular input system. In related work, Voronon (23) has found that use of a compound US (cortical plus hypothalamic stimulation vs cortical stimulation alone) increased the tendency for neurons to show associative conditioning. Thus, a simple pairing theory of conditioning in which any two pathways to a given neuron can be used as the CS and US does not appear to be generally valid. Rather, the activation of different types of input pathways in a particular pattern appears to be a necessary feature for the occurrence of conditioning.

ACKNOWLEDGEMENTS

This work was supported by a grant from the Whitehall Foundation, an NSF Predoctoral Fellowship and an N. L. Tarter Research Fellowship.

REFERENCES

1. Doty, R. W. Electrical stimulation of the brain in behavioral context. Ann Rev Psychol 20: 289-230, 1969.
2. Cohen, D. H. Development of a vertebrate experimental model for cellular neurophysiologic studies of learning. Cond Reflex 4: 61-80, 1969.
3. Thompson, R. F., Berger, T. W., Cegavske, C. F., Patterson, M. M., Roemer, R. A., Teyler, T. J., & Young, R. A. The search for the engram. Am Psychol 31: 209-227, 1976.
4. Woody, C. D. Aspects of the electrophysiology of cortical processes related to the development and performance of learned motor responses. The Physiologist 17: 49-69, 1974.
5. Olds, J., Disterhoft, J. F., Segal, M., Kornblith, C. L., & Hirsh, R. Learning centers of rat brain mapped by measuring latencies of conditioned unit responses. J Neurophysiol 35: 202-219, 1972.
6. Segal, M., & Olds, J. Behavior of units in hippocampal circuit of the rat during learning. J Neurophysiol 35: 680-690, 1972.
7. Black-Cleworth, P., Woody, C. D., & Niemann, J. A conditioned eyeblink obtained by using electrical stimulation of the facial nerve as the unconditioned stimulus. Brain Res 90: 45-56, 1975.
8. Woody, C. D., & Black-Cleworth, P. Differences in excitability of cortical neurons as a function of motor projection in conditioned cats. J Neurophysiol 36: 1104-1115, 1973.
9. Woody, C. D., Vassilevsky, N. N., & Engel, J. Jr. Conditioned eye blink: unit activity at coronal-precruciate cortex of the cat. J Neurophysiol 33: 851-864, 1970.
10. O'Brien, J. H. & Fox, S. S. Single-cell activity in cat motor cortex. I. Modifications during classical conditioning procedures. J Neurophysiol 32: 267-284, 1969.

11. O'Brien, J. H., & Fox, S. S. Single-cell activity in cat motor cortex. II. Functional characteristics of the cell related to conditioning changes. J Neurophysiol 32: 285-296, 1969.
12. O'Brien, J. H., Wilder, M. B., & Stevens, C. D. Conditioning of cortical neurons in cats with antidromic activation as the unconditioned stimulus. J Comp Physiol Psychol 91: 918-929, 1977.
13. Rosenblum, S. M. & O'Brien, J. H. A cryogenic study of cortical conditioning changes. J Neurophysiol 40: 957-967, 1977.
14. Quinn, K. J. & O'Brien, J. H. Neuronal responses during classical conditioning using central stimulation as the CS and US. Manuscript in preparation, 1981.
15. Quinn, K. J. Responses of pyramidal tract cells during a differential classical conditioning paradigm using central stimulation as the conditioned and unconditioned stimuli. Unpublished PhD Dissertation, University of Oregon Health Sciences Center, 1981.
16. Baranyi, A. & Feher, O. Conditioned changes of synaptic transmission in the motor cortex of the cat. Exp Brain Res 33: 283-298, 1978.
17. Baranyi, A. & Feher, O. Intracellular studies on cortical synaptic plasticity. Exp Brain Res 41: 124-134, 1981.
18. Baranyi, A. & Feher, O. Synaptic facilitation requires paired activation of convergent pathways in the neocortex. Nature 290: 413-414, 1981.
19. Bindman, L. J., Lippold, O. C. J., & Milne, A. R. Prolonged changes in excitability of pyramidal tract neurones in the cat: a postsynaptic mechanism. J Physiol 286: 457-477, 1979.
20. Martin, G. K., Land, T., & Thompson, R. F. Classical conditioning of the rabbit (oryctolagus cuniculus) nictitating membrane response, with electrical brain stimulation as the unconditioned stimulus. J Comp Physiol Psych 94: 216-226, 1980.
21. Mis, F. W., Gormezano, I., & Harvey, J. A. Stimulation of abducens nucleus supports classical conditioning of the nictitating membrane response. Science 206: 473-475, 1979.
22. Powell, G. M. & Moore, J. W. Conditioning of the nictitating membrane response in rabbit (oryctolagus cuniculus) with electrical brain-stimulation as the unconditioned stimulus. Physiol & Behav 25: 205-216, 1980.
23. Voronin, L. L. Microelectrode analysis of the cellular mechanisms of conditioned reflex in rabbits. Acta Neurobio Exp 40: 335-370, 1980.
24. O'Brien, J. H. & Packham, S. C. Conditioned leg movement in the cat with massed trials, trace conditioning and weak US intensity. Cond Reflex 8: 116-124, 1973.

ASSOCIATIVE PROCESSES IN SPINAL REFLEXES

Michael M. Patterson, Joseph E. Steinmetz
Alvin L. Beggs, and Anthony G. Romano

College of Osteopathic Medicine and
Department of Psychology
Ohio University, Athens, Ohio 45701

SUMMARY

Acute, paralyzed, spinal cats were used to examine extinction and retention parameters as well as the involvement of cutaneous afferent terminals in classical conditioning of a hindlimb flexor nerve response. The CS consisted of a train of pulses delivered to the superficial peroneal (sensory) nerve and the UCS was a 50 V shock delivered to the ankle skin of the same hind leg. Conditions was measured as an increase in the response amplitude of the deep peroneal (motor) nerve. First, the effects of presenting massed vs. distributed extinction trials were explored. Conditioned response amplitude decrements were found when 60 extinction trials were administered immediately after aquisition at a rate of one per minute (massed condition). These decrements were not apparent when one extinction trial was delivered every ten minutes (distributed condition). From this data it is apparent that the conditioned response increase does not fall off spontaneously over a two hour period. In the second experiment, significant differences were not found between groups of animals allowed 1/2, 1, 2, 3, or 4 hr. between acquisition and extinction trials. These results were interpreted to indicate that response amplitude increases noted during acquisition were not the product of simple sensitization. Finally, excitability changes involving cutaneous afferent terminals were studied using the antidromic invasion technique. No tonic or phasic excitability changes were found over the course of training. This finding indicates that presynaptic facilitation is not involved in response amplitude increases observed during classical conditioning of the cat hindlimb flexor nerve response.

INTRODUCTION

Initial attempts to classically condition spinal reflexes using a spinalized preparation were undertaken by Culler and Shurrager (e.g., Shurrager & Culler, 1938). In these studies, the investigators reported successful conditioning of reflex leg flexion in acute spinal dogs when a tail shock or leg touch conditioned stimulus (CS) was paired with a leg shock unconditioned stimulus (UCS). The results were interpreted as showing the establishment of a "substitute response which was not reflexly present after transection" (Shurrager & Culler, 1940). In another series of studies, however, Kellogg and associates generally failed to find changes in spinal reflex responses with stimulus pairing (e.g., Kellogg, Pronko, & Deese, 1946). These researchers contended that the response alterations obtained by the Culler group were simply changes involving pre-existing responses, thus not associative "learning". Since these early studies many successful (e.g., Durkovic, 1975) as well as unsuccessful (e.g., Lloyd, Wikler, & Whitehouse, 1969) reports of classical conditioning involving the spinal reflexes have surfaced. See Patterson (1976) for a comprehensive review of the spinal conditioning literature.

Our work in spinal conditioning procedures evolved from a preparation initially described by Fitzgerald and Thompson (1967). These authors utilized electrical stimulation of the thigh skin as a CS and shock to the footpad as a US to classically condition the hindlimb flexion reflex in acute spinal cats. Paired CS-UCS trials resulted in conditioning of the flexion reflex in response to the CS as measured by an increase in the magnitude of contraction of the tibialis anterior muscle. In an initial series of studies, Patterson, Cegavske, and Thompson (1973) used a similar isolated cat spinal cord preparation to measure response alteration to CS-UCS pairings as compared to control conditions. In this preparation stimulation of the superficial peroneal (sensory) nerve constitutes a CS and a standard 50 volt pulse train delivered to the skin of the ankle of the same leg serves as the UCS. Conditioning is measured as an increase in the response amplitude of the deep peroneal (motor) nerve. The first study used a co-terminating 750 msec CS and 500 msec UCS with a fixed 60 sec intertrial interval (ITI) and a 250 msec interstimulus interval (ISI). Under these conditions, response to the CS increased over trials when the CS and UCS were paired, but not when the stimuli were presented 30 sec apart in an unpaired manner. Most of the response increase occurred in the first 20-25 trials and response amplitude decreased with CS-alone presentations (extinction). In a second study, a CS-alone control group was added and the length of the ITI randomized (i.e., mean 60 sec. paired; 30 sec. unpaired). Pairing the CS and UCS resulted in response increases whereas cats that received unpaired or CS-alone trials failed to demonstrate conditioning. Finally, an estimation of the amount and duration of response alterations produced by the UCS alone was made by presenting the CS at various times following the UCS. The results indicated a general response increase beginning almost immediately following the UCS, but disappearing before the 30 or 60 sec. ITI of the unpaired and paired conditioning groups. These findings show that the results of pairing are not simply due to sensitization effects produced by UCS presentations.

Patterson (1975a) utilized a backward conditioning paradigm to study the effect of CS-UCS overlap that occurs during pairing. In this study, the CS and UCS were paired normally and at 100 msec and 250 msec backward intervals (i.e., UCS onset preceded CS onset). The results indicated normal conditioning when forward pairing was utilized but no response increase when either backward interval was used. Thus, response increases noted in the paired animals are not the result of additive effects initiated by stimulus overlap. Patterson (1975b) varied the ISI to find an optimal stimulus asynchrony for producing response alterations in the spinal conditioning preparation. Nine groups of cats were presented the CS and UCS at 0, 20, 60, 125, 250, 500, 1000, 2000, and 4000 msec ISIs. The greatest response increase was seen with a 250 msec ISI, lesser at 60, 125, 500, and 1000 msec, and little at 20, 2000, and 4000 msec. Simultaneous CS and UCS presentation resulted in a slight decrease or inhibition of response. The results are very similar to results obtained by ISI manipulations in conditioning studies involving intact subjects (e.g., Smith, Coleman, & Gormezano, 1969).

The present paper provides additional information regarding retention and extinction parameters and the neurophysiology of spinal conditioning procedures. Three studies recently completed or currently underway are presented here: 1) An examination of the effects of presenting massed versus distributed extinction trials, 2) An analysis of conditioned response retention as a function of varying time intervals allowed between acquisition and extinction, and 3) An examination of the excitability of the cutaneous afferent terminals during spinal conditioning procedures.

EXPERIMENT 1

Methods

Forty-two adult male and female cats purchased from local animal suppliers were used in this experiment. The apparatus used in the present series of experiments as well as general surgical procedures have been detailed elsewhere (Patterson, 1975a; Patterson, Cegavske, & Thompson, 1973). Briefly, a three-channel film reader programmed ITIs and gated the presentation of the CS and UCS. Grass S88 and S48 stimulators were used to initiate the stimuli which were delivered to the animals through Grass SIU5 stimulation-isolation units. Bipolar platinum-iridium wire electrodes were used to deliver the CS and record the amplified gross nerve volleys. The nerve responses were photographed automatically with a Grass C4 kymograph camera. The surgically prepared animals were held in a rigid frame on a Kopf spinal investigation table. Expired CO2 levels were constantly monitored by a Beckman CO2 analyzer and a CO2 level of about 5% was maintained in the paralyzed cat by adjusting respiratory volume of a Harvard small animal respirator. An infusion pump was utilized for long-term iv injections while a thermostatically controlled heating pad maintained the animals body temperature.

Following etherization and endotracheal intubation, a spinal transection at the 12th thoracic vertebra was performed on each subject. Subsequently, ether was removed, Flaxedil injected iv for paralysis, and respiration begun. The superficial peroneal sensory and deep peroneal motor nerves of the left leg were dissected free, the cut ends of the nerves crushed, and subsequently tied to the distal electrodes. The UCS, a 500 msec train of 25 Hz, 2 msec, 50 v pulses delivered through stainless steel wound clips to the left ankle skin, was given and subjects showing a nerve response of less than 0.08 mv were discarded as damaged. Intensity of the CS, a train of 10 Hz, 1 msec pulses which was coterminous with the UCS, was set to give a response about .02-.04 mv. Each subject was then allowed to rest for a period of time until the response to the CS was stable to infrequent test pulses.

Subjects were next randomly assigned to one of six experimental conditions (n=7). The six groups differed in the number of paired acquisition trials they received as well as the manner and number of extinction (CS-alone) trials that followed acquisition. All subjects were given 15 CS-alone trials to establish a baseline response amplitude and these trials were followed immediately by either 20, 40, or 60 acquisition trials. An average ITI of 60 sec. was used during acquisition while the ISI was maintained at 250 msec. Each acquisition group was further subdivided into two groups that received either massed or distributed extinction trials immediately after acquisition. Animals in the massed condition were given a total of 60 CS-alone presentations with an average ITI of 60 sec. Animals in the distributed condition received one CS-alone presentation every 10 min. until a total of 12 extinction trials were administered over a 2 hr. period.

Results

For each subject, peak response amplitude of the motor nerve volley to the initial CS pulse was measured. The average pulse amplitude on the last 10 CS-alone trials served as the baseline to which later acquisition and extinction trials were compared. Percent of this baseline was calculated over blocks of five trials for acquisition and extinction. In addition, the average of the baseline CS-alone pulses was subtracted from the average response amplitude over blocks of five trials in acquisition and extinction to give a corrected mean amplitude.

The percent baseline responses for acquisition trial blocks were analyzed with three separate mixed factor analyses of variance (Type SPF-p.q; Kirk, 1968). In these analyses, comparisons of individual trial number groups separated on the basis of subsequent extinction conditions served as the between variable (e.g., 20-massed versus 20-distributed) while trial blocks served as the repeated variable. Significant blocks effects were noted when the 20 trial ($F = 6.29$, $p < .01$), 40 trial ($F = 4.71$, $p < .01$), and 60 trial ($F = 2.87$, $p < .01$) acquisition data were analyzed. There were no acquisition differences apparent within any one level of number of acquisition trials. Analyses of the corrected mean data revealed significant block effects for the 20 trial ($F = 6.16$, $p < .01$), 40 trial ($F = 6.13$, $p < .01$), and 60 trial ($F = 2.81$, $p < .01$) acquisition groups. Unlike the percent baseline analyses of acquisition differences within the individual levels of number of acquisition trials, a significant difference between the 40 trial-massed extinction and 40 trial-distributed extinction groups was discerned when corrected means were analyzed ($F = 4.54$, $p < .05$). Subsequent Tukey analysis ($Q = 9.85$, $p. < .05$) showed that that the 40-distributed group ($M = 84.87$) had a greater average block acquisition measure than did the 40-massed group ($M = 47.73$).

The extinction data were analyzed with three factor mixed design analyses of variance (Kirk, 1968). Number of acquisition trials and extinction condition served as the between variables while trial blocks (in the massed condition) and trial number (in the distributed condition) constituted the repeated variable. Significant differences between the two extinction conditions were noted when both percent of baseline response ($F = 15.13$, $p < .01$) and corrected means ($F = 15.84$, $p < .01$) were examined. (See Figure 1) No significant blocks or trial number effects were found. However, significant Blocks X Extinction condition interactions were present when the percent baseline ($F = 2.78$, $p. < .01$) and corrected means ($F = 2.49$, $p < .01$) were analyzed.

The above data indicate that conditioning took place in animals that received either 20, 40, or 60 acquisition trials and, in general, no differences in conditioning could be found within the individual groups when they were compared on the basis of subsequent assignment into massed versus distributed extinction conditions. Analysis of the extinction data, however, revealed large

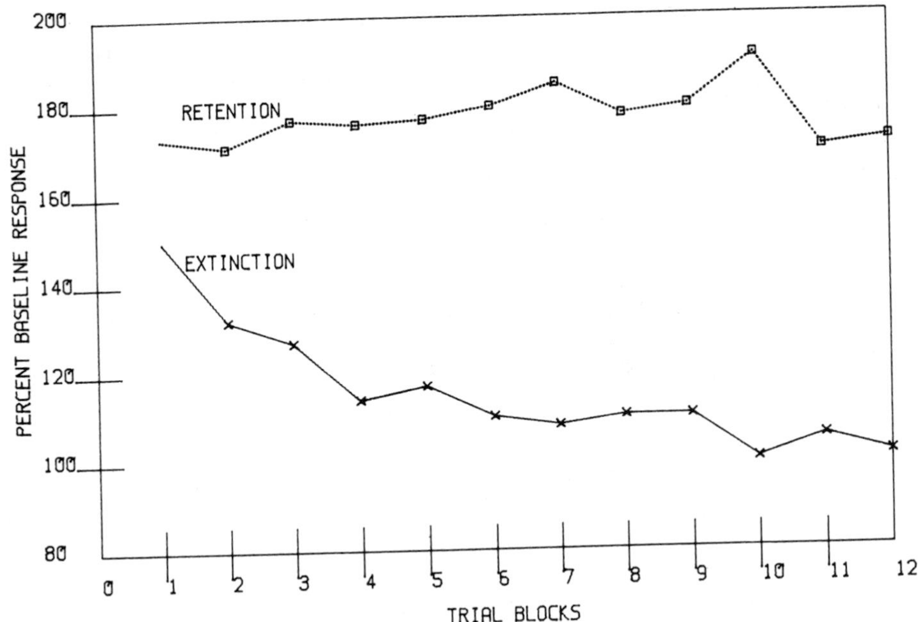

Fig. 1. Mean response amplitudes in extinction over individual trials (distributed condition) or five trial blocks (massed condition) as a percentage of CS-alone response amplitude averaged over groups. The distributed condition animals (dotted line) received 1 CS-alone trial per 10 min. while the massed condition animals (solid line) received 1 CS-alone trial every minute.

differences between the two extinction procedures. Those animals given the probe-CS once every 10 min. showed greater responses to the CS than did those animals that received CS-alone trials at a rate of one per minute. The significant interaction can be explained when the relative performance of the two extinction conditions are compared. Those animals receiving 60 extinction trials showed a response decrease to base levels within 1 hr. Conversely, animals that received 12 probe-CS presentations showed complete retention of the conditioned response at the end of the 2 hr. period. It is obvious that in this study, numbers of extinction trials are confounded with extinction time. However, there is evidence that the response increase due to pairing does not fall off spontaneously over a two hour period, but will decline if a certain number of CS-alone trials are presented in a massed fashion.

EXPERIMENT 2

Methods

Subjects, apparatus, surgical procedures, and response specifications were the same as in Experiment 1. Thirty-five cats were used in this experiment. Subjects were randomly assigned to one of five groups (n=7). All animals received 50 paired acquisition trials with an ISI of 250 msec and an average ITI of 60 sec. After acquisition, the animals were allowed either a 1/2, 1, 2, 3, or 4 hr. wait before 50 extinction (CS-alone) trials were administered.

Results

Two-way mixed factor analyses of variance were used to examine acquisition and extinction in this study. For these analyses, assignment into groups on the basis of the various time periods allowed between acquisition and extinction served as the between variable while block averages of five trials constituted the within factor. Significant acquisition block effects were obtained when percent of baseline ($F = 2.13$, $p < .01$) and corrected means ($F = 3.54$, $p < .01$) were examined. Significant differences between waiting period groups were not present when either measure was analyzed. Significant extinction block effects were also obtained when percent baseline ($F = 2.51$, $p < .01$) and corrected means ($F = 3.73$, $p < .01$) data were examined. As in the acquisition analyses, no significant between group effects were apparent.

These data indicate the presence of acquisition and extinction but no differences in retention of the conditioned response when various time intervals are allowed to elapse between acquisition and extinction. This study provides additional evidence that simple sensitization of the spinal response system is not an adequate explanation of neural response increases seen during spinal conditioning procedures. If sensitization were responsible for response increases, one would expect to see less retention with increasing time intervals allowed between acquisition and extinction. The present data clearly show a lack of these retention differences.

EXPERIMENT 3

This experiment was conducted to test the excitability of the afferent terminals for possible presynaptic alterations that could affect response output during spinal conditioning procedures. Possible tonic excitability changes involving the cutaneous afferent nerve terminals were explored using Wall's (1958) antidromic test technique.

Methods

In this study, cats underwent a spinal transection, were paralyzed, and the hindlimb nerve dissected as described in Experiment 1. Next, the spinal cord was exposed by performing a laminectomy between L-4 and L-6. The cats were then mounted in a cat spinal stereotaxic device, electrodes tied to the distal ends of the sensory and motor hindlimb nerves, and the dura opened between L-4 and L-6 to allow access to the spinal cord. Gross cord dorsum potentials were recorded from the left side of the exposed cord and the area producing the maximum cord dorsum potential was determined. At this point, a microelectrode was lowered into the region of the superficial peroneal afferent terminals (Layer IV). Single shocks were delivered through the microelectrode to evoke an antidromic volley recorded monophasically from electrodes tied to the distal end of the superficial peroneal nerve. The amplitude of the antidromic response was maximized by vertical movement of the electrode. Shock intensity was adjusted to yield an intermediate antidromic volley. Oscilloscope tracings of the afferent nerve volley were photographed for subsequent data analysis on the same Grass Kymograph camera used to photograph records of the motor nerve response. In this study, the CS was delivered to the superficial peroneal nerve at a point proximal to the antidromic recording electrode.

The area under the antidromic response evoked in the cutaneous nerve following an orthodromic volley in the same nerve was determined to insure the above techniques could detect changes in afferent terminal excitability. This procedure was carried out both before and after conditioning procedures were administered. Animals that failed to show the characteristic antidromic response - stimulus interval function were not used in the study.

Fifteen cats served as subjects in this study. The animals were randomly assigned in two groups; a paired group (n=9) that received 60 paired acquisition trials followed by 40 extinction (CS-alone) trials and a CS-alone group (n=6) that received 100 CS-alone trials. Both groups were given an initial 20 CS-alone presentations to establish a baseline response level. Sixty second ITIs were allowed for both groups. Before the initial baseline CS-alone trial and at the end of every 10 trials that followed, an antidromic test series was administered. The test series consisted of an antidromic volley followed by a CS test pulse which in turn was followed by a second antidromic volley. Five seconds elapsed between the two antidromic stimulations and the presentation of the orthodromic pulse. These procedures resulted in 13 total test series; three during the baseline CS-alone period, six during the acquisition period, and four during the extinction period. Area under the antidromic response was measured for the 13 test series. Averages of the three test series given during the baseline CS-alone period served as the baseline response level to which acquisition and extinction test series were compared.

Results

Percent baseline response data from this experiment were analyzed with nine separate two factor-mixed-design analyses of variance. Trial presentation condition (i.e., paired vs. CS-alone) was the between factor and trials or trial blocks constituted the within factor. An analysis of acquisition trials revealed a significant trial blocks effect ($F = 2.83$, $p < .01$) indicating that conditioning had occurred as well as a significant group effect ($F = 5.32$, $p < .05$). More specifically, the paired group ($M = 134.68\%$) demonstrated a greater baseline response amplitude than the CS-alone group ($M = 112.69\%$). Analysis of extinction trial data revealed no significant differences over trial blocks or between paired and CS-alone animals. The antidromic excitability test series administered before and after each animal received acquisition and extinction trials were also analyzed. Significant trial block effects were noted when both pre-conditioning ($F = 30.98$, $p < .01$) and post-extinction ($F = 17.03$, $p < .01$) excitability series were examined. In both series the greatest percent baseline responses were found when the orthdromic volley preceded the antidromic volley by 20 msec. Finally, the antidromic response trials administered during acquisition and extinction were analyzed. No significant group differences in the antidromic responses recorded before and after the orthodromic test volley were present either during acquisition or extinction. Additionally, the antidromic responses did not significantly change as a function of training nor as a result of position relative to the interspersed orthodromic volley (See Fig. 2).

The data from this experiment indicate that although a significant response amplitude increase was evident in animals that received paired presentations of the CS and UCS, tonic changes in excitability of the afferent terminals were not observed. This suggests that presynaptic facilitation did not occur at the terminals. This mechanism can therefore be excluded as an explanation of response amplitude increase observed during spinal conditioning procedures. In addition, significant differences were not evident when antidromic responses obtained before and after an orthodromic test volley were compared over the course of training. Thus, phasic excitability changes involving the afferent terminals can also be excluded as a factor involved in spinal conditioning.

DISCUSSION

The results of the studies outlined here suggest that the effect of a classical conditioning operation on excitability of spinal reflex pathways is not a transient alteration and that the process occurs within the spinal interneuron fields or at the motoneurons. The first study showed that the response increase produced by various numbers of paired trials persisted for two hours

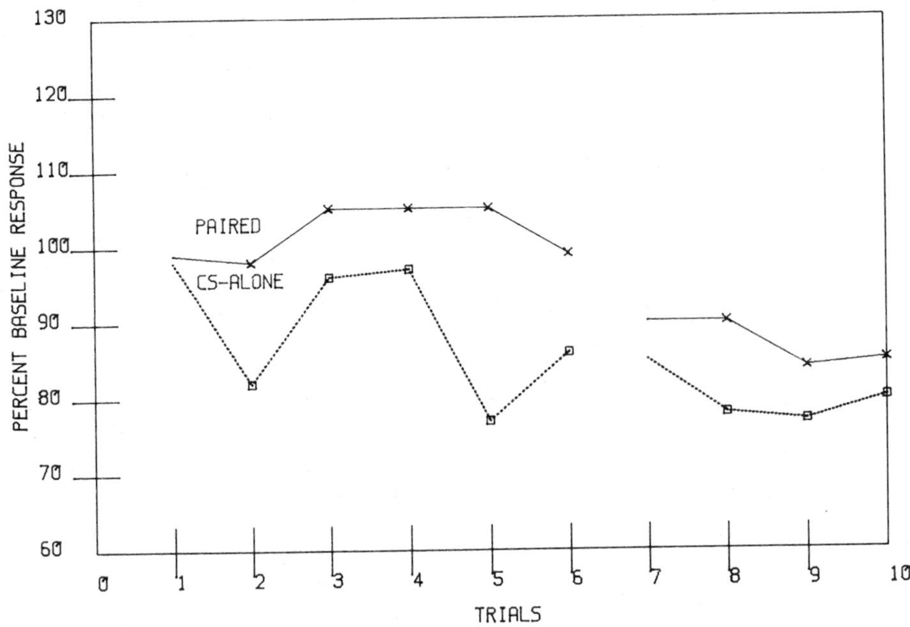

Fig. 2. Area under antidromic volley evoked by stimulation recorded in the superficial peroneal nerve for paired (solid line) and CS-alone (dotted line) animals. The data points are percents of baseline responses and are collapsed over the pre- and post-orthodromic volley responses. Trials 1-6 were obtained during the acquisition period and trials 7-10 were obtained during extinction.

without significant change while massed extinction trials over one hour produced a significant decrease in the response amplitude. While confounding time and trial presentations, the study strongly suggested that the response would generally decrease only under the active effects of CS-alone trials. The second study held acquisition time constant but varied the time allowed between acquisition and extinction from 1/2 to 4 hours. Here, the extinction data were the same for all groups, showing that the response increase with pairing was not subject to spontaneous decay over a period of up to four hours, but then underwent a decrease with the active CS-alone extinction trials. Together the two studies strongly indicate that the process responsible for the response increases during CS-UCS pairing is a fairly long-lasting alteration rather than a phasic alteration. The site of the change has been limited to the spinal cord by the experimental design and the third study suggests that afferent terminal excitabilities are not changed by the paired trials despite increased motor responses. Thus the site of the observed alteration is most probably within the interneuron paths. These studies, along with our previous work (e.g., Patterson, 1975a, b, 1980; Patterson, Cegavske, & Thompson, 1973) and the elegant work of Durkovic (1975) strongly support the operation of a unique effect of stimulus pairing in the isolated cat spinal reflex circuits which closely parallels that seen in classical conditioning studies with intact subjects.

As Walters, Carew, and Kandel (1979) have recently noted, one of the central problems confronting the study of behavior is the analysis of the neural mechanisms underlying learning. Implicit here is the assumption that "learned" behaviors can be distinguished from behaviors which are not considered under the rubric of "learning". The distinction has always been difficult and some of the traditional means often used to distinguish "real learning" from other kinds of behavioral changes are being called into question. For example, the demonstration of long-term habituation blurs one distinction between learned and other behavioral changes, that of retention. Thus, it is important to differentiate behavioral changes according to the operations producing the alteration. In this regard the operations of classical conditioning produce an associative behavioral change as opposed to the behavioral alterations of habituation and sensitization caused by stimulus repetition.

Interest in the classical conditioning paradigm as a tool for elucidating the neural mechanism of associative behavioral change has increased substantially over the past few years. Building upon Gormezano's (e.g., 1966) early efforts to closely define the classical conditioning paradigm and its control procedures, Thompson and his colleagues first called for (Thompson, Patterson, & Teyler, 1972) then began an analysis of the neural underpinnings of classical conditioning of the nictitating membrane response in the rabbit (e.g., Thompson, Berger, & Berry, 1980). This research has proven remarkably fruitful and interesting. More recently, Kandel and his associates have identified an effect of the classical conditioning paradigm on the aplysia (Walters, Carew, & Kandel, 1979). The delineation of unique effects of CS-UCS pairing in the aplysia has already led to the beginning of a cellular analysis of the effect (Carew, Walters, & Kandel, 1981). Both the rabbit and aplysia preparations are elegant preparations, one for the behavioral control in an intact animal and the other for the potential ease of cellular analysis. It is obvious from the demonstrations of CS-UCS pairing effects in both rabbit and aplysia, that the operation of stimulus association occurs over a wide range of neural complexity. Within the mammalian species, stimulus pairing effects have been shown in preparations ranging from intact to far from intact. Russell and his colleagues have shown classical nictitating membrane conditioning in neodecorticate rabbits (e.g., Oakley & Russell, 1972), Norman et al. have found classical eyeblink conditioning in bilaterally hemispherectomized cats (Norman et al., 1974) while Schmaltz and Theios (1972) have shown rabbit nictitating membrane conditioning in bilaterally hippocampectomized rabbits. As indicated previously, our own work builds on and extends data showing effects of stimulus pairing in spinal reflex pathways.

These studies, showing stimulus pairing effects over a wide range of nervous system types and at various levels of the mammalian nervous system strongly suggest that stimulus pairing has quite pervasive effects at all levels of the central nervous system. Our studies, as well as some of the others noted (e.g., Schmaltz & Theios, 1972) have begun to note differences in the effects of stimulus pairing at various levels of the CNS. In our studies, we have failed to note the characteristic latency shifts in the response so pervasively seen in intact animal conditioning. These response timing shifts, such as decreased onset latency and progressive centering of the peak amplitude of the conditioned response at the time of unconditioned response onset are among the most visible aspects of the adaptiveness of learning mechanisms. It is reasonable to assume, however, that such adaptive aspects of the response to stimulus pairing should not be seen in the spinal preparation. The process of even simple association formation in the intact animal is a vastly complex process, geared to adapt the organism to its environment. The full nervous system is utilized to achieve that adaptive ability. When the nervous system is truncated, some of that adaptive ability is lost, as for example, the loss of post-extinction savings during reacquisition in the Schmaltz and Theios hippocampectomized animals.

It is increasingly evident that the reflex paths of the cat spinal cord are able to respond to the pairing of two stimuli in a specific manner which has many of the formal characteristics of response development seen during classical conditioning in the intact animal. However, this response development appears to be the product of a cellular mechanism which does not have the capability of adapting the response further to the demands of the situation. Thus the spinal preparation appears to be demonstrating the raw associative mechanism at a cellular level devoid of the powerful adaptive mechanisms available with full brain systems. The further elucidation of these cellular mechanisms should thus provide valuable insights into the associative process produced by stimulus pairing.

REFERENCES

Carew, T.J., Walters, E.T., & Kandel, E.R., 1981, Associative learning in aplysia: Cellular correlates supporting a conditioned fear hypothesis. Science, 211:501.

Durkovic, R.G., 1975, Classical conditioning, sensitization, and habituation of the flexion reflex of the spinal cat. Physiol. Behav., 14:297.

Fitzgerald, L.A., & Thompson, R.F., 1967, Classical conditioning of the hindlimb flexion reflex in the acute spinal cat. Psychon. Sci., 8:213.

Gormezano, I., 1966, Classical conditioning. In Experimental Methods and Instrumentation, J. Sidowski (Ed.), McGraw-Hill:NY.

Kellogg, W.N., Deese, J., & Pronko, N.H., 1946, On the behavior of the lumbo-spinal dog. J. Exp. Psych., 36:503.

Kirk, R.E., 1968, Experimental Design: Procedures for the Behavioral Sciences. Wadsworth: Belmont, California.

Lloyd, A.J., Wikler, A., & Whitehouse, J.M., 1969, Nonconditionability of flexor reflex in the chronic spinal dog. J. Comp. Physiol. Psychol., 68:576.

Norman, R.J., Villablanca, J.R., Brown, K.A., Schwafel, J.A., & Buchwald, J.S., 1974, classical eyeblink conditioning in the bilaterally hemispherectomized cat. Exper. Neurol., 44:363.

Oakley, D.A., & Russell, I.S., 1974, Differential and reversal conditioning in partially neodecorticate rabbits. Physiol. Behav., 13:221.

Patterson, M.M., 1975a, Effects of forward and backward classical conditioning procedures on a spinal cat hind-limb flexor nerve response. Physiol. Psychol., 3:86.

Patterson, M.M., 1975b, Interstimulus interval effects on a classical conditioning paradigm in the acute spinalized cat. Paper presented at the Society for Neuroscience, New York, November.

Patterson, M.M., 1976, Mechanisms of classical conditioning and fixation in spinal mammals. In Advances in Psychobiology, Vol III. Riesen,A., & Thompson, R.F. (Eds.), Wiley: NY.

Patterson, MM., 1980, Mechanisms of classical conditioning of spinal reflexes. In Neural Mechanisms of Goal-directed Behavior and Learning. R.F. Thompson, L.H. Hicks and J.B. Shvyrkov (Eds), Academic Press: NY.

Patterson, M.M., Cegavske, C.F., & Thompson, R.F., 1973, Effects of a classical conditioning paradigm on hind-limb flexor nerve response in immobilized spinal cats. J. Comp. Physiol. Psychol., 84:88.

Schmaltz, L.W., & Theios, J., 1972, Acquisition and extinction of a classically conditioned response in hippocampectomized rabbits (Oryctolygus cuniculus). J. Comp. Physiol. Psychol., 79:328.

Shurrager, P.S., & Culler, E.A., 1938, Phenomena allied to conditioning in the spinal dog. Amer. J. Physiol., 123:186.

Shurrager, P.S., & Culler, E.A., 1940, Conditioning in the spinal dog. J. Exp. Psychol., 26:133.

Smith, M., Coleman, S., & Gormezano, I., 1969, Classical conditioning of the rabbit's nictitating membrane response at backward, simultaneous, and forward CS-UCS intervals. J. Comp. Physiol. Psychol., 69:226.

Thompson, R.F., Berger, T.W., & Berry, S.D., 1980, Brain mechanisms of learning. In R.F. Thompson, L.H. Hicks and V.B.Shvyrkov (Eds), Neural Mechanisms of Goal-directed Behavior and Learning, Academic Press: NY.

Thompson, R.F., Patterson, M.M., & Teyler, T., 1972, Neurophysiology of learning. Annual Review of Psychology, 23:73.

Wall, P.D., 1958, Excitability changes in afferent fibre terminations and their relation to slow potentials. J. Physiol. (Lond.), 142:1.

Walters, E.T., Carew, T.J., & Kandel, E.R., 1979, Classical conditioning in aplysia californica. Proc. Natl. Acad. Sci., 76(12):6675.

ACKNOWLEDGEMENTS

The research discussed here was generously supported by NINCDS Grants NS10647 and NS14545, the American Osteopathic Association Bureau of Research and the Ohio University College of Osteopathic Medicine.

PLASTICITY, EXPERIENCE AND RESOURCE ALLOCATION IN MOTOR CORTEX AND HYPOTHALAMUS

D. Nico Spinelli and Frances E. Jensen

Departments of Computer and Information
Science and Psychology
University of Massachusetts
Amherst, MA 01003

SUMMARY

Training kittens to avoid an "unsafe" visual stimulus by flexing one forearm has major effects on visual and somatic cortex adult organization (4). Here we show that two important interfaces to the world, motor cortex and the hypothalamus, are similarly affected. Punctuate stimulation of the motor cortex reveals a four-fold increase in the diameter of the area allocated to the control movement of the trained forearm relative to the untrained one. Some of the motor responses in the animals resembled elementary movements in comprising correct responses during training. Cellular responses in the hypothalamus showed a shift toward cells with selectivity for the trained forearm; some of these cells showed the additional characteristic of selective responsivity to the visual stimuli used in training. It appears that the partitioning of the motor cortex and the repertoire of responses available to it are substantially influenced by early experience. The access that sensory stimuli have to the hypothalamus is also modified, possibly changing the way in which the adult will later cope with demanding tasks. The results dramatically demonstrate that simple early experience exerts widespread effect on structures which will later prove critical in setting the limits of individual potential.

We have recently demonstrated that if an unusually large amount of information is presented to a patch of skin on one side of the body during development, a reallocation of resources takes place in somatosensory cortex such that the cortical area allocated to that patch of skin becomes many times larger than normal.

We have also shown that in this cortical area dendritic branching (1) and bundling (2) are considerably greater than in the corresponding area in the contralateral hemisphere where the untrained forearm is represented.

The procedure we used to bring about these changes consisted of a simple avoidance procedure in which a "safe" or an "unsafe" visual stimuli was presented to a kitten through goggles and the kitten was required to flex one of the forelegs to the "unsafe" stimulus or receive a mild shock on that foreleg. Such a discrete response was chosen to facilitate investigating the effect of the training on motor cortex to determine if a reallocation similar to that in somatosensory cortex had occurred. Penfield and others (3) have shown that parts of the body which have greater sensory and motor sophistication have larger cortical representations in general.

We show in this report that early experience has a significant effect on the final size of the representation areas within the motor cortex. Further, while the brain interacts with the outside world through the motor system, it exercises control over the internal milieu through an interface which is largely contained within the hypothalamus. We also show in this report that in the hypothalamus polymodal responses to visual and somatic stimuli have been modified in accordance to the stimuli used during training.

Behavioral

Six kittens were trained to a simple avoidance conditioning task which required the animal to lift one of its forearms to avoid a mild electrical shock on that arm in response to an "unsafe" visual stimulus. Correct response caused the appearance of a "safe" visual stimulus. A mild shock (1.2 mA pulses, 4/sec. constant current) was delivered through stimulating electrodes placed on the skin of one forearm. Good contact was obtained by shaving the skin and moistening skin with saline solution. Visual displays were generated by goggles which were fastened on the head of the kitten with an elastic band. The stimuli consisted of vertical and horizontal black lines on a white background and were placed on the focal plane of convex lenses so that they would appear at infinity and therefore in focus to the kittens. Each pair of goggles could generate 2 stimuli, one for each eye. The stimuli were turned on separately by small light bulbs. Only one stimulus was presented at any one time. We will refer to the unsafe stimulus as that which was associated with the shock. The other stimulus was therefore only presented in the safe condition.

Safe and unsafe stimulus lines were orthogonally oriented to each other. Thus for any kitten during training, a stimulus of specific orientation was always presented to the same eye and would be followed by a shock to a specific forearm. Flexion of that forearm terminated the unsafe condition and activated the safe stimulus for the other eye. Kittens were trained for 8 minutes a day for 12-15 weeks.

To investigate the neural changes produced by the training procedure, the animals were prepared for single cell recording (see 4 for details) and then placed in a stereotaxic apparatus that left the visual field free and also enabled us to observe limb movements. The skin on the scalp was then incised and the cruciate gyrus of both hemispheres was exposed. For microelectrode penetrations in the hypothalamic area, a small area of skull was removed bilaterally at AP 7.0-12.0 mm, L: 0-5.0 mm. The dura was then removed to expose all cortical areas and Gelfoam moistened in saline was applied as temporary protection. Stimulation of motor cortex was preformed after moving the Gelfoam while carefully maintaining the level of anesthesia as specified below. After mapping motor responses, an agar gel was used to prevent brain pulsation and protect all cortical areas. Contact lenses were used to correct for accommodation. Electrophysiological recordings of somatosensory cortex were carried out under conditions specified in previous report (4).

Motor Cortex Stimulation

As the level of anesthesia is critical for motor cortex stimulation (5, 6), it was carefully maintained at a constant level by small controlled injections of sodium pentothal. Anesthetic depth was such that all spontaneous movements were abolished but good cortical excitability was maintained.

The type of stimulation used was a simple isolation transformer driven at 60 Hz. A resistor in series with the secondary of the transformer allowed current control. While more sophisticated methods are available for cortical stimulation, we found that the isolation transformer was most convenient and effective, and intensity could be varied most easily. The stimulus was delivered using concentric electrode with an outer diameter of 0.7 mm and an inner core of 0.2 mm in diameter.

We obtained a definition of the motor map by using bipolar and monopolar stimulation and by using different current intensities. The motor map was generated by stimulating on a grid of points 1 mm apart from each other. The grid was started from the sagittal fissure and proceeded laterally to the edge of the cruciate gyrus 1 mm anterior and 2 mm posterior to the cruciate sulcus. Stimulus intensity was adjusted by placing the tip of the concentric electrode on the temporal muscle and increasing the current until threshold was reached. Motor maps were then made at twice and four times the threshold intensity. In the bipolar condition, the output wires from the transformer were connected one to the core of the concentric microelectrode and one to the tubing.

In the monopolar condition one of the output wires was connected to the temporal muscle of the cat and the second output wire was connected to the core of the concentric electrodes (7).

Electrophysiological Recording

The sensory representation was mapped using tungsten microelectrodes in the postcruciate gyrus on a grid of penetrations spaced mediolaterally 0.5 and 1 mm apart and the boundaries of the representation of the contralateral forearm were mapped by identifying the position of receptive fields of adjacent body areas. Cell responses were obtained by stroking the skin, hair bending, and pressure and joint movements. Cells were also tested for auditory and visual polymodal responses. Various sounds were used to determine auditory responses and visual responses were elicited by displaying a moving black bars and edges against a white background. Special attention was paid to orientation sensitivity and ocular dominance of any visual response obtained.

Behavior

The 6 kittens were trained for 12-15 weeks before recording. Three kittens started training between 5 and a half and 6 weeks of age and the remaining kittens between 6 to 8 weeks of age. Kittens rapidly reached a high success rate in making a correct response to avoid shock and by the sixth week of training all kittens were responding correctly 98% of the time. There was no significant difference between the performance curves of the younger and older kittens.

Motor Cortex

In general, bipolar and monopolar stimulation of motor cortex yielded comparable results, the only difference being that the intensity of the monopolar stimulation required more careful control. For each hemisphere we constructed a motor map of the contralateral body similar to Penfield's method (8). We were thus able to compare quantitatively the extent of cortical surface dedicated to the trained forearm versus that dedicated to the untrained one. Responses were tabulated in terms of flexion or extension of specific joints and muscle groups.

The enlargement of the trained area was highly significant ($p < .001$, $t = 11.68$, $df = 5$) and consisted of a four-fold increase in the diameter of the cortical area dedicated to the trained forearm. Motor maps for the two hemispheres are shown in Figure 1. Furthermore, the response threshold of the trained forearm was lower relative to areas concerned within other body parts within the same and opposite hemispheres. This was especially true in the postcruciate gyrus, where often the trained forearm was the only body part that could be induced to respond to cortical stimulation. Monopolar stimulation elicited responses at lower thresholds than did the bipolar. A remarkable observation was that the

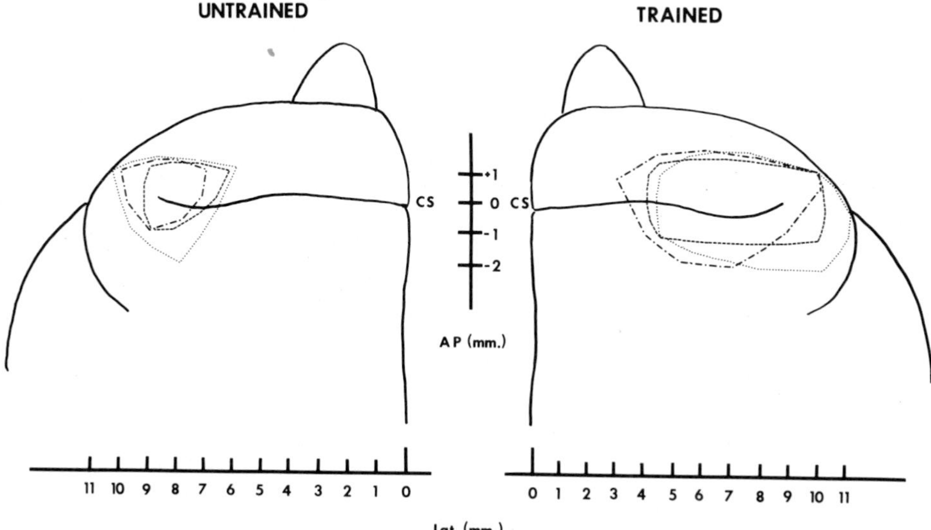

Figure 1. Varied line boundaries show the representational areas in motor cortex of 3 cats in which forearm movement could be induced by cortical stimulation. Hemispheres contralateral to the untrained and trained forearm are shown. The area allocated to the control of movement in the trained forearm was enlarged an average of 30% over that area concerned with movement of the untrained forearm.

type of movement elicited by cortical stimulation was characteristic of the individual behavior of the animal during training. Thus, in most animals a large amount of cortex would produce flexion, but in one animal which had learned to lift the lever by extending and abducting its forearm, a large cortical area was found that would produce the same movement when stimulated.

Hypothalamus

A total of 160 units were bilaterally recorded from the dorsal, lateral, and ventromedial hypothalamic nuclei of 5 cats. No major differences were found between these areas and therefore all cells were pooled for analysis. Upon identifying a cell, we tested it for somatic, visual, and auditory responsivity, as described: 78% of the cells responded to somatic stimulation, 54% to visual, and 13% to auditory stimulation. Somatic receptive fields for neurons in the hypothalamus were found to be often large, ill-defined, and were either bilaterally, ipsilaterally, or contralaterally located. We did not try to systematically build body maps; rather we concentrated on those cells that could be activated by stimulation of the trained forearm versus those that were excited by stimulation of the untrained one. In all cats, a significantly greater percentage of cells ($x = 33\%$) exhibited a somatic response to the trained forearm as compared to the average of 19% which could be found to be responsive to somatic stimulation of the untrained forearm ($p < .005$, $t = 5.78$, $df = 4$).

Visual responsivity of cells in the hypothalamus also appeared to be affected by the training procedure. Cells with orientation sensitivity identical to the unsafe stimulus were found approximately three times as frequently as other types ($p < .001$, $\chi = 67, 3$, $df = 4$). Further, a number of cells were found that responded to stimulation of the traine forearm in addition to the visual stimuli which were presented in the training situation. The location of the cells recorded from was histologically verified (Figure 2).

Somatosensory Cortex

Somatic and polymodal responses were recorded from a total of 203 units in 6 cats, 126 units from the hemisphere contralateral to the trained forearm and 79 units from that contralateral to the untrained arm. Comparison reveals that the cortical area in which cells were found responsive to the trained forearm was significantly larger than that of the other hemisphere in which cells were found responsive to the untrained forearm ($p < .001$, $t = 9.04$, $df = 5$). Figure 3 illustrates that in general the cortical representation for the untrained forearm spanned about 0.5 mm on the mediolateral axis in the postcruciate cortex. However, on the opposite hemisphere, an area of 2.5 - 3.0 in diameter was found as the representation of the trained forearm, indicating a four-fold enlargement. In addition, the percentage of visually responsive cells was larger in this area and particularly many more responded to the training stimuli when presented to the eye to which they

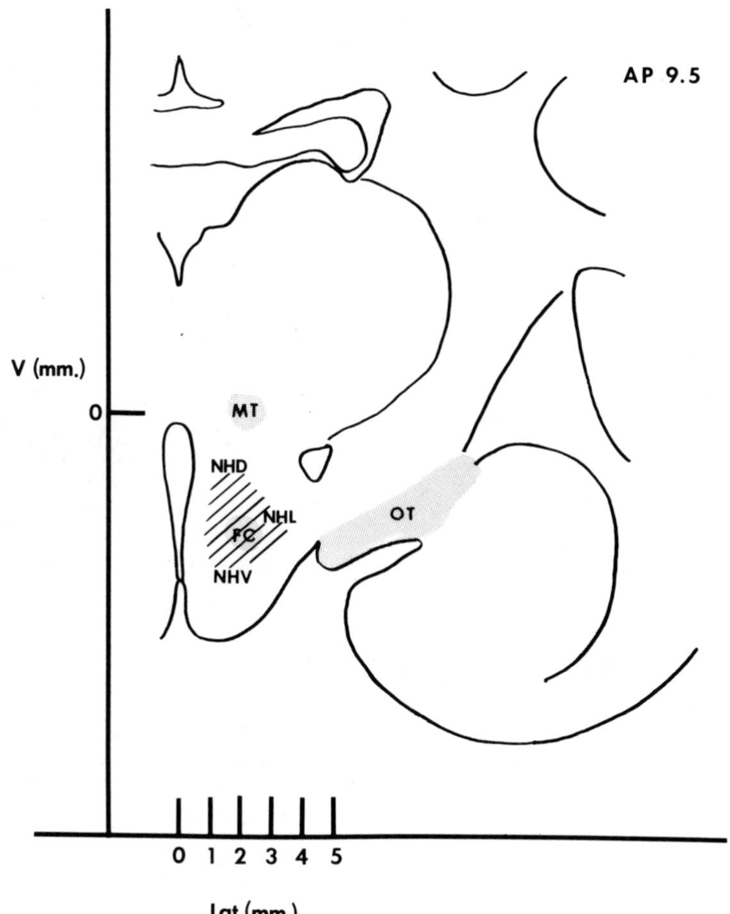

Figure 2. Diagrammatic representation of a section taken through the cat's brain at AP: +9.5. Striped area represents regions where cells were marked after recording and verified histologically. The ventral, lateral, and dorsal hypothalamic nuclei have been labeled NVL, NHL, NDL, respectively, according to the atlas of Snider and Niemer (13). Lateral and ventral stereotaxic axes are also shown.

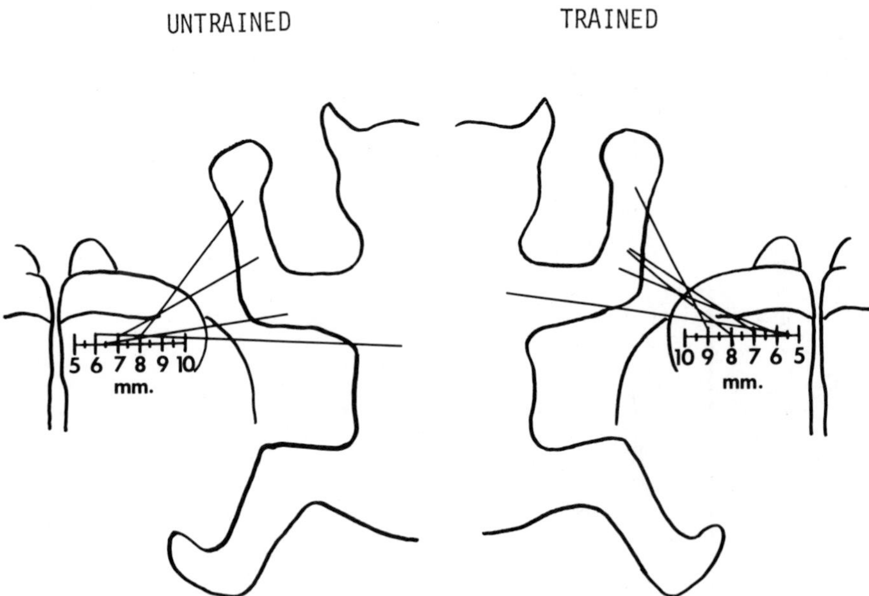

Figure 3. Representation of the trained and untrained sides of the body on somatosensory cortex as averaged from 3 cats. Penetrations are indicated in mm lateral to the sagittal sulcus at 1.5 mm posterior to the cruciate sulcus. Lines are drawn from the penetration location on the cortex to the part of the body to which cells within that penetration responded to stimulation. The area allocated to the trained forearm was enlarged an average of 350% over that of the untrained area.

appeared during training ($p < .005$, $t = 6.75$, $df = 5$). As these results are essentially similar to those reported in a previous paper (4), we will not discuss them further at this time.

These experiments confirm our previous findings (4) that a simple experience during development leads to a substantial enlargement of the somatic cortical representation of the somatic trained forearm. We now extend our investigation to the motor cortex and the hypothalamus. We find that the motor representation of the trained forearm is also greatly enlarged; that is, early experience can reallocate cortical resources in the motor strip as well. The magnification of a cortical sensory area seems easier to explain in terms of enhanced sensitivity due to the larger number of cells dedicated to that function. This is the case for such areas as those dedicated to the finger tips. Magnification of motor areas could be understood by noting that a greater number of cells is required for finer movements and that "muscles...are represented again and again and again, in different combinations" (8). In a way, the greater the number of possible combinations in which cells appear the greater the intelligence of that area. Further, the types of elementary movements available in motor cortex seem to be determined in part by early experience, just as the types of elementary feature detectors available in visual cortex are strongly influenced (and permanently so) by the visual environment present during early development (9). These considerations seem to be supported by our findings that dendritic branching and bundling of the cells have been affected in a way which is suggestive of greater connectivity in the area representing the trained forearm (1, 2). The size of a cortical area seems directly related to the sophistication of the function performed (10). Clearly then, the adaptive value of plasticity must be that the size, i.e., the intelligence, of a cortical area can be tuned up or down from the genetic endowment by early experience. There is much evidence that early experience can affect the response of organisms to stressful situations (11). Sensory activity in the hypothalamus is a reflection of the fact that this part of the brain needs to know about the outside world to adjust the internal milieu to cope with external events. These results show that early experience modifies hypothalamic access to sensory events as well, a finding which could explain the literature referred to above.

In conclusion, results from sensory and motor cortices indicate that the enlargement of forearm representations through early training is at the expense of adjacent representational areas (12). As we believe that these changes are permanent (9), the results show that relatively simple experiences during development could have far-reaching consequences in determining how the brain allocates resources which are clearly responsible for the way in which the adult organism will adapt to demands imposed by the environment. Further research is clearly needed; however, a useful hypothesis at this time might be that the structural and functional changes observed could provide the foundations for understanding how learning predispositions evolve as a consequence of early experience.

REFERENCES

1. D. N. Spinelli, F. E. Jensen, and G. Viana Di Prisco. Early Experience effect on dendritic branching on normally reared kittens. Experi. Neurol., Vol. 68, No. 1, 1980.

2. F. E. Jensen and D. N. Spinelli. Early experience effect on dendritic bundles. Society for Neuroscience Abstracts, Vol. 5, 1979.

3. For example, W. G. Penfield and E. Boldrey. Somatic motor and sensory representation in the cerebral cortex of amn as studied by electrical stimulation. Brain 60: 389, 1937; C. N. Woolsey and D. Fairman. Contralateral, ipsalateral and bilateral representations of cutaneous receptors in somatic areas I and II of the cerebral cortex of pig, sheep, and other animals. Surgery 19: 684, 1946; C. N. Woolsey. Organization of somatic sensory and motor areas of the cerebral cortex. In H. F. Harlow and C. N. Woolsey (Eds.) Biological and biochemical bases of behavior. Madison, 1958, Univ. of Wisc. Press; and L. I. Malis, K. H. Pribran and L. Kruger. Action potentials in "motor" cortex evoked by peripheral nerve stimulation. J. Neurophysiol. 16: 161, 1953.

4. D. N. Spinelli and F. E. Jensen. Plasticity: The mirror of experience. Science 203: 75-79, 1979.

5. O. A. M. Wyss and S. Obrador. Adequate shape and rate of stimuli in electrical stimulation of the cerebral motor cortex. Am. J. Physiol. 120: 42, 1937.

6. C. Cure and T. Rasmussen. Effects of altering parameters electrical stimulating currents upon motor responses from precentral gyrus of the Macaca mulatta. Brain 77: 18, 1954.

7. The rationale for bipolar stimulation is that in this case the current propagation path is between the tubing and the inner core and produces the least current spread. Because the current path is localized on the surface of the cortex, stimulation is of decreased intensity in the deeper cortical layers. In the monopolar condition, there is probably better conduction to the deeper layers. In the monopolar condition, there is probably better conduction to the deeper layers but current spread is greater and stimulus localization is dependent upon careful adjustment of current intensities so that the current should exceed threshold only in close proximity of the electrode tip.

8. E. V. Evarts. Feedback and corollary discharge: A merging of concepts. Neurosci. Res. Program Bull. 9: 86, 1971.

9. D. N. Spinelli, H. V. B. Hirsch, R. W. Phelps, and J. Metzler. Visual experience as a determinant of the response characteristics of cortical receptive fields in cats. Exp. Brain Res. 15: 289, 197

10. W. G. Penfield and E. Boldrey. Somatic motor and sensory representation in the cerebral cortex of man as studied by electrical stimulation. Brain 60: 389, 1937.

11. For example, J. V. Brady, Ulcers in "executive" monkeys. Sci. Amer. 199: 95, 1958; and W. J. H. Nauta, (Eds.) The Hypothalamus. Springfield, Ill., 1969, C. C. Thomas, publisher.

12. In fact, the work of Penfield has shown similar phenomena of variation in humans even though lack of developmental data makes it impossible to determine the relative contribution of early experience of each subject, as can be seen from the following: "The (cortical representational) fields...overlap each other because of the great variability in individual cases. If arm and hand extend unusually high, then the lower extremity may have its representation only in the fissure," from Epilepsy and Cerebral Localization, by Wilder, Penfield, and P. C. Ericson, (Eds.) Springfield, Ill., 1941 p. 45, C. C. Thomas, Publisher.

13. R. S. Snider and W. T. Niemer. A Stereotaxic Atlas of the Cat Brain. Third Printing. Chicago, Ill., 1970, Univ. of Chicago Press.

This research was funded in part by Grant #2ROIMH25329-05 and by AFOSR Contract "F33615-80-C-1088.

A NEURAL ANALOG OF CONDITIONING: MODIFICATIONS OF PYRAMIDAL TRACT RESPONSE

L.L. Voronin and V.A. Markevich

Brain Institute, Academy of Medical Sciences, Moscow 107120, and Institute of Higher Nervous Activity and Neurophysiology, Academy of Sciences, Moscow 117485 (USSR)

INTRODUCTION

Two basic explanations of conditioning at neurophysiological levels are known (see Kandel 1976; Voronin, 1976, 1980a with references). The first one postulates changes in synaptic efficacy and the second one presumes modifications in neuronal postsynaptic properties (membrane threshold, endogeneous pacemaker and the like). We shall refer to these two classes of hypotheses as "synaptic" and "membrane" hypotheses, correspondingly. Most theorists favour synaptic hypotheses, although it has been strongly supported only for the most simple type of learning - i.e. habituation of defensive reflex in invertebrates (Kandel, 1976; Zucker, 1972). In conditioning experiments Woody et al. (1970) and Woody and Engel (1971) found that thresholds for direct electrical stimulation in motor areas projecting to the target muscle of the conditioned response (CR) were lower in conditioned than in naive animals. These data were not supported for other types of CRs (Kotlyar et al., 1979). Nevertheless some measurements, especially those of Woody and Black-Cleworth (1973), with intracellular recordings may be interpreted as an indication of a decrease in membrane thresholds as a postsynaptic mechanism underlying the elaboration of the CR. Long lasting postsynaptic resistance shifts of cortical neurons have been found in experiments (Woody et al., 1978) which imitated some features of conditioning procedures and might be termed "cellular analogs" of CRs (see Kandel, 1976). On the other hand, changes in amplitude of excitatory postsynaptic potentials (EPSP) have been found in motor cortical neurons in our experiments (Voronin and Kozhedub, 1971; Voronin, 1976, 1980a) and by other authors (Baranyi and Feher, 1978) on cellular analogs of CRs. Moreover, short latency EPSPs were found to appear in neurons of sensorimotor cortex after elaboration of a behavioral CR - a so called "local conditioned startle response" (Voronin and Ioffe, 1974; Voronin, 1976, 1980a). These data have been considered as the experimental support of the idea that an increase in the efficacy of excitatory synapses underlies behavioral conditioning.

More direct consideration of synaptic hypotheses demands an analysis of identified monosynaptic responses. With this aim in mind, the experimental situation that was used for elaboration of the "local conditioned startle response" (Voronin et al., 1975; Voronin, 1976, 1980a) was modified in the present study. Peripheral (light or sound) conditional stimuli (CS) were substituted for direct stimulation of the motor cortex. Neuronal "conditioned" changes were evaluated by recording the pyramidal tract response (PTR) as evoked by the cortical CS. It is known (Patton and Amassian, 1965) that PTR consists of an early deflection ("direct" or D wave) followed by a series of later deflections ("indirect" or I waves). The D wave most probably results from direct excitation of pyramidal neurons whereas I waves represent indirect trans-synaptic discharges and include monosynaptic discharges. It was suggested that analysis of PTR changes during "conditioning" procedure allowed to choose between synaptic and membrane hypotheses because modifications of D wave should indicate changes in excitability of pyramidal tract neurons itself whereas modifications of I components might reflect additionally, changes in efficacy of intracortical synapses.

METHODS

Experiments were done on white rats (250-300 g body weight) freely moving in a 30 sm χ 30 sm χ 35 sm box. Sufficiently long (about 80 sm) flexible wires were used to connect electrodes to stimulators and amplifiers during the experiment. In the first series of experiments without stimulus pairings, PTR recordings were done in locally anaesthetized subjects with tubocurarine injection and artificial respiration. In all cases preliminary operation was carried out under Nembutal anaesthesia (35-40 mg/kg intraperitoneally) 3-5 days before the basic experiment. The operation included exposing the skull of the animal and stereotaxic (Fifkova and Marsala, 1962) insertion of bipolar stimulating electrodes in the lateral hypothalamus (LH) (P 2; L 2; H 8.2). Two bipolar electrodes were inserted in the motor cortex (P 1; L 3). The motor cortical electrodes were placed on the exposed cortical surface or inserted about 1 mm deep. Recording electrodes were placed in the bulbar pyramids (P 10.7; L 0.4; H 8.3-8.5). Inter-electrode distance for every bipolar pair was 1-2 mm for stimulating electrodes and about 3 mm for recording ones. Parameters of the LH stimulation (a train of 300 ms duration of 0.07-0.6 mA, 0.1-0.3 ms pulses at 100 Hz) were chosen 1-3 days before the basic experiment as supporting stable self-stimulation (25-44 trains per minute). The basic experiment began with control applications of CS pulses (0.3-4.0 mA; 0.05-0.5 ms). From 3 to 5 series of the CSs were delivered, single series consisting of 8 or 16 CS presentations. Parameters of the CS were selected in order to evoke at one I wave and D wave with amplitude about two times less than maximal D wave amplitude in the same preparation (see Fig. 1A and Results for I and D wave definitions). Afterwards, the pairing procedure began. Single CS applied through one pair of cortical electrodes was combined with stimulation applied through the adjacent (within 1-2 mm) pair of cortical electrodes (unconditional stimulus - US) and with stimulation of LH ("additional reinforcement", see Voronin et al., 1975). Cortical US was a train of 4-8 pulses at 100 Hz with other parameters within the range of the above mentioned parameters of the CS. As a rule, US parameters were selected in order to cause a distinct movement of the contralateral forelimb parameters of the LH stimulation were those chosen during self-stimulation session, but in some experiments current strength was increased from 30 to 50%. A self-stimulation pedal was not available to the subject during the basic experiment. The interval between CS and US was 150 ms; between US and LH stimulation it was 100 ms. After 2-4 series of parings, an "extinction" procedure (presentation of isolated CS) was done. Pairings were repeated after 3-5 extinction series. Intertrial intervals during the pairing procedure were 100 s. During control and extinction series, the intertrial interval was 10 s. There were pauses of 1.5 to 20 min between series of stimuli. Continuous extinction (up to 99 isolated CSs) was practiced in some experiments.

Two types of control procedures were used. In 6 experiments, only cortical CS and US were paired without LH reinforcement. In 5 other experiments (a group of 4 additional animals), LH stimulation was applied 100-700 ms before single cortical stimulus. Single PTRs evoked by the CS were recorded in most experiments. In all experiments PTRs within each series were averaged (8 or 16 stimuli) during the experiment using the analyzer F-37. Amplitudes were measured between zero line or "initial point" of the corresponding wave and the peak of the wave (see Fig. 3B, a triangle). "Initial point" of D or I wave was chosen as a deflection on the descending limb of stimulus artifact or of D wave correspondingly (arrows in Fig. 1A). Different methods of the measurements (from zero line or from the "initial point") provided quantitatively similar results. Evaluation of the results was carried out by non-parametric statistical methods (Gubler and Genkin, 1973).

RESULTS

PTRs in Unanaesthetized Rats

Bearing in mind that previous recordings of PTR (Patton and Amassian, 1954; Bindman et al., 1979) have been done on restrained cats and monkeys, a group of 11 subjects was used (1) to study

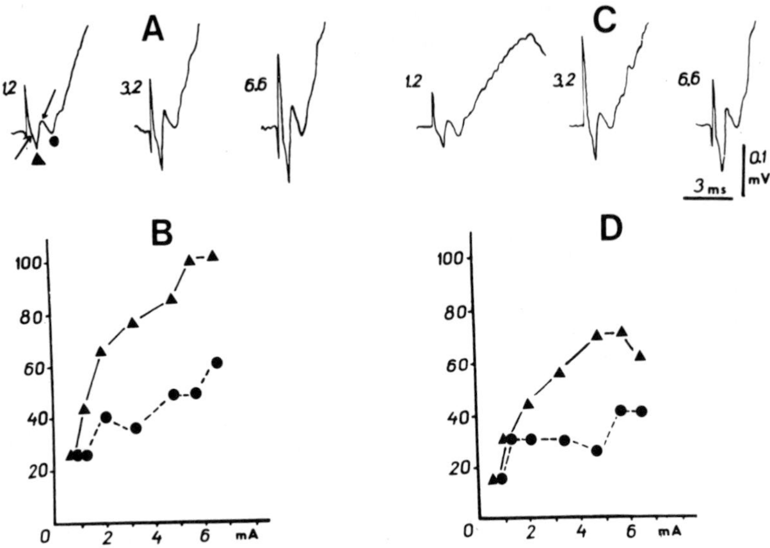

Fig. 1. PTRs in freely moving (A, B) and restrained (C, D) rats. A, C - examples of averaged responses to stimulation with various currents (numbers - current strength in mA). B, D - dependence of amplitude of D (triangles) and I (dots) waves (ordinate, mcV) from the stimulating current strength (abscissa, mA). Arrows denote "initial points" for D and I wave amplitude measurements.

waveform and latency of the PTR in freely moving rats and (2) to compare the PTR in freely moving and in restrained animals. Examples of PTRs recorded in freely moving rats are shown in Fig. 1A, and Fig. 2-4; PTRs recorded in curarized rats are shown in Fig. 1B. Monopolar (with reference electrode in the scalp bone) or bipolar recordings were made. In all figures positivity of exploring electrode (or of "more active" lower electrode in case of bipolar recording) is signalled by downward deflection. In most cases it was possible with proper stimulus and electrode adjustment to distinguish a positive early wave (Fig. 1A, a triangle) with a latency of 0.5 to 1.3 ms (mean 0.8 + 0.3 ms, n = 11) and a later wave (Fig. 1A, a dot) with a latency of 1.5 to 3.3 ms (mean 1.8 - 0.5 ms). The waveform and latency distributions were not significantly different for freely moving and curarized rats. Amplitudes of PTRs (from 40 to 200 muV for most experiments) were also in the same range in these groups, being slightly higher in freely moving rats (compare Fig. 1B and D). Two early components were similar to D and I waves in anaesthetized cats and monkeys (Patton and Amassian, 1954) and will be termed correspondingly. The difference between peaks of these D and I waves was 1-2 ms (mean 1.5 ± 0.5 ms). More late components (with latency of more than 4-5 ms) were different

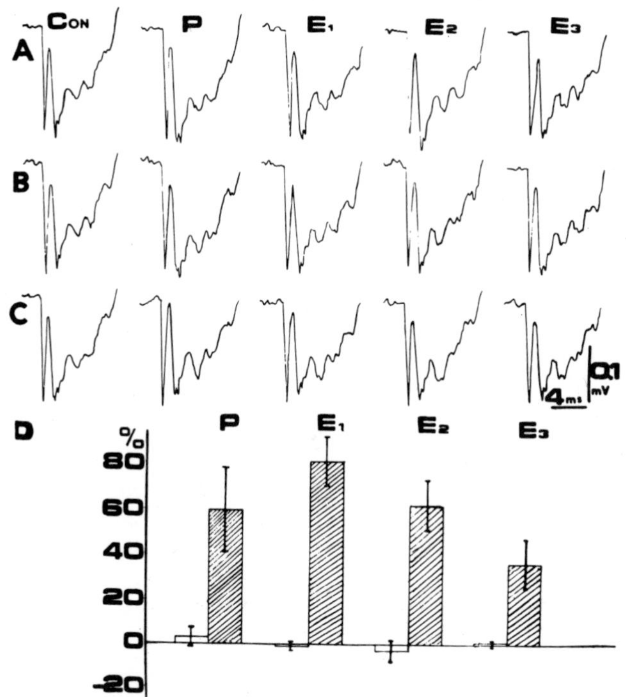

Fig. 2. "Conditioned" PTR changes. A-C examples of averaged PTRs. Con - control series (in A) or the last extinction series before the next pairings (in B, C); P - pairings; E_1, E_2, E_3 - responses from three consecutive periods of extinction; D - mean changes in amplitudes of direct (empty columns) and indirect wave (stippled columns) relative to the mean control before pairings calculated from measurements of 5 (P), 9 (E_1 and E_2) and 8 (E_3) averaged responses. Error bars represent $\pm$ 1S.E.

in some cases in curarized and freely moving animals and in the latter they probably included movement artifacts. Thus, only early components with latencies in above mentioned ranges were measured

Table 1. Amplitude of D (digits above the lines) and I Wave (digits under the lines) During and After Three Different Procedures

Procedure	Number of Experiments	During Procedure[a]	Aftereffects[b] 1	2	3
Pairings of Cortical and Hypothalamic Stimulations	11	97 ±6 121*±8	100 ±4 123*±11	100 ±7 116*±10	99 ±7 107*±7
Backward Pairings	5	106±5 88±5	78±2 92±5	81±17 96±9	- -
Cortical Stimulation Without Hypothalamic Reinforcement	6	87±17 90±18	95±6 91±7	95±12 89±10	- -

[a]The table lists percentages of mean amplitudes (± S.E.) relative to control series in the same experiment.
[b]Three extinction periods after pairings and two periods of CS presentations after two control procedures are denoted as "Aftereffects".
*Significant difference (P<.05, criteria of Signs) from the control series in the same experiments.

as D and I waves. The amplitudes of D and I waves were stable or tended to decrease during long-lasting (several hours) experiments without stimulus pairings. Amplitudes increased with increase in the strength of stimulation, dependence of D wave amplitude being steeper than that of I wave (Fig. 1B, D).

Changes in Amplitude of D and I Waves

A total of from 48 to 176 pairings of CS, US, and LH stimulation (in one case 272 pairings) was performed in 14 basic experiments (8 subjects). These experiments could be divided into two groups. In the first group amplitudes of D and I waves with relatively constant interpeak separation of 1-2 ms could be measured for the entire experiment. In 7 of these 11 experiments (6 subjects), mean I wave amplitude increased during paired series in comparison with the control series before the pairings. The increase was from 10 to 60%. Fig. 2 illustrates the experiment with maximal mean increase (compare control I wave in Fig. 2A with that in

B and C during pairings). The first stippled column in Fig. 2D represents mean change in I wave amplitude calculated for all 5 series of pairings performed in this experiment. All extinction series were divided into three groups. Amplitude of I wave in the first extinction group (Fig. 2D, column E_1) is slightly greater than that during pairings (the difference is statistically non-significant, $P<0.1$, t-test). The amplitude tended to restore in the subsequent extinction series (Fig. 2D, columns E_2, E_3). A similar tendency to amplitude restoration during extinction was observed in 6 of 7 experiments.

As shown in Fig. 2D, no changes in mean D wave amplitude were observed in this experiment. In general, mean amplitudes of D waves increased during pairing series in 4 of 11 experiments, this increase being from 3 to 38%. Amplitudes of I waves were also increased in all these 4 experiments. However, in distinction from I waves, D waves were not decreased during extinction trials in most experiments. Pooled data for all 11 experiments are summarized in Table 1. Increases in amplitudes of I waves during pairing and the tendency to diminution during late extinction trials are evident. Mean data show no changes in amplitude of D wave.

Appearance of an "Additional" Wave During Pairings

In 3 of 14 basic experiments (2 subjects) in addition to the above quantitative changes in I wave amplitude, qualitative changes were observed in later pairing series. These changes could be described as appearance of an additional positive-negative wave (Fig. 3B, 4A, arrows) with a latency 0.6 to 1.3 ms more than that of the D wave, which is intermediate between latencies of D and I waves. Isolated CS presentations resulted in diminution of the amplitude of the additional component (Fig. 3C, 4A) and decrease in frequency of its occurrence (Fig. 4B). The frequency (up to 80-100% as calculated from 16 consecutive CS presentations) could be restored readily using a procedure analogous to instrumental conditioning as in (Fig. 4B). During such a procedure every "additional wave" was followed by LH stimulation, CSs being presented every 15-30 s.

D wave amplitudes were significantly modified in one of these animals, but the time course of the modification was not in full accordance with expected changes during conditioning - extinction sequences (Fig. 3C). Indeed, approximately a twofold increase in D wave amplitude was observed before the last two pairing series (compare Fig. 3A and B). This increase persisted up to the end of the experiment in spite of extinction procedures (Fig. 3C, continuous line). In contrast, mean amplitude of the additional component (Fig. 3C, stippled line) increased as a result of the pairings and decreased during extinction series. Appearance of the new wave precluded exact measurements of the initial I wave

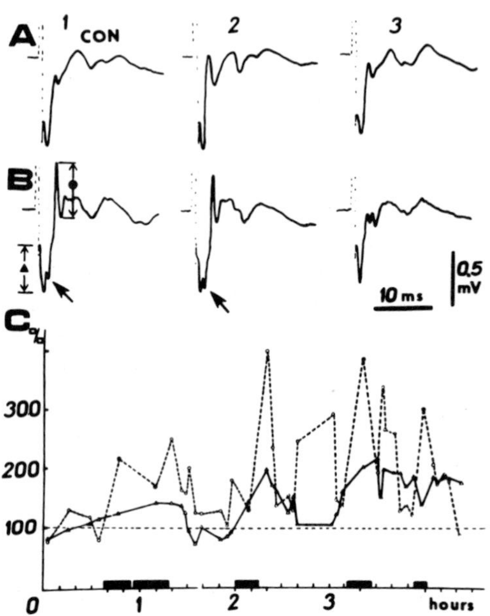

Fig. 3. PTR modifications with appearance of an additional wave. A, B - examples of averaged responses from the control (A1), pairing (A2, B1) and extinction (A3, B2, B3) trials; oblique arrows denote the positive peak of the additional component; C - time courses of amplitudes of D (continuous line) and I wave (stippled line). Ordinate: percentage of amplitude relative to the mean of 4 control averages before pairings. Amplitudes were measured between vertical arrows as shown in B1. Abscissa: time in hours. Black bars denote pairing periods.

amplitude. With this in mind, the results of these experiments were not included in Table 1. If it is assumed that the additional wave represents a modified I wave (see Discussion) and corresponding measurements are incorporated in Table 1, mean increase in amplitude of I wave would be even more significant.

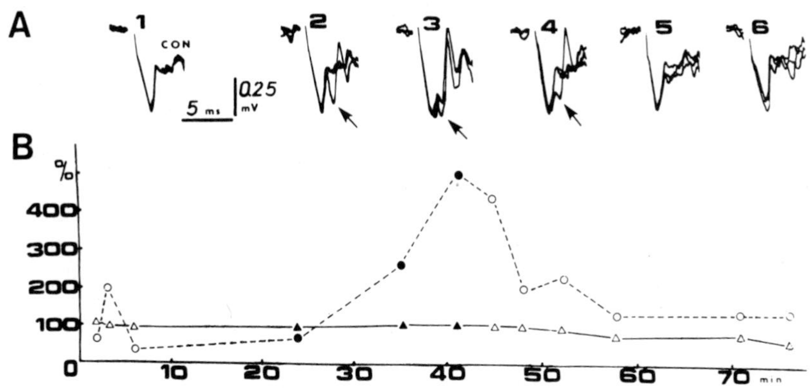

Fig. 4. Restoration of the additional wave during "instrumental conditioning" procedure. A - superposition of last 4 responses from extinction (1, 4-6) and "conditioning" series (2, 3); B - time courses in the same experiment. Ordinate: continuous line - amplitude of D wave; stippled line - frequency of the occurrence of an additional component with amplitude of at least 0.15 mV in 16 consecutive trials. Both measurements are done relative to the 3 extinction series (white symbols) immediately before "conditioning" procedure (black symbols). Remaining conventions as in Fig. 3.

Control Procedures

5 experiments were done to check upon influences of LH stimulation which could be unspecific for pairings. LH stimulation was applied 0.1-0.7 s before single cortical stimuli and these "backward pairings" were repeated for 80 to 176 times in every experiment. Averaged responses to cortical stimulation were recorded during these procedures, about 1-2 min (the first period of aftereffects in Table 1) and 3-6 min after LH stimulation (the second aftereffect period in Table 1). As is evident from Table 1, a tendency for a slight decrease in the PTR amplitude resulted from this procedure. Similar insignificant decreases were found in a control experiment with pairings of two cortical stimuli (single one and a train) without LH stimulation (Table 1, third procedure).

DISCUSSION

Modifications of I waves during "conditioning" and "extinction" procedures occurred in most cases in a direction predicted by synaptic hypotheses. Measured I waves have a latency (1-2 ms more than D wave latency), which assumes a monosynaptic activation of pyramidal tract neurons. Interpretation of the "additional wave" is somewhat less certain. It has a latency, which is intermediate between that of D and I waves. A clearer biphasic waveform may indicate involvement of other fibres than those mediating both D and I waves. However, it seems improbable that the additional wave reflects direct activation of slow conducting neurons because (1) experiments with direct stimulation of white matter in cats and monkeys indicate that slow conducting fibres make negligible contribution to PTR (Patton and Amassian, 1954); (2) there is no separation of pyramidal tract neurons into two distinct groups according to conduction velocities in rats (Shulgovski and Moskvitin, 1972); and (3) we never observed additional waves of similar latencies in many experiments without pairings even after very strong stimuli (as in Fig. 1). In view of sufficient delay between peaks of D wave and "additional wave" and variability (within 0.5 ms) of the latency of the later, one may suggest that the latter represent an additional I component arising from essential increases in efficacy of intracortical synapses. Explanation based on increased excitability of interneurons seems less probable because it demands an additional suggestion about essential differences in properties of pyramidal tract neurons and interneurons in regard to conditioned modifications.

All these considerations demand more direct tests in future experiments. Independently of interpretation of the nature of the "additional wave", our data raise a question about a mechanism, which provides synchronization of discharges of many pyramidal tract neurons. In fact, the "additional component" could arise almost in an all-or-none manner in the "conditioned" state (Fig. 4A).

In general, our measurements seem to support synaptic hypotheses of conditioning. On the other hand, our data indicate that in some cases changes in D waves were also observed, though not so prominent and reversible as changes of I waves and especially of additional waves. Thus our and literature data (Woody et al., 1970-73) allow to suggest that synaptic and membrane mechanisms are not contradictory and both of them may take part in learning processes.

Further indirect support of synaptic hypotheses is provided by studies of long-term hippocampal potentiation (LTP) discovered by Bliss and Lomø (1973). It was suggested (Voronin et al., 1974; Voronin and Kudryashov, 1977; Douglas and Goddard, 1975) that elementary cellular mechanisms of LTP are similar to those of CRs. This suggestion was based on properties of LTP such as longevity (Douglas and Goddard, 1975), specificity for stimulated pathway (Andersen et al., 1977; Lynch et al., 1977; Sharonova et al., 1976), "extinction" and self-restoration (Voronin et al., 1974). "Specificity" of LTP as well as data received with intracellular recordings (Andersen et al., 1977; Voronin and Kudryashov, 1977; 1979; Skrebitski and Vorobyev, 1979) and with quantal analysis (Voronin, 1981) suggest the synaptic nature of LTP. As shown by our data, no similar LTP and only short-term posttetanic potentiation (Voronin, 1970) was produced in motor cortex after tetanization. It was shown here that repeated tetanizations should be paired with additional hypothalamic stimulation to produce long-lasting facilitation of neocortical responses. Reproducible long-lasting potentiation of PTR was found as an increase in D wave amplitude in acute preparations in special conditions of depressed synaptic transmission (Bindman et al., 1979).

The developed paradigm is suitable for single neuron recordings. Future experiments could be aimed at a more detailed analysis of changes in synaptic efficacy or postsynaptic excitability. For the latter, changes in synaptic bombardment could be separated from possible endogeneous postsynaptic changes. To study changes in synaptic efficacy, cortical "minimal" and "unitary" postsynaptic potentials (Voronin, 1980b) could be analysed within the frame of quantal hypothesis of Katz (see Voronin, 1979 for references and methods and Voronin, 1981 for above mentioned data on quantal analysis of LTP). With slight modifications of the experimental situation, the studied neural analog could possibly be converted into a behavioral conditioned reflex with recording of peripheral motor effects (e.g. foreleg movement).

SUMMARY

Average pyramidal tract response (PTR) was recorded in moving rats after direct cortical stimulation. Direct (D) waves with 0.5-1.3 ms latency and presumably monosynaptic indirect (I) waves with 1.5-3.3 ms latency were distinguished. Cortical stimulation (as a conditional stimulus) was paired with reinforcing stimulation of the lateral hypothalamus in a neuronal analog of conditioning. A statistically significant increase in I wave amplitude was found after pairings without significant mean changes in D wave amplitude. I wave amplitude tended to restore to the control level as a result of "extinction" procedure. An additional wave of presumably transsynaptic origin with a latency which was intermediate between that of D and I waves appeared in two animals. The changes in D waves were not so reproducible and reversible as changes in the additional waves in the same animals. The additional wave is considered to appear due to enormous increase in efficacy of intracortical synapses during pairing procedure. In general, the results are considered to support synaptic hypotheses of conditioning. The studied paradigm seems to be promising in further study of synaptic and postsynaptic mechanisms of conditioning.

REFERENCES

Andersen, P., Sunberg, S.H., Sveen, O., and Wigstrom, H., 1977, Specific long-lasting potentiation of synaptic transmission in hippocampal slices, Nature, 266:736.

Baranyi, A., and Feher, O., 1978, Conditioned changes of synaptic transmission in the motor cortex of the cat. Exp. Brain Res., 33:283.

Bindman, L.J., Lippold, O.C.J., and Milne, A.R., 1979, Prolonged changes in excitability of pyramidal tract neurones in the cat: a post-synaptic mechanisms, J. Physiol., 286:457.

Bliss, T.V.P., and Lomø, T., 1973, Long-lasting potentiation of synaptic transmission in the dentate area of the anaesthetized rabbit following stimulation of the perforant path, J. Physiol., 232:334.

Douglas, M.R., and Goddard, G.V., 1975, Long-term potentiation of the perforant path-granule cell synapse in the rate hippocampus, Brain Res., 86:205.

Eccles, J.C., 1953, "The Neurophysiological Basis of Mind", Clarendon Press, Oxford.

Fifkova, E., and Marsala, J., 1962, Stereotaxic brain atlases of cat, rabbit and rat, in: J. Bures, M. Petran, and J. Zachar "Electrofiziologicheskie Metody Issledovania" (in Russian), Inostrannaya Literatura, Moscow.

Gubler, E.W., and Genkin, A.A., 1973, "Primenenie Neparametricheskikh Kriteriev Statistiki v Mediko-biologicheskikh Issledovaniyakh" (in Russian), Meditsina, Leningrad.

Kandel, E.R., 1976, "Cellular Basis of Behavior", W.H. Freeman and Co., San Francisco.

Lynch, G.S., Dunwiddie, T., and Gribkoff, V., 1977, Heterosynaptic depression: a postsynaptic correlate to long-term potentiation, Nature, 266:737.

Patton, H.D., and Amassian, V.E., 1954, Single- and multiple-unit analysis of cortical stage of pyramidal tract activation, J. Neurophysiol., 17:345.

Sharonova, I.N., Voronin, L.L., and Skrebitski, V.G., 1976, Long-lasting posttetanic potentiation of hippocampal evoked potentals to the stimulation of Schaffer collaterals (in Russian), Zh. Vyssh. Nervn. Deyat., 26:214.

Shulgovski, V.V., and Moskvitin, A.A., 1972, Sensorimotor area of the white rat's cerebral cortex: Motor projection (in Russian), Biol. Nauki, N 10:24.

Skrebitski, V.G., and Vorobyev, V.S., 1979, A study of synaptic plasticity in hippocampal slices, Acta Neurobiol. Exp., 39:632.

Voronin, L.L., 1970, Posttetanic changes in intracellular response to direct cortical stimulation, Neurophysiology, 2:454 (Translated from Neirofiziologiia, 2:601).

Voronin, L.L., 1976, "Microelectrode study of Neurophysiological Mechanism of Conditioning, Soviet Research Reports, Vol. 2," C.D. Woody, ed., BIS/BRI, USLA, Los Angeles.

Voronin, L.L., 1978, Involvement of cortical neurones in conditioned and unconditioned startle reflex, Neuroscience, 3:133.

Voronin, L.L., 1979, Quantum analysis of postsynaptic potentials, Neurophysiology, 11:366 (Translated from Neirofiziologiia, 11:491).

Voronin, L.L., 1980a, Microelectrode analysis of the cellular mechanisms of conditioned reflex in rabbits, Acta Neurobiol. Exp., 40:335.

Voronin, L.L., 1980b, Unitary and minimal postsynaptic potentials (in Russian), Usp. Fiziol. Nauk, 11:19.

Voronin, L.L., 1981, Cellular mechanisms of long-term posttetanic potentiation in the hyppocampus, in: "Adv. Physiol. Sci., vol. 36, Cellular Analogues of Conditioning and Neural Plasticity," O. Feher, F. Joo, ed., Pergamon Press and Akademiai Kiado, Budapest.

Voronin, L.L., Gerstein, G.L., Kudryashov, I.E., and Ioffe, S.V., 1975, Elaboration of a conditioned reflex in single experiment with simultaneous recording of neural activity, Brain Res., 92:385.

Voronin, L.L., and Ioffe, S.V., 1974, Changes in unit postsynaptic responses at sensorimotor cortex with conditioning in rabbits, Acta Neurobiol. Exp., 34:505.

Voronin, L.L. and Kozhedub, R.G., 1971, Analysis of postsynaptic potential changes in a cellular analog of conditioned reflex (in Russian), Zh. Uyssh. Nervn. Deyat., 21:997.

Voronin, L.L., and Kudryashov, I.E., 1977, Long-lasting hippocampal posttetanic potentiation with particular reference to mechanisms of conditioned reflex, in: "Proc. of IUPS, vol. XIII, 27 Intern. Congr. Physiol. Sci.", Paris.

Voronin, L.L., and Kudryashov, I.E., 1979, Unit responses in hippocampus during long-lasting posttetanic potentiation (in Russian), Zh Uyssh. Nervn. Deyat., 29:141.

Voronin, L.L., and Kudryashov, I.E., and Ioffe, S.V., 1974, Posttetanic potentiation in hippocampus and its relation with mechanisms of conditioned reflex (in Russian), Dokl. Akad. Nauk SSSR, 217:1453.

Woody, C.D., and Black-Cleworth, P., 1973, Differences in excitability of cortical neurones as a function of motor projection in conditioned cats, J. Neurophysiol., 36:1104.

Woody, C.D., and Engel, J.Jr., 1972, Changes in unit activity and thresholds to electrical microstimulation at coronal-pericruciate cortex of cat with classical conditioning of different facial movements, J. Neurophysiol., 35:230.

Woody, C.D., Swartz, D.E., and Gruen, E., 1978, Effects of acetylcholine and cylic GMP on input resistance of cortical neurons in awake cat, Brain Res., 158:373.

Woody, C.D., Vassilevsky, N.N., and Engel, J.Jr., 1970, Conditioned eye blink: unit activity at coronal-precruciate cortex of the cat, J. Neurophysiol., 33:851.

Zucker, R.S., 1972, Crayfish escape behavior and central synapses, II. Physiological mechanisms underlying behavioral habituation, J. Neurophysiol., 35:621.

CLASSICAL CONDITIONING IN *APLYSIA*:

NEURONAL CIRCUITS INVOLVED IN ASSOCIATIVE LEARNING

E.T. Walters*, T.J. Carew, R.D. Hawkins, E.R. Kandel

Center for Neurobiology and Behavior
College of Physicians and Surgeons
Columbia University
New York, New York 10032

SUMMARY

Recent analyses of the neural control of learning and memory suggest that one needs to identify and examine the neuronal circuitry specific to the behavior that is modified by the learning in order to study the cellular mechanisms underlying these processes. In this paper we describe an example of a simple form of classical conditioning in the gastropod mollusk *Aplysia californica*. This example of associative learning offers considerable promise for a cellular analysis because it involves relatively simple and well-analyzed neuronal circuits. Knowledge of the neuronal circuits involved in the conditioning pathways is reviewed, and a preliminary hypothesis for the mechanisms of this form of classical conditioning is considered.

INTRODUCTION

Evidence from a variety of vertebrate and invertebrate animals indicates that behavior is generated and controlled by specific patterns of activity in precisely organized neural circuits (for reviews see Kandel, 1976; Kennedy and Davis, 1977; Tsukahara, 1981). These results indicate that an analysis of the neuronal

*Department of Physiology
School of Medicine, University of Pittsburgh
Pittsburgh, PA 15261

mechanisms of different forms of learned modifications of behavior will require knowledge of the underlying neuronal circuitry in order to identify the particular cellular alterations responsible for the behavioral modifications. This view has recently been supported by cellular analyses of nonassociative forms of learning (habituation and sensitization) in simple preparations which indicate that these forms of learning involve modifiable synapses at specific loci within the neural circuit (Castellucci et al., 1970; Castellucci and Kandel, 1974; 1976; Klein and Kandel, 1980; Krasne, 1969; Zucker, 1972).

The success of studies which have examined synaptic alterations underlying nonassociative learning in gastropod mollusks has encouraged the search for associative learning capabilities in these animals. This search has in turn led to the discovery that gastropods have rather considerable associative learning capabilities (Mpitsos and Collins, 1975; Gelperin, 1975; Crow and Alkon, 1978; Walters et al., 1979; 1981a; Davis et al., 1980; Sahley et al., 1981; Lukowiak and Sahley, 1981). However, the neural analysis of associative learning in gastropods has been limited by the complex nature of the behavioral and neural systems involved in the forms of associative learning that have been demonstrated in these animals (Davis and Gillette, 1978; Crow and Alkon, 1980; Chang and Gelperin, 1980; Carew et al., 1981a). This limitation can be reduced by examining associative learning in very simple behaviors mediated by restricted neuronal circuits whose components are accessible for cellular study. We here discuss classical conditioning of an elementary reflex in *Aplysia* made up of well characterized neuronal elements. The simplicity of this reflex may enable the identification and characterization of the synaptic alterations supporting associative learning. Our emphasis here is two-fold. One, we will describe our present knowledge of the neuronal circuits involved in the conditioning, and two, we will outline an analytic strategy designed to facilitate the elucidation of the critical neuronal alterations involved in the learning.

A SIMPLE REFLEX IS CAPABLE OF BEING MODIFIED BY CLASSICAL CONDITIONING

The gill and siphon withdrawal reflex is an attractive system for examining classical conditioning because it has been extensively analyzed on the cellular level. This cellular analysis has been essential for the systematic investigation of two forms of nonassociative learning, habituation and sensitization (see below). The gill lies beneath the mantle shelf within the mantle cavity formed by the wing-like parapodia on the animal's back (Fig. 1). The posterior end of the mantle shelf projects up as an exhalant funnel -- the siphon. The tail projects behind the siphon and

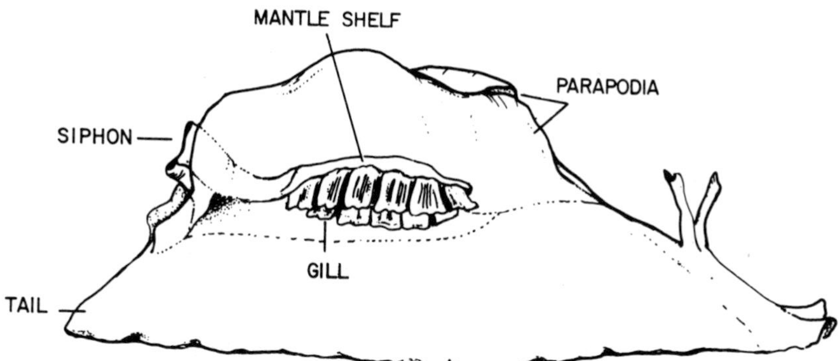

Fig. 1. Organs involved in classical conditioning of gill and siphon withdrawal in *Aplysia*. The mantle organs are viewed through the right parapodium (normally opaque). The conditioned stimulus is delivered to the siphon and the unconditioned stimulus to the tail.

posterior parapodial region. Tactile stimulation of either the siphon or tail elicits the siphon and gill withdrawal reflex -- the gill contracts beneath the mantle shelf and the siphon withdraws out of sight between the parapodia. We found that the gill and siphon withdrawal reflex to siphon stimulation could become dramatically enhanced by pairing a very weak conditioned stimulus (CS) to the siphon with a strong unconditioned stimulus (US) to the tail (Carew et al., 1981b).

Animals were trained with a light tactile stimulus to the siphon as CS (a nylon bristle applied briefly to the siphon), and a strong electric shock to the tail as US. Animals were tested with the CS alone after the first and then every fifth trial. To assess whether changes in response to the CS were due to the temporal association of the two stimuli, several control groups were run receiving either: (1) explicitly unpaired CS-US presentations, (2) random CS-US presentations, (3) CS alone, (4) US alone, or (5) no stimulation. After 16 training trials the paired animals showed significantly longer siphon withdrawals in response to the CS alone than did all other groups and this difference increased with continued training (Fig. 2). After 31 trials extinction was begun by giving a series of 10 CS-alone tests to all groups. During extinction the paired group's responses decreased but remained

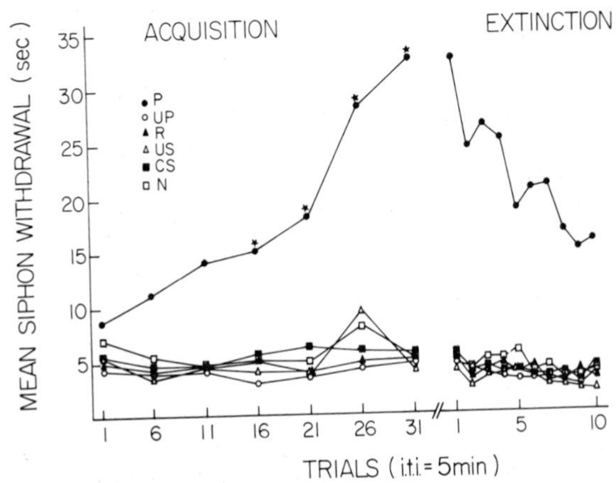

Fig. 2. Classical conditioning of siphon withdrawal in *Aplysia*. Trials were given every 5 minutes. After the first and then every 5 training trials a test was given by applying the CS alone. P-paired group (CS-US interval about 0.5 seconds); UP-unpaired group (CS-US interval 2.5 minutes); R-random group (CS-US interval randomly varied); US-US alone group; CS-CS alone group; N-naive (no training) group. Following training (31 trials) extinction was begun by applying the CS alone to all groups at 5 minute intervals for 10 trials. Only the paired group showed significantly enhanced siphon withdrawal during acquisition or extinction. (From Carew, Walters, and Kandel, 1981c)

significantly higher than all controls. When animals were retested 24 hours later (Fig. 3) the paired group's responses were still significantly higher than all others. However, now the animals that had been trained with the US alone showed significant sensitization of siphon withdrawal compared to the other groups. Thus the siphon withdrawal reflex can express both classical conditioning and sensitization, but the effects of classical conditioning are significantly stronger than those of sensitization and take less time to become manifest.

In a separate experiment (Carew et al., 1981b) retention was examined by giving 30 training trials and then testing with the CS alone at 24 hr intervals (Fig. 4). Paired animals showed significant retention of the conditioned siphon withdrawal response for three days. The US-alone group showed significant sensitization for two days. The sensitization was, however, significantly less than the conditioned effect. Thus this simple form of classical conditioning is rapidly acquired (within 15 trials) and is retained for several days.

NEURONAL CIRCUITS IN THE ABDOMINAL GANGLION ARE INVOLVED IN THE CONDITIONED RESPONSE

Removal of the abdominal ganglion after training eliminated differences between paired and unpaired groups, indicating that conditioning is mediated by the central rather than the peripheral nervous system (Carew et al., 1981b). Much is now known about the central circuits within the abdominal ganglion that mediate gill and siphon withdrawal in response to siphon stimulation, and recently some of the neural circuitry mediating input to the abdominal ganglion from the tail has been delineated. Because the siphon and tail pathways mediate the CS and US, as well as the conditioned and unconditioned responses (CR and UR), we will first review what is known about these circuits, and then pinpoint areas in need of further study. In addition, we will review what is presently known of the plastic properties of neuronal elements in these circuits because these may suggest some mechanisms of modifiability available to mediate conditioning.

The CS Pathway Involves Known Sensory Neurons

The CS pathway from the siphon has been extensively analyzed (Castellucci et al., 1970; Byrne et al., 1974). Mechanical or electrical stimuli to the siphon activate members of an identified cluster of about 24 mechanoreceptors (the LE cells, siphon S.N. in Fig. 5) whose somata are located in the abdominal ganglion. These sensory neurons synapse onto both motor neurons and interneurons and their synaptic terminals are a major locus for the physiological alterations underlying habituation and

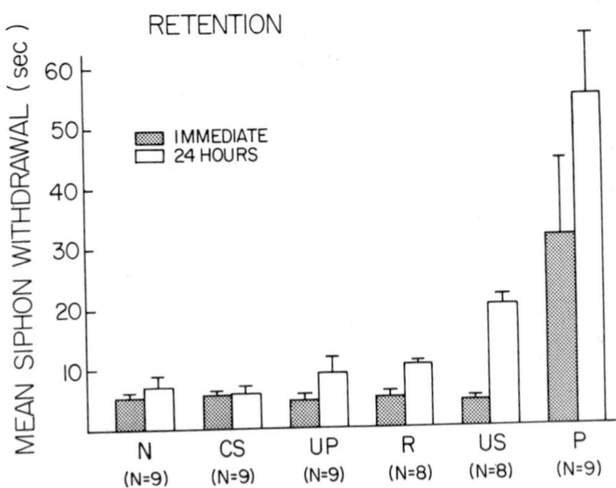

Fig. 3. Comparison of immediate and 24 hour retention of conditioning. The groups shown in Figure 1 were retested 24 hours later. Shaded bars are scores from the first extinction test in Figure 1. Open bars are scores obtained 24 hours later. The paired group was still significantly higher than all other groups after 24 hours, but new differences emerged among the control groups. The US-alone group was significantly higher than the other controls, and the unpaired and random groups were significantly higher than the CS-alone and naive groups. (From Carew, Walters, and Kandel, 1981c)

Classical Conditioning in Aplysia

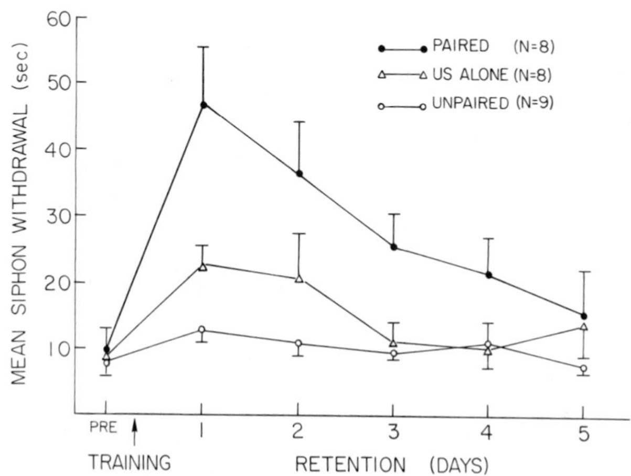

Fig. 4. Retention of the conditioned response. After a pretraining test (PRE) 3 groups were trained for 30 trials with paired, unpaired, or US-alone stimulation. Each group was then tested with the CS alone once every 24 hours. The enhancement of the paired group was retained for 3 days while the enhancement of the US-alone group (sensitization) was retained for 2 days. The paired scores were significantly higher than the US-alone scores on days 1 through 3. (From Carew, Walters, and Kandel, 1981c)

sensitization. During habituation EPSPs from the sensory neurons show a progressive homosynaptic depression and a reduction in the amount of transmitter released, caused by a decrease in Ca^{++} influx (Castellucci et al., 1970; Castellucci and Kandel, 1974; Klein and Kandel, 1978). During sensitization the presynaptic terminals show an increase in Ca^{++} influx and heterosynaptic facilitation of transmitter release (Castellucci et al., 1970; Castellucci and Kandel, 1976; Klein and Kandel, 1978, 1980). The biophysical and biochemical mechanisms of habituation and sensitization have now been explored in considerable detail at these synapses (Brunelli et al., 1976; Klein and Kandel, 1978; 1980; Castellucci et al., 1980; 1981; Camardo et al., 1981).

The CR and UR Pathways Involve Known Motor Neurons

Both unconditioned and conditioned responses to the CS (siphon and gill withdrawal) are mediated by a group of individually identified siphon and gill motor neurons in the abdominal ganglion (Frazier et al., 1967; Kupfermann and Kandel, 1969; Kupfermann et al., 1974). The gill component is mediated by six motor neurons, three of which (L7, LDG1, and LDG2; Gill MN in Fig. 5) account for 75% of the gill withdrawal reflex (Kupfermann et al., 1974). The motor control of siphon withdrawal is not as completely worked out but there are about 15 central siphon motor neurons, of which 10 can be individually identified (Perlman, 1979; and unpublished observations). In addition there are about 30 peripheral siphon motor neurons (Bailey et al., 1979). The central and peripheral siphon motor neurons, like the gill motor neurons, receive monosynaptic excitatory postsynaptic potentials (EPSPs) from the LE sensory neurons. In the case of the gill motor neurons these monosynaptic connections account for about 60% of the synaptic response to weak siphon stimulation (Byrne et al., 1978). As described above, these monosynaptic connections are a major locus for the mechanisms of nonassociative learning; they also constitute an attractive, and easily examined, potential locus for the physiological alterations produced by classical conditioning.

An interesting feature of the conditioned response is that it lasts about three to five times longer than the brief withdrawal to the CS prior to training. This prolongation of the gill and siphon withdrawal response could be produced in part by an increase in the firing of the sensory neurons and by an increase in the strength of the connections made by the sensory neurons on their central target cells (see Discussion). However, another mechanism that might prolong the conditioned withdrawal response is recruitment of additional excitatory interneurons that can maintain the excitation of the motor neurons beyond the initial burst of activity in the sensory neurons. Two classes of interneurons have been described in the abdominal ganglion which could contribute to the prolongation of the response. First, excitatory interneurons (such

Classical Conditioning in *Aplysia*

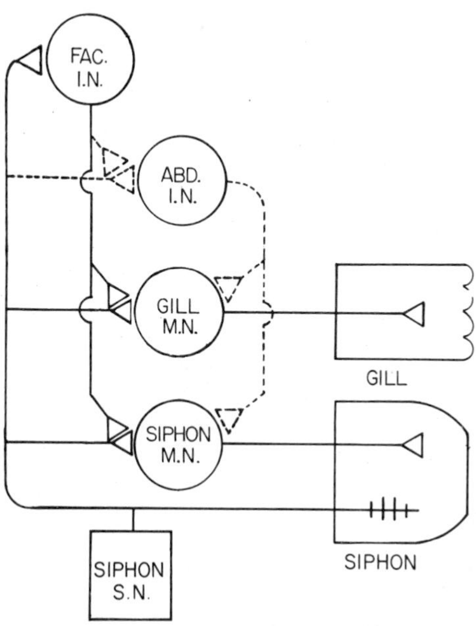

Fig. 5. CS and CR pathways in the abdominal ganglion. Mechanical or electrical stimulation of the siphon skin activates siphon sensory neurons (siphon S.N.) which make monosynaptic connections to gill and siphon motor neurons (Gill M.N. and Siphon M.N.) as well as to excitatory interneurons (ABD. I.N.) and facilitatory interneurons (FAC. I.N.). The facilitatory interneurons cause presynaptic facilitation of transmission at the siphon sensory neuron terminals. Although respiratory pumping interneurons are activated by siphon stimulation and, in turn, excite gill and siphon motor neurons (Byrne, unpublished observations), it is not yet known how they are connected to other neurons in this circuit and so they are not shown.

as L22 and L23) are directly excited by the siphon sensory neurons and in turn make direct projections to the motor neurons (Hawkins et al., 1981a; ABD. I.N. in Fig. 5). Second, a group of interneurons (e.g., L26) has recently been identified which also receive connections from the siphon sensory neurons and which can generate respiratory pumping activity in gill and siphon motor neurons (Byrne and Koester, 1978; Byrne, unpublished observations). Respiratory pumping involves withdrawal of the mantle organs and can be elicited by siphon stimulation (Kupfermann and Kandel, 1969; Kupfermann et al., 1974; Kanz et al., 1979). Thus the network of interneurons that generates this motor output would seem to be a good candidate for contributing to the prolongation of gill and siphon withdrawal to the CS. Finally, the CS can also produce a very long lasting slow depolarization in the motor neurons (Hawkins, unpublished observation) which could be enhanced by the conditioning procedure.

Sensory Neurons In the US Pathway Have Recently Been Identified

We have recently identified a cluster of mechanoreceptor neurons in each pleural ganglion that innervate the tail and are activated by the US (Walters et al., 1981b). These sensory neurons have not been observed to make monosynaptic connections to cells in the gill and siphon withdrawal circuits of the abdominal ganglion, but they do connect to interneurons in the pleural ganglia (Fig. 6) which in turn have powerful excitatory actions on gill and siphon motor neurons (Walters and Byrne, in preparation). While these pleural interneurons make some monosynaptic connections to gill and siphon motor neurons, their actions are largely relayed by additional interneurons in the abdominal ganglion (Walters, Hawkins, and Byrne, unpublished observations). Some abdominal interneurons, including identified tail-sensitive facilitatory interneurons (Hawkins et al., 1981a; Hawkins, 1981b; Fig. 7) receive strong connections in the pleural ganglia from the tail sensory neurons (Walters, Hawkins, and Byrne, unpublished observations). These connections could be monosynaptic but, because of the long distance from the synapse to the postsynaptic cell body (where the intracellular recording is made) morphological rather than electrophysiological techniques will probably be necessary for evaluating monosynapticity. Thus the pathway from the US to the abdominal motor neurons mediating gill and siphon withdrawal comprises several parallel paths that involve at least two and often three or more synaptic relays (Fig. 8). Although this pathway is complex compared to the CS and CR pathways, the progress thus far in characterizing the pleural and abdominal interneurons in the US pathway suggests that many of these cells will be individually identifiable, and that their roles during conditioning can be evaluated.

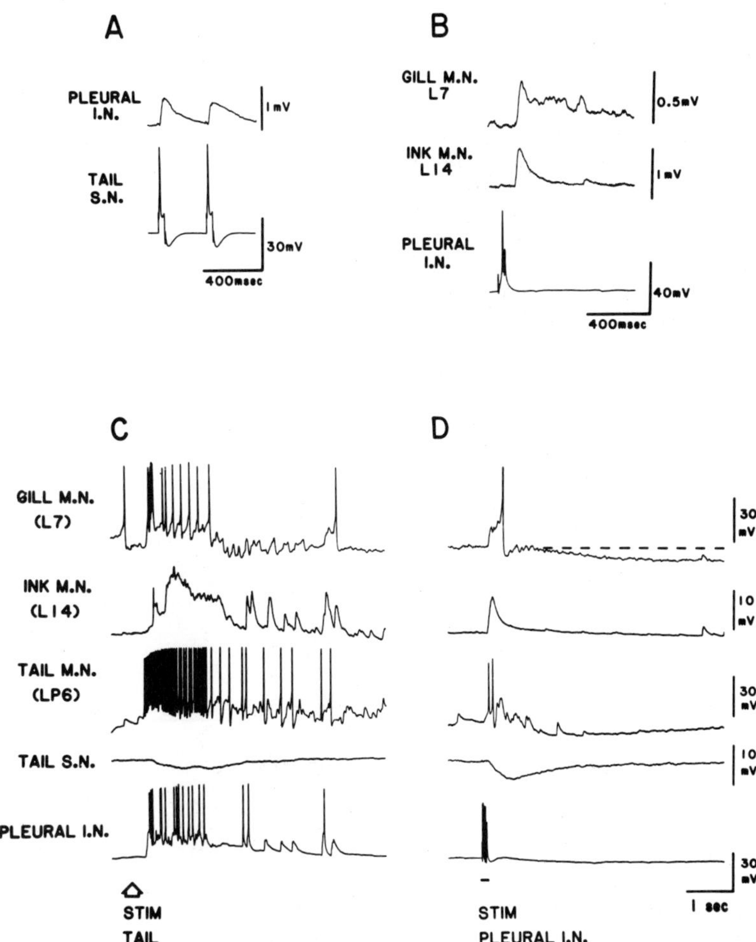

Fig. 6. A pleural ganglion interneuron in the US pathway. (A.) Monosynaptic connections from a tail sensory neuron (S.N.) to a pleural interneuron (I.N.). (B.) Monosynaptic connection of the same pleural interneuron to ink motor neuron (M.N.) L14 in the abdominal ganglion, and polysynaptic connection to gill motor neuron L7. (C.) Activation of the pleural interneuron by noxious tail stimulation and simultaneously recorded responses of a tail sensory neuron, tail motor neuron, ink motor neuron, and gill motor neuron. (D.) Responses in the same neurons shown in part C to intracellular stimulation of the pleural interneuron. This pleural interneuron appears to mediate a significant part of the noxious tail input to neurons in the abdominal ganglion. (From Walters and Byrne, in preparation)

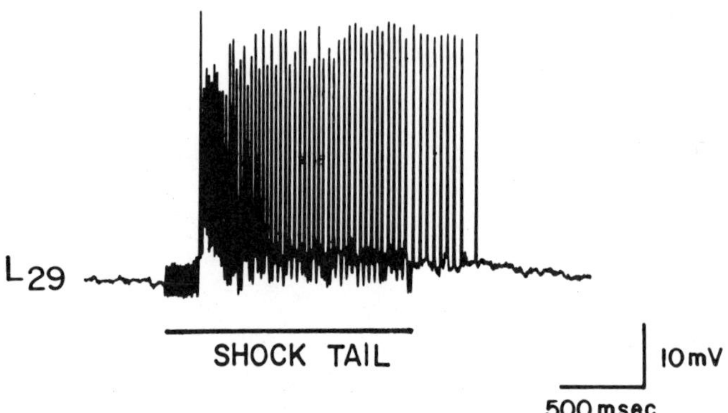

Fig. 7. Activation of identified facilitatory interneuron by noxious tail stimulation in a semi-intact preparation. A.C. electric shock was applied to the tail during the period indicated by the bar (from Hawkins, in preparation).

The CS and US Pathways Converge on Several Types of Interneurons

If the conditioned enhancement of the strength and duration of the response to the CS involves the facilitation of synaptic connections in the CS pathway, a third class of interneurons in the abdominal ganglion, the "facilitatory interneurons" (L29) seems particularly likely to have an interesting role. The activity of the L29 interneurons is responsible for a significant component of the presynaptic facilitation of the siphon sensory neurons and interneurons during sensitization (Hawkins, 1981). These interneurons are excited by both siphon and tail stimulation (see Fig. 7), pathways which produce presynaptic facilitation of the siphon sensory neurons (Hawkins et al., 1981a,b; FAC IN in Fig. 5). Since these interneurons receive convergent input from the CS and US, and since their activity can result in powerful enhancement of the first and perhaps some subsequent synapses in the CS pathway, it seems possible that they may be involved in the temporal integration of the CS and US input which leads to acquisition of the conditioned response (see Discussion).

DISCUSSION

The pathways involved in conditioning of siphon and gill withdrawal in *Aplysia*, although simple even by gastropod standards,

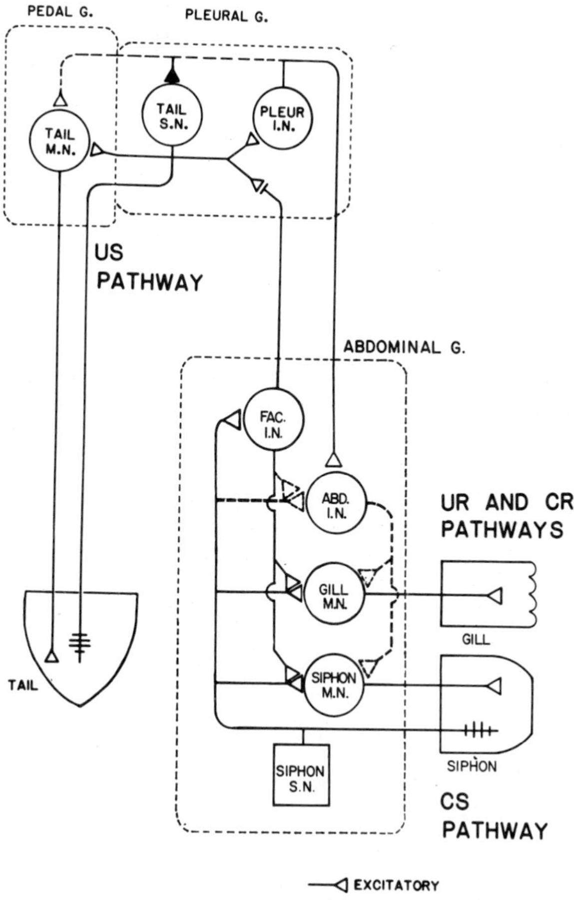

Fig. 8. Schematic wiring diagram of major pathways involved in the conditioning of gill and siphon withdrawal. The CS and CR pathways in the abdominal ganglion are shown in greater detail in Figure 5. The US from the tail is mediated by a population of sensory neurons (S.N.) in the pleural ganglion that make monosynaptic connections to tail motor neurons (M.N.) in the pedal ganglion and interneurons (I.N.) in the pleural ganglion. These interneurons send axons to the abdominal ganglion and make polysynaptic connections (via as yet unidentified abdominal ganglion interneurons, ABD I.N.) to gill and siphon motor neurons. A parallel pathway to the abdominal ganglion is made by connections from the tail sensory neurons to the facilitatory interneurons. These connections appear to be made in the pleural ganglion and, as discussed in the text, might be monosynaptic. (From Walters, Hawkins, and Byrne, in preparation)

nevertheless involve a variety of neuronal elements. Thus, guidelines for selecting neurons that are most likely to play critical roles in the conditioning are useful for efficiently undertaking an analysis of the mechanisms underlying conditioning.

An initial, easily tested guiding hypothesis that can account for the results reviewed above is that conditioning causes a temporally specific increase in the strength of the synaptic connections from the siphon sensory neurons to their follower cells (see also Kandel and Schwartz, 1982; Carew and Kandel, 1982; Klein and Kandel, 1982). Thus the effective intensity of the CS would be increased during training by an increase in the effectiveness of the primary afferents in the CS pathway. This increase would be reflected in enhanced synaptic input to the gill and siphon motor neurons, which could come about in at least two ways. First, the monosynaptic EPSPs from the siphon sensory neurons to the motor neurons would be larger and longer-lasting, and thus would directly enhance the response of the motor neurons to siphon stimulation. Second, the increased effectiveness of the sensory neuron connections to the various excitatory interneurons (and possibly to respiratory pumping interneurons as well) would be expected to result in the enhanced recruitment of these interneurons which can then maintain excitation of the siphon and gill motorneurons following termination of activity in the sensory neurons. A third potential mechanism, increased firing of the sensory neurons to the CS, is discussed below.

The idea that conditioning involves a pairing specific increase in the connections between the siphon sensory neurons and the motor receptors is particularly interesting because these synapses are known to be capable of heterosynaptic facilitation, and the cellular mechanisms underlying this facilitation have been explored in detail (see "CS Pathway" above). These mechanisms are thought to underlie behavioral sensitization but could also be utilized during classical conditioning. The utilization of a common locus (the siphon sensory neuron presynaptic terminals) and mechanism (presynaptic facilitation) to express both classical conditioning and sensitization would be of additional interest in light of theories that have postulated close mechanistic and evolutionary relationships between these associative and nonassociative forms of learning (Kandel, 1967; Wells, 1968; Razran, 1971). In addition, if the memory for classical conditioning involves the cellular mechanisms for sensitization, these mechanisms might be expected to result in a third form of enhanced input to gill and siphon motor neurons after conditioning -- increased firing of the sensory neurons to the CS. The decreased potassium conductance that occurs in the siphon sensory neurons during heterosynaptic facilitation decreases the threshold for firing action potentials (Klein and Kandel, 1980). Such a decrease in threshold has recently been seen in response to both injected current and cutaneous stimulation in another population of primary mechanoreceptors in _Aplysia_ during sensitization (Walters and Byrne, unpublished observations), and might be expected to occur in the siphon sensory neurons as well.

Thus far this hypothesis can account for the memory for classical conditioning but not for the temporally specific acquisition process -- the mechanisms that differentiate conditioning from general sensitization. Kandel and Schwartz (1982) have recently proposed that, while the memory for conditioning and sensitization could be stored at the siphon sensory neuron synapses, the temporal specificity underlying conditioning could be determined by the integration of convergent input from the CS and US by the identified facilitatory interneurons (Hawkins et al., 1981a,b; Hawkins, 1981b). Specifically, temporal and spatial summation of paired input from the siphon and tail at these interneurons could in principle be expected to produce considerably more presynaptic facilitation of the siphon sensory neurons than occurs during unpaired stimulation of these pathways (for details see Klein and Kandel, 1982).

The hypotheses presented here are preliminary and will certainly need revision. For example, in view of the number and variety of interneurons that have been described in these circuits, it would not be surprising to find additional interneuronal loci that have critical roles in conditioning. Even simple brains such as that of _Aplysia_ may depend upon redundancy and a multiplicity of mechanisms for classical conditioning. However, whether or not the hypotheses discussed above ultimately prove to be correct, their value is that they can be precisely formulated and directly tested, a process which can bring us closer to understanding the neuronal mechanisms of conditioning.

REFERENCES

Bailey, C.H., Castellucci, V.F., Koester, J., and Kandel, E.R., 1979, Cellular studies of peripheral neurons in siphon skin of _Aplysia californica_, _J. Neurophysiol._, 42:530.

Brunelli, M., Castellucci, V., and Kandel, E.R., 1976, Presynaptic facilitation as a mechanism for behavioral sensitization in _Aplysia_, _Science_, 194:1176.

Byrne, J.H., and Koester, J., 1978, Respiratory pumping: Neuronal control of a centrally commanded behavior in _Aplysia_, _Brain Res._, 143:87.

Byrne, J.H. Castellucci, V., and Kandel, E.R., 1974, Receptive fields and response properties of mechanoreceptor neurons innervating siphon skin and mantle shelf in Aplysia, J. Neurophysiol., 37:1041.

Byrne, J.H., Castellucci, V., and Kandel, E.R., 1978, Contribution of individual mechanoreceptor sensory neurons to defensive gill-withdrawal reflex in Aplysia, J. Neurophysiol., 41:418.

Camardo, J.S., Klein, M., and Kandel, E.R., 1981, Sensitization in Aplysia: Serotonin elicits a decrease in sensory neuron K^+ current not related to I_K early or I_K Ca^{++}, Soc. Neurosci. Abstr., 7:836.

Carew, T.J., Walters, E.T., and Kandel, E.R., 1981a, Associative learning in Aplysia: Cellular correlates supporting a conditioned fear hypothesis, Science, 211:501.

Carew, T.J., Walters, E.T., and Kandel, E.R., 1981b, Associative learning in a simple reflex in Aplysia, Soc. Neurosci. Abstr., 7:353.

Carew, T.J., Walters, E.T., and Kandel, E.R., 1981c, Classical conditioning in a simple withdrawal reflex in Aplysia californica, J. Neurosci., in press.

Carew, T.J. and Kandel, E.R., 1982, Some conceptual issues in the study of simple forms of learning, in Princeton Symposium on Primary Neural Substrates of Learning and Behavior Change, in preparation.

Castellucci, V.F. and Kandel, E.R., 1974, A quantal analysis of the synaptic depression underlying habituation of the gill-withdrawal reflex in Aplysia, Proc. Natl. Acad. Sci. USA, 71:5004.

Castellucci, V.F. and Kandel, E.R., 1976, Presynaptic facilitation as a mechanism for behavioral sensitization in Aplysia, Science, 194:1176.

Castellucci, V.F., Pinsker, H., Kupfermann, H.I., and Kandel, E.R., 1970, Neuronal mechanisms of habituation and dishabituation of the gill-withdrawal reflex in Aplysia, Science, 167:1745.

Castellucci, V., Schwartz, J.H., Kandel, E.R., Nairn, A., and Greengard, P., 1981, Protein inhibitor of the cyclic AMP-dependent protein kinase can block the onset of, as well as reverse the electrophysiological correlates of sensitization of the gill-withdrawal in Aplysia, Soc. Neurosci. Abstr., 7:836.

Chang, J.J. and Gelperin, A., 1980, Rapid taste aversion learning by an isolated molluscan central nervous system, Proc. Natl. Acad. Sci. USA, 77:6204.

Crow, T. and Alkon, D.L., 1978, Retention of an associative behavioral change in Hermissenda, Science, 201:1239.

Crow, T.J. and Alkon, D.L., 1980, Associative behavioral modification in Hermissenda: Cellular correlates, Science, 209:412.

Davis, W.J. and Gillette, R., 1978, Neural correlate of behavioral plasticity in command neurons of Pleurobranchaea, Science, 199:801.

Davis, W.J., Villet, J., Lee, D., Rigler, M., Gillette, R., and Prince, E., 1980, Selctive and differential avoidance learning in the feeding and withdrawal behavior of Pleurobranchaea californica, J. Comp. Physiol. A, 138:157.

Frazier, W.T., Kandel, E.R., Kupfermann, I., Waziri, R., and Coggeshall, R.E., 1967, Morphological and functional properties of identified neurons in the abdominal ganglion of Aplysia californica, J. Neurophysiol., 30:1288.

Gelperin, A., 1975, Rapid food-aversion learning by a terrestrial mollusk, Science, 189:567.

Hawkins, R.D., 1981, Identified facilitating neurons are excited by cutaneous stimuli used in sensitization and classical conditioning of Aplysia, Soc. Neurosci. Abstr., 7:354.

Hawkins, R.D., Castellucci, V.F., and Kandel, E.R., 1981a, Interneurons involved in mediation and modulation of the gill-withdrawal reflex in Aplysia. I. Identification and characterization, J. Neurophysiol., 45:304.

Hawkins, R.D., Castellucci, V.F., and Kandel, E.R., 1981b, Interneurons involved in mediation and modulation of the gill-withdrawal reflex in Aplysia. II. Identified neurons produce heterosynaptic facilitation contributing to behavioral sensitization, J. Neurophysiol., 45:315.

Kandel, E.R., 1967, Cellular studies of learning, in: "The Neurosciences: A Study Program," G.C. Quarton, T. Melnechuk, F.O. Schmitt, ed., Rockefeller Univ. Press, N.Y.

Kandel, E.R., 1976, "Cellular Basis of Behavior," Freeman and Co., San Francisco.

Kandel, E.R. and Schwartz, J.H., 1981, Molecular biology of an elementary form of learning in Aplysia: Modulation of transmitter release by cyclic nucleotides, Science, in press.

Kanz, J.E., Eberly, L.B., Cobbs, J.S., and Pinsker, H.M., 1979, Neuronal correlates of siphon withdrawal in freely-behaving Aplysia, J. Neurophysiol., 42:1538.

Kennedy, D. and Davis, W.J., 1977, Organization of invertebrate motor systems, in "Handbook of Physiology: The Nervous System I," E.R. Kandel, ed., Williams and Wilkins, Baltimore.

Klein, M. and Kandel, E.R., 1978, Presynaptic modulation of voltage-dependent Ca^{++} current: Mechanism for behavioral sensitization in Aplysia californica, Proc. Natl. Acad. Sci. USA, 75:3512.

Klein, M. and Kandel, E.R., 1980, Mechanism of calcium current modulation underlying presynaptic facilitation and behavioral sensitization in Aplysia, Proc. Natl. Acad. Sci. USA, 77:6912.

Klein, M. and Kandel, E.R., 1982, On the mechanistic relationship of sensitization to classical conditioning, in Princeton Symposium on Primary Neural Substrates of Learning and Behavioral Change, in preparation.

Krasne, F.B., 1969, Excitation and habituation of the crayfish escape reflex: The depolarizing response in lateral giant fibres of the isolated abdomen, J. Exp. Biol., 50:29.

Kupfermann, I. and Kandel, E.R., 1969, Neuronal controls of a behavioral response mediated by the abdominal ganglion of Aplysia, Science, 164:847.

Kupfermann, I., Carew, T.J., and Kandel, E.R., 1974, Local, reflexive and central commands controlling gill and siphon movements in Aplysia californica, J. Neurophysiol., 37:990.

Lukowiak, K. and Sahley, C., 1981, The in vitro classical conditioning of the gill withdrawal reflex of Aplysia californica, Science, 212:1516.

Mpitsos, G.J. and Collins, S.D., 1975, Learning: rapid aversion conditioning in the gastropod mollusc Pleurobranchaea, Science, 188:954.

Perlman, A.J., 1979, Central and peripheral control of siphon-withdrawal reflex in Aplysia californica, J. Neurophysiol., 42:510.

Razran, G., 1971, "Mind in Evolution: An East-West Synthesis of Learning Behavior and Cognition," Houghton Mifflin, Boston.

Sahley, C.L., Gelperin, A., and Rudy, J.W., 1981, One-trial associative learning in a terrestrial mollusc, Proc. Natl. Acad. Sci. USA, 78:640.

Tsukahara, N., 1981, Synaptic plasticity in the mammalian central nervous system, Ann. Rev. Neurosci., 4:351.

Walters, E.T., Carew, T.J., and Kandel, E.R., 1979, Associative learning in Aplysia californica, Proc. Natl. Acad. Sci. USA, Vol. 76, No. 12:6675.

Walters, E.T., Carew, T.J., and Kandel, E.R., 1981a, Associative learning in Aplysia: Evidence for conditioned fear in an invertebrate, Science, 211:504.

Walters, E.T., Carew, T.J., and Kandel, E.R., 1981b, Identification of sensory neurons involved in two forms of classical conditioning in Aplysia, Soc. Neurosci. Abstr., 7:353.

Wells, M.J., 1968, "Lower Animals," McGraw-Hill, New York.

Zucker, R.S., 1972, Crayfish escape behavior and central synapses. II. Physiological mechanisms underlying behavioral habituation, J. Neurophysiol., 35:621.

SENSORY PLASTICITY AND LEARNING: THE MAGNOCELLULAR MEDIAL GENICULATE NUCLEUS OF THE AUDITORY SYSTEM

Norman M. Weinberger

Department of Psychobiology
University of California
Irvine, CA

SUMMARY

The magnocellular medial geniculate nucleus (MGm) is a non-lemniscal component of the thalamo-cortical auditory system. It develops discharge plasticity rapidly during behavioral conditioning, in contrast to the ventral medial geniculate, the lemniscal and non-plastic component. Continual recordings from single cells during the acquisition of the pupillary conditioned response reveals an exceptionally high proportion of plastic neurons, the most plastic of which have a pronounced onset discharge to initial presentation of acoustic stimuli. Facilitation of monosynaptic field potentials in MGm lasts for several hours following brief high-frequency stimulation of its major afferent, with respect both to increased amplitude and decreased latency. Responses of single units are also facilitated for hours, as indexed by increased probability of discharges and decreased latency and latency variability. Together, these findings suggest a functional relationship between conditioning and long-lasting facilitation. Moreover, they underscore the capacity of the auditory system to express physiological plasticity under a variety of circumstances.

INTRODUCTION

Every scientific discipline can be characterized by its "paradigms", or implicit ways of viewing its practice and its data (Kuhn, 1962). So it is with neurobiology, and thus with the neurobiology of learning. Nervous systems are seen as comprised of three major components--sensory, motor, and intermediate. The sensory systems provide accurate input, the motor systems create appropriate behavior, while the intermediate systems, often referred to in part as "associative" systems, are thought to perform the vital and central function of learning. This seems to make good sense. Memories should be stored elsewhere than sensory and motor systems, and they are vital for learning. When common sense is reinforced by science, and vice versa, can the truth be far behind? Perhaps.

In recent years, there has been an accumulation of findings that suggest the inadequacy of this standard paradigm of learning. For example, on the motor side, Woody and his associates (1974) have presented a strong case for plasticity induced by behavioral conditioning in projection neurons of the motor cortex of the cat. On the sensory side, one might first point to the findings of Kandel and his associates (1978) that the critical events in habituation occur in sensory neurons. In mammals, there is a very large body of findings indicating the development of physiological plasticity in sensory systems, especially the auditory system, during habituation and also during associative learning (Buchwald et al., 1966; Olds et al., 1972; Oleson et al., 1975; Disterhoft and Stuart, 1976; Gabriel et al., 1976). This body of data has not been incorporated, or even much noticed, in the literature on sensory physiology.

Among the disquieting implications of these findings are (1) the active involvement of all three major components of nervous systems in learning and (2) a particular paradox, often expressed teleologically, about the role of sensory systems. How can a sensory system simultaneously provide an accurate representation of the world (reflect the physical parameters of stimuli) and also change its responses according to the meaning or signal value of a stimulus (reflect the psychological parameters of stimuli)? We and others have suggested that, at least in the case of the auditory thalamo-cortical system, two separate components are responsible for these two functions (Ryugo and Weinberger, 1976, 1978). We have identified these as the lemniscal, non-plastic, ventral medial geniculate nucleus (MGv) and the non-lemniscal, plastic, magnocellular medial geniculate nucleus (MGm). Our findings to date are described briefly below.

GENERAL APPROACH

In order to study plasticity in the auditory system, it is essential to eliminate extrinsic sources of physiological change, principally alterations in sound level peripheral to the cochlea. This is best done by neuromuscular paralysis, so we developed a chronic cat preparation which could develop all the major features of Pavlovian conditioning under paralysis and artificial respiration. In this preparation, the pupillary dilation conditioned response, developed by the pairing of an acoustic with an electrocutaneous stimulus, satisfies these requirements. Thus, the pupillary response exhibits habituation, rapid (10-20 trials) systematic growth during

CS-US pairing, discrimination between reinforced and non-reinforced stimuli, discrimination reversal, repeated discrimination reversal (Oleson et al., 1972), inhibition of delay (Oleson et al., 1973) and inhibitory control of the pupillary conditioned response by a non-reinforced stimulus (Weinberger et al., 1973). The cochlear microphonic does not change systematically during training (Ashe et al., 1976).

Initial neurophysiological studies employed the recording of more than one cell at a time (so-called "multiple unit" or "unit cluster" activity) in order to locate regions of the auditory system in which neuronal learning occurred. We found cellular conditioning in the auditory cortex (and in the cochlear nucleus following cortical learning), plus discrimination and discrimination reversal of the enhanced cellular response to the conditioned stimulus, as well as pupillary conditioning (Oleson et al., 1975). Due to space limitations, relationships between behavioral conditioning and neural plasticity will not be considered here; see Weinberger, 1980, 1981, for details.

THE MAGNOCELLULAR MEDIAL GENICULATE NUCLEUS (MGm)

The possibility of correlating structure with cellular plasticity became obvious in light of increasing anatomical and physiological evidence that sensory systems in general and the auditory system in particular are comprised of both highly specific, spatially organized regions and less specific cell groups; Graybiel (1972) has termed these "lemniscal line" and "lemniscal adjunct" systems or channels, respectively. The coalescence of these systems in cortex suggested that analysis of these sensory components be investigated at the level of the thalamus. The medial geniculate nucleus (thalamic auditory system) has been particularly well characterized both anatomically and physiologically. It is actually comprised of three major subdivisions, the ventral, dorsal, and magnocellular (medial) subnuclei, on the basis of cyto- and myeloarchitectonics, Golgi impregnation, afferents, and efferents (Morest, 1964; Ramon y Cajal, 1966; Oliver and Hall, 1975; Ryugo and Killackey, 1974) (Fig. 1). Both anatomical and physiological evidence indicate that the ventral division is lemniscal, while the magnocellular division is not (see Ryugo and Weinberger, 1978, for detailed discussion and references).

THE COMPARTMENTALIZATION OF PLASTICITY DURING BEHAVIORAL CONDITIONING

An investigation of neural plasticity within the medial geniculate nucleus revealed that only the MGm neurons learned during classical conditioning (Ryugo and Weinberger, 1976, 1978). The specificity of this result is clear because MGm cells also exhibited differential conditioning between the reinforced condition-

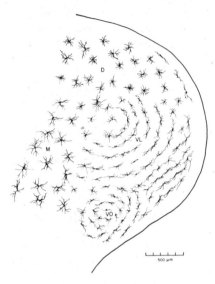

Figure 1: Camera lucida reconstruction of the MGB from Golgi material. Typical distribution of neuronal types through the middle of the medial geniculate body of the adult cat. Coronal section, Golgi-Cox. Abbreviations: D, dorsal division; M, magnocellular division; VL, ventral division, pars lateralis; VO, ventral division, pars ovoida.

ed stimulus and another acoustic stimulus that was not reinforced. Furthermore, recordings were obtained simultaneously from learning cells in the MGm division and non-plastic cells in the ventral division (Fig. 2).

These results have been replicated in two other laboratories. Miller (1979) has found multiple-unit conditioned responses in the medial but not in the ventral division of the medial geniculate of the rabbit during instrumental conditioning. Birt et al. (1978) reported similar findings in the rat using a training regimen that is a hybrid classical-instrumental conditioning situation. Together, these findings indicate that plasticity in the MGm is not confined to certain species or training regimens. It is also of interest that the tripartate organization of the medial geniculate nucleus is essentially the same across a very wide and diverse range of mammals. In addition to the rat, cat, and rabbit, there are the tree shrew (Oliver and Hall, 1975), the squirrel monkey (Jordan, 1973), the owl monkey (Fitzpatrick and Imig, 1978) and the opossum (RoBards, unpublished data). It appears that the magnocellular medial geniculate nucleus constitutes an especially conditionable substrate of an evolutionarily conservative nature, i.e., one which was attained early in mammalian evolution and thereafter maintained.

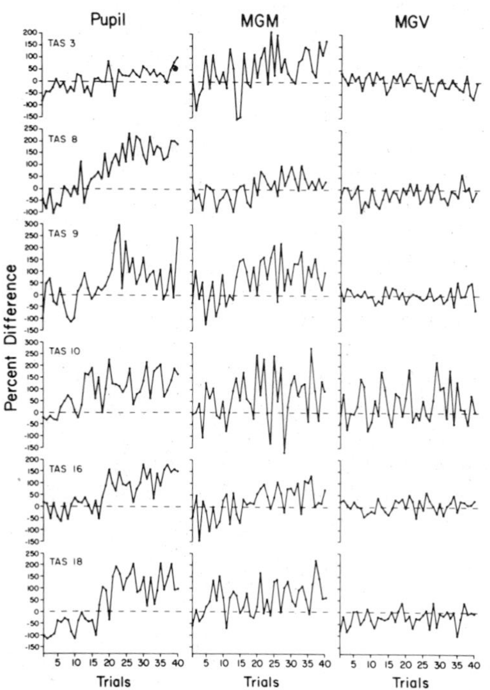

Figure 2: Trial-by-trial functions of pupillary, MGm, and MGv responses during conditioning. Each point represents the normalized response to the CS+ during its 1.0 sec. presentation, expressed as a percent difference score relative to its mean sensitization value (dashed line). Both pupil and MGm neuronal activity exhibit a systematic growth of responsivity during conditioning. MGv neuronal activity fails to demonstrate such conditioned response enhancement. Data are from 6 animals that developed pupillary conditioning and had placements in MGm and MGv of the same medial geniculate body.

CHARACTERISTICS OF SINGLE NEURON DISCHARGES IN MGm

Single cell recordings concurrent with formation of the pupillary dilation conditioned reflex were obtained from 34 cells in 34 cats. As one goal of these experiments was to seek discharge characteristics predictive of conditionability, the data from only one cell per animal were suitable. Thus, while it was technically feasible to run a second training series, recording from a second cell after completion of the initial training, the cat was no longer naive; neither were its neurons.

Of 34 cells, 24 (71%) developed a significant change in evoked discharge. The total were divided into four groups: (A) cells with increased response meeting a rigorous criterion ($p < .001$), n=8; (B) cells with increased response meeting a less severe criterion ($p < .05$), n=9; (C) cells failing to meet significance at the 5% level (n=10); (D) cells developing a significant decrease ($p < .05$) in response during conditioning (n=7) (Fig. 3). Group A shows pronounced habituation during the sensitization phase followed by an increased response which is clearly present by trials 8-10, and which has not reached asymptote by the end of the first twenty conditioning trials. There is no pronounced change in background activity. Group B, which met a less severe statistical criterion, has a less pronounced habituation function but also does exhibit rapid learning. In contrast to Group A, this potentiated evoked discharge reaches asymptote quickly (trial 12) and returns to baseline at the end of twenty trials. Background activity is also more variable for these cells, and there is an indication of a slight increase in background discharges during conditioning. [However, the nature of this increase could not account for the incremental learning curve for evoked activity.] Cells which failed to meet statistical significance (Group C) have a poor habituation function and no clear learning function. Of interest, there is a significant

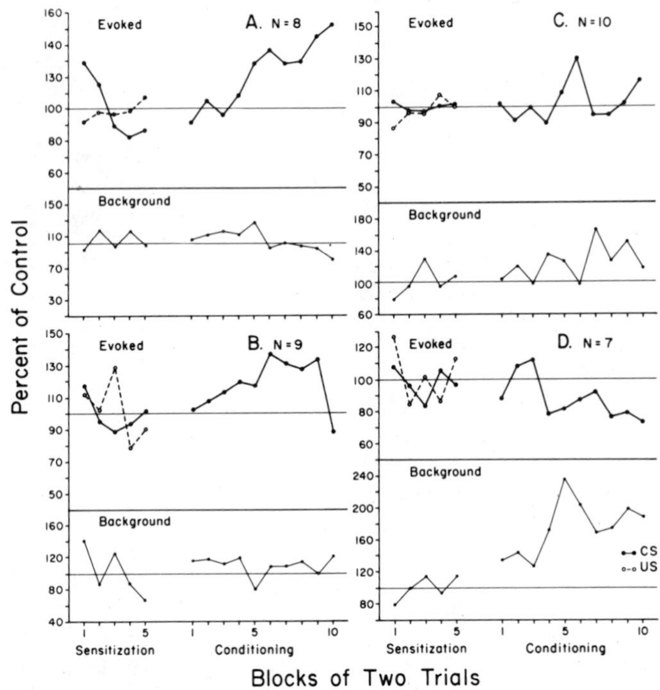

Figure 3: Learning curves for four cell groups according to learning criteria.

increase in background discharge during conditioning. Cells developing a decrease in response to the conditioned stimulus (D) also develop a significant increase in background activity. The functions for evoked and background discharges are almost mirror images; thus, the apparent decremental learning is due to the increase in background activity rather than to an actual decrease in the number of spikes evoked by the conditioned stimulus. The conditioning procedure has in effect converted cells which initially had little response to the CS into cells with an inhibitory response.

The different learning functions of the groups probably account for the modest slopes of learning curves seen in the previous experiment, in which multiple-unit recordings were used. Thus, addition of the single unit data from all four groups of neurons would yield only a modest positive slope. Also, it is clear that MUA data do not reflect the underlying heterogeneity of single unit data.

Several parameters of spontaneous discharges (from the period preceding the start of training) and evoked discharges (during the first few sensitization trials) were calculated for each cell, in order to determine whether there was a physiological characteristic predictive of subsequent discharge plasticity. None of these measures differentiated among or between the four groups of cells. Inspection of the histograms for each cell suggested that the pattern of response to the conditioned stimulus was different among the groups. Specifically, it appeared that cells exhibiting a large onset response were also those which conditioned rapidly and persistently (Fig. 4), i.e., Group A, in contrast to cells which had an equal or larger overall response to the CS, but without a pronounced "onset" response. The data were reanalyzed on the basis of the first 100 msec. of CS presentation. Indeed it was found that Group A had a significantly larger onset response, relative to background activity, than any of the other three groups ($p < .001$) (Fig. 5).

Thus, overall responsiveness to the conditioned stimulus does not predict rapid and persistent cellular learning whereas the presence of a large onset response does predict response plasticity (for further details, see Weinberger, 1981).

LONG-LASTING FACILITATION - MONOSYNAPTIC RESPONSES

Long-term potentiation (LTP) is characterized by the elicitation of a persistent (minutes to hours or days) enhancement of an electrically evoked potential by a brief (hundreds of milliseconds to several seconds) stimulus train. These characteristics have aroused interest in LTP as a possible mechanism for the long-term storage of information in the brain and as an analogue, or even a possible mechanism for learning (Bliss and Lømo, 1973). Heretofore, LTP has been reported only within the hippocampus.

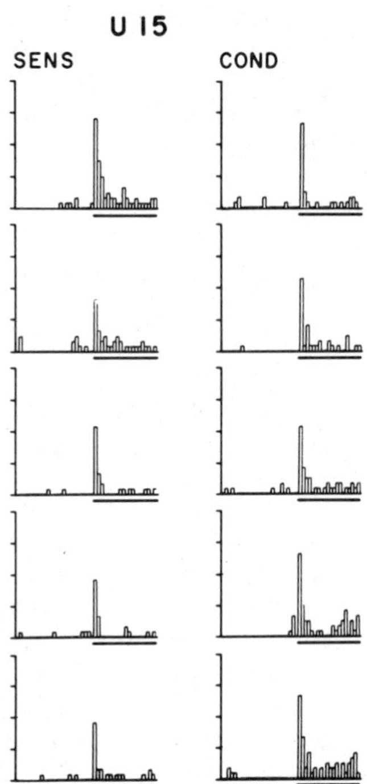

Figure 4: Histograms and pupillary records for a Group A cell, CS = one sec. (horizontal line). Each histogram is the sum of two consecutive trials, each bar represents 50 msec. Data for the ten trials of sensitization (CS and US presented randomly) and the first ten trials of conditioning (CS and US paired) are presented. Note the decrement during sensitization and the extremely rapid increment during conditioning. Calibration: 6 spikes per division; horizontal bar, 1 sec.

In view of the plastic properties of the MGm during behavioral learning and the putative importance of LTP for learning, we investigated the possibility that the MGm could develop an LTP-type phenomenon in response to stimulation of its major input path, the brachium of the inferior colliculus (BIC) (Moore and Goldberg, 1963; Morest, 1964). Cats were prepared under barbiturate anesthesia, with a bipolar stimulating electrode in the BIC and a tungsten recording electrode in the MGm. The basic experimental protocol was as follows. Single test stimuli (0.2 Hz, 0.1 - 0.3 ms) were presented at various voltages (current levels of 0.1 - 0.9 mA). Next, a sub-maximal voltage was selected and stimuli were presented thereafter at 0.2 Hz, for a period of at least 20 minutes, by which time responses to this baseline stimulation were stable. One to three consecutive trains of high frequency stimulation (100-300 Hz, 285

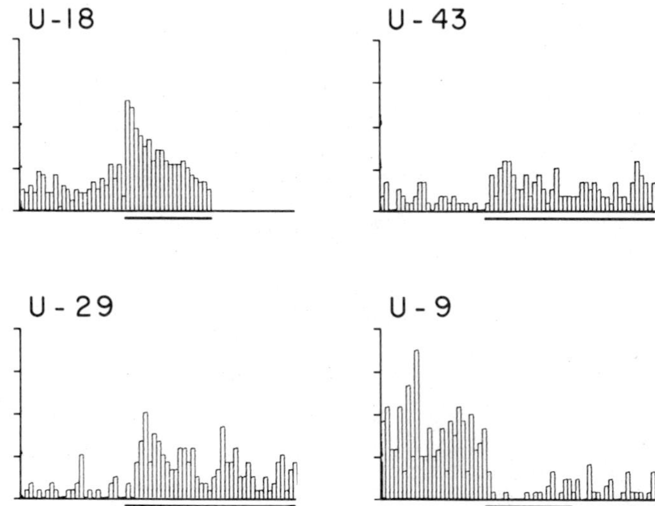

Figure 5: Representative histograms from the entire sample of 34 cells for the first five sensitization trials. U-18, from Group A, has a large response at the onset of the CS (horizontal bar, 1 sec.). Other types of histograms were not found in Group A.

ms) were then presented without interruption of the test stimuli, and test stimuli were continued for at least 30-40 min. A post-train voltage series was then run, followed by the resumption of test stimuli for periods up to four hours. We report here the results of experiments with 11 animals in which the electrode tips were histologically verified to have been in the BIC and the MGm.

The response of the MGm to single BIC stimuli consists of a biphasic wave with a latency of approximately 0.94 $\pm$ 0.08 msec. to onset and amplitudes of 50 to 200 microvolts. The presynaptic volley was usually partially obscured by the stimulus artifact and so could not be measured consistently. Transient facilitation ("frequency facilitation") of the response was present during and sometimes for about 30 sec. following the high frequency train. In some instances, initial depression of the response was present for about 15 sec. following the high frequency train. Regardless of the initial change, there was a gradual potentiation of the response in all animals (average maximum of 145% of baseline). The duration of facilitation was as long as 4-1/2 hours; most experiments were terminated before the response had returned to baseline values, so that no upper limit has been determined yet. In addition to enhancement of amplitude, reduction of latency was routinely obtained (Figs. 6-7). Amplitude facilitation was also evidenced by voltage functions obtained at least 30-40 min. after high frequency

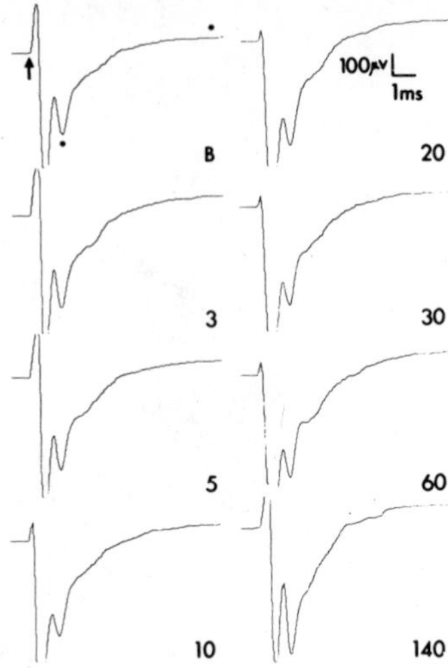

Figure 6: Monosynaptic potentials (average of 6 responses) for one cat, illustrating amplitude facilitation relative to baseline values (B) during 140 minutes following high frequency stimulation. Arrow indicates beginning of single test stimulus; dots denote peak-peak amplitude measure.

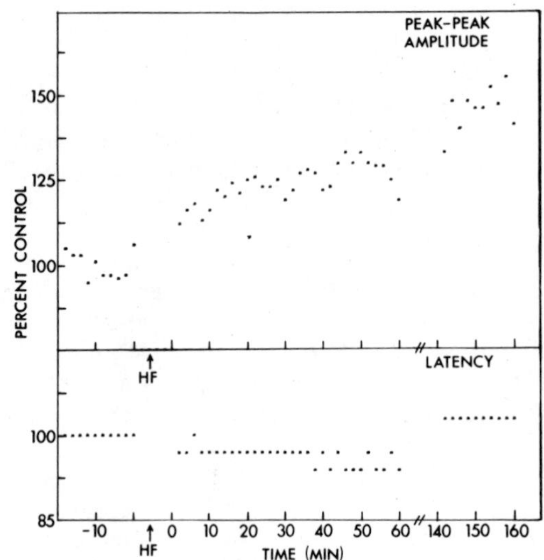

Figure 7: Summary data for the same subject whose records are in Fig. 6. Each point is the average of 24 responses (2 min. periods). Note the gradual increase in amplitude, still evident at termination of experiment after 160 minutes, and reduction in latency, to onset of the monosynaptic response.

stimulation (Fig. 8). We term this phenomenon "long-lasting facilitation" (LLF) because, at this time, no claim is made that it is identical to that seen in the hippocampus.

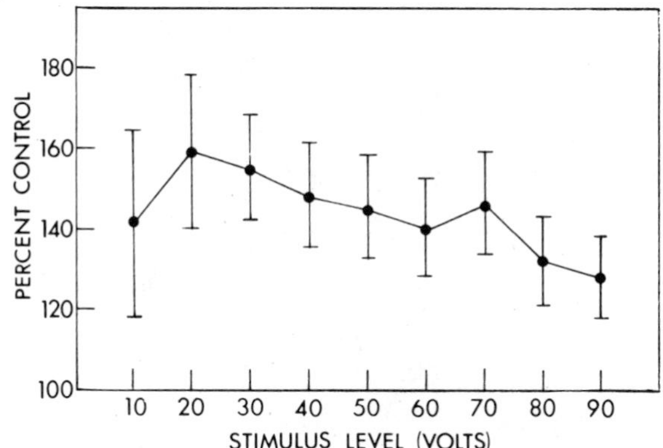

Figure 8: Group data (N=11) showing facilitation of monosynaptic responses as a function of voltage. Vertical bars = + 1 S.E.

LONG-LASTING FACILITATION - SINGLE CELL RESPONSES

We have recorded from single units in the MGm (1 per cat) using the same preparation and general paradigm as in the study of monosynaptic responses. After high frequency stimulation, neurons developed a variety of long-lasting changes in their firing patterns: (1) a decrease in spike latency, (2) an increase in the number of evoked spikes, (3) a decrease in the variability of spike onset, and (4) a decrease in interspike interval variance (Fig. 9). The observed changes lasted for up to 128 minutes (the longest interval over which we could monitor single unit activity). The neurons were localized histologically in the MGm. Neurons which did not demonstrate discharge plasticity were localized in the ventral and dorsal divisions. These findings indicate that potentiation of the monosynaptic response is most likely due to increased excitability of single cells within the MGm, and supports the view that synapses in MGm are involved.

CONCLUSION

The focus of research on the neurobiology of learning, particularly in vertebrates, has been on those neural systems which are neither sensory nor motor. This has been based, I think, on an implicit belief that plasticity underlying behavioral adaptations, as seen in learning, is a property of these "intermediate" or

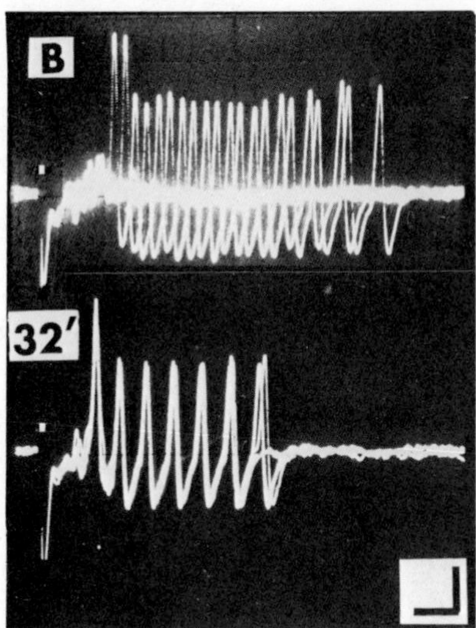

Figure 9: Unitary discharges to single stimuli before (top) and 32 minutes following brief high frequency stimulation of the brachium of the inferior colliculus. Each record is the superimposition of 5 consecutive test stimuli. Note the reduction in latency, latency variability and increase in discharges (top = 21, bottom = 34 spikes). Calibrations: 1 msec., 100 uV.

"associative" regions, but not of sensory or motor systems. It now appears that all three of the major components of nervous systems are intimately involved in learning. We have presented evidence that, within the thalamo-cortical auditory system, specific physiological plasticity develops in the magnocellular medial geniculate nucleus during behavioral conditioning. Moreover, "long-lasting facilitation", another form of physiological plasticity, can be induced in this structure. That such a form of plasticity occurs in a sensory system, as well as in an intermediary structure as central as is the hippocampus, suggests the need to question fundamental assumptions about the neural bases of learning. That the involvement of sensory systems complicates our task might also be expected, because the field of learning is an extremely difficult one. Even after the cellular events underlying plasticity are understood, it will still be necessary to determine how the various sub-systems of the nervous system participate and cooperate to yield integrated adaptive behavior based upon learning.

ACKNOWLEDGMENTS

Research reported here was supported by BNS76-81924 from the National Science Foundation, NIMH Predoctoral Fellowship No. MH

05440-02, NIMH Predoctoral Fellowship No. MH 05424, NIMH Predoctoral Fellowship No. MH 51324, and NS16108 from the National Institute of Neurological and Communicative Disorders and Stroke. Thanks are also due to Richard Gerren and William Hopkins for their work on long-lasting facilitation and to Elaine Hackelman for secretarial services.

REFERENCES

Ashe, J. H., Cassady, J. M., and Weinberger, N. M., 1976, The relationship of the cochlear microphonic potential to the acquisition of a classically conditioned pupillary dilation response, Behav. Biol., 16:45.

Birt, D., Nienhuis, R., and Olds, M., 1978, Separation of associative from non-associative short latency changes in medial geniculate and inferior colliculus during differential conditioning and reversal in rats, Soc. Neurosci. Abst., 4:255.

Bliss, T. V. P. and Lømo, T., 1973, Long lasting potentiation of synaptic transmission in the dentate area of the anaesthetized rabbit following stimulation of the perforant path. J. Physiol., 232:331.

Buchwald, J. S., Halas, E. S., and Schramm, S., 1966, Changes in cortical and subcortical unit activity during behavioral conditioning, Physiol. Behav., 1:11.

Disterhoft, J. F. and Stuart, D. K., 1976, Trial sequence of changed unit activity in auditory system of alert rat during conditioned response acquisition and extinction, J. Neurophysiol., 39: 266.

Fitzpatrick, K. A. and Imig, T. J., 1978, Projections of auditory cortex upon the thalamus and midbrain in the owl monkey. J. Comp. Neurol., 177:537.

Gabriel, M., Miller, J. D., and Saltwick, S. E., 1976, Multiple unit activity of the rabbit medial geniculate nucleus in conditioning, extinction, and reversal, Physiol. Psychol., 4:124.

Graybiel, A. M., 1972, Some fiber pathways related to the posterior thalamic region in the cat, Brain Behav., Evol., 6:363.

Jordan, H., 1973, The structure of the medial geniculate nucleus (MGN): A cyto- and myeloarchitectonic study in the squirrel monkey, J. Comp. Neurol., 148:469.

Kandel, E. R., 1978, A cell-biological approach to learning, Soc. Neurosci., Bethesda, Md.

Kuhn, T. S., 1962, The Structure of Scientific Revolutions, University of Chicago Press, Chicago, Illinois.

Miller, J. D., 1979, Multiple unit activity in the rabbit thalamus and inferior colliculus during differential avoidance conditioning and reversal, Unpublished doctoral thesis, University of Texas.

Moore, R. Y. and Goldberg, J. M., 1963, Ascending projections of the inferior colliculus in the cat, J. Comp. Neurol., 121:109.

Morest, D. K., 1964, The neuronal architecture of the medial geniculate body of the cat, J. Anat. (Lond.), 98:611.

Olds, J., Disterhoft, J. F., Segal, M., Kornblith, C. L., and Hirsh, R., 1972, Learning centers of rat brain mapped by measuring latencies of conditioned unit responses, J. Neurophysiol., 35: 202.

Oleson, T. D., Ashe, J. H., and Weinberger, N. M., 1975, Modification of auditory and somatosensory system activity during pupillary conditioning in the paralyzed cat, J. Neurophysiol., 38:1114.

Oleson, T. D. Vododnick. D. S., and Weinberger, N. M., 1973, Pupillary inhibition of delay during Pavlovian conditioning in paralyzed cat, Behav. Biol., 8:337.

Oleson, T. D., Westenberg, I. S., and Weinberger, N. M., 1972, Characteristics of the pupillary dilation response during Pavlovian conditioning in paralyzed cats, Behav. Biol., 7:829.

Oliver, D. L. and Hall, W. C., 1975, Subdivisions of the medial geniculate body in the tree shrew (Tapaia glis), Brain Res., 86:217.

Ramon y Cajal, S., 1966, Studies on the Diencephalon, Trans. by E. Ramon-Moliner, Charles C. Thomas, Springfield, Ill.

Ryugo, D. K. and Killackey, H. P., 1974, Differential telencephalic projections of the medial and ventral divisions of the medial geniculate body of the rat, Brain Res., 82:173.

Ryugo, D. K. and Weinberger, N. M., 1976, Differential plasticity of morphologically distinct neuron populations in the medial geniculate body of the cat during classical conditioning, Soc. Neurosci. Abst., 2:435.

Ryugo, D. K. and Weinberger, N. M., 1978, Differential plasticity of morphologically distinct neuron populations in the medial geniculate body of the cat during classical conditioning, Behav. Biol., 22:275.

Weinberger, N. M., 1980, Neurophysiological studies of learning in association with the pupillary dilation conditioned reflex, in: Neural Mechanisms of Goal-Directed Behavior and Learning, R. F. Thompson, L. H. Hicks, and V. B. Shvyrkov, eds., Academic Press, New York, pp. 241-261.

Weinberger, N. M., 1981, Effects of conditioned arousal on the auditory system, in: The Neural Basis of Behavior, A. L. Beckman, ed., Spectrum Publishing Co., Jamaica, N.Y.

Weinberger, N. M., Oleson, T. D., and Haste, D., 1973, Inhibitory control of conditional pupillary dilation response in the paralyzed cat, Behav. Biol., 9:307.

Woody, C. D., 1974, Aspects of the electrophysiology of cortical processes related to the development and performance of learned motor responses, The Physiologist, 17:49.

APPENDIX

The following figures pertain to latencies of transmission through neural networks involved with conditioning. They illustrate material apart from that included in the earlier manuscripts.

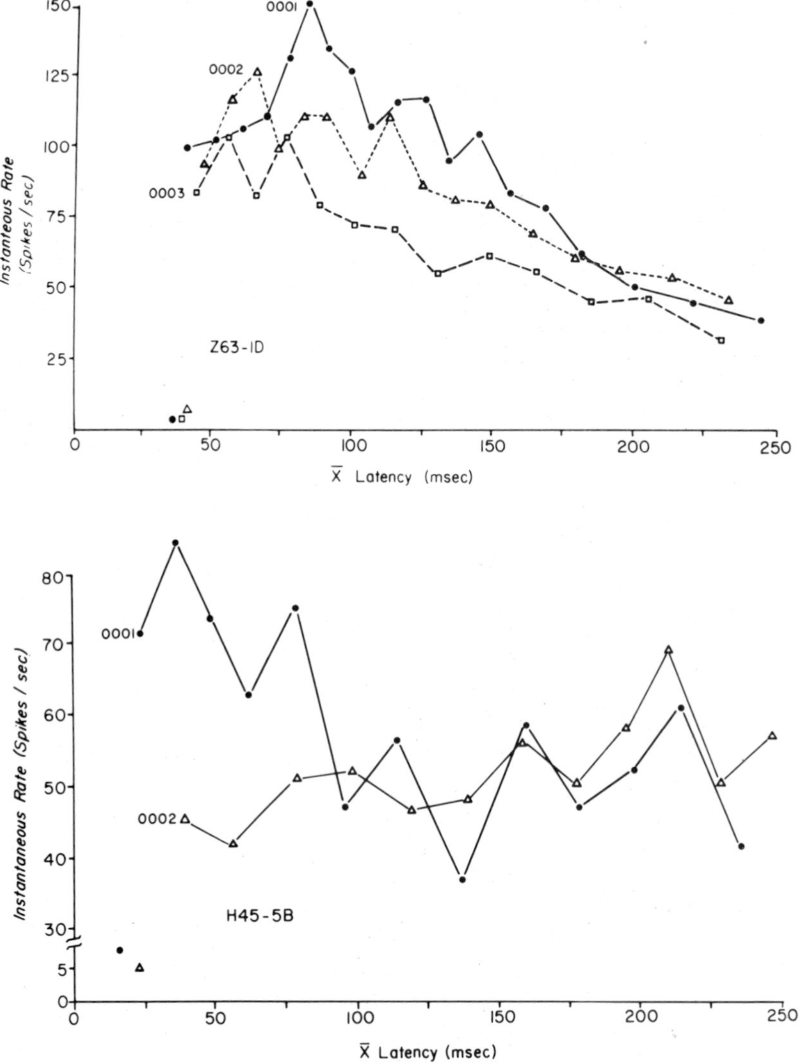

Fig. 1. Instantaneous discharge rate (computed from interspike intervals) versus time after auditory stimulus onset for two units (Z63-1D and H45-5B) recorded under three different behavioral conditions: 0001 (filled circles) = auditory reaction time with background visual stimuli, 0002 (open triangles) = visual reaction time with background auditory stimuli, and 0003 (open squares) = nonperformance with background auditory stimuli. (From Miller et al., Amer. J. Otolaryng., 1980, 1, 119=130.)

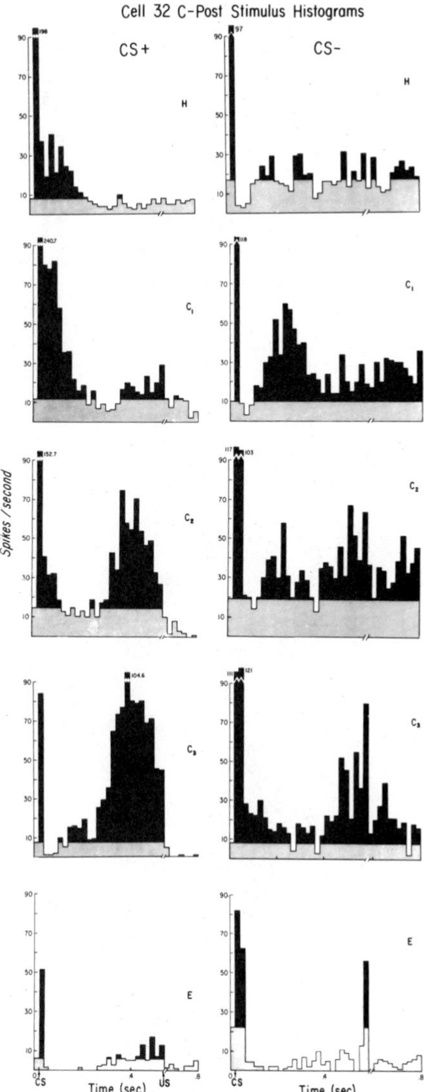

Fig. 2. PSTHs of CS+ and CS- responses of an individual neuron for an habituation-conditioning-extinction sequence. Each histogram sum of 75 trials. Stimuli (3 0.2 ms pulses, 250 Hz, 5 volts) through sc needles in left (CS+) and right (CS-) hindpaws were CSs. The pyramidal tract US was a 100 ms train of 25 0.5 ms pulses at a voltage (10 v) just above threshold to elicit an antidromic response in the recorded neuron (postcruciate cortex of unanesthetized, flaxedilized cat). ITI randomized with mean of 12 sec (range 6-18) and sequence of CS+ and CS- randomized within a set of 50 trials. Average background rate coded gray. Note excitatory change in response to CS+ at 300-550 ms. (O'Brien et al. JCPP, 1977).

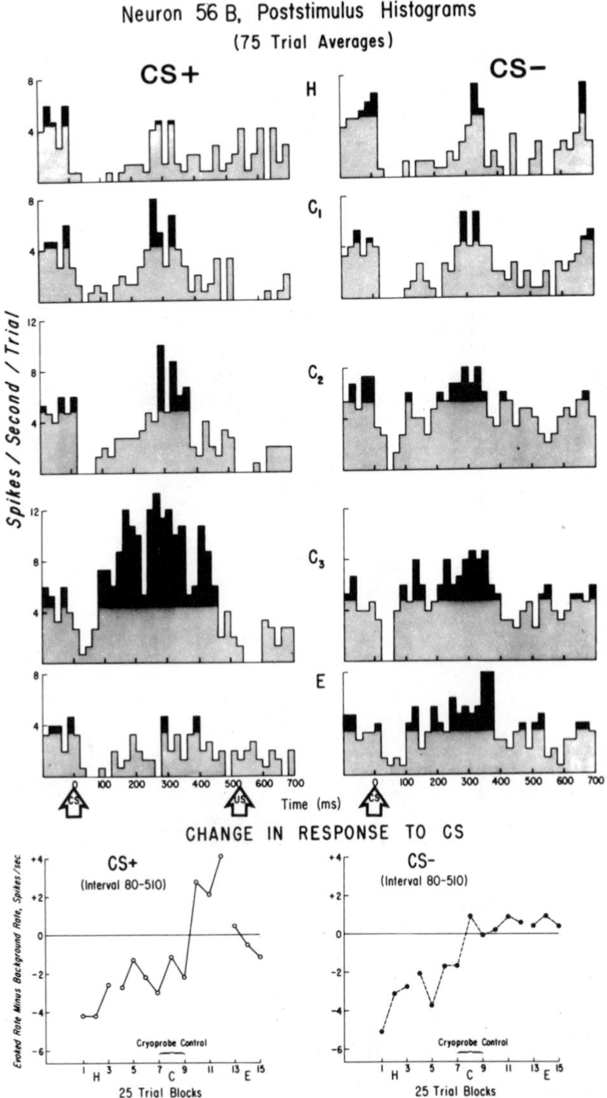

Fig. 3. PSTHs of CS+ and CS- responses of an individual neuron for an habituation-conditioning-extinction sequence. Each histogram sum of 75 trials. Stimuli (3 0.2 ms pulses, 250 Hz, 4 volts) through subcutaneous needles in right (CS+) and left (CS-) forepaws were CSs, and simultaneous stimulation (8 volts) of both hindpaws was the US. Neuron recorded from right postcruciate cortex of unanesthetized, flaxedilized cat. ITI randomized with mean of 12 sec (range 6-18) and sequence of CS+ and CS- randomized within a set of 50 trials. Average background rate is stippled gray area. Note excitatory change in response to CS+ at 80-510 ms. (Rosenblum & O'Brien, J. Neurophysiol., 1977).

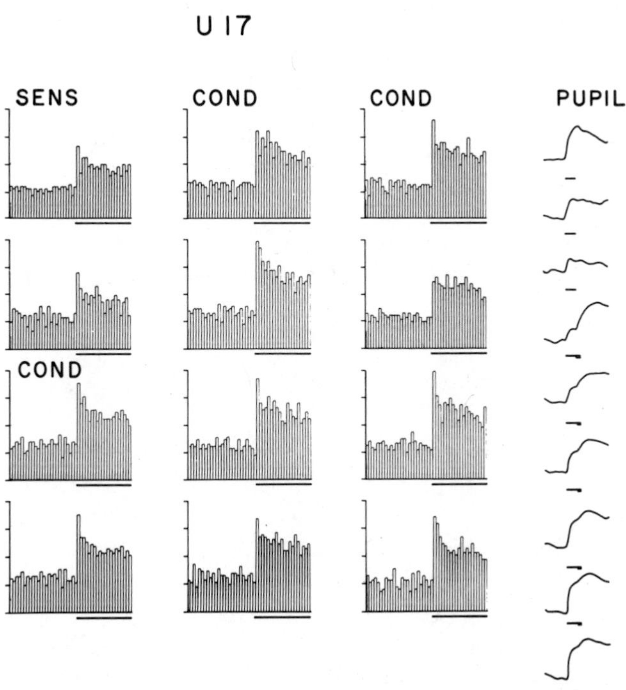

Fig. 4. Histograms and pupillary records for cell U-17 from Group A, the most plastic cells in the magnocellular medial geniculate nucleus. Each histogram is the sum of five consecutive trials; each bar represents 50 msec. Note the largest evoked discharge is at stimulus onset (1st 50 msec.), and the neuronal responses have been increased within the first five trials of conditioning. The effect is persistent through the tenth block (trials 46-50) of training. Calibration: 12 spikes/division; horizontal bar = 1 sec. CS (white noise). Sample pupillary records, top to bottom: sensitization trials 1,7,10 and conditioning trials 1,5, 10,20,30,45. Note decrement in pupillary response during sensitization and subsequent development of the CR during stimulus pairing. Horizontal bar = CS; downward marker = US. (From N.M. Weinberger).

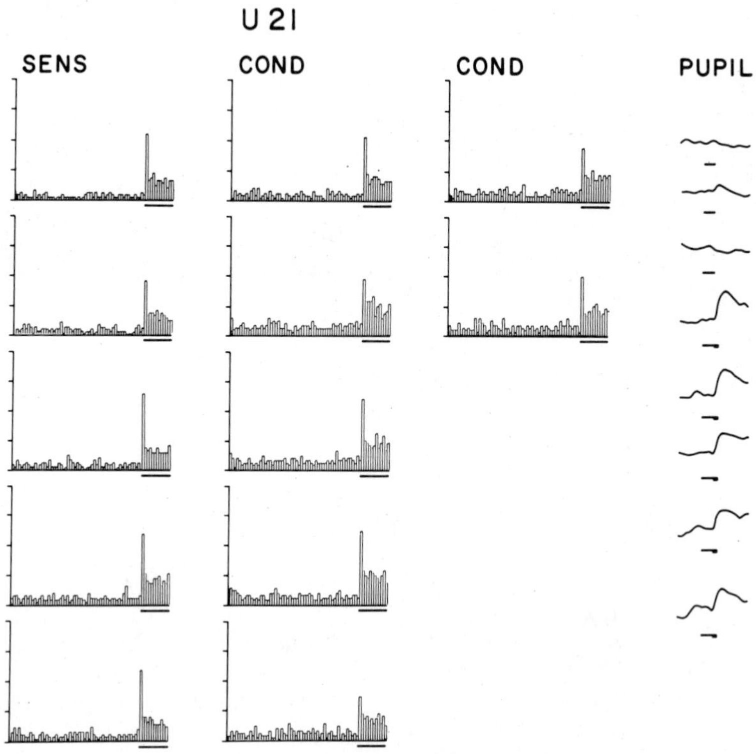

Fig. 5. Histograms and pupillary records for cell U-21. Each histogram is the sum of 5 consecutive trials. Note the largest evoked discharge is at stimulus onset (first bar) but the cell failed to develop systematic change in the response during training. However, this animal also failed to develop a pupillary conditioned response, although an unconditioned response was in evidence during stimulus pairing. These data illustrate a non-plastic unit in a non-learning animal; therefore these neural data cannot be interpreted as a counter example to the finding that a pronounced onset response predicts neuronal plasticity in the magnocellular medial geniculate, as there is no independent behavioral evidence of the adequacy of the preparation. Large onset responses appear necessary but not sufficient for the later rapid development of persistent neuronal plasticity in the MGm. Calibrations: 12 spikes per division. Pupillary records (top to bottom), sensitization trials 1,3, 10 and conditioning 1,6,16,26,35. (From N.M. Weinberger).

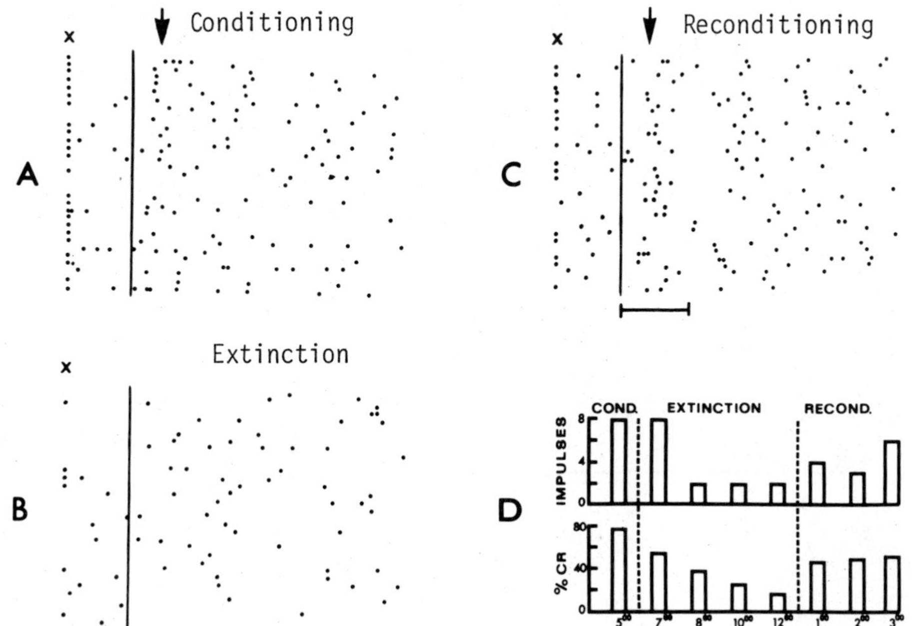

Fig. 6. Study of a single unit through extinction and reconditioning of blink. A: 32-sweep raster of evoked activity in conditioned animal. B: activity after extinction. C: activity after reconditioning. Initial bars designate conditioned blink response on that sweep. Solid line corresponds to click presentation. Arrows show increased unit response. 40-msec time calibration as shown in C. D: number of impulses above spontaneous rate per 32 sweeps in 8- to 28-msec period after click, averaged and shown at real time intervals during extinction and reconditioning (above), and compared with corresponding percent conditioned response performance (below). (From Woody et al., J. Neurophysiol. 1970).

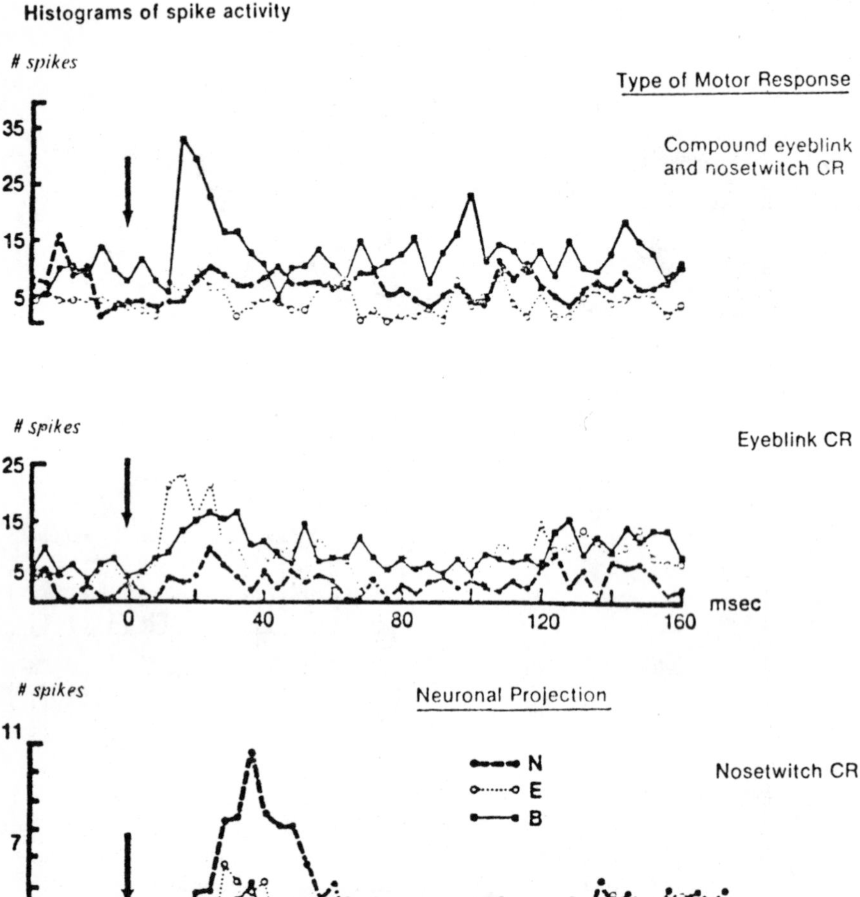

Fig. 7. Patterns of activity evoked in the motor cortex of cats trained to perform different conditioned movements. Unit activity is divided according to the projection of the area from which it was recorded: B, with eyeblink and nosetwitch muscles; E, eyeblink muscles. The traces are the averages of recordings from many single units. (Woody and colleagues, unpublished.)

CONTRIBUTORS

Daniel L. Alkon
Section on Neural Systems
Laboratory of Biophysics
Marine Biological Laboratory
Woods Hole, Massachusetts 02543

Craig D. Applegate
Department of Psychology
University of Vermont
Burlington, Vermont 05401

Alvin L. Beggs
College of Osteopathic Medicine
and Department of Psychology
Ohio University
Athens, Ohio 45701

L.S. Benardo
Department of Neurology
Stanford University Medical Ctr.
Stanford, California 94305

D.A. Benson
Department of Biomedical Eng.
John Hopkins University,
School of Medicine
Baltimore, Maryland 21205

Theodore W. Berger
Psychobiology Program
Dept. of Psychology & Psychiatry
University of Pittsburgh
Pittsburgh, Penn. 15260

Federico Bermudez-Rattoni
Department of Psychology and
Mental Retardation Research Center
University of California
Los Angeles, California 90024

Stephen D. Berry
Department of Psychology
Miami University
Oxford, Ohio 45056

Neil E. Berthier
Department of Psychology
University of Massachusetts
Amherst, Massachusetts 01003

Phillip J. Best
Department of Psychology
University of Virginia
Charlottsville, Virginia 22901

Lynn J. Bindman
Department of Physiology
University College London
London, WC1E 6BT, England

Dorwin Birt
Division of Biology 216-76
Calif. Institute of Technology
1201 E. California Boulevard
Pasadena, Calif. 91125

Jennifer S. Buchwald
Mental Retardation Research Center
Brain Research Institute & Dept of
Physiology, Univ. of Calif., Med. Ctr.
Los Angeles, Calif. 90024

Y. Burnod
INSERMU3 CNRS
Hospital Salpetriere
47 Bd Hospital
Paris, France

J. Calvet
INSERMU3 CNRS
Hospital Salpetriere
47 Bd Hospital
Paris, France

T.J. Carew
Center of Neurobiology and
Behavior College of Physicians
and Surgeons
Columbia University
New York, New York 10032

Edward P. Christian
Dept. of Physiology and
Pharmacology
Bowman Gray School of Medicine
Winston-Salem, North Carolina 27103

G.A. Clark
Stanford University
Stanford, California 94305

David H. Cohen
Dept. of Neurobiology and Behavior
State Univ. of New York at
Stony Brook
Stony Brook, New York 11790

John A. Conner
University of Illinois
Urbana, Illinois and
Bell Telephone Laboratories
Murray Hill, New Jersey

Carl W. Cotman
Department of Psychobiology
University of California
Irvine, California 92717

Sam A. Deadwyler
Dept. of Physiology & Pharmacology
Bowman Gray School of Medicine
Winston-Salem, North Carolina 27103

John E. Desmond
Department of Psychology
University of Massachusetts
Amherst, Massachusetts 01003

John F. Disterhoft
Dept. of Cell Biology and Anatomy
Northwestern Univ. Medical School
Chicago, Illinois 60611

R.J. Elble
Dept. of Neurobiology & Neurology
Washington Univ. School of Medicine
Saint Louis, Missouri 63130

Graham E. Fagg
Department of Psychobiology
University of California
Irvine, California 92717

Eberhard E. Fetz
Dept. of Physiology & Biophysics
and Regional Primate Research Ctr.
University of Washington
Seattle, Washington 98105

Kent Foster
Department of Psychology
University of Texas at Austin
Austin, Texas 78712

Robert C. Frysinger
Department of Psychology
University of Vermont
Burlington, Vermont 05401

Joaquin M. Fuster
Dept. of Psychiatry & Brain Research
Institute, School of Medicine
University of California at
Los Angeles
Los Angeles, California 90024

Michael Gabriel
Department of Psychology
University of Texas at Austin
Austin, Texas 78712

Michela Gallagher
Department of Psychology
University of North Carolina
Chapel Hill, North Carolina 27514

John Garcia
Dept. of Psychology and Mental
Retardation Research Center
University of California
Los Angeles, California 90024

P.F.C. Gilbert
Dept. of Neurobiology and
Neurology
Washington Univ. School of Medicine
Saint Louis, Missouri 63130

M.H. Goldstein, Jr.
Dept. of Biomedical Engineering
Johns Hopkins University
School of Medicine
Baltimore, Maryland 21205

R.D. Hawkins
Center for Physicians and Surgeons
Columbia University
New York, New York 10032

R.D. Heinz
Dept. of Biomedical Engineering
Johns Hopkins University
School of Medicine
Baltimore, Maryland 21205

Alvin J. Hill
Department of Psychology
University of Virginia
Charlottsville, Virgina 22901

Philip E. Hockberger
University of Illinois
Urbana, Illinois and
Bell Telephone Laboratories
Murray Hill, New Jersey

Graham Hoyle
Department of Biology
University of Oregon
Eugene, Oregon 97403

Masao Ito
Dept. of Physiology
Faculty of Medicine
University of Tokyo
7-3-1 Hongo, Bunkyoku
Tokyo 113, Japan

Herbert Jasper
Centre de recherche en sciences
neurologiques
Université de Montréal and
The Montreal Neurological Institute
4501 Sherbrooke St. W.
Montreal H3Z 1E7

Frances E. Jensen
Dept. of Computer and Information
Science and Psychology
University of Massachusetts
Amherst, Massachusetts 01003

E.R. Kandel
Center for Neurobiology and Behavior
Columbia University
New York, New York 10032

Bruce S. Kapp
Department of Psychology
University of Vermont
Burlington, Vermont 05401

Raymond P. Kesner
Department of Psychology
University of Utah
Salt Lake City, Utah 84112

R.N. Kettner
Stanford University
Stanford, California 94305

Stephen W. Kiefer
Dept. of Psychology and Mental
Retardation Research Center
University of California
Los Angeles, California 90024

Nina Kraus
Department of Cell Biology
Northwestern Univ. Medical School
Chicago, Illinois 60611

John L. Kubie
Department of Physiology
Downstate Medical Center
State University of New York
Brooklyn, New York 11203

Kisou Kubota
Primate Research Institute
Kyoto University
Inuyama, Aichi, 484, Japan

Richard W. Lambert
Department of Psychology
University of Texas at Austin
Austin, Texas 78712

Thomas H. Lanthorn
Department of Psychobiology
University of California
Irvine, California 92717

D.G. Lavond
Stanford University
Stanford, California 94305

O.C.J. Lippold
Department of Physiology
University College London
London, WCIE 6BT, England

V.A. Markevich
Brain Institute, Academy of
Medical Sciences, Moscow 107120
and Institute of Higher Nervous
Activity and Neurophysiology
Academy of Sciences
Moscow 117485 (USSR)

Joe L. Martinez, Jr.
Psychobiology Department
School of Biological Sciences
University of California
Irvine, California 92717

B. Maton
INSERMU3 CNRS
Hospital Salpetriere
47 Bd Hospital
Paris, France

Michikazu Matsumura
Department of Anatomy and
Psychiatry, M.R.R.C.
UCLA Medical Center
Los Angles, California 90024

M.D. Mauk
Stanford University
Stanford, California 94305

D.A. McCormick
Stanford University
Stanford, California 94305

Josef M. Miller
Department of Otolaryngology
and Regional Primate Research Center
University of Washington
Seattle, Washington 98105

Alex R. Milne
Department of Physiology
University College London
London, WC1E 6BT, England

John W. Moore
Department of Psychology
University of Massachusetts
Amherst, Massachusetts 01003

James H. O'Brien
Department of Medical Psychology
The Oregon Health Sciences University
Portland, Oregon

M.E. Olds
Division of Biology 216-76
California Institute of Technology
1201 E. California Boulevard
Pasadena, California 91125

David S. Olton
Department of Psychology
The Johns Hopkins University
Baltimore, Maryland 21218

Edward Orona
Department of Psychology
University of Texas at Austin
Austin, Texas 78712

William B. Orr
Psychobiology Program
Dept. of Psychology and Psychiatry
Univeristy of Pittsburgh
Pittsburgh, Pennsylvania 15260

Michael M. Patterson
College of Osteopathic Medicine
and Department of Psychology
Ohio University
Athens, Ohio 45701

Bryan E. Pfingst
Department of Otolaryngology
and Regional Primate Research Ctr.
University of Washington
Seattle, Washington 98105

D.A. Prince
Department of Neurology
Stanford University Medical Ctr.
Stanford, California 94305

Kevin J. Quinn
Department of Medical Psychology
Oregon Health Sciences University
Portland, Oregon

James B. Ranck, Jr.
Department of Physiology
Downstate Medical Center
State University of New York
Brooklyn, New York 11203

Edmund T. Rolls
Oxford University
Dept. of Experimental Psychology
South Parks Road
Oxford, U.K.

Anthony G. Romano
College of Osteopathic Medicine
and Department of Psychology
Ohio University
Athens, Ohio 45701

Kenneth W. Rusiniak
Dept. of Psychology and Mental
Retardation Research Center
University of California
Los Angeles, California 90024

Allen F. Ryan
Department of Otolaryngology
and Regional Primate Research Center
University of Washington
Seattle, Washington 98105

M.H. Schieber
Dept. of Neurobiology and Neurology
Washington University School of
Medicine
Saint Louis, Missouri 63130

John Schlag
Dept. of Anatomy and Brain
Research Institute
UCLA Medical School
Los Angeles, California 90024

Madeline Schlag-Rey
Dept. of Anatomy and Brain
Research Institute
UCLA School of Medicine
Los Angeles, California 90024

Michael T. Shipley
Dept. of Cell Biology and Anatomy
Northwestern Univ. Medical School
Chicago, Illinois 60611

Paul R. Solomon
Department of Psychology
Williams College
Williamstown, Massachusetts 01267

D. Nico Spinelli
Dept. of Computer and Information
Science and Psychology
University of Massachusetts
Amherst, Massachusetts 01003

Nancy S. Squires
Mental Retardation Research Center
Brain Research Institute and
Department of Physiology
University of California
Medical Center
Los Angeles, California 90024

Joseph E. Steinmetz
College of Osteopathic Medicine
and Department of Psychology
Ohio University
Athens, Ohio 45701

W.T. Thach
Departments of Neurobiology and
Neurology
Washington University
School of Medicine
Saint Louis, Missouri 63130

Richard F. Thompson
Department of Psychology
Stanford University
Stanford, California 94305

Nakaakira Tsukahara
Dept. of Biophysical Engineering
Faculty of Engineering Science
Osaka University
Toyonaka, Osaka and National
Institute for Physiological Sciences
Okazaki, Japan

L.L. Voronin
Brain Institute
Academy of Medical Sciences
Moscow 107120 and
Institute of Higher Nervous Activity
and Neurophysiology
Academy of Sciences
Moscow 117485 (USSR)

E.T. Walters
Department of Physiology
School of Medicine
University of Pittsburgh
Pittsburgh, Pennsylvania 15261

Norman M. Weinberger
Department of Psychobiology
University of California
Irvine, California 92717

D.J. Weisz
Stanford University
Stanford, California 94305

Mark O. West
Dept. of Physiology and Pharmacology
Bowman Gray School of Medicine
Winston-Salem, North Carolina 27103

Charles D. Woody
Depts. of Anatomy and Psychiatry,
M.R.R.C.
UCLA Medical Center
Los Angeles, California 90024

Bo-yi Yang
Department of Psychology
Stanford University
Stanford, California 94305

Robert S. Zucker
Physiology-Anatomy Department
University of California
Berkeley, California 94720

INDEX